LUNG FUNCTION

UNIVERSITY *of* LIMERICK

TELEPHONE: 061 202158 / 202172 / 202163

Items can be renewed from BORROWER INFO on the Library Catalogue
www.ul.ie/~library

PLEASE NOTE: This item is subject to recall after two weeks if required by another reader.

Lung Function

Assessment and Application
in Medicine

J.E.COTES
DM, DSc, FRCP, FFOM
Visitor, University Department of Physiological Sciences
Formerly Reader in Respiratory Physiology,
External Scientific Staff of Medical Research Council, and
Honorary Consultant in Clinical Respiratory Physiology
Newcastle upon Tyne

With the editorial collaboration of
G.L.LEATHART
MD, FRCP, DIH, FFOM
Formerly Senior Lecturer
in Occupational Health, and
Honorary Consultant Physician
Newcastle upon Tyne

FIFTH EDITION

OXFORD
BLACKWELL SCIENTIFIC PUBLICATIONS
LONDON EDINBURGH BOSTON
MELBOURNE PARIS BERLIN VIENNA

© 1965, 1968, 1975, 1979, 1993 by
Blackwell Scientific Publications
Editorial Offices:
Osney Mead, Oxford OX2 OEL
25 John Street, London WC1N 2BL
23 Ainslie Place, Edinburgh EH3 6AJ
238 Main Street, Cambridge
  Massachusetts 02142, USA
54 University Street, Carlton
  Victoria 3053, Australia

Other Editorial Offices:
Librairie Arnette SA
2, rue Casimir-Delavigne
75006 Paris
France

Blackwell Wissenschafts-Verlag GmbH
Meinekestrasse 4
D-1000 Berlin 15
Germany

Blackwell MZV
Feldgasse 13
A-1238 Wien
Austria

First published 1965
Second edition 1968
Third edition 1975
Fourth edition 1979
Polish edition 1969
Italian edition 1978
Fifth edition 1993

Set by Setrite Typesetters, Hong Kong
Printed and bound in Great Britain
by Butler & Tanner Ltd,
Frome and London

DISTRIBUTORS

Marston Book Services Ltd
PO Box 87
Oxford OX2 ODT
(*Orders*: Tel: 0865 791155
      Fax: 0865 791927
      Telex: 837515)

USA
Blackwell Scientific Publications, Inc.
238 Main Street
Cambridge, MA 02142
(*Orders*: Tel: 800 759-6102
      617 876-7000)

Canada
Times Mirror Professional Publishing, Ltd
130 Flaska Drive
Markham, Ontario L6G 1B8
(*Orders*: Tel: 800 268-4178
      416 470-6739)

Australia
Blackwell Scientific Publications Pty Ltd
54 University Street
Carlton, Victoria 3053
(*Orders*: Tel: 03 347-5552)

A catalogue record for this title
is available from the British Library

ISBN 0-632-03526-9

Library of Congress
Cataloging in Publication Data

Cotes, J.E.
  Lung function:
  assessment and application in medicine/
  J.E. Cotes, in collaboration with
  G.L. Leathart. — 5th ed.
      p.   cm.
  Includes bibliographical references
  and indexes.
  ISBN 0-632-03526-9
  1. Pulmonary function tests.
  2. Respiration. I. Leathart, G.L.
  II. Title.
  [DNLM: 1. Lung — physiology.
  2. Respiratory Function Tests.
  WF 600 C843]
  RC734.P84C68 1993
  616.2'4075 — dc20

Contents

Preface

This book describes the respiratory function of the lungs in a variety of circumstances and indicates how the function can be assessed. The function includes lung ventilation, gas exchange and lung perfusion with their respective physiological control mechanisms. The circumstances include the resting state, sleep, exercise, abnormal environments and diseases of the lung and other organs. The applications are in respiratory medicine including lung function laboratories and in paediatrics, geriatrics, environmental, occupational and sports medicine and medico-legal work. The material that has been assembled is also likely to be of use to non-respiratory physiologists, bioengineers, ergonomists, anthropologists and other scientists.

The present edition incorporates most of the advances of the past 12 years. These include internationally agreed conventions for standardising many measurements of lung function; better understanding of forced expiratory flow and the indices which describe it; advances in knowledge of pulmonary ventilation and perfusion in different circumstances; new methods for measuring the transfer factor (diffusing capacity); better understanding of breathlessness, factors which limit exercise and how disability can be assessed; more accurate reference values for indices of lung function in infants, children and adults (including better understanding of ethnic variation); improvements in the methods for measuring the mechanical properties of the lungs (particularly in infants); clarification of the mechanisms of asthma and pulmonary hypertension; improved ways of interpreting the lung function in clinical and occupational medicine and in epidemiology; new discoveries about the diaphragm and the mechanisms of upper airway obstruction; the introduction into respiratory medicine of sleep studies (polysomnography) and long-term oxygen therapy. In addition many recent and some historical references have been added to the section on references. These changes have entailed extensive revision to the book, which still retains its original format. Thus it should continue to be of use to all who have an interest in lung function and the normal and clinical physiology of respiration.

J.E. Cotes

Acknowledgements

In the preparation of this edition I have again received much help and encouragement from colleagues who have kindly supplied material or commented on the manuscript. They include Dr G.R. Barer (Sheffield, pulmonary circulation), Dr C. Borland (Papworth, transfer factor), Dr S. Capewell (Cardiff, collection and storage of blood), Dr D.J. Chinn, (Newcastle, ventilatory capacity, indices of gas mixing, reference values), Dr P. Corris (Newcastle, lung function in disease), Dr J.M.B. Hughes (London, radio-isotopes), Mrs K. O'Donovan (Newcastle, references), Dr S.J. Pearce (Durham, clinical aspects), Dr N.B. Pride (London, lung mechanics), Professor Ph.H. Quanjer (Leiden, specifications for equipment), Dr J.W. Reed (Newcastle, ventilation–perfusion relationships, control of breathing, exercise), Dr J. Stocks (London, neonates and infants), Dr P. Valabhji (Cardiff, case of asthma). Dr G.L. Leathart (Newcastle) scrutinised the completed manuscript and read the proofs. Professor G. Berry (Sydney) and the late Professor P.D. Oldham (Cardiff), prepared or advised on the nomograms.

Many authors have kindly allowed me to reproduce their published diagrams; their authorship is acknowledged on the captions. Additional unattributed material has been compiled with help from members of the laboratory including Dr D.J. Chinn, Mr C. Elliott, Dr I.L. Mortimore and Miss K. Simper. Mr M.F. Clay (Edinburgh) drew the cartoon.

Several illustrations are reproduced by kind permission of the copyright holders of books or scientific journals. These sources are indicated in the captions; they include *Acta Physiologica Scandinavica, American Journal of Medicine,* American Physiological Society, *American Review of Respiratory Diseases, Anaesthesia,* Blackwell Scientific Publications Ltd, *British Journal of Diseases of the Chest, British Journal of Industrial Medicine, British Medical Journal, Bulletin Européan de Physiopathologie Respiratoire, Clinical Allergy, Clinical Science,* Commonwealth Book Fund Program of Memorial Sloan-Kettering Cancer Center, *Diseases of the Chest, European Respiratory Journal, Journal of Clinical Investigation, Journal of Applied Physiology, Journal of Physiology,* Oxford University Press, W.W. Norton & Co, *Physiological Reviews, Respiration Physiology, Respiration Medicine, Thorax.*

The text and the author index were prepared by Mrs A.B. Blackhall. Some of the figures were prepared by the Audio-Visual Centre of the University of Newcastle upon Tyne, Mr S.B. Pearce and his fellow trainee librarians scrutinised the references and Mrs A. Marks helped with the proof-reading. The printing was overseen by Mr E. Wates and Miss J. Elliott, and the publication by Mr Peter Saugman, of Blackwell Scientific Publications. The subject index was prepared by Mrs C. Sheard.

The book is a collaborative venture to which many persons have contributed. To all of them I am grateful, as I am to the individuals and publishing companies who kindly allowed the reproduction of material for which they hold the copyright. In this respect as in the preparation of the text a strenuous attempt has been made to achieve accuracy and completeness. However, some lapses are inevitable and for all of these I both accept responsibility and ask indulgence. A letter pointing out any error or omission would be welcomed.

Finally, I am indebted to my wife for her encouragement, to the University of Newcastle upon Tyne for access to their facilities, and to the Medical Research Council, Wellcome Foundation, Health and Safety Executive and European Coal and Steel Community for research funds; this support has enabled the laboratory to contribute to the world-wide research upon which the present account is based.

J.E. Cotes

1: Early Developments and Future Prospects

The gaseous environment

The atmosphere is the result of processes taking place on the surface of the earth. Initially the processes were physical, then biological. Now man's activity is contributing as well. As a result the ozone layer, which provides a shield against ultraviolet light, is shrinking. At the same time carbon dioxide is accumulating and this prevents the escape of radiant heat received from the sun. The changes have stimulated interest in the work of Berkner, Marshall, Lovelock and others on the evolution of the gaseous environment. The latter developed the Gaia hypothesis that the composition of the atmosphere has been determined largely by biological activity.

Before the advent of living organisms, the atmosphere included approximately 10% carbon dioxide which was released from the earth's crust as it cooled. There was no free oxygen. This gas probably first appeared some 3.5×10^9 years ago either as a result of or coincidental to the development of organisms capable of photosynthesis. The organisms multiplied and their activity reduced significantly the atmospheric concentration of carbon dioxide; the oxygen was initially taken up by combination with iron and other elements so the atmospheric concentration remained less than one part per million. According to the Gaia hypothesis an increase in the accumulation of organic matter led to the development of methanogens and related organisms which liberated methane into the atmosphere, and this provided some shielding against ultraviolet light. The shielding made possible a rise in the concentration of ammonia gas which provided a substrate for the growth of photosynthesising organisms; as a result the atmospheric concentration of oxygen began to rise. Subsequently the concentration rose rapidly, by geological standards, from 0.1% to 1% over about one million years (Fig. 1.1).

When the ambient oxygen concentration reached 0.2% aerobic organisms became abundant in the surface layers of lakes and oceans and at 2% life began to move onto the land. A concentration of 3% appears to have been attained approximately 1.99×10^9 years ago. At a concentration of 10% photosynthesis was at its peak; this further

I

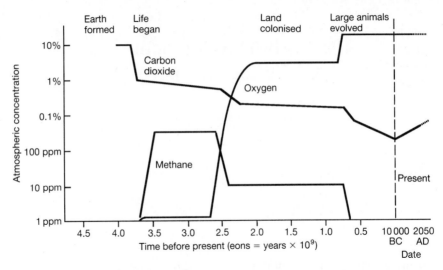

Fig. 1.1 Approximate time scale for the evolution of the gaseous environment. (After Lovelock J. *The Ages of Gaia: (C)*. Commonwealth Book Fund Program of Memorial Sloan-Kettering Cancer Center, 1988.)

raised the oxygen concentration and lowered the concentration of carbon dioxide. The changes reduced the available substrate (carbon dioxide) and increased the formation of hydrogen peroxide, superoxide ions and atomic oxygen which were potentially lethal to cells. Photosynthesis was reduced in consequence. The balance between promotion and inhibition of photosynthesis formed a feedback loop which, with other factors, led to the atmospheric concentration of oxygen stabilising at its present level. Stabilisation appears to have been achieved at the start of the phanerozoic era some 6×10^8 years ago and led to the evolution of animals with skeletons, including the dinosaurs. Subsequently, the oxygen concentration may have changed transiently, for example as a result of dust clouds from the impact of large meteors but so far the equilibrium level has always been restored. Now further changes appear imminent as a result of human activities. Chorofluro-carbon compounds from aerosol sprays and refrigeration systems are entering the upper atmosphere and destroying ozone which at present screens out much ultraviolet light. Carbon stored in fossil fuels is being re-oxidised to carbon dioxide which enters the atmosphere, where the concentration is rising. The concentrations of sulphur components and oxides of nitrogen are rising as well. Tropical forests with their attendant rain clouds are being destroyed and the sun, due to its internal nuclear energy, is progressively emitting more heat. At the same time the earth's internal radioactivity is diminishing. The changes are affecting the earth's climate but not yet the atmospheric oxygen concentration where any shift in the equilibrium is likely to occur slowly. Meanwhile, the evidence for biological activity contributing to the evolution of the physical environment is now overwhelming. Living organisms first appeared in an anaerobic environment which they helped to convert to an aerobic one whilst all the time adapting to the new conditions as they were creating them. On this account the capacity to tolerate conditions of hypoxia and to a lesser extent hypercapnia are part of man's heritage; the physiological mechanisms are described in subsequent chapters. The evolutionary history also points to a need for protection against oxygen radicals. However, there is only limited evidence for Berkener and Marshall's suggestion that the latter mechanisms emerged during periods of what we would now regard as hyperoxia.

Functional evolution of the lung

Aerobic organisms developed in an aqueous medium where the amount of oxygen is determined by its partial pressure and by the solubility; this is such that, at 37°C, the concentration in water is only about one-fortieth of that in air (Table 1.1). By contrast carbon dioxide is highly soluble so at physiological partial pressures the concentration in water is nearly as great as in air. The consequences for gas exchange of these differences in solubility have been investigated by Rahn, Dejours, Piiper and their collaborators amongst others.

For fish the problem of obtaining sufficient oxygen was solved by the evolution of the gill system. This organ is perfused by a large volume of water from which almost all the oxygen is extracted; the blood leaving the bronchial clefts contains oxygen in a concentration equal to that in blood leaving the lung in man. However, the water perfusing the gill takes with it carbon dioxide in solution and this lowers the CO_2 tension in the blood to less than 0.7 kPa (5 mmHg). Mainly on this account the blood pH is relatively high, approximately 8.0 pH units at a temperature of 20°C. At higher temperatures the pH falls to approach that in the blood of man. Concurrently, the solubility of oxygen in water and hence the amount delivered to the gill clefts is reduced. In the tropics a high ambient temperature might also cause the drying up of streams and to meet this hazard some freshwater fish developed lung-like pouches in the back of the pharynx; they also developed primitive limbs with which to crawl along the stream beds in search of water. For this type of existence a gill for the exchange of carbon

Table 1.1 Atmospheric concentrations and solubilities in water of oxygen and carbon dioxide

	Units	Oxygen	Carbon dioxide
Atmospheric concentration	vol/vol	0.2093	0.0003
Solubility in water at 1 atm and 20°C*	$\dfrac{\text{vol. of gas (STPD)}}{\text{vol. of water}}$	0.031	0.88
Solubility in water at 1 atm and 37°C*	$\dfrac{\text{vol. of gas (STPD)}}{\text{vol. of water}}$	0.024	0.55

* Solubility in blood plasma is approximately 10% less.

dioxide and a primitive lung for the exchange of oxygen formed a life-saving combination. The lung was further developed in reptiles, whilst in birds the pouches were adapted as reservoirs from which air was pumped through parabronchi; these supplied air to the diffusive zone where the whole of the available surface was lined with capillaries. This arrangement resulted in a very compact lung with a high capacity to transfer gas. The amphibians developed in a different way by shedding their scales to leave a soft vascular skin which replaced the gill as a means of exchanging carbon dioxide with the surrounding water. Somewhere between these diverging species emerged the primitive mammal and eventually man.

Early studies of lung function

Erasistratus (*c*. 280 BC) and Galen (131−201) demonstrated the role of the diaphragm as a muscle of respiration, the origin and function of the phrenic nerve and the function of the intercostal and accessory muscles. The function of the diaphragm was further explored by da Vinci (1452−1519) who observed that during inspiration the lung expanded in all directions following the movement of the thoracic cage. The collapse which followed puncture of the pleura was described by Vesalius (1514−1564).

The need for fresh air was recognised by Galen who believed it reacted with the blood in the left heart and arteries to produce the 'vital spirit'. The absence of a visible communication between the pulmonary artery and the pulmonary vein led him to suggest that blood passed through invisible pores between the two sides of the heart; thus he failed to comprehend the function of the lung. This was surmised by Ibn-al-Nafis (*c*. 1210−1289) and by Servetus (1511−1553) who separately recognised the impermeability of the interventricular septum and proposed that blood passed from the pulmonary artery through the lung to the pulmonary vein. Harvey (1578−1657) demonstrated that blood circulated through the lung and Malpighi (1628−1694) showed that the blood capillaries were in close proximity to the smallest air spaces. These observations prepared the way for a correct understanding of lung function.

The role of ventilation in maintaining life was demonstrated by Vesalius who was able to restore the activity of the heart in an apnoeic dog by insufflating air into the trachea through a reed. Hooke (1635−1703) subsequently showed that the essential factor was the supply of fresh air which he allowed to escape through puncture holes in the pleura after the lung had been exposed. Boyle (1627−1691) and to a lesser extent Mayow (1643−1679), demonstrated that the constituent of air which supported combustion also supported life. Lower (1631−1691) further showed that the uptake of air in the lung caused the blood to change colour. These discoveries laid the foundations for subsequent studies of gas exchange but their importance was not immediately apparent. The confusion was such that on 22 January

1666, after a meeting of the Royal Society on the subject of respiration, Samuel Pepys wrote in his diary, 'it is not to this day known, or concluded on among physicians ... how the action is managed by nature, or for what use it is'.

The past 300 years

The information about the lung which was necessary for the birth of respiratory physiology was available by about the year 1667. Thereafter aspects of the subject developed at different rates, reflecting their immediate interest and the techniques which were available for their investigation.

Lung volumes

The volume of air which a man can inhale during a single deep breath was first measured by Borelli (1679). Subsequent work established that this quantity in an average adult is about 200–300 in^3 (3.3–4.9 l) at ambient temperature. The need for a temperature correction was pointed out by Goodwyn (1788). Thackrah (1831) showed the volume of air to be less in women than in men and to be reduced amongst workers in flax and other occupations due to the inhalation of dust. The measurement was put on a quantitative basis by Hutchinson (1846). Hutchinson defined the vital capacity as 'the greatest voluntary expiration following the deepest inspiration' and designed a spirometer for its estimation. He showed that the vital capacity is related to the height such that 'for every inch of height (from 5 ft to 6 ft) eight additional cu. inches of air at 60°F are given out by forced expiration'. He further showed that the vital capacity decreased with age and was reduced by excess weight and by disease of the lung. The measurement of the residual volume by a gas dilution method was first performed by Davy (1800). The method using whole body plethysmography was developed by DuBois and colleagues (1956).

Lung mechanics

The role of the elastic recoil of the lung in causing expiration was demonstrated by Donders (1853) who was the first to measure the retractive force. This work was extended by Dixon and Brodie (1903) and by Cloetta (1913). At about the same time Rohrer (1915) was applying the concepts of Newtonian mechanics to explain the relationship between the force exerted by the respiratory muscles and the rate of air flow. This approach was extended by his successors. Neergaard and Wirz (1927) who used the pneumotachograph of Fleisch (1925). Neergaard also demonstrated the role of surface forces in the lung by comparing the relationship of the lung volume to the retractive force when the air in the lung was replaced by water. This work was repeated independently by Radford (1954) who with Pattle (1955), Clements

5

(1956) and Avery and Mead (1959), established the physiological and chemical significance of lung surfactant. Knowledge of the visco-elastic properties of the lung was extended by Bayliss and Robertson (1939), Dean and Visscher (1941), Rahn, Otis, Chadwick and Fenn (1946), Mead and Whittenberger (1953) and their many collaborators; a seminal review was prepared by Mead (1961). The role of antitrypsin in protecting the lung from proteolytic enzymes was discovered by Eriksson (1964).

Ventilatory capacity

The relationship of the vital capacity to breathlessness was considered by Peabody (1915) who also compared the ventilation during the inhalation of carbon dioxide with that during exercise. The use of the forced vital capacity was advocated by Strohl (1919). The role of changes in lung distensibility in causing breathlessness was explored by Christie (1934). The maximal breathing capacity was introduced as a dynamic test of lung function by Jansen, Knipping and Stromberger (1932), who calculated it from the forced vital capacity. The maximal voluntary ventilation was first measured by Hermannsen (1933). The use of the proportion of the vital capacity which could be expired in one second as a guide to airways obstruction was introduced by Tiffeneau (1948). The measurement was facilitated through the addition of a timing device to the spirometer by Gaensler (1951) and subsequently by McDermott and colleagues (1960). A convenient and reasonably accurate peak flow meter was developed by Wright (1959) and other instruments followed.

Blood chemistry and gas exchange in the lung

During the eighteenth century the role of the lung as an organ of gas exchange was obscured by the belief of Lavoisier (1777) and others that it was the site of combustion. This was disproved by Magnus (1837) who used an extraction technique to analyse the gases in the arterial and venous bloods. The use of such data for the calculation of cardiac output was proposed by Fick (1870), whilst the true site of oxidation was demonstrated by Pflüger (1872). The techniques for analysing gases were improved by Haldane and described in *Methods of Air Analysis* (1899); an improved method for determining the concentrations in the blood was described by Haldane and Barcroft (1902). The tonometer methods for measuring the blood gas tensions were developed by Bohr (1890) and Krogh (1910) and further technical advances were reported by Peters and Van Slyke in *Quantitative Clinical Chemistry* (1932). The application of these and other techniques to human arterial blood was made possible through the introduction by Hürter (1912) of the procedure of arterial puncture.

The relationship of the pressure to the content of oxygen in the blood was explored by Paul Bert and described in *La Pression Baro-*

métrique (1878); in this he showed that the pressure and not the concentration of gases in the atmosphere is of physiological significance. The oxygen dissociation curve was described by Bohr (1904). With Hasselbalch and Krogh (1904), Bohr showed that its shape is greatly influenced by the coexisting tension of carbon dioxide. Further advances were made by Barcroft and summarised in *The Respiratory Function of the Blood* (1914). The dissociation curve for carbon dioxide was described by Christiansen, Douglas and Haldane (1914) and the chemical reactions were further explored by Hasselbalch, Hastings, Roughton, Sendroy, Stadie and others. Some of this work is described by L.J. Henderson in *Blood: a Study in General Physiology* (1928).

The exchange of gas across the alveolar capillary membrane was considered by Bohr (1891). He found that the tension of oxygen was sometimes higher in the arterial blood than in the alveolar gas and concluded that oxygen was secreted by the alveolar cells. The measurements were in error but the hypothesis was supported by Haldane and Smith (1896–1898) who during inhalation of gas containing carbon monoxide, obtained differences between the observed and expected tensions of carbon monoxide in the blood which could best be explained by the secretion of oxygen. This view was opposed by Krogh (1910) and Barcroft, who believed correctly that the transfer of oxygen took place solely by diffusion. The controversy led Bohr (1909) to develop his integration method for determining the mean tension of oxygen in the pulmonary capillaries and to calculate the diffusing capacity of the lung for carbon monoxide. It also stimulated physiological expeditions to high altitudes, including those to Pikes Peak, described by Douglas, Haldane, Y. Henderson and Schneider (1913), and Cerro de Pasco, described by Barcroft in the second edition of *The Respiratory Function of the Blood*. Studies of conditions at high altitude were also undertaken by Dill, Christensen and Edwards (1936), and by Houston and Riley (1947). Subsequently interest shifted to the Himalayas where the physiological adaptations necessary for the ascent of Mount Everest were investigated by Pugh (1964) and West (1983), amongst others. Meanwhile, the transfer of oxygen from alveolar gas to pulmonary capillary blood was explored by Lilienthal and Riley (1946) and Piiper (1961). Understanding of the transfer of carbon monoxide was advanced by Roughton and Forster (1957). The single-breath method for the measurement of transfer factor (diffusing capacity) for carbon monoxide was developed by Marie Krogh (1915) and improved under Comroe's guidance by Forster, Fowler and colleagues (1954). The anatomical basis of gas exchange was described in quantitative terms by Weibel (1963).

The distribution of gas in the lung was considered by Zuntz (1882) who introduced the concept of deadspace; this was first measured at post-mortem by Loewy (1894). The deadspace for carbon dioxide was measured during life by Bohr (1891) as well as by Haldane and others who used the method of sampling the alveolar gas devised by Haldane and Priestley (1905). By this method Douglas and Haldane (1912) showed that the deadspace increased with the depth of inspiration, but the magnitude of the increase was disputed by Krogh and Lindhard (1913–1914) who sampled the end tidal gas. Part of the increase was believed by Haldane to represent ventilation of the alveolar ducts and atria where the ventilation per unit of perfusion (i.e. the ventilation–perfusion ratio) was higher than in the alveoli. Haldane, Meakins and Priestley (1918–1919) explored the effects of uneven lung function upon the composition of alveolar gas and arterial blood. The application of these concepts to patients with lung disease was described by Meakins and Davies in *Respiratory Function in Disease* (1925).

The role of the pulmonary circulation was clarified through the practical exploration of the technique of cardiac catheterisation by Cournand (1942) and by McMichael and Sharpey-Schafer (1944). The mechanisms underlying uneven lung function were further illuminated by the development of bronchospirometry by Jacobaeus (1932), the concept of regional inhomogeneity by Rauwerda (1945), the respiratory mass spectrometer by Fowler (1957), the oxygen electrode by Clark (1953) and radio-isotope assay methods by Knipping (1955). These techniques were used to good effect by Rahn and Fenn (1955) and by West (1969) who, with Wagner (1974), developed the multiple inert gas elimination technique for describing ventilation–perfusion inequality.

Control of respiration

Knowledge of the central nervous regulation of respiration stems from the observations of Legallois (1812) and Flourens (1824) that a lesion in a small area of the medulla oblongata caused cessation of breathing. The location of the respiratory region was defined with increasing precision by many workers, including Lumsden (1923) and Pitts, Magoun and Ranson (1939). At an early stage Hering and Breuer (1868) separately showed that the region received, via the vagi, sensory information on the distension of the lung. This provides the basis for a mechanism of self-regulation whereby the inflation of the lung tends to terminate inspiration and to initiate expiration whilst deflation of the lung has the opposite effect. Activity in single vagal fibres was recorded by Adrian (1933) and others; their work paved the way for dramatic advances in understanding the role of pulmonary receptors which are now being made by, amongst others, the colleagues and pupils of Whitteridge (1950) including Paintal, Widdicombe and Guz. Sears (1963) showed that the muscle spindles in the respiratory muscles also contributed to regulation, whilst Campbell and Howell (1963) explored the part they might play in the sensation of dyspnoea. The Hering–Breuer centenary symposium provided a seminal review (Porter 1970); it also introduced respiratory physiologists to some psychological techniques for the quantification of breathlessness.

The stimulant effects upon respiration of both a deficiency of oxygen and a moderate excess of carbon dioxide were known to Pflüger (1868)

8

who believed the former to be the more important factor. In this he was in agreement with Rosenthal (1862). Evidence for the role of carbon dioxide was provided by Miescher-Rüsch (1885), whilst Geppert and Zuntz (1888) demonstrated the stimulant action of other products of metabolism. The action of carbon dioxide in man was investigated quantitatively by Haldane and Priestley (1905) who, over a wide range of barometric pressures, demonstrated that the ventilation was adjusted to maintain the alveolar carbon dioxide tension at a constant level.

J.S. Haldane's great contribution is summarised in *Respiration* (1922). It was republished jointly with Priestley in 1935. The role of the blood hydrogen ion concentration in controlling breathing was suggested by Winterstein (1911) and elaborated, amongst others, by Yandell Henderson in *Adventures in Respiration* (1938). Gesell (1923) believed the response of the respiratory region to be affected by the metabolism of the sensitive cells. The role of hypoxaemia was advanced through the identification by Heymans (1926) and De Castro (1928) of the chemoreceptors in the carotid and aortic bodies; their function was further studied by Comroe and Schmidt (1938). The interdependence of the responses of ventilation to hypercapnia and hypoxaemia was demonstrated by Nielsen and Smith (1951), whilst the effects of inhalation of oxygen were studied by Leonard Hill and Flack (1910), A.V. Hill, Long and Lupton (1924), Asmussen and Nielsen (1946), Comroe and Dripps (1950), Dejours (1966) and others. The combined effects on respiration of these and other factors were synthesised into a multiple theory of respiratory regulation by Gray in *Pulmonary Ventilation and its Physiological Regulation* (1950).

Energy expenditure during exercise

The rates of exchange of oxygen and carbon dioxide in the lung were measured by Lavoisier (1784) who showed that they varied with the level of activity. The relationship of the resting metabolism to the body surface area was demonstrated by Robiquet and Thillaye (1839). The underlying biochemical processes were investigated by Liebig (1842), Voit (1857), Rubner (1883) and others. One important landmark was the demonstration by Fletcher and Hopkins (1907) that lactic acid was produced in muscles during anaerobic contractions.

The extensive documentation of human metabolism by indirect calorimetry was made possible through the development by Zuntz (1891) of a portable apparatus; the method was compared against direct human calorimetry by Atwater and Rosa (1897). Other equipment was introduced by Tissot (1904), Douglas (1911), Benedict and Roth (1922), Kofranyi and Michaelis (1940), Müller and Frantz (1952) and Wolff (1958). The need to relate the results to the body weight of the subjects was recognised by Frentzel and Reach (1901). The energy expenditure during activity was measured by many workers, including Benedict (1915), whilst the relationship to the speed of locomotion was analysed in detail by Magne (1920), A.V. Hill and his colleagues,

9

including Lupton (1922), Atzler and Herbst (1927), Fenn (1930), Margaria (1939) and others.

Future prospects

The mechanisms which underlie the respiratory function of the lung are now quite well understood. The practical assessment of lung function is an accepted part of clinical medicine, occupational medicine and epidemiology. The techniques for assessment are in the process of standardisation internationally and computerised equipment is available in bewildering variety; thus the subject has matured.

New discoveries continue to be made; this process is helped by the relative accessibility of the lung, the versatility of the many tools which are available for its investigation and the dedication of investigators. Their enthusiasm is often a response to the deceptive simplicity of the respiratory system, its central role in human experience and the excitement of discovery! Some aspects of lung function which are now in course of study are listed in Table 1.2. The diversity of the topics is evidence that the prospects for research into lung function both within the discipline and in collaboration with others is as exciting now as formerly. The realisation of these prospects is likely to be helped by

Table 1.2 Some aspects of lung function now in course of study

Category	Sub-division	Topics of research interest
Anatomy	Topography	Influence on regional expansion and gas distribution
	Lung tissue	Collateral and anastomotic pathways, receptors, diffusion, lung elasticity
Biochemistry	Metabolism	Production of mucus, surfactant and proteolytic enzymes. Ageing
	Genetics	Atopy, α_1 antitypsin, DNA, ethnic factor in lung function
Pharmacology	Bronchomotor tone	Determinants, mechanisms, relation to immunity
Mechanics	Chest wall	Properties of respiratory muscles
	Lung	Determinants of volume changes
Distribution	Gas and blood	Factors affecting. Consequences
	Particles	Distribution, deposition, clearance
	Acinus	Diffusion in gas phase: relation to structure
Gas exchange	Lung membrane	Structure, area, permeability, water content
	Reaction with blood	Structure and reactivity of haemoglobin 2,3-diphosphoglycerate, other metabolites

Table 1.2 *Continued*

Guide to references

Category	Sub-division	Topics of research interest
Control of respiration	Central nervous system	Activity of respiratory neurones, central receptors, vagal afferents Spinal mechanisms Nature of breathlessness
	Peripheral receptors	Activating factors, mechanisms, function
	Effects on ventilation	Respiratory drive and sensitivity. Pattern of breathing
	Sleep apnoea	Incidence, mechanisms, consequences
Response to exercise	Ventilation	Determinants. Contribution to exercise limitation
	Circulation	O_2 delivery to muscles. Cardiac output and underlying factors
	Metabolism	Aerobic and glycolytic pathways, relation to fibre type
	Physical training	Mechanisms, limiting factors
Abnormal function	Applied physiology	Abnormal barometric pressures and temperatures, anaesthesia, heart and lung transplantation, respiratory distress syndrome
	Structure and function	Lung diseases, inhaled noxious agents, drugs, systemic disorders
	Pathology	Cleansing mechanisms. Determinants of altered structure
	Therapy	Broncho- and vasoactive drugs. Immunosuppressants. Long-term and hyperbaric oxygen. Assisted ventilation. Breathing exercises
Epidemiology	Normal function	Growth and ageing. Reference values
	Inhaled substances	Occupational and environmental pollutants, smoking. Prophylaxis
Methodology	Standardisation	Techniques. Quality control
	Laboratory safety	Good practises. Preventing cross infection

the present book which describes the techniques of the respiratory physiologist and the results of their application in man.

Guide to references

The references (Chapter 18) are classified under subject headings of which the following are particularly relevant to the present chapter:

2: Terminology

Glossary of terms

The terms used in respiratory physiology are defined in the text and listed in the index. Some general terms which are not specific to respiratory physiology are defined in Table 2.1.

Table 2.1 General terms which are used in respiratory physiology

Term	Description*
Acidaemia	A relative excess of hydrogen ions in blood (vs alkalaemia)
Airways obstruction	Narrowing or occlusion of airways (often inferred from airflow limitation which is then the correct usage)
Anoxia	Absence of oxygen
Apnoea	Cessation of breathing
Asphyxia	Hypoxia and hypercapnia due to severe diminution in ventilation
Bradypnoea	Decreased frequency of breathing (vs tachypnoea)
Bronchoconstriction	Airways obstruction due to increased tone of bronchial smooth muscle (vs bronchodilatation)
Cyanosis	Lips or buccal mucous membrane a bluish colour
Dyspnoea	A consciousness of difficulty in breathing
Hypercapnia	A relatively high tension of carbon dioxide in blood (vs hypocapnia)
Hyperinflation	An increase in functional residual capacity (measured or inferred)
Hyperpnoea	An increase in ventilation relative to the metabolic rate (vs hypopnoea)
Hyperventilation	An increase in ventilation sufficient to cause hypocapnia (vs hypoventilation)
Hypoxaemia	A relative deficiency of oxygen in blood
Hypoxia	A relatively low tension of oxygen at a specified site
Lactacidaemia	Acidaemia due to a raised concentration of lactic acid
Metabolic acidosis	An increase in blood non-volatile acids or reduction in basic substances; if compensated the blood HCO_3 is reduced and the pH normal (vs metabolic alkalosis)
Orthopnoea	Dyspnoea ameliorated by an upright posture
Reference values	Values with which the results under consideration may be compared

Table 2.1 *Continued*

Term	Description*
Respiratory acidosis	An increase in blood carbon dioxide tension; if compensated the blood HCO_3^- is increased and the pH normal (vs respiratory alkalosis)
Steady state	The condition of equilibrium for a particular variable

* In these descriptions the term 'relative' is used with respect to a healthy person breathing air at sea level. The blood concentrations relate to the systemic arterial circulation.

Abbreviations and primary symbols

Some lung function indices are designated by abbreviations and others by symbols. The former are made up of the initial letters of the words which describe the measurements. Examples are given in Table 2.2 together with the pages in the text where the indices are defined.

Table 2.2 Abbreviations used to indicate some respiratory indices; the indices are commonly reported in standard international units (SI) except in USA where traditional units are used (page 16)

Abbreviation	Index	SI units*	Page
Lung volume			
CC	Closing capacity	l (or % TLC)	219
CV	Closing volume	l (or % VC)	219
ERV	Expiratory reserve volume	l	105
FRC	Functional residual capacity	l	104
IC	Inspiratory capacity	l	105
IRV	Inspiratory reserve volume	l	105
IVC	Inspiratory vital capacity	l	105
RV	Residual volume (symbol V_R)	l	105
RV%	$100 \times RV/TLC$	%	
TGV	Thoracic gas volume	l	157
TLC	Total lung capacity	l	104
Ventilatory capacity			
VC	Vital capacity	l	106
T	Forced expiratory time	s	140
FEF	Forced expiratory flow (or MEF)	$l s^{-1}$	123
FEV_t	Forced expiratory volume†	l	122
$FEV_t\%$	Percentage expired† (i.e. $100 \times FEV_t/FVC$)		139
FIV	Forced inspiratory volume†	l	122
FMF	Forced mid-expiratory flow (alternatively $FEF_{25-75\%}$ or MMF)	$l s^{-1}$	122
FVC	Forced vital capacity	l	135
IMBC	Indirect maximal breathing capacity (estimated from FEV_1)	$l \, min^{-1}$	392
IPF	Inspiratory peak flow	$l s^{-1}$	124
IVPF	Isovolume pressure flow curve	—	117
MBC	Maximal breathing capacity	$l \, min^{-1}$	134
MEF	Maximal expiratory flow†	$l s^{-1}$	123

Continued p. 14

Table 2.2 *Continued*

Abbreviation	Index	SI units*	Page
MEFV	Maximal expiratory flow volume curve	–	123
MMF	Maximal mid-expiratory flow (symbol FMF)	ls^{-1}	122
MTT	Mean transit time	s	123
MVV	Maximal voluntary ventilation‡	$l\,min^{-1}$	122
PEF	Peak expiratory flow	ls^{-1}	123
PEFV	Partial expiratory flow volume curve	–	123
SDTT	Standard deviation of transit times	s	141
TVC	Timed vital capacity (now replaced by FEV_t)	l	135
Lung mechanics			
AWR	Airway resistance (symbol *R*aw)	$kPa\,l^{-1}s$	108
EPP	Equal pressure point	–	117
Gas exchange			
A-aD	Alveolar–arterial tension difference (e.g. for O_2)	kPa	204
RER	Respiratory exchange ratio	–	36
RQ	Respiratory quotient	–	36
TF	Transfer factor (symbol *T*l)	$mmol\,min^{-1}\,kPa^{-1}$	292
Response to exercise			
AT	Anaerobic threshold§	$mmol\,O_2\,min^{-1}$	427
EEV	Excess exercise ventilation	l	355
PFI	Physical fitness index	–	437
SV	Stroke volume	ml	187
VE	Ventilation equivalent¶	–	370
Other			
CNLD	Chronic non-specific lung disease	–	515
COPD	Chronic obstructive pulmonary disease	–	515
FFM	Fat free mass	kg	56
PEEP	Positive end-expiratory pressure	–	649

* Volumes are in l BTPS (page 18). The SI unit of time is the second but min are permitted and are often more appropriate. For other units see Table 2.5.
† The time in s or the segment of the forced expiratory spirogram should be indicated e.g. FEV_1, $FEF_{25-75\%\ FVC}$, $FEF_{75-85\%\ FVC}$, $FEF_{200-1200FVC}$. Flow rates measured after the expiration from TLC of a specified volume of gas (expressed as % of FVC) are designated $FEF_{x\%FVC}$ (where $x = TLC - x\%$ FVC, e.g. $FEF_{75\%\ FVC}$). The volume can also refer to the gas remaining in the lung at the instant of measurement, for example RV + 25% FVC or 60% TLC; the corresponding flow rates are designated respectively: $MEF_{25\%\ FVC}$ and $MEF_{60\%\ TLC}$. From this it follows that $FEF_{75\%\ FVC} = MEF_{25\%\ FVC}$; the latter usage is recommended.
‡ The frequency of breathing should be indicated, e.g. MVV_F, if uncontrolled, MVV_{40}, if controlled at $40\,min^{-1}$.
§ Owles' point or Wassermann's point is preferable (page 427).
¶ Also called ventilatory equivalent of oxygen.

The symbols come mainly from biochemistry and biophysics: their use in respiratory physiology was codified in 1950 by Pappenheimer and colleagues. A major revision was made in 1980 by the Commission of Respiratory Physiology of the International Union of Physiological Sciences and refinements have been introduced by the American Physiological Society and by a working group of the European Coal and Steel Community. Symbols are printed in italics (Table 2.3).

Table 2.3 Primary symbols used in respiratory physiology *Suffixes*

Table 2.3 Primary symbols used in respiratory physiology

Primary symbols	
C	Concentration in blood, also compliance
sC	Specific compliance
D	Diffusing capacity*
E	Elastance
F	Fractional concentration in dry gas
f	Frequency
G	Conductance
sG	Specific conductance
K	Krogh factor (Tl/V_A)
k	Coefficient of lung distensibility
$\dot{n}$ (n')	Amount of substance per unit time
P	Pressure
Q	Volume of blood
$\dot{Q}$ (Q')	Volume of blood per unit time
R	Respiratory exchange ratio, also resistance
S	Saturation, also ventilatory response to CO_2
T	Transfer factor
t	Time
V	Volume of gas
$\dot{V}$ (V')	Volume of gas per unit time
$\dot{v}$ (V'')	Instantaneous flow rate of gas

* D symbolises the rate constant for movement of substances by diffusion, e.g. across the alveolar capillary membrane. It can represent the rate constant for transfer of substances by multiple processes which include both diffusion and chemical reaction, e.g. transfer from alveolar gas to red cells in alveolar capillaries, but for this application the term transfer factor (symbol T) is more appropriate (page 277).

Derivatives with respect to time are portrayed in a traditional manner. Volume per unit of time (i.e. $V \div t$) is $\dot{V}$ in the gas phase and $\dot{Q}$ in the blood phase; the units are $1\,\text{min}^{-1}$. The rate of change of volume with time, i.e. dV/dt is represented by $\dot{v}$ in the units $1\,\text{s}^{-1}$. This usage is adopted for the present account. Alternatively a mathematical notation may be used as in Table 2.3 which lists the primary symbols and, where appropriate, their mathematical equivalents.

Suffixes

A primary symbol is usually qualified by suffixes which define the anatomical site or substance to which the measurement refers, as well as other information which clarifies the meaning of the symbol in the context in which it is used. Suffixes are printed in Roman type. The anatomical site is usually represented by the first letter of its name; this is usually written in lower case except when the measurement refers to the gas phase. The mean or average value at a particular site is represented by a bar over the corresponding suffix. Thus the partial pressure of oxygen in alveolar gas is P_{A,O_2}; in mixed venous blood the oxygen tension is $P\bar{\text{v}},\text{O}_2$ and in systemic arterial blood it is P_{a,O_2}. Other suffixes are listed in Table 2.4. The concepts *partial pressure* and *gas tension* are considered below.

Table 2.4 Some suffixes used in respiratory physiology

A	alveolar (e.g. V_A)
a	arterial (e.g. $Pa,_{O_2}$)
an	anatomical (e.g. Van,ds)
aw	airway (e.g. Raw)
B	barometric (e.g. P_B)
C	cardiac (e.g. fc)
c	capillary (e.g. $Pc,_{O_2}$)
c'	end capillary (e.g. $Pc',_{CO_2}$)
di	diaphragm (e.g. Pdi)
ds	deadspace (e.g. Vds)
dyn	dynamic (e.g. $Cdyn$)
E	expired (e.g. $\dot{V}_E$)
el	elastic
ex	exercise (e.g. $\dot{V}_E$ ex)
I	inspired (e.g. ti)
iso-$\dot{v}$	isoflow (e.g. V iso-$\dot{v}$)
l	lung (e.g. Tl)
m	alveolar capillary membrane (e.g. Dm)
max	maximal (e.g. $\dot{n}_{O_2}$ max)
PA	pulmonary artery (e.g. P_{PA})
pl	pleural (e.g. Ppl)
R	respiration (e.g. f_R)
rb	rebreathing (e.g. S_{CO_2}, rb)
s	shunt (e.g. $\dot{Q}s$)
sb	single breath (e.g. $Tl,_{CO}.sb$)
ss	steady state (e.g. $Tl,_{CO}.ss$)
st	static (e.g. Cst)
th	thoracic (e.g. Rth)
ti	tissue (e.g. Rti)
tm	transmural (e.g. Ptm)
tot	total (e.g. $ttot$)
$\bar{v}$	venous (e.g. $P\bar{v},_{CO_2}$)
va	venous admixture (e.g. $\dot{Q}va$)

Units

The units used in respiratory physiology have evolved in line with scientific practice. However, the rate of change has been uneven and this has led to the present unsatisfactory situation in which many countries including all European countries have adopted standard international units (SI units) for most indices whilst others including the United States have continued to use more traditional units. The two conventions have in common the litre as the unit of volume, degrees celsius for temperature and seconds or minutes as units of time. Blood pressure is still in millimetres of mercury even though for most applications within the traditional system of units the mmHg has been replaced by the torr (after Torricelli). The SI system differs from the traditional in using metric units for length, mass and their derivatives including pressure (where the appropriate unit is the kilopascal), energy (joules) and power (watts). The amount of a chemical substance is in molar units, usually millimoles. SI units are used in the present account together with some commonly used traditional equivalents. Of these the mmHg has been retained as a unit of pressure or gas tension in

Table 2.5 Derivation of SI from traditional units

Category	SI unit	Conversion factor
Temperature	celsius (°C, i.e. °K − 273)	(°F − 32) × 5/9
Pressure	kilopascal (kPa, i.e. kilonewton per m^2)	mmHg* × 0.1333 (or ÷ 7.50) cmH$_2$O × 0.0981 (or ÷ 10.2) atmos × 101.3 (or bar × 100)
Length	centimetre (10^{-2} m) metre (m) kilometre (10^3 m)	inch × 2.54 (or ÷ 0.394) inch ÷ 39.37 (or × 0.0254) miles × 8/5 (or × 1.609, or ÷ 0.621)
Mass	gram (10^{-3} kg) kilogram (kg)	oz × 28.3 lb ÷ 2.2 (or × 0.4536)
Volume	litre (dm^3)	ft^3 × 28.316
Velocity	metre s^{-1} metre min^{-1}	mph ÷ 2.23 ft/s ÷ 3.28 × (or × 0.3048) mph × 26.8
Energy	joule (J, i.e. kg m^2 s^{-2})‡	cal × 4.184
Power	watt (W, i.e. J s^{-1})‡	kp† m min^{-1} × 0.163 (or ÷ 6.12) horse power × 745.7, or for metric hp × 745.5
Frequency	hertz (Hz, i.e. s^{-1})	—
Amount of substance in gaseous form	millimole (mmol)§	for most gases ml STPD ÷ 22.4 but for CO$_2$ ÷ 22.26
Compliance	l kPa^{-1}	l cmH$_2$O^{-1} × 10.2 (or ÷ 0.098)
Resistance	kPa l^{-1} s	cmH$_2$O l^{-1} s × 0.098 (or ÷ 10.2)
Conductance	l s^{-1} kPa^{-1}	l s^{-1} cmH$_2$O^{-1} × 10.2 (or ÷ 0.098)
Ventilatory response to CO$_2$	l min^{-1} kPa^{-1}	l min^{-1} mmHg^{-1} × 7.5
Transfer factor	mmol min^{-1} kPa^{-1}	ml min^{-1} mmHg^{-1} × 0.335 (or ÷ 2.986)

* 1 mmHg is approximately 1 torr.
† kilopond (page 417).
‡ See also page 417.
§ Molar concentration (mol l^{-1}) = P (atmos)/RT(°K) where R (gas constant) = 0.0821 l atmos K^{-1} mol^{-1}.

preference to the torr which appears not to be widely known in medicine. The conversion factors between SI and traditional units are given in Table 2.5.

Partial pressure and gas tension

Partial pressure is the subject of Dalton's law which describes the pressure exerted by an individual gas present in a mixture. For example, gas present in the lung (alveolar gas) comprises oxygen (O_2), carbon dioxide (CO_2), inert gases which are mainly nitrogen, hence are designated (N_2) and water vapour (H_2O). When the airways are open to the atmosphere the sum of the partial pressures is equal to the barometric pressure: thus

$$P_B = P_{A,O_2} + P_{A,CO_2} + P_{A,N_2} + P_{A,H_2O} \qquad (2.1)$$

The partial pressure of water vapour is that for gas at body temperature, saturated with water vapour. When body temperature is 37°C the aqueous vapour is 6.3 kPa (47 mmHg or torr). The pressure of dry gas is obtained by subtracting the water vapour pressure from the barometric pressure. Hence from equation 2.1:

$$P_B - P_{H_2O}(37) = P_{A,O_2} + P_{A,CO_2} + P_{A,N_2} \qquad (2.2)$$

When a gaseous substance is in solution in a liquid, for example blood, the effective partial pressure or tension is that which the substance would exert in gas in equilibrium with the liquid in question. This is irrespective of whether or not a stable gaseous phase is present. In its absence, the sum of the tensions of all gases present in the liquid need not add up to the barometric pressure. For example, in the mixed venous blood the tensions of oxygen, carbon dioxide and nitrogen are on average, 5, 6 and 77 kPa (40, 46 and 574 mmHg) respectively. The sum of these tensions is 88 kPa (660 mmHg) which is less than the average pressure of dry gas in the lung at sea level, i.e. $(101.3 - 6.3) = 95$ kPa $(760 - 47 = 713$ mmHg). This has the effect that a small bubble of air introduced into the venous blood will come to have this relative composition and will be reabsorbed (page 627).

Standardisation of volumes for temperature and pressure

Measurements of gas volume are made at the temperature and pressure of the recording equipment where the gas molecules are at ambient temperature and pressure (ATP); expired gas is usually also saturated with water vapour and in these circumstances its condition is designated ATPS. Ambient conditions vary so the volumes need to be converted to a standard condition, which for most purposes is that obtaining in the lung; here the gas is at body temperature and pressure and saturated with water vapour (BTPS). In other circumstances, for example when reporting the volume of oxygen or other gas exchanged between lungs and blood, the standard conditions are for temperature 0°C and for pressure one atmosphere (P_B, = 101.3 kPa or 760 mmHg of dry gas designated STPD). However, the reporting of the amount of a gas as a volume at STPD is now replaced by the quantity of substance in mmol (page 16).

The relationship of gas volume to pressure is an inverse one; it is described approximately by Boyle's law which has the form $PV = K$. The relationship of volume to ambient temperature is the subject of Charles' law which states that the volume is proportional to the absolute temperature in degrees kelvin (T), hence $V = K'T$; this can be rewritten as $V = K'(273 + t)$, where t is temperature in degrees celsius. The two equations are combined in the general gas equation; this represents that for a given mass of gas under two sets of conditions $P_1V_1/T_1 = P_2V_2/T_2$. The equation is used to convert gas volumes to BTPS or STPD from measurements made at ATP. For this purpose:

$$V_{BTPS} = V_{ATP} \times \frac{273 + 37}{273 + t} \times \frac{P_B - P_{H_2O}(t)}{P_B - P_{H_2O}(37)} \qquad (2.3)$$

$$V_{STPD} = V_{ATP} \times \frac{273}{273 + t} \times \frac{P_B - P_{H_2O}(t)}{P_B, \text{ standard}} \qquad (2.4)$$

where V is gas volume under the conditions specified, t is ambient temperature and 37 is body temperature in degrees celsius, P_B is

Standardisation of volumes for temperature and pressure

Table 2.6 Factors for conversion of volumes from ATPS to STPD and BTPS

Ambient temperature (°C)	Aqueous vapour pressure		Factor to convert to:	
	kPa	mmHg	STPD	BTPS
10	1.23	9.2	0.952	1.153
11	1.31	9.8	0.949	1.148
12	1.40	10.5	0.945	1.143
13	1.49	11.2	0.940	1.138
14	1.60	12.0	0.936	1.133
15	1.71	12.8	0.932	1.128
16	1.81	13.6	0.928	1.123
17	1.93	14.5	0.924	1.118
18	2.07	15.5	0.920	1.113
19	2.20	16.5	0.916	1.108
20	2.33	17.5	0.911	1.102
21	2.49	18.7	0.906	1.096
22	2.64	19.8	0.902	1.091
23	2.81	21.1	0.897	1.085
24	2.99	22.4	0.893	1.080
25	3.17	23.8	0.888	1.075
26	3.36	25.2	0.883	1.069
27	3.56	26.7	0.878	1.063
28	3.77	28.3	0.874	1.057
29	4.00	30.0	0.869	1.051
30	4.24	31.8	0.864	1.045
31	4.47	33.7	0.859	1.039
32	4.76	35.7	0.853	1.032
33	5.03	37.7	0.848	1.026
34	5.32	39.9	0.843	1.020
35	5.62	42.2	0.838	1.014
36	5.95	44.6	0.832	1.007
37	6.28	47.1	0.826	1.000
38*	6.63	49.7	0.821	0.994
39*	6.99	52.4	0.816	0.987
40*	7.37	55.3	0.810	0.980

* At above body temperature gas in a bellows or other waterless spirometers is not fully saturated with water vapour. The appropriate factor is then midway between the value quoted and that for body temperature.

Terminology   barometric pressure and P_{H_2O} is aqueous vapour pressure at the temperature indicated. Values for P_{H_2O} in saturated gas are listed in Table 2.6, together with factors for converting gas volumes from ATPS to BTPS and STPD. They have been calculated for standard barometric pressure and may be used when the actual pressure deviates by less than 2.5%. In other circumstances conversion should be made using the equations. When this is done on a computer the aqueous vapour pressure over the range 10°C to 40°C may be represented by the following equation due to Berry:

$$P_{H_2O},\ t = 0.1333\ (9.993 - 0.3952t + 0.03775t^2) \qquad (2.5)$$

where 0.1333 converts from mmHg to kilopascals and t is as defined above. The error in P_{H_2O} derived in this way is less than 0.09 kPa (0.7 mmHg).

Guide to references

The references (Chapter 18) are classified under subject headings of which the following are particularly relevant to the present chapter:

3: Basic Equipment and Methods

Introduction

The basic measurements required are the volume, flow rate, pressure and chemical composition of the respired gas, in a variety of circumstances. The measurements are usually made using transducers sensitive to linear displacement, or physical gas analysers. The sensors are incorporated in semi-automatic or automatic types of apparatus which are often relatively simple to use and yield fully processed results on-line or with only minimal delay. However, the conventions adopted by the manufacturer when programming the equipment need to be known and accepted and the setting up and calibration must be followed meticulously. By contrast traditional methods were slower, often required manipulative skill and in the case of gas sampling and analysis entailed exposure to mercury vapour and corrosive chemicals; some examples of such equipment are illustrated in Fig. 3.1. The traditional methods usually measured the required attributes directly and when properly set up by dedicated personnel could yield very accurate results. Most laboratories have some traditional items in reserve for occasional use or for teaching so their features are touched on in the present account.

Measurement of gas volumes and flow rates

Connecting the subject to the equipment

The majority of procedures entail making measurements on respired gas via a mouth piece and two-way valve box. The nasopharynx is sealed off either reflexly as when exhaling forcibly through the mouth or by use of a nose clip. The mouth piece may be a rigid circular tube of diameter at least 2.5 cm (1 in) or a flattened tube of equivalent cross-sectional area fitted with a gum shield to ensure an airtight fit. Subjects unable to tolerate a mouth piece can use a well-fitting oro-

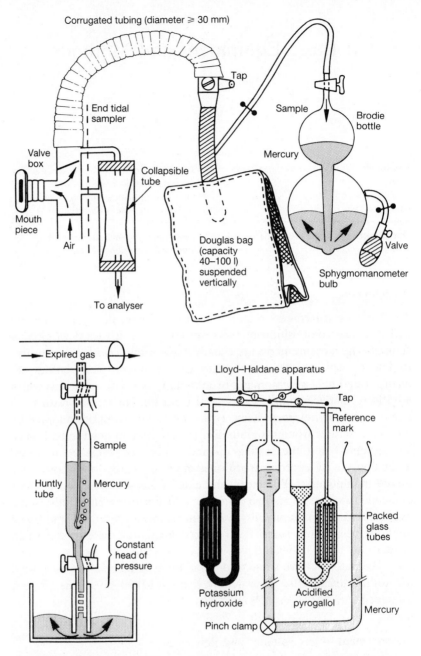

Fig. 3.1 Douglas bag, mouth piece, valve box and tubing for the collection of the
expired gas. After pummelling the bag and flushing the side tube, a sample can be
transferred to a Brodie bottle (capacity 50 ml). For operation of an end-tidal sampler the
pressure changes in the valve box are transmitted to the space round the collapsible tube
which acts as a reservoir; the end-tidal gas is drawn from here into the analyser at a rate
of 50–200 ml min^{-1}. The Huntly tube (capacity 50 ml, lower left) permits collection of a
representative sample of the gas expired over a period of 1 or 2 min. The gas can be
analysed using a Lloyd–Haldane apparatus (lower right and page 33).

Table 3.1 Inspiratory flow resistances which do not themselves reduce the ventilation minute volume ($\dot{V}E$), expressed as suction at a flow rate of $85\,l\,min^{-1}$ ($3\,ft^3\,min^{-1}$)

$\dot{V}E$ ($l\,min^{-1}$)	Suction (kPa)	(cmH_2O)
<10	0.5	5.0
10–30	0.25	2.5
30–100	0.10	1.0
>100	0.07	0.7

Note: Expiratory flow resistances should not exceed twice these levels. For protective respirators in order to avoid undue discomfort (but not hypoventilation) Bentley and others recommend a maximal peak pressure of $1.7\,kPa$ ($17\,cmH_2O$).

nasal mask. The fit is achieved by selecting one from a number of semi-rigid face pieces or by using a face piece with a soft inflatable edge and fastening it using a relatively tight harness. Volume or flow-measuring devices can be attached to the inspiratory or expiratory ports of the valve box or mask and the expired gas can be channelled past a sampling point or a mixing chamber if a representative sample is required (Fig. 14.5, page 426).

The respiratory equipment should not itself hinder the flow of gas into or out of the lungs and on this account should have an acceptably low flow resistance (Table 3.1). However, despite this precaution the use of a mouth piece or oro-nasal mask can alter the pattern of breathing; under resting conditions the principal change is an increase in tidal volume of approximately 30%. The distortion can be avoided by abandoning the mouth piece and instead using a ventilated canopy or recording the respiratory excursion of the thorax and abdomen. The excursion can be recorded photographically, or by magnetometers, strain gauges or other sensors applied to the torso or by plethysmography. These methods are only suitable for a few applications; for the majority a mouth piece is used and any interaction with breathing is ignored.

Measuring devices

A volume of gas is usually best measured with a spirometer or gas meter and a flow rate with a flow-measuring device. However, flow rate can also be obtained from volume by differentiation with respect to time and volume from flow rate by integration in a similar manner. Thus the distinction between volume- and flow-measuring devices has been reduced but neglect of the difference can still lead to error because not all instruments are suitable for all applications. The instrument which is chosen should conform to internationally agreed standards of accuracy for volume and dynamic characteristics (Table 3.2).

Spirometry. Gas volume is usually measured in a spirometer. This can take the form of a cylinder, piston, wedge or bellows of known dimensions; for use by adults it should have a volume displacement of at

Table 3.2 *Minimal* standards for equipment used for measurement of gas volumes and flow rates: recommendations of European Coal and Steel Community (ECSC) and American Thoracic Society Epidemiology Standardisation Project (ESP)

	ECSC	ESP
Volume range	0–8 l	0–7 l
Volume accuracy	$\pm 3\%$ or ± 50 ml[x]	3% or 50 ml
Reading accuracy	25 ml	50 ml
Driving pressure	<0.03 kPa	Not stated
Paper speed	0.02 m s^{-1}	0.02 m s^{-1}
Recording time	14 s accurate to $\pm 1\%$	15 s[‡]
Flow range	1–15 l s^{-1}	0.2–12 l s^{-1}
Flow accuracy	$\pm 4\%$ or ± 0.07 l s^{-1}	Not stated
Dynamic resistance	<0.05 kPa l^{-1} s	0.15 kPa l^{-1} s
Inertia	<0.001 kPa l^{-1} s^2	Not stated
Maximal mouth pressure	<0.6 kPa	Not stated
Dynamic response	3–20 Hz[†]	Not stated

[x] Whichever is greater.
[†] The response should be flat (within 5%) at 3 Hz for FEV_1, MMEF and $MEF_{25\%\ FVC}$, 5 Hz for $MEF_{50\%\ FVC}$, and 20 Hz for PEF.
[‡] 30 s for VC (ATS 1987 update)

least 8 l. The container is sealed by either a trough of water as in a gasometer, or by an expansile bellows or rolling seal. Where water is used the level should be maintained constant by regular checking. The displacement of the spirometer should be linear with volume and the equipment should comply with the standards indicated in Table 3.2. Some of the common features and uses of the different types of spirometer are indicated in Table 3.3. Procedures for calibration are given on page 50.

The volume recorded by a spirometer is that of gas at the pressure and the temperature of the gas-containing chamber. The pressure will

Table 3.3 Some types of spirometers

Type	Shape	Seal	Common features	Applications
Benedict, Roth	Long cylinder (dia. approx. 20 cm)	Water	Water oscillation, low deadspace	Closed circuit
Tissot	Large cylinder	Water	High inertia	Storing gas
Mendel, Bernstein	Wide	Water	Small displacement	Dynamic volumes
Krogh	Wedge	Water	Small displacement	Dynamic volumes
Vitalograph	Wedge	Bellows	High inertia	FEV_1 and FVC
McDermott	Cube	Bellows	Low resistance and inertia	Dynamic volumes and flow rates
Modern	Wide piston	Rolling seal	High performance	All

normally be atmospheric. The temperature will vary with circumstances so should be recorded. It is likely to be close to ambient temperature and lower than body temperature, hence the exhaled gas cools as it enters the spirometer. If the materials used for the spirometer conduct heat and have a high thermal capacity, the exhaled gas rapidly achieves thermal equilibrium and this is also the case if the exhalation is slow. However, equilibrium may not be achieved following a rapid exhalation into a spirometer made entirely of components having a low thermal conductivity: a situation where this occurred has been described by Perks and colleagues.

Spirometers are used for measurement of vital capacity, dynamic lung volumes and flow rates (page 134) and for measurement of total lung capacity and its subdivisions (page 149). For the latter application the subject rebreathes from the spirometer for up to 20 min so the contained gas should be conditioned by the absorption of exhaled carbon dioxide and the replenishment of oxygen which is taken up. Carbon dioxide is absorbed using soda lime granules in a vertical canister of wide cross-sectional area; these features ensure that the distribution of the granules is uniform and the resistance to airflow is not material. The granules should be renewed after 2 h of regular use or when the fractional concentration of carbon dioxide exceeds 0.005. Oxygen should be added at a rate which is adjusted to maintain a constant volume of gas in the spirometer at the end of expiration (page 152). To ensure that the conditioning is uniform and to overcome the flow resistance of the soda lime the gas is circulated by a fan; the flow rate should be approximately $100 \, l \, min^{-1}$ and the circuit adjusted so that the pressure at the mouthpiece is atmospheric. This can be checked by noting that when the mouthpiece is open to air there is no movement of gas into or out of the circuit. There should also be no leaks as assessed by observing that after closing the mouthpiece there is no loss of volume over 20 min following applying a weight to the spirometer. A method for measuring the volume of gas in the circuit is described on page 152 and a routine for checking that all is working satisfactorily on page 72.

In some spirometers the volume signal is differentiated to yield flow rate. The method is acceptable provided that the spirometer has an adequate frequency response (preferably 10 Hz), the output is linear, and the differentiator is accurate to 1% of the signal. Methods of calibration are described on page 52. Alternatively the signal from the spirometer can be expressed as volume per 10 ms, which is in effect flow rate; volumes are then obtained by summation.

Gas meters. Traditional gas meters measure volume by displacement. In wet gas meters the blades of a paddle wheel dip into a trough of water which should be level; the wheel is rotated by gas delivered at a steady rate. The meters can be accurate but have a high resistance. They were formerly used for measuring the volume of gas contained in Douglas bags. Dry gas meters comprise two inter-connected bellows which fill alternately. The resistance can be low enough for use in a breathing circuit and the accuracy can be 1% over complete cycles of the mechanism. Over segments of the cycle the calibration is alinear. Dry gas meters were formerly used on-line in exercise studies. The Kofranyi Michaelis dry gas meter, which incorporates a mechanism for collecting a representative sample of respired gas, is sometimes used for monitoring respiration during daily activities. It has a relatively high flow resistance.

Impedance plethysmograph. In this instrument which was developed by Milledge and Stott, the sensor is an expansile wire coil round the torso. The coil acts as the inductive element in an oscillatory circuit. Changes in torso diameter with respiration alter the inductance and hence the frequency of the oscillator and this is detected as a direct current (d.c.) signal. In the commercial model (Respitrace) two sensors are used respectively to monitor expansion of the upper chest and abdomen and the signals are summed after calibration to ensure that they are comparable. Then:

$$\Delta V_m = a\ \Delta RC + b\ \Delta Abd \qquad (3.1)$$

where ΔV_m is volume change at the mouth, ΔRC and ΔAbd are the changes in the signals respectively from the rib cage and the abdominal transducers, a and b are calibration factors also called volume−motion coefficients.

This two compartment model developed by Konne and Mead is adequate for tidal breathing but not for vital capacity manoeuvres. Calibration is done by one of several methods including voluntarily altering the position of rib cage and diaphragm during breathholding (iso-volume method) and fractionating the tidal breaths into segments. The variability under favourable conditions is approximately 6% but is more during deep breathing. Recalibration is advisable following body movement. The instrument is used for monitoring ventilation during sleep and when the nose and mouth are involved with other activity, for example phonation or assisted ventilation.

Respiratory anemometers. Anemometers monitor airflow. In hot wire anemometers the airflow cools the wire and this causes a change in electrical resistance. In the rotating vane anemometer developed by Wright, the vane is mounted in a tube and the air enters through oblique slots cut in its wall. The characteristics of the anemometer are determined by the shape and size of the slots. In both types of instrument the calibration curve can be alinear, and in the latter, at very low flow rates, some air can pass the vane before it starts to rotate. These difficulties have now largely been overcome, for example, by programming a microprocessor to construct a calibration curve. The calibration signal can be a standard volume of gas delivered from a syringe with different amounts of force (e.g. Morgan ventilometer). The signal from the anemometer can be used to drive a trigger device for sampling the respired gas; this instrument (Miser) is suitable for field studies of energy expenditure.

In constant pressure, variable orifice anemometers such as the *Wright peak flow meter*, a slot aperture in communication with a mouthpiece is initially sealed off by a moveable vane or piston restrained by a constant tension spring. Forcible exhalation into the instrument enlarges the aperture to the extent needed to maintain a constant pressure in the mouthpiece. The maximal enlargement and associated excursion of the vane reflect the peak expiratory flow. The initial calibration of the Wright peak flow meter (original version) was performed biologically using subjects whose peak flow was also registered using a pneumotachograph: the relationship of this calibration to that obtained using steady flows from a rotameter is given by equation 3.2:

$$\text{PEF } (\text{ls}^{-1}) = 0.017 \, (0.95 \, \dot{V} \, (\text{l min}^{-1}) + 47) \qquad (3.2)$$

where PEF is the corrected peak flow reading, $\dot{V}$ is the rotameter reading and 0.017 converts from l min^{-1} to ls^{-1} (see also page 139). Other versions of the meter can be calibrated against the original, which is held by the manufacturer, or against an appropriate pneumotachograph using a group of subjects whose PEF values cover the range of the instrument under test. Provided the resistance of the meter does not affect the peak flow the calibration can also be performed with a computer-controlled pump. Using this approach Miller and colleagues have observed deficiencies in some currently available peak flow meters including alinearity (e.g. mini-Wright meter) and inappropriate damping (e.g. Ferrasis meter). To reduce error the meter should be linear over the range $0-14\text{ls}^{-1}$ and the frequency response should be flat up to a frequency of 20 Hz. The measurement of peak expiratory flow has been reviewed by Quanjer, Lebowitz and Gregg on behalf of the European Respiratory Society. The measurement is described on page 139.

Pneumotachograph. A pneumotachograph monitors airflow; this is usually done in terms of the reduction in pressure which occurs across a resistance, either a wire grid or a bundle of parallel small tubes; these types were introduced by Lilly and by Fleisch respectively (Fig. 3.2). The changes in electrical resistance of a heated wire and the Doppler shift induced by the flow of gas can also be used as a signal. In the pressure pneumotachograph the temperature of the resistance should preferably be maintained at the temperature of expired gas leaving the mouth (approximately 32°C). This reduces condensation of water vapour which otherwise increases the resistance of the detector. Any additional condensate can be vapourised by periodically drying the pneumotachograph using a fan. Heating the pneumotachograph also minimises fluctuations in temperature between inspired and expired gas; these can affect the pressure drop across the resistance by altering the viscosity of the gas. However minor fluctuations in temperature still occur as a result of changes in flow rate; these can be allowed for electronically.

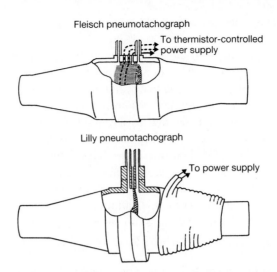

Fig. 3.2 Fleisch- and Lilly-type pneumotachographs each fitted with thermostat and heater (Hewlett Packard).

The pressure drop is registered using a differential strain gauge manometer. The Fleisch pneumotachograph has the advantage of compactness because even relatively short capillary tubes rapidly eliminate turbulence in the air-stream. In the Lilly type the turbulence is controlled by using a tapered tube. The dimensions determine the range over which the instrument is linear; for a pressure drop of up to 0.1 kPa (1 cmH$_2$O) the range in air at sea level can be from zero to 16 l s^{-1} but 0 to 6 l s^{-1} is adequate for monitoring tidal breathing. Compared with a pressure pneumotachograph a hot wire pneumotachograph is usually linear over a smaller range of flow rates whilst the sonic pneumotachograph can be linear over a larger range. Calibration is carried out using rotameters supplied with ambient air (Fig. 3.8, page 49). A calibration curve which is alinear but stable can be linearised by electronic means; the resulting calibration curve should be checked for linearity and stability. The calibration curve is sensitive to changes in gas density during a period of measurement, for example during an exhalation following inhalation of a single breath of 80% helium in oxygen. This source of error can be avoided by interposing a bag-in-box (Donald, Christie box) between the mouthpiece and the pneumotachograph. Alternatively the flow rate can be measured using a spirometer (page 25). The signal from the pneumotachograph is sometimes integrated to yield volume. The accuracy of integration can readily be checked using a one litre gas syringe but drift in the integrator is often a problem. It can be corrected by automatic re-zeroing but it is preferable to avoid this by using an instrument of high quality.

Respiration counters. Respiratory frequency per min can be obtained from inspection of the chest wall or from any instrument which responds to a movement of the chest or the resulting airflow. Thus use has been made of a microswitch attached to a band round the chest, a light beam interrupted by a breathing valve, a thermistor in the nose, an impedance jacket and other instruments. The principal error is from irregularities in the signal; these can be identified by adopting criteria for what constitutes reversal of movement of the chest wall or of air flow.

Transducers and amplifiers

Simple manometers

A pressure which is constant or only changing very slowly can be measured directly with a U-tube manometer containing a liquid of known density; the pressure is given by the product of the density and the height of the column of the liquid which the unknown pressure will support. Water and mercury manometers are commonly used in this way both for calibrating other pressure recorders and for measuring the resistance characteristics of physiological equipment. The method is illustrated in Fig. 3.3.

Electric manometers

Pressure transducers convert a change in pressure or other variable into an electrical signal. The pressure is applied to one side of a diaphragm, crystal, or other device of which the other side is at atmospheric pressure, except when it is proposed to measure the differential pressure between two sites; in these circumstances the pressure at the second site is applied to the other side. The movement of the diaphragm or the distortion of the crystal lattice is detected as a change in electrical resistance, capacitance or inductance. For measurement of the pressure drop across a pneumotachograph, use is made of a low-pressure differential transducer, whilst for the pressure at the tip of a long catheter of small internal diameter there is need for a high-pressure low-volume-displacement transducer.

For the measurement of velocity and of linear movement, including that of the chest wall, use may be made of a differential transformer-type transducer. Displacement of the core of the transducer produces a proportional change in the output voltage. Where two or more pressure transducers are used concurrently they should preferably be of the same type in order that their outputs can be synchronised.

The electromanometers which are used for recording pressure should have an accuracy and resolution of less than 2% of the maximal pressure which it is proposed to measure. The pressure range should be for maximal respiratory pressure $\pm 30\,$kPa and for whole body plethysmography $\pm 2\,$kPa (mouth pressure) and $\pm 2 \times 10^{-2}\,$kPa (plethysmograph pressure). The response should be a linear function of the pressure to within 2% of the full-scale deflection and the time required for 95% response should be of the order of 0.01 s. With

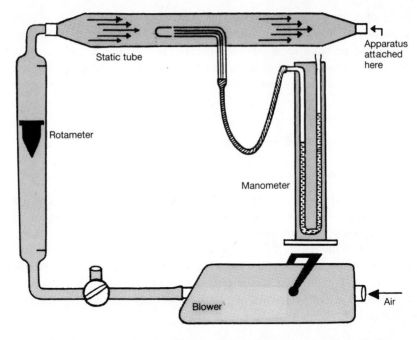

Static tube

Rotameter

Manometer

Apparatus attached here

Blower

Air

Fig. 3.3 Static tube and other equipment for determining the resistance to air flow imposed by items of physiological apparatus. The outer tube has an internal diameter of 5 cm and the angle of the cones is 7°. The inner tube is of diameter 8 mm and length 10.5 cm; it is perforated by 7 holes (diameter 0.97 mm) located 3.2 cm down-stream from the hemispherical head. The outer tube should ideally extend for 1 m on either side of the static tube. The pressure is recorded at selected flow rates before and after connection of the apparatus to be tested; the resistance at these flow rates is then obtained by difference.

The method is satisfactory when, as is usually the case, the back pressure is less than 0.2 kPa (2.0 cmH$_2$O). For higher pressures the reading on the rotameter should be adjusted for the change in the density of the gas according to the following relationship:

$$\dot{V} = \dot{V}_0 \sqrt{\frac{(P_B + P)}{P_B}}$$

where $\dot{V}_0$ and $\dot{V}$ are the initial and corrected readings on the rotameter, P_B is barometric pressure and P is the pressure difference registered by the manometer.

appropriate damping and suitable recording equipment most mano-meters can be used to follow cyclical fluctuations in pressure occurring with a frequency of up to about 40 Hz; this is adequate for most purposes (e.g. Table 3.2, page 24). Manometers which would meet a more stringent specification are also available.

Electronic amplifiers

The output from the transducer is coupled to an amplifier, which should have characteristics that match both the transducer and the recorder which it is proposed to use. These requirements are now best met by semiconductor integrated circuit amplifiers; they combine a high gain (amplification) with a high input resistance and operate at a low d.c. voltage and current which makes for electrical safety. This class of amplifiers includes integrated circuit operational amplifiers which may be used with glass electrodes for the measurement of pH and $P\text{CO}_2$ where an input resistance in excess of 10^{11} ohms is required.

New families of integrated circuits are now becoming available including complementary metal oxide semiconductors (C-MOS); these have a very low power consumption so are suitable for portable equipment which runs off batteries.

As well as their use in amplifiers, integrated circuit chips now have applications as counters, timers, voltage to frequency converters, waveform generators, zero voltage switches, memories, analogue to digital converters and many other functions.

Recorders for use with electronic equipment

Digital displays

These may take the form of light emitting diodes, liquid crystals or gas discharge tubes; they have the advantages of being relatively robust and cheap and of minimising errors in reading.

Cathode-ray oscilloscope coupled to a recording camera

A cathode-ray oscilloscope, when it is coupled with amplifiers which are appropriate for respiratory physiology, usually has a flat frequency response from d.c. to about 1 mHz; however, if it is required, a response of up to 50 mHz can be obtained at relatively low cost. Oscilloscopes with plug-in facilities for both the vertical and the horizontal axes are extremely versatile and can be used to record one or several signals simultaneously with respect to time or to provide accurate X–Y displays. In a storage oscilloscope the image is retained on the screen for subsequent inspection and photography. The use of a polaroid camera then permits early verification of the result. The oscilloscope has the disadvantages of not providing a permanent record except with photography, and the definition is not as good as with the other systems. Permanent records can also be obtained using fibre-optic recording oscilloscopes.

A mirror galvanometer shining on photographic paper

The most satisfactory instrument of this type is the ultraviolet galvanometer recorder in which use is made of pencil-type plug-in galvanometers; these have a frequency response which is flat over the range from d.c. to 5 kHz and one recorder can accept as many as 25 channels. Each channel may, if necessary, occupy the whole width of the light-sensitive paper. The recorders are robust and portable and the record does not require processing, unless it is to be exposed to bright sunlight, or stored for a long period of time.

Direct writing chart recorders

With these instruments, the signal is relayed by either a milliammeter
or a potentiometer and the record is inscribed on moving paper by a
marking device. The milliammeter swivels about a central point so the
record is relatively narrow. It can be subject to arc distortion, especially
when the distance from the point of rotation to the paper is relatively
short. In addition, the accuracy of the milliammeter recorders, whilst
sufficient for most purposes, is seldom better than 1% of the full-scale
deflection. The main advantages of these recorders are their small size,
so that a number of records may be obtained simultaneously, and their
frequency response, which is usually flat from d.c. to about 1 kHz
depending on the mass of the stylus (see below).

The recorder is usually equipped with a fibre tip pen which is less
liable to clog or blot than is an ink pen. Heated filaments, when they
write on a knife-edge, have little arc distortion but they require specially
treated paper which is expensive. The excursion of these systems is
limited both because the styluses cannot be allowed to cross and
because the records may only be linear over a relatively narrow width
of paper. The frequency response is usually satisfactory up to 100 Hz.
Ink jets can cross without interference and are usually independent of
frequency over a wide range (up to 1000 Hz); they are satisfactory
when properly maintained.

The potentiometric recorders are null-point instruments in which the
potential to be measured is balanced against a reference potential by a
process of successive approximations in which the marking device is
moved by a servo-operated electric motor into the position of equilibrium. These devices have no distortion: their accuracy is of the order
of 0.1% of the full-scale deflection. They provide a wide chart record.
However, they have a relatively slow frequency response, which is
usually less than 10 Hz.

Direct-writing recorders are widely used on account of their convenience, especially when an instantaneous record of events is required
for continuation of an investigation. Twin co-ordinate chart recorders
in which two variables are recorded simultaneously along two axes at
right angles are also of value for some applications; the frequency
response of these instruments is in most instances only satisfactory up
to about 1 Hz but recorders with a more rapid response are now
available. The relatively low frequency response of chart recorders is
due mainly to the inertia of the moving parts. This limitation can be
overcome by the use of microcircuits to store the incoming signals
which may then be replayed at a slower rate. In this way signals with
respect to time may be recorded over a deflection of 250 mm with an
accuracy of 0.2%, and a frequency response of up to 20 kHz. For $X-Y$
displays similar advantages can be obtained.

Electromagnetic tape readers permit the storage of several channels of information on reels or cassettes. By the use of integrated circuit techniques the data may be pre-processed into a form suitable for direct input into a small desk top computer or into a calculator with provision for electrical input. The results of individual measurements may then be displayed via a graph plotter, a digital display or a printer; the last is particularly suitable for measurements made on epidemiological surveys. The results for series of subjects may be similarly stored, then for purposes of statistical analysis, fed into a computer with a large memory.

Microprocessors are based on a read-only-memory (ROM); this is programmed to the requirements of a particular task. Extra memories together with input and output devices, including a printer or graph plotter, form a microcomputer which can be used on-line during experimental measurements. Microprocessors now form an integral part of most equipment for the assessment of lung function. They oversee the intermediate stages of the measurement, and tabulate, calculate and annotate the results. Through their use many errors are eliminated and the results can be made available in the form in which they are to be used almost as soon as all the data have been collected.

Analysis of gases

Chemical methods

The concentrations of oxygen and carbon dioxide in the respired gas were traditionally determined by volumetric methods which depended upon chemical absorption. The procedures require a delicate touch but are accurate when undertaken by a skilled operator. Using these methods the gas is drawn into a graduated burette over mercury and its initial volume is recorded at barometric pressure. The carbon dioxide is then absorbed by exposure of the gas to potassium hydroxide, after which the measurement of volume is repeated. The volume of carbon dioxide in the initial sample is obtained by difference. This procedure is repeated for oxygen, which is absorbed by either pyrogallol or anthraquinone and sodium hydrosulphite made up in potassium hydroxide. The Lloyd–Haldane apparatus is illustrated in Fig. 3.1. The micro-Scholander apparatus can also be used. Some suitable reagents are given in Table 3.4.

Physical methods

These methods utilise some physical property of gases in order to analyse the constituents of a mixture. Some examples are given in Table 3.5. In most instances the property is not unique to an individual gas so the presence of other gases must be allowed for. One convenient

Table 3.4 Reagents for use with the chemical absorption methods of gas analysis at or above 20°C

Acid rinse		Glycerol	21 ml
		H_2SO_4 (conc.)	1 ml
		Na_2SO_4 (anhydr.)	66.4 g
		H_2O	400 ml

40 mg of pulverized $K_2Cr_2O_7$ are added to 50 ml of this solution immediately before use

Absorber for CO_2		KOH	8.86 g
		$K_2Cr_2O_7$	40 mg
		H_2O	100 ml
Absorber for O_2	A	KOH	5 g
		H_2O	100 ml
	B	$Na_2SO_4 \cdot 2H_2O$	24 g
		Anthraquinone	0.1 g

The oxygen reagent is made up by dissolving 1.3 g of B in 10 ml of A. In this form it will only keep for a few days but the components will keep indefinitely

Table 3.5 Physical methods for analysis of gases

Physical attributes	Gases for which appropriate	Other gases which interfere
Differential absorption (gas chromatography)	All	—
Flame conductivity	C_2H_2 and other hydrocarbons	O_2, CO_2
Gamma emission	^{85}Kr, $^{15}O_2$, $^{17}O_2$, ^{133}Xe	—
Infrared absorption	CO_2, CO, N_2O, C_2H_2	H_2O*
Kinematic viscosity	He, H_2, SF_6	†
Mass	All	See text
Paramagnetic properties	O_2, NO	—
pH in solution	CO_2	†
Photo-ionisation	O_2	†
Polarographic potential	O_2	†
Refraction index	He	—
Sound transmission	He, H_2	O_2, CO_2, H_2O
Thermal conductivity	He, CO_2, N_2O, H_2	O_2, H_2O
Ultraviolet emission	N_2	CO_2, H_2O, SF_6

* Other gases including oxygen, can give rise to collision broadening of the absorption bands for the gas to be analysed; the broadening alters the calibration.
† Variable depending on conditions.

attribute is mass, which for most purposes is equal to the gram molecular weight; this is the basis for resolution in respiratory mass spectrometers such as that originally developed by Fowler. Most instruments are able to analyse simultaneously up to four gases having molecular weights in the range 1–200. The response time is about 0.1 s. The resolution is normally to one mass unit. It is then not possible to distinguish between carbon monoxide and nitrogen, since both have molecular weights of about 28. The overlap can cause a small error when measuring nitrogen in the presence of carbon dioxide since up to 0.6% of the CO_2 can be reduced to carbon monoxide in the instrument. Carbon monoxide can be analysed in the form $C^{18}O$. Nitrous oxide overlaps with carbon dioxide, since both have a mass of approximately 44, but the former gas is oxidised to nitric oxide which can be detected separately. In addition the concentration of water vapour may not be accurately assessed and may cause other artifacts if it condenses to form water droplets in the sampling tube. The errors can usually be allowed for by computation. Calibration is considered subsequently (page 50).

Measurement of oxygen consumption and respiratory exchange ratio

Oxygen consumption

The consumption of oxygen by a subject can be measured by closed-circuit spirometry (page 152) but is more often calculated from the volume and composition of the respired gas. The analysis is usually performed on gas which has been dried, using a paramagnetic analyser for oxygen and infrared analyser for carbon dioxide. The remainder is then nitrogen plus the rare gases (98.9% and 1.1% respectively). The consumption of oxygen per min is the difference between the amounts of oxygen which enter and leave the lung. Thus:

$$\dot{n}_{O_2} = 1000/22.4\,[\dot{V}_I \times F_{I,O_2} - \dot{V}_E \times F_{E,O_2}]\ \text{mmol}\,\text{min}^{-1} \quad (3.3)$$

where $\dot{n}_{O_2}$ is the consumption of oxygen in $\text{mmol}\,\text{min}^{-1}$, $\dot{V}_I$ and $\dot{V}_E$ are the volumes of gas which are respectively inspired and expired per min in l STPD and the remaining symbols are defined in Table 3.6. The numerical ratio converts the term within the bracket from $\text{l}\,\text{min}^{-1}$ to $\text{mmol}\,\text{min}^{-1}$. This derivation entails measuring the volumes of both the inspired and expired gas since the two differ on account of the oxygen which is absorbed seldom being replaced by an exactly equal volume of carbon dioxide. However, under stable conditions breathing air the difference does not extend to nitrogen. This gas with or without the rare gases can therefore be used to correct for the change in volume. To this end the volume of nitrogen entering and leaving the lung per min is represented as follows:

$$\dot{V}_I \times F_{I,N_2} = \dot{V}_E \times F_{E,N_2} \quad\quad (3.4)$$

Table 3.6 Symbols for quantities used in the calculation of consumption of oxygen

	Inspired concentration*	Expired concentration
Oxygen	F_{I,O_2} (0.2093)*	F_{E,O_2}
Carbon dioxide	F_{I,CO_2} (0.0003)	F_{E,CO_2}
Nitrogen (including rare gases)	F_{I,N_2} (0.7904)	F_{E,N_2}

* These fractional concentrations are for breathing air.

This relationship is then restated:

The volume of gas inspired per l of gas expired

$$= \dot{V}_I/\dot{V}_E = F_{E,N_2}/F_{I,N_2}$$

The volume of O_2 inspired per l of gas expired

$$= F_{I,O_2} \times F_{E,N_2}/F_{I,N_2}$$
$$= 0.2648 \times F_{E,N_2} \text{ (including rare gases)}$$

The volume of O_2 absorbed per l of gas expired

$$= 0.2648 \times F_{E,N_2} - F_{E,O_2}$$

O_2 consumption per min

$$= (1000/22.4)\dot{V}_E \times (0.2648 \times F_{E,N_2} - F_{E,O_2}) \text{ mmol min}^{-1} \quad (3.5)$$

When, instead of the expired minute volume, the inspired minute volume is recorded it may be converted into the corresponding expired minute volume via equation 3.4. Thus:

$$\dot{V}_E = \dot{V}_I \times F_{I,N_2}/F_{E,N_2} \quad (3.6)$$

If it is convenient to analyse only one gas, the concentration of oxygen should be obtained and used in an empirical equation such as proposed by Musgrove and Doré. Alternatively the analysis may be performed before and after the absorption of carbon dioxide.

Respiratory exchange ratio

The respiratory exchange ratio is the ratio of the rate of appearance of carbon dioxide in the lung to the rate of disappearance of oxygen. Under steady state conditions the ratio is representative of the metabolism of the subject and is called the *respiratory quotient*. It is calculated in the following manner:

$$R = \dot{n}_{CO_2}/\dot{n}_{O_2} = F_{E,CO_2}/(0.2648 F_{E,N_2} - F_{E,O_2}) \quad (3.7)$$

where R is the respiratory exchange ratio and $\dot{n}CO_2$ and $\dot{n}O_2$ are respectively the rates of evolution of carbon dioxide and of consumption of oxygen per min.

Collection and storage of blood

Choice of site

If the patient has a good peripheral blood flow, capillary blood samples accurately reflect the composition of the circulating blood. The samples are analysed by techniques which require not more than 0.1 ml of blood. These can be used to estimate the capillary blood pH, the tensions of carbon dioxide and oxygen, the bicarbonate concentration, the saturation of haemoglobin with oxygen or carbon monoxide and the concentration of lactic acid. The sample may be obtained anaerobically, via a small capillary tube, from the heel in infants, and in older subjects from the ear lobe or the pulp of a finger. The part is first rendered hyperaemic by local heat and a rubefacient cream (e.g. Transvasin, Reckitt & Colman, or Algipan, Wyeth Laboratories, Maidenhead). After cleansing the skin with alcohol, a stab incision is made 3 mm above the lower border of the ear lobe through to a sterile rubber bung or cork behind the ear. Free flow of blood is essential to permit rapid collection into a heparin coated 100 µl glass capillary tube. However, if accurate or repeated estimates are required, the arterial blood should be sampled directly.

Arterial puncture sites, in order of preference, are the radial, brachial, dorsalis pedis and femoral. In neonates an umbilical artery catheter may be used. With practice, the radial artery is satisfactory in most patients, usually has good collateral circulation, and produces the lowest incidence of complications. The technique is easily taught to doctors, nurses and other medical personnel.

Procedure for arterial puncture (single sample)

For radial artery puncture, the supinated wrist is supported in a hyper-extended position by an assistant or by micropore tape. The radial artery pulsation is located proximal to the flexor skin crease, and 1–2 ml of local anesthetic (lignocaine 2%) is then injected beneath the skin and subcutaneous tissues and 2 min allowed to take effect. Few doctors now use the traditional siliconised glass syringe and large (green) needle. Most prefer a 23SWG (blue) or 25SWG (orange) needle or winged IV cannula (Butterfly, Abbot Laboratories, Maiden-head). This is connected to a 2 ml or 5 ml plastic syringe and the deadspace filled with 0.25 ml of 1000 units per ml heparin. A small air bubble is left in the distal plastic IV cannula tubing to permit 'flash back' and visualisation of pulsation to confirm successful arterial puncture. This is invaluable when using arteries adjacent to large veins at the brachial or femoral sites.

To make the insertion the operator fully cleanses the skin with alcohol then palpates the radial artery pulsation with the fingers of one hand. The steel needle is inserted at an angle of approximately 60° to the skin surface and advanced until pulsating arterial blood appears. If the needle passes too deeply and touches the radius, the likely position of the radial artery is reassessed. The needle is partially withdrawn and then advanced once more. When it is placed correctly the arterial blood sample should aspirate almost effortlessly into the syringe. However, the radial artery is often small, and a high success rate is achieved only with practice.

The brachial artery site is easier but complications more frequent. The arm should be hyper-extended at the elbow and supported on a pillow. Again the pulsation is palpated with the fingers of one hand, the needle guided with the other.

Procedure for arterial cannulation

This permits both repeated arterial blood sampling and also direct
blood pressure monitoring. The radial artery site in the non-dominant
arm is again preferred, and local anaesthetic used even for apparently
comatose patients in intensive care units. Percutaneous cannulation
produces less complications than surgical 'cut downs'. Allen's test is
recommended to ensure adequate collateral blood flow from the ulnar
artery.

A standard 20SWG IV, Teflon, parallel sided cannula, such as a
Venflon (Viggo Laboratories, Helsingborg, Sweden) is satisfactory.
Alternatively, indwelling flexible IV cannulae (20 or 22SWG) can be
inserted over their own steel cannulae, or using a standard Seldinger
technique with a guide wire. Meticulous skin preparation is essential,
and a small skin incision facilitates subsequent insertion of the cannula.
The needle tip is held at 30° to the skin and advanced until a 'flash
back' of blood is seen. The plastic cannula is then advanced over the
steel needle a further 2 or 3 cm along the arterial lumen and the steel
needle (or guide wire) is then removed. The resulting blood flow can
usually be controlled by firm pressure on the vessel proximally. The
cannula hub is then fixed via a 3-way tap to a continuous flushing
device and, if required, to a continuous pressure monitoring system by
monometer tubing. The cannula should be firmly secured by transparent
adhesive dressings or skin sutures and sterile dressings. The cannula
site should be inspected frequently for bruising or infection.

If difficulties arise, consider transfixing the artery and then slowly
withdrawing the needle until 'flash back' is seen, at which point the
plastic cannula can then be advanced. The Seldinger technique can be
used in the same way.

Haemostasis after arterial puncture

Firm digital pressure should be applied to the puncture site for 5 min
by the patient, the doctor or an assistant. A firmly wrapped crepe
bandage appears less effective. Prolonged pressure should be used in
patients with bleeding diatheses or those on anticoagulants. In addition
specific antidotes should be available, including protamine sulphate for
patients receiving heparin and fresh frozen plasma for those on warfarin.
Patients on long-term prednisolone almost always bruise.

Contra-indications and complications

Arteries should never be punctured through infected or broken skin.
Complications following simple arterial puncture are rare, particularly
at the radial site. They have been reviewed by Williams. Short-term
local pain and tenderness occur in about 25% of patients and, after
24 hours, bruising in 40% or even 90% if on long-term prednisolone. If
a plastic cannula of the Venflon type is left *in situ* the injection portal

must be taped over to avoid inadvertent intra-arterial injection of noxious drugs.

Complications following cannulation increase with duration and include bruising and haematomas, arterio-venous fistulae or false aneurysms, air embolism and infection. Although thrombosis and occlusion of the radial artery is common, recanalisation usually occurs and ischaemic damage is rare. Common sense precautions are reviewed by Runcie. Bleeding from the puncture site may occur up to 48 h after removal of the cannula. The patient should be alerted to the possibility, and instructed to apply firm digital pressure and summon help.

Collection and storage of blood

Two to five millilitres of arterial blood are aspirated with minimum effort into a syringe containing less than 0.25 ml of 1:1000 units per ml of heparin; excess heparin can produce an artificial metabolic acidosis in the sample. A small air bubble almost invariably appears during aspiration; the cannula or needle should be disconnected and the bubble promptly expelled (into a cotton wool ball) and an airtight cap then applied to the syringe. If several air bubbles are present the sample should be discarded.

The arterial blood gas sample is stable for less than 5 min at room temperature; over longer periods white cell metabolism will reduce the Po_2 and raise the Pco_2 by approximately $1-5$ kPa per hour. If routine blood gas analysis is likely to be delayed the sample should be stored on ice at 0°C. The analyses of Po_2 and Pco_2 should be performed within an hour. Samples for lactate or pyruvate analysis should be delivered immediately into trichloroacetic acid at 0°C, centrifuged and stored at -10°C.

Analysis of blood for oxygen

The amount of oxygen in the blood may be reported as the content in volumes per cent, as the saturation (which is the content expressed as a percentage of the capacity when the blood is exposed to a high tension of oxygen) or as the tension of oxygen. The saturation can be deduced from the tension by reference to the blood dissociation curve (e.g. Fig. 9.3 on page 280); conversely, the tension of oxygen can be deduced from the saturation over the range where there is a linear relationship between these variables. Outside this range the tension of oxygen can only be determined by a direct method.

Content of oxygen and saturation of haemoglobin

Volumetric method. Oxygen saturation is calculated as follows:

$$\text{Saturation} = \frac{\text{content of oxygen}}{\text{capacity of oxygen}} \times 100\% \qquad (3.8)$$

39

The content of oxygen was formerly determined from the volume which is liberated when potassium ferricyanide solution is added to a measured amount of blood in a closed container. The volume is estimated either from the change in pressure at constant volume by the method of Van Slyke, or the change in volume at constant pressure by the method of Haldane. The capacity is determined by similar analysis of blood which has been saturated with oxygen; an allowance is then made for the volume of oxygen which is dissolved in the plasma. At a tension of oxygen of 13.3 kPa (100 mmHg) this is $0.13 \, \text{mmol} \, \text{l}^{-1}$ (0.3 ml per 100 ml) whilst at a tension of 93 kPa (700 mmHg) it is $0.9 \, \text{mmol} \, \text{l}^{-1}$ (2.0 ml per 100 ml).

Spectrophotometric methods. The oxygen saturation of haemoglobin is estimated from the proportion which is present in a reduced form. It is obtained by passing a ray of light through the haemoglobin in solution, then measuring the absorption at two wavelengths. These are: (i) an isobestic point where the absorption is the same for the oxygenated and the reduced haemoglobin, e.g. 805 nm (8050 Å); (ii) a wavelength where the absorption is very different for the two haemoglobins, e.g. 650 nm (6500 Å). Other combinations of wavelengths can also be used. Triton X100 is used to secure haemolysis of the blood before analysis.

The capacity of haemoglobin for oxygen is a simple function of the amount of haemoglobin present (see page 278). The amount can be determined after its conversion to cyanmethaemoglobin by the method of Drabkin. This technique is adequate for most purposes. However, it also detects methaemoglobin and this may lead to the oxygen capacity of blood being overestimated in patients with polycythaemia, in whom some haemoglobin is present in this form.

The spectrophotometric methods are most accurate when applied to haemolysed blood *in vitro*; they are less accurate when applied to whole blood because the light beam is then partly scattered by the red cells. *In vivo* a further error can occur, on account of variation in the degree of dilatation of blood vessels affecting the amount of blood in the light path. The error is reduced by securing maximal vasodilatation, for example by massaging the part with Ralgex (Beecham Proprietaries), and by using a microprocessor to confine the measurements to the time when the vessels are distended by the pulse wave. This *pulse oximetry* is carried out using light which is either transmitted through the lobe or pinna of the ear or reflected from a finger, heel or other part. The former method is commonly used for exercise studies and the latter for sleep studies and measurements in infants. An earpiece should not be applied at the site of a perforation made for cosmetic purposes. The device should be protected from extraneous light, maintained at a constant temperature and attached securely. As an additional precaution, the instrument can be set at 100% after the subject has breathed oxygen for 10 min. However, this is not now considered necessary; the procedure is invalid for some patients with congenital heart disease. The accuracy is usually better than ±4% except when the saturation is greatly reduced (<65%); it can then be improved by performing an *in vivo* calibration against samples of arterial blood analysed in the laboratory.

Polarographic method. The quantity of oxygen in a measured volume of blood can be deduced from the change in oxygen tension which occurs when the oxygen is liberated from combination with haemoglobin by potassium ferricyanide or carbon monoxide in solution. The tension is measured by polarography (see below) which can also be used to construct the haemoglobin dissociation curve. For this purpose oxygenated blood and blood previously equilibrated with 100% nitrogen are mixed in known proportions; the concentration of red cells should be the same in both and the reservoirs in which the bloods are contained should be agitated before the blood is withdrawn. Alternatively the content of oxygen may be increased progressively by electrolysis. A procedure is described by Longmuir and Chow.

Tension of oxygen in blood

The tension of oxygen in the blood may be determined in several ways, each of which, in skilled hands, has a standard deviation of approximately 0.25 kPa.

Dissociation curve method. Over the range 2.5–9 kPa (20–70 mmHg) the tension of oxygen can be determined from the saturation of haemoglobin by means of the blood dissociation curve for oxygen (Fig. 9.3, page 280); a correction should be made if the body temperature departs to a material extent from 37°C or the pH of the blood is other than 7.4.

Riley bubble method. When the tension of oxygen does not exceed about 13 kPa (100 mmHg) it can be determined by a volumetric equilibrium method such as that evolved by Riley from the earlier method of Krogh. Success with the method depends upon the correct manipulation of a Roughton–Scholander syringe and requires a delicate touch. This is best learnt in a laboratory where the method is used. The method takes 20–25 min per sample, employs inexpensive apparatus which is simple to maintain and also yields the tension of carbon dioxide; it is suitable for field laboratories or when the electrical supply is variable.

Polarography. For most applications the tension of oxygen is best determined by polarography. By this method the oxygen in a sample of gas or in solution in blood at 37°C is brought into contact with a platinum electrode to which an e.m.f. of −0.6 V is applied (Fig. 3.4). The current which flows is then a function of the rate of reduction of oxygen at the tip of the electrode; the rate depends upon the diameter of the electrode and the tension of oxygen in the solution. An electrode of diameter 0.025 mm is commonly used because measurements can then

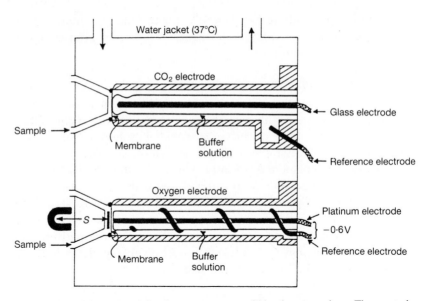

Fig. 3.4 Electrode analysers for the measurement of blood—gas tensions. The gas to be analysed diffuses through the semipermeable membrane of polyethylene or other material into the buffer solution which bathes the electrode. For carbon dioxide, the change in pH is measured with a glass electrode. The electrode is calibrated with gas or water containing carbon dioxide at a known tension. For oxygen, the current which flows between the platinum and reference electrodes is passed into an electrometer amplifier coupled to a recorder of the potentiometer type. When the diameter of the platinum electrode exceeds about 0.025 mm the blood is agitated by rotating the magnetically coupled stirring bar (S) at about 25 Hz. Calibration is usually carried out with gas or with blood equilibrated with oxygen at known tensions.

be made on unstirred capillary blood. As a result of the work of Clark the electrode is protected by a membrane made of polyethylene or polytetrafluoroethylene (PTFE) (thickness 0.025 mm); this permits the access of molecules of oxygen and carbon dioxide but not those of other substances whose presence could interfere with the response. Routine calibration is carried out with gases containing oxygen at known tensions: the gases are humidified and heated to 37°C by bubbling through water. When setting up the equipment and for greater accuracy on individual subjects, calibration should also be performed using blood. This is equilibrated with the gas in a swirling or a rotating-disc tonometer or by bubbling, using an anti-foam agent and a vessel coated with silicone. To avoid cooling of the blood during bubbling, the rate of flow of the gas should be relatively slow ($<$100 ml min^{-1}) and to avoid a rise in the tension of oxygen due to surface forces in the bubbles their diameters should be relatively large (2—7 mm). The calibration of the polarograph is linear for both water and blood, the coefficient of proportionality varying between 0.93 and 1.0, depending on the electrode. The method is suitable for gaseous oxygen as well as for oxygen in blood or other fluid. Alternative electrode systems include one based on a silver—lead galvanic cell. The cell is used for *in vitro* measurement. The polarograph electrode can be incorporated in a syringe or arterial catheter or applied to the skin for measurement of

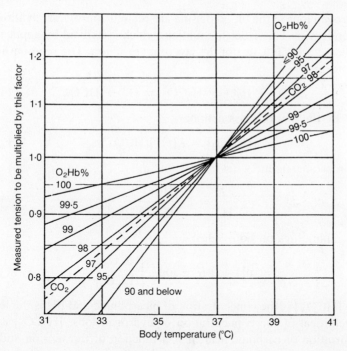

Fig. 3.5 Nomogram showing the factors by which the blood−gas tensions obtained by measurement at 37°C should be multiplied in order to obtain the correct tensions at body temperature; the factors for oxygen are a function of the saturation of haemoglobin. (Source: Kelman GR, Nunn JF. *J Appl Physiol* 1966; **21**: 1484−1490.)

transcutaneous oxygen tension. The electrode should then be heated to promote vasodilatation. The transcutaneous method is suitable for newborn infants and most patients in intensive care. It can also be used for respiratory patients amongst whom Hutchinson and colleagues observed the following relationship of transcutaneous to arterial oxygen tension:

$$Pa,o_2 = 1.14 \, (Ptc,o_2 - 0.67) \qquad \text{SEE } 0.69 \qquad (3.9)$$

where Pa,o_2 and Ptc,o_2 are respectively arterial and transcutaneous oxygen tension (kPa). The standard error of the estimate (SEE) can be reduced if, concurrent with one of the measurements, a sample of arterial blood is drawn and then analysed in the laboratory.

When the temperature of the equipment (usually 37°C) differs from that of the blood at the time of collection the measured tensions also differ from those which obtain in the body; a correction for this effect of the difference in temperature can be made given the factors in Fig. 3.5. Calibration is considered subsequently (page 50).

Analysis of blood for carbon dioxide

Direct methods

The tension and the content of carbon dioxide and the concentration of hydrogen ions in the blood plasma are related approximately through the Henderson–Hasselbalch equation, which is derived by application to carbonic acid (H_2CO_3) of the law of mass action. The relationship is of the form:

$$CO_2 + H_2O \rightleftharpoons H_2CO_3 \rightleftharpoons H^+ + HCO_3^- \qquad (3.10)$$

Hence by the law of mass action:

$$[H_2CO_3] = K[H^+][HCO_3^-] \qquad (3.11)$$

or on rearrangement:

$$\frac{I}{H^+} = K\frac{[HCO_3^-]}{[H_2CO_3]} \qquad (3.12)$$

Then, taking logs on both sides:

$$pH = pK + \log_{10}\frac{[HCO_3^-]}{[H_2CO_3]} \qquad (3.13)$$

where $[HCO_3^-]$ is the concentration of bicarbonate and pH is the log of the reciprocal of the concentration of hydrogen ions. $[H_2CO_3]$ is the concentration of carbonic acid: it is a function of the tension and the solubility of the carbon dioxide in human plasma, such that:

$$[H_2CO_3] = S/1000 \times P_{CO_2}\ mol\,l^{-1} \qquad (3.14)$$

where S is a modified Bunsen absorption coefficient, which, for plasma at 37°C is in SI units 0.231 and in traditional units 0.0306, pK is the dissociation exponent and is usually assumed to have a constant value of 6.10. The assumption is adequate in normal circumstances but very different values for pH have been obtained in subjects in whom the acid–base balance was disturbed. The variation has been explained by Covington and colleagues as being due to the presence in plasma of the ionic species $H_2CO_3.HCO_3^-$ which is not represented in the equation. Neglect of this substance effectively invalidates the equation in abnormal circumstances.

For describing the *in vitro* relationship between the tension of carbon dioxide in blood and the plasma pH, allowance should be made for the concentrations of haemoglobin and titratable non-carbonic acid (base); the latter is called base excess. It may be subdivided into two components, one reflecting endogenous metabolic processes including the production and oxidation of lactic acid (page 518) and the other associated with the transport, storage and control activities of the kidneys, the gastro-intestinal tract and the skeleton. The resulting Van Slyke equation has been arranged in a form suitable for a programmable calculator by Siggaard–Andersen:

$$[HCO_3^-] - 24.4 = -(2.3[Hb] + 7.7) \times (pH - 7.40) + \frac{BE}{1 - 0.023[Hb]} \qquad (3.15)$$

where $[Hb]$ is blood concentration of haemoglobin in $mmol\,l^{-1}$ and BE is base excess in the same units; the other terms are as defined above.

44

When some of the variables in equations 3.13 and 3.15 are known, the remainder may be obtained by calculation or by use of the equivalent nomogram (Fig. 3.6). Usually the pH is measured with a glass electrode and the tension of carbon dioxide with a CO_2 electrode such as that described below. The method then yields the plasma bicarbonate concentration, the base excess and the total CO_2 content of plasma. Alternatively the bicarbonate concentration can be obtained from the volume of carbon dioxide gas which is liberated from plasma by the addition of acid. The volume is measured directly in a Van Slyke or Haldane apparatus or indirectly by subsequent titration of the acid. The method then yields the tension of carbon dioxide.

From the Henderson–Hasselbalch relationship by substitution in equation 3.13 of measured values for the pH and the concentration of bicarbonate.

By interpolation using the Astrup technique. For this purpose three measurements of pH are made at 37°C, (i) on the sample of blood to be analysed, (ii) and (iii) on samples of the same blood after they have been equilibrated at 37°C with saturated gas containing respectively lower and higher tensions of carbon dioxide than the unknown sample;

Analysis of
blood for
carbon dioxide

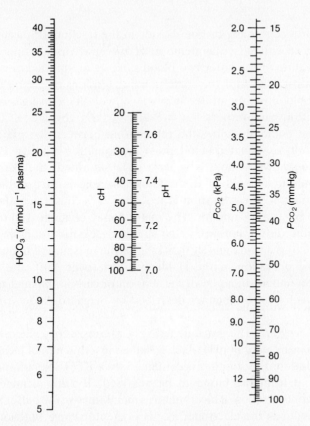

Fig. 3.6 Graphical solution of the Henderson–Hasselbalch equation for blood at 38°C. (Source: Siggaard-Andersen O. *Scand J Clin Lab Invest* 1963; **15**: 211–217.)

45

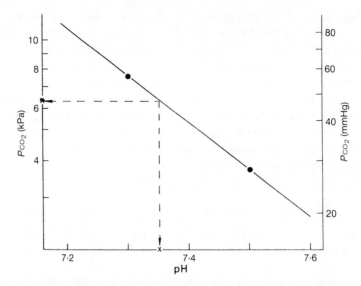

Fig. 3.7 Interpolation method for estimating the tension of carbon dioxide in blood. The pH, log P_{CO_2} relationship for the unknown sample is constructed from measurements of the pH of two aliquots of blood equilibrated respectively with appropriate mixtures of carbon dioxide in air (e.g. F_{CO_2} 0.04 and 0.08, closed circles). X is the pH of the unknown sample before equilibration. For oxygenated blood * indicates the corresponding P_{CO_2}.

gas mixtures containing carbon dioxide in the fractional concentrations 0.04 and 0.08 with the remainder in air or oxygen are usually appropriate. The pH values of the latter two blood samples are plotted on semi-log paper against values for the corresponding tensions of carbon dioxide; when the blood is equilibrated at sea level with the above gas mixtures these tensions are respectively 3.8 and 7.6 kPa (Fig. 3.7). The line joining the points describes the relationship between the pH and the P_{CO_2} for fully oxygenated blood under the condition of study. Provided that the unknown sample is at least 90% saturated, the P_{CO_2} which corresponds to the pH of the unknown sample is then obtained by interpolation; if the saturation is less than 90% this value should be corrected by a small amount. The method may be applied to 0.1 ml of blood when, during normoxia, the standard deviation of a single estimate of P_{CO_2} is approximately 0.25 kPa. In the presence of hypoxaemia, due to the operation of the Haldane effect (page 289), the method leads to an underestimation of the tension of carbon dioxide; this may be allowed for in the manner described by Siggaard-Andersen.

The CO_2 electrode. The instrument (Fig. 3.4) consists of a glass electrode for the measurement of pH, which is bathed in a thin film of bicarbonate buffer solution; the solution is contained by a PTFE membrane which separates it from the blood to be analysed. By this arrangement a constant concentration of bicarbonate is maintained in the buffer solution which surrounds the electrode; its pH is then a simple function of the tension of carbon dioxide in the solution, which, as a result of diffusion

Table 3.7 Factors for correcting the blood pH to the temperature of the body (t_b°C) when the measurements are made at 38°C (pH_{38}). They are derived for a CO_2 content in plasma of 25 mmol l^{-1} and are used in the form: $pH_b = pH_{38} - factor\ (t_b - 38)$

pH_{38}	Factor
7.00−7.15	0.0127
7.16−7.30	0.0136
7.31−7.45	0.0142
7.46−7.60	0.0149

(Source: Adamson K Jr, Daniel SS, Gandy D, James LS. *J Appl Physiol* 1964; **19**: 897−900.)

across the membrane, is equal to that in the unknown sample. The electrode is calibrated with either humidified gas containing a known partial pressure of carbon dioxide or water with which the gas has been equilibrated. The method was developed initially by Severinghaus and his colleagues; it is now standard in most laboratories.

Correction factors for use when the temperature of the blood at the time of the analysis differs from that at which it is collected are shown in Fig. 3.5. The corresponding factors for blood pH are listed in Table 3.7.

The Riley bubble method. By this method the tensions of carbon dioxide and oxygen in blood are determined concurrently; the procedure is described on page 41.

Indirect methods

The tension of carbon dioxide in the mixed venous blood is similar to that in the tissues and, at rest, exceeds the tension in the arterial blood by approximately 0.8 kPa (6 mmHg).

The tension of carbon dioxide in the subcutaneous tissue may be obtained by injecting under the skin 50 ml of gas containing carbon dioxide in a fractional concentration of 0.06. At the end of an hour a sample is withdrawn and analysed for carbon dioxide.

The tension of carbon dioxide in the mixed venous blood can be obtained by a rebreathing method in which the lung is used as a tonometer. The expired gas is then analysed for carbon dioxide either breath by breath (page 252) or after collection in a bag. The method for exercise is described on page 241 and that for rest, due to Campbell and Howell, below. It requires a three-way tap which communicates with both a bag of about 2 l capacity and a mask or mouthpiece by which the bag is connected to the subject. The bag is fitted with a small-bore side connection from which a sample of gas can be drawn off for analysis. The bag initially contains 1.0 or 1.5 l of oxygen. To make the measurement the subject first rebreathes from the bag for a period of 1.5 min or until the ventilation begins to rise. This manoeuvre raises the tension of carbon dioxide in the lung−bag system to near the level of the mixed venous blood but at the expense of some retention in the body of carbon dioxide; the latter is then eliminated by allowing the subject to breathe air for a period of 3 min. After this time, the rebreathing is repeated for 20 s or five breaths: this manoeuvre raises the tension of carbon dioxide in the bag to the level of the mixed venous blood when it is fully saturated with oxygen. A sample of the gas is then analysed for carbon dioxide to an absolute accuracy of 0.1% in a simplified Haldane gas-analysis apparatus. Subsequently the rebreathing is repeated to confirm that equilibrium has in fact been achieved. The tension of carbon dioxide is calculated by use of the following relationship:

$$P\bar{v},\text{co}_2 \text{ (indirect)} = F_{A,\text{co}_2} \times (P_B - P_{H_2O}) \qquad (3.16)$$

where $P\bar{v},\text{co}_2$ is the tension of carbon dioxide in the mixed venous blood when it is saturated with oxygen, F_{A,co_2} is the fractional concentration of carbon dioxide in the bag, and $(P_B - P_{H_2O})$ is the pressure of dry gas in the lungs at 37°C. The tension of carbon dioxide in the arterial blood is less than that in the mixed venous blood by, on average, 0.8 kPa (6 mmHg).

Success with the method depends on the volume of oxygen in the bag being no larger than is necessary to permit rebreathing. The connection between the bag and the subject should be gas-tight and the tap should only be turned in the intervals after the subject has completed an expiration and before the start of the next inspiration. The method is useful for the study of subjects with normal lungs, for the screening of out-patients and for hospital in-patients who have been fitted with a tracheotomy tube (page 649). In other acutely ill patients spuriously low values are sometimes obtained, especially when the tidal volume is small or the subject is restless or semi-conscious. In such circumstances the P_{a,co_2} should be measured directly.

Quality control

Preparation of gas mixtures and calibration procedures are described in this section. Minimal standards for equipment used for measurement of gas volumes and flow rates are given in Table 3.2 (page 24). Some aspects of the equipment, the training of technicians and laboratory routines are considered in Chapter 4. The operational features of equipment for assessing the cardiorespiratory response to exercise are summarised in Table 14.7 (page 427).

Preparation of gas mixtures

Special gas mixtures are expensive to buy and need to be ordered well in advance of the time when they are required. Alternatively, they can be prepared in the laboratory using some of the equipment illustrated in Fig. 3.8. Mixtures needed only occasionally can be prepared by volumetric dilution or mixed as they are required using a set of calibrated

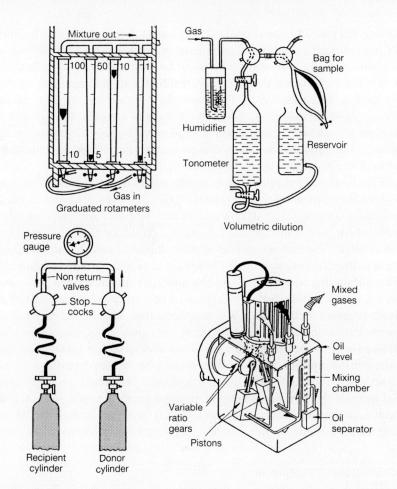

Fig. 3.8 Equipment for making up gas mixtures. *Upper right.* Preparation by volumetric dilution when only a small quantity is required. The bag should be evacuated initially, then the deadspace of the apparatus should be flushed before each gas is added. *Upper left.* Graduated rotameters can be used to prepare gas mixtures for immediate use. *Lower left.* Gas mixtures prepared in high-pressure cylinders. The pressure gauge should be of high quality and for convenience have a dial of diameter at least 12.5 cm (5 in). *Lower right.* The Wösthoff pump mixes two gases in predetermined proportions using two pistons of fixed volume driven by variable ratio gears.

rotameters. The range of flow rates should reflect the intended gas concentrations in the final mixture; ranges for air of $0.1-1.0 \, \mathrm{l\,min^{-1}}$, $1.0-10.0 \, \mathrm{l\,min^{-1}}$ and $10.0-100 \, \mathrm{l\,min^{-1}}$, with additional calibration charts for oxygen, nitrogen and carbon dioxide, are adequate. For other gases it is usually better to make up mixtures in high-pressure cylinders by a process of decanting. To this end, the final pressure in the cylinder is decided on and is then apportioned between the different gases according to their intended concentrations in the final mixture. The gases are added to the recipient cylinder through an appropriate adaptor. Either the gas from the master cylinder having the lowest pressure is delivered first or a compression pump is used. The pump should be lubricated with water and fitted with a means for subsequently drying the gas. The gas should be transferred slowly to prevent heating of the recipient cylinder and cooling of the donor. This is important as any difference in temperature between the two cylinders will affect the relationship between the pressure readings and the quantity of gas which has been transferred. Alternatively the quantity can be assessed by weighing the cylinders. When the process is complete the cylinder is laid on its side for 24 h to allow complete mixing of the gases to take place. The mixture should not subsequently be stored at below its critical temperature which for carbon dioxide is $-78.5°C$.

This method of preparation is widely used but is not free from risk, especially when potentially explosive gases are used. The risk is minimised by ensuring that all connectors and adaptors are clean and that non-return valves are operating correctly. No oil or grease should ever be applied. The copper tubing of the adaptor should be annealed by heat at internals of approximately 5 years to reduce the risk of cracking. In addition, the equipment should be operated only by trained personnel in a place set aside for this purpose. The gas cylinders are tested at high pressure before they are supplied; they should be retested at intervals to detect any deterioration with use. They should also be treated with respect; for example, all cylinders should be labelled and when in an upright position they should be clamped to the wall or otherwise supported. Leakage of gas should be looked for using soap solution or the sampling probe of an appropriate gas analyser. A leak which cannot be controlled by screwing a valve fingertight or by tightening a retaining nut should be referred for specialist scrutiny.

Calibration of equipment

On two occasions 18 years apart standard gas mixtures were circulated to a number of lung function laboratories; on both occasions the results of the analysis varied by up to 10%, yet the instruments were capable of a 1% accuracy (Table 3.8). Similarly for patients studied in several laboratories; the variability between the laboratories greatly

Table 3.8 Variability in gas analysis between 57 lung function laboratories in the UK

Gas	Concentrations (%)	Reproducibility* (%)	Percentage of samples accurate to 1%	Main fault in instrument calibration
Oxygen	11−18	1.8−5.3	48	Zero error
Carbon dioxide	3.8	8.9	28†	Curvilinearity
Carbon monoxide	0.1−0.3	3.2−4.9	14	Curvilinearity
Helium	8−14	3.0−3.2	37†	

* Based on analysis of gas in small cylinders; the gas concentration as assessed in the reference laboratory varied by less than 0.6%.
† The resulting errors in the calculated respiratory exchange ratio and transfer factor exceeded 5% in respectively 28% and 20% of instances.
(Source: Chinn DJ, Naruse Y, Cotes JE. *Thorax* 1986; **41**: 133−137.)

exceeded that when the measurements were repeated in the same laboratory.

Such studies have amply demonstrated the importance of all aspects of calibration yet the subject continues to have a low priority and to be an important cause of discrepant results. Calibration of equipment is considered here and standardisation of procedures in the sections where the tests are described.

Faults in equipment can arise during manufacture or transit; they can also occur from the ageing of the components, or their interaction with other equipment. In addition, the performance may be affected by the temperature, humidity, or magnetic field in the laboratory as well as by the manner of use, which will also vary. The effect of these factors upon the performance of the instrument should be established by accurate calibration which should be carried out both when the equipment is received and at appropriate intervals thereafter. The calibration should be performed in circumstances which simulate as closely as possible the actual conditions of use. The properties of the instruments which should be investigated include reproducibility, accuracy or linearity and response time.

Reproducibility reflects the extent to which a result varies when it is repeated. The variability is described by the standard error of the estimate or, where the error is a proportional one, by the coefficient of variation. For physical measurements the latter is normally less than 0.5%. Biological measurements are rather less reproducible with co-efficients of variation of the order of 2% for stature and forced expiratory volume, 5% for transfer factor and 15% for compliance. The variability of biological measurements is greater between sessions and from day to day compared with measurements made at a single session. A high level of reproducibility is of particular importance when serial measurements of lung function are used to assess the changes over time in groups of subjects (page 58). The reproducibility will normally be assessed when a new measurement is introduced into the laboratory and as part of the training programme for new staff.

Accuracy reflects the extent to which a result deviates from an absolute standard. The standard will normally be defined in terms of length, mass and time from which can be derived volume, concentration, flow rate, resistance (or conductance) and elastance. Examples of laboratory standards are given in Table 3.9; they include a 1 l or 3 l gas syringe, flow–volume simulator, and calibration gas mixtures; the latter can be purchased or prepared in the laboratory (Fig. 3.8). The tolerance on the standard should be established. For physical measurements the accuracy should normally be better than 1%. The minimal standards for equipment used for measurements of gas volume and flow are given in Table 3.2 (page 24). A procedure for calibrating a spirometer is illustrated in Fig. 3.9.

The standard is used to construct a calibration graph in which the correct result on the Y-axis is related to the observed result on the X-axis. The relationship should lie on the line of identity which for

Table 3.9 Calibration of laboratory equipment

Feature	Equipment	Standard
Permeability	Douglas bag	Calibration gas
Linearity	Volume recorders	Gas syringe (1 l or 3 l)
	Flow recorders	Calibrated rotameters
		Flow−volume simulator
	Peak flow meter	See page 27
	Pressure transducer	Mercury or water manometer
	Gas analyser	Calibration gas
Resistance	Volume and flow measuring devices	Static tube (Fig. 3.3)
Paper speed	Chart recorder	Stop watch
Response time	Flow and pressure recorders	Square wave impulse*
Frequency response	Flow and pressure recorders	Sinusoidal wave impulse†

* A square wave can be generated by the abrupt release of gas previously stored in a drum or a balloon at a known pressure. When the gas is released manually or by bursting the balloon with a pin the rise time is of the order of 0.01 s. The volume which is released is closer to that which is calculated from the adiabatic than from the isothermal relationship for gases, i.e. $PV^{\gamma} = RT$, where γ is the ratio of the specific heats of a gas at constant pressure and constant volume (Cp and Cv respectively). Thus $\gamma = Cp/Cv = 1.4$ for air.
† A sinusoidal wave form can be generated by a piston-type pump. A wave form which more nearly resembles normal breathing may be produced using an appropriate cam.

equal scales on the two axes is a straight line at an angle of 45° to both axes and passing through the origin. Alternatively, there may be a proportional or zero error or the relationship may be alinear (Fig. 3.10).

Causes for some of these deviations are indicated in Table 3.8; their detection requires that the calibration should be performed at a minimum of three points and not two or even one as is built into some physical gas analysers. The calibration will normally be undertaken at the beginning and end of each measurement session but for instruments which are subject to drift an appropriate check should be performed for each patient. Conversely very stable instruments, including most helium katharometers, can be calibrated once a month.

Response time includes the *delay time* between application of the signal and the start of the response and the *rise time* to 95% of the final response. In the case of a gas analyser both the delay and the rise time vary over a wide range reflecting the gas sampling system and the type of analyser (Table 3.5). For pressure transducers and pneumotachographs the two times should be short and there should be no overshoot (page 29); this aspect should form part of the calibration. For other instruments the response time will normally be assessed when the equipment is set up and if there is reason to believe that it may be faulty. Some features of calibrations are summarised in Table 3.9.

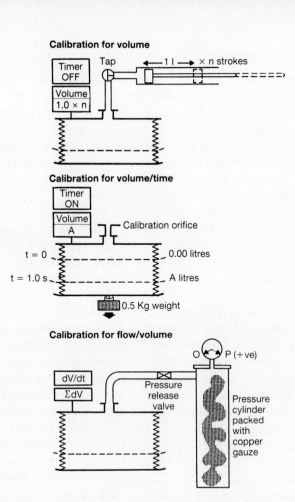

Fig. 3.9 Calibration of a McDermott bellows spirometer showing the use of a calibrated syringe, a standard orifice and weight and a flow volume simulator.

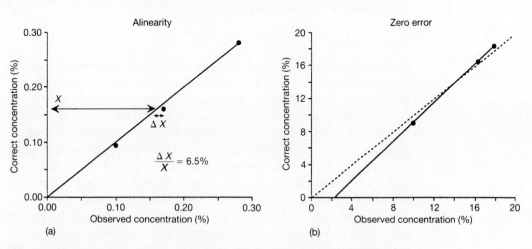

Fig. 3.10 Examples of faulty calibration. (a) Alinearity, which in this example is 6.5%; (b) zero error, in this case more than 2% absolute concentration. See also Table 10.3, page 311. (Source: Chinn DJ, Naruse Y, Cotes JE. *Thorax* 1986; **41**: 133–137.)

Sterilisation of equipment

The equipment used for assessment of lung function should be free
from respiratory hazards including accumulated secretions and potentially harmful bacteria. This requirement is usually met by washing in
antiseptic detergent solution (e.g. Cetavlon) and by using disposable
mouthpieces and valve boxes. Sterile equipment should be used for
manoeuvers which entail forced inspiration and for high risk patients
e.g. those who may have infective hepatitis or whose immunological
defence mechanisms are impaired (page 586).

After each test the mouthpiece, mask and rubber breathing valves
should be either discarded or scrubbed in the chosen detergent, then
dried and lightly dusted with chalk. The connecting tubes, valve
box and rebreathing bags should be rinsed and drained. The other
components should be dismantled for cleaning at weekly or monthly
intervals depending on the frequency of use. The closed breathing
circuits may also be sterilised using formaldehyde gas or hydrogen
peroxide mist; the former is obtained by bubbling air through a 40%
aqueous solution of formaldehyde (formalin), the latter by use of an
ultrasonic aerosol generator. The equipment is subsequently flushed
with air. However, except for equipment which has been designed with
the needs of sterilisation in mind these methods are seldom completely
effective. Thus the ease with which any new equipment can be sterilised
should be noted prior to purchase. High risk patients should be isolated
from those parts of the equipment which cannot be cleaned effectively.
This is best done by using a biological filter or interposing a disposable
bag-in-box assembly. However, for tests where these measures may
impair the accuracy and reproducibility of the measurement, traditional
methods of achieving sterility should be used instead.

Anthropometric measurements

Stature and sitting height

Stature, also called standing height, is an important reference variable
for the description of lung function as to a lesser extent is sitting height
(page 456). Stature should be measured using a stadiometer (e.g.
Harpenden) as this leaves the observer with both hands free to position
the subject. The heels should be together and the subject as tall as
possible with the heels, calf, buttocks and back preferably touching the
stadiometer. When this position is achieved the observer cups the
angles of the mandible in his two hands, tilts the subject's face so that
the lower orbital margin is level with the external auditory meatus and
applies gentle upward traction to the head. Compared with subjects
who are standing erect but unsupported this procedure may increase
the apparent height by up to 5 cm (Fig. 3.11). It also improves the
reproducibility of the measurement which is then less than 2 mm. For
the measurement of the sitting height a similar procedure is used

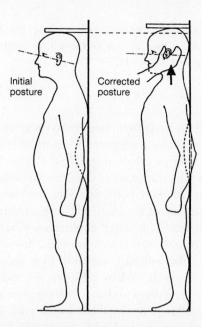

Initial
posture

Corrected
posture

Fig. 3.11 Procedure for measurement of stature showing the effects of moving the head into the Frankfort plane (dotted and dashed line horizontal) and then applying traction. For details, see text.

except that the subject should be seated on a high flat-topped stool. The muscles of the buttock should be relaxed and to achieve this the feet may be supported on an adjustable foot rest (e.g. Holtain sitting height stool).

Span

The span from the finger tip to finger tip with the arms and fingers horizontally abducted can be used as an estimate of biological stature when there is spinal deformity. Godfrey and colleagues found the two dimensions to be interchangeable in children but in adults Tweeddale found less good agreement (95% confidence limits ±8.14 cm). To make the measurement the subject stands with the left arm fully extended and abducted. The demi-span is the length from the tip of the longest finger to the centre of the sternal notch. The distance is measured with a tape then doubled to give the span.

Body mass

Body mass, also called body weight. The body mass is widely available and has a high accuracy (<0.01 kg) provided the weighing machine is properly calibrated. The subject should be lightly clad without footwear and the weight of the clothes or representative garments should be recorded. Body mass is correlated with stature but in adults and some children the correlation is eliminated by expressing the mass per metre squared of stature (BM/St^2). This body mass index, also called *Quetlet's index*, is widely used as a measure of fat-free mass and/or obesity; however, more specific indices are obtained by partitioning the mass into fat and non-fat components.

Fat-free mass

The fat-free mass of the body (lean body mass) is an important reference variable for the physiological response to exercise (page 431) and also contributes to the lung function (page 492). It may be deduced from the body weight and the thickness of the skin-plus-subcutaneous tissues which provide a measure of body fat. The thickness is measured at four sites on the left side of the body using an ultrasonic probe or skin callipers (e.g. Holtain). The latter equipment is recommended. The sites are over the biceps and triceps muscles, below the angle of the scapula and above the anterior superior iliac spine. The sites are marked with a skin pencil. When callipers are used the skinfold is picked up between the thumb and the forefinger and the readings are taken 2 s after the callipers are applied. In the case of the upper arm, the olecranon process is marked with the elbow flexed and the arm then hangs free; the measurements are made at a level mid-way between this point and the acromion process with the skin fold in the long axis of the limb (Fig. 3.12). The measurement below the angle of the scapula is made in the line of the muscle and that just above and medial to the anterior superior iliac spine in a line parallel to the external oblique muscle. The percentage of body mass which is fat is calculated from the sum of two or more skinfold thicknesses using empirical relationships; for children and adolescents those of Slaughter and colleagues are recommended (Table 3.10) and for adults the equations of Durnin and Womersley (Fig. 3.13). Fat-free mass (FFM) is estimated from the percentage fat using the following relationship:

$$\text{FFM (kg)} = \text{body mass} \times (100 - \%\text{fat}) \div 100 \qquad (3.17)$$

In the derivation of % fat the body density obtained by under-water weighing was used to partition the body weight into a fat component and a fat-free mass component using arbitrary values for their respective densities. The derivation neglects differences between individuals in the proportions of muscle to bone; this has not proved to be a disadvantage except in the case of adult Negroes whose fat-free mass is underestimated by, on average, 3 kg. A similar error might be expected for Australian Aboriginals. The subject is reviewed by Norgan and Jones.

Numerical treatment of results

The incorporation of microprocessors and computers into respiratory apparatus (page 33) has revolutionised the calculation and interpretation of numerical results. The results are now usually presented to the operator as a digital display, a print out and/or a graph drawn by an

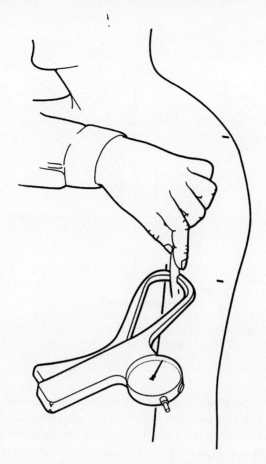

Fig. 3.12 Measurement of skinfold thickness. (Source: Cotes JE, Steel J. *Work-related Lung Disorders*. Oxford: Blackwell Scientific Publications, 1987, 93.)

Table 3.10 Equations relating % fat (y) to the sum of the triceps and subscapular skin fold thickness (x) in children and adolescents (age range 8–17 yrs). The equations have the form $y = ax + bx^2 + c$

| | Regression Coefficients | | | |
	a	b	Constant	SEE
Males				
$x < 35$ mm	1.21	−0.008	See below	3.6%
$x > 35$ mm	0.783	—	1.6	
Females				
$x < 35$ mm	1.33	−0.013	−2.5	3.9%
$x > 35$ mm	0.546	—	9.7	

Constant term for males in relation to puberty and ethnic group ($x < 35$ mm)

Ethnic group	Before	At	After puberty
Caucasian	−1.7	−3.4	−5.5
Negro	−3.5	−5.2	−6.8

(Source: Slaughter MH, Lohman TG, Boileau RA *et al. Hum Biol* 1988; **60**: 709–723.)

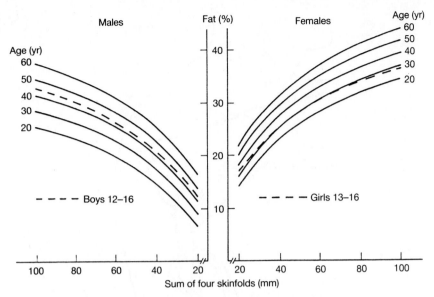

Fig. 3.13 Graphical representation of the equations of Durnin and Womersley relating the sum of four skinfold thicknesses to percentage of body mass which is fat. The coefficient of variation of the estimate is of the order of 6%. For details see text. (Source: Durnin JVGA, Womersley J. *Br J Nutr* 1974; **32**: 77−99.)

X−Y plotter. The processing can usually incorporate any conventions recommended in this or other sources. The operator should be aware of how the results have been obtained and of the decision tree used for their interpretation (page 79). The scrutiny and interpretation of results are discussed in Chapter 4. The numerical treatment is described by Oldham and in textbooks of statistics, for example, by Fisher, by Bradford Hill and by Armitage and Berry. Some aspects are reviewed here.

Differences between serial measurements

Strategy. The index which is chosen should preferably have a good reproducibility (page 51) and, if only a limited number of observations can be made, these should be concentrated at the beginning and end of the period of observation. However, when following up groups of subjects over a period of years the collection of intermediate results both provides a reason for the observer keeping in touch with the subjects and can lead to the detection of bias which might otherwise influence the result (Fig. 3.14). The minimal number of subjects needed to achieve a meaningful result can be calculated in terms of the standard deviation of the measurement, the degree of certainty which is required and the change which is considered meaningful. Then:

$$n = 2 \left(\frac{\text{factor} \times \text{SD between days}}{\bar{x}_1 - \bar{x}_2} \right)^2$$

where the denominator is the minimal change which it is proposed to

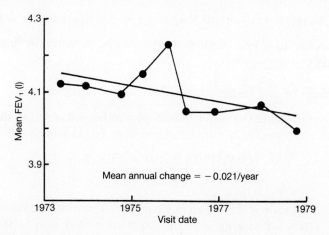

Fig. 3.14 Mean levels of FEV_1 for 33 subjects assessed on nine occasions between April 1973 and October, 1978. The downward trend was interrupted by one anomalous result. (Source: Diem JE, Jones RN, Hendrick DJ *et al. Am Rev Respir Dis* 1982; **126**: 420–428.)

detect. The factor has components for the risk of both a false positive result (usually taken as 0.05) and a false negative result (which can be between 0.05 and 0.2). For these two circumstances the value of the factor are respectively 3.6 and 2.8. Then in the case of FEV (SD ≈ 0.5 l), if the meaningful difference is 0.25 l the number of subjects (n) is between 104 and 63 depending on the degree of certainty. For further details Armitage and Berry should be consulted.

Reporting a difference. Longitudinal changes over periods of years can yield longitudinal reference values. These are seldom used at present but in future will be of practical importance for the long term surveillance of respiratory health. Changes over short periods of time are of interest in relation to clinical management and intervention studies and are commonly expressed as a percentage; thus

$$\text{percentage change} = 100(x_1 - x_2)/x_1\% \qquad (3.18)$$

where x_1 and x_2 are the initial and final values. However, the difference term $(x_1 - x_2)$ is inevitably correlated with the initial level (x_1) and this may lead to error in the interpretation. Examples are given by Oldham and by Rossiter. The error is avoided when the change is expressed in natural logarithms* or is related to the mean level: thus

* When the rate of change of a variable is proportional to its magnitude, then $dx/dt = kx$, where k is the constant of proportionality and is the proper measure of the proportional changes. Integrating gives $\ln x = \ln x_0 + kt$ where x_0 is the value of x at time zero and ln indicates the natural logarithm. With observations x_1, at times t_1 and x_2 at time t_2:

$$\ln x_1 = \ln x_0 + kt_1 \quad \text{and} \quad \ln x_2 = \ln x_0 + kt_2$$

so that

$$k\% = (\ln x_1 - \ln x_2)/(t_1 - t_2)$$

Equation 3.19 (overleaf) differs from this to an extent which in practice is negligible.

59

$$\text{Change} = (x_1 - x_2)/0.5(x_1 + x_2) = \Delta x/\bar{x} \text{ or } 100\Delta x/\bar{x}\% \quad (3.19)$$

The response to a bronchodilator drug can be reported in this form (page 145).

Relationship of one variable to another

Where one variable (y) is dependent on another variable (x) the two are often expressed as a ratio or percentage, for example

$$[\text{FEV}_1/\text{FVC}] \times 100 = \text{FEV}_1\% \quad (3.20)$$

$$\dot{V}\text{E}/\dot{V}\text{O}_2 = \text{VE} \quad (3.21)$$

where the notation is that given in Chapter 2. The resulting ratio (y/x) can be a way of making y independent of x, but only when y is proportional to x, i.e. the graph of y on x is a straight line through the origin. This is the case for FEV% which is therefore a valid index. By contrast the ventilation equivalent (VE) (i.e. $\dot{V}\text{E}/\dot{V}\text{O}_2$) is mathematically unsound because the ratio is not independent of the denominator (in this case $\dot{V}\text{O}_2$). Other examples are given in Table 3.11. The error is avoided by reporting y at a standard value of x, preferably the mean value. This is best done by interpolation using the relationship of y on x which usually has a linear form, i.e.

$$y = mx + c \quad (3.22)$$

If the relationship is curvilinear it should be transformed into a linear form by taking reciprocals or using logarithms. An example of the former conversion is shown in Fig. 5.12 (page 111). For the latter an example is the regression of lung function on stature in children as in Fig. 15.4 (page 455); here the curves can be linearised by the use of natural logarithms, i.e.

$$\ln y = m \ln x + c \quad (3.23)$$

hence

$$y = e^c.x^m \quad (3.24)$$

Table 3.11 Examples of ratio indices which are mathematically unsound because they are correlated with their denominators (i.e. they exhibit colinearity (page 63))

Original form	Alternative
Body mass/stature	Body mass/(stature)x*
FEV$_1$/stature	FEV$_1$/(stature)x*
Ventilation equivalent ($\dot{V}\text{E}/\dot{V}\text{O}_2$)	Use linear regression or $\dot{V}\text{E}_{45}$‡
Oxygen pulse ($\dot{V}\text{O}_2/fc$)	Use linear regression or fc_{45}§
Aerobic power ($\dot{V}\text{O}_2$/body mass)	$\dot{n}\text{O}_2$ max/(body mass)$^{0.67}$
Kco($T\text{l}/V_\text{A}$)†	Tl

* x is usually 2 but 3 is preferable in some circumstances.
† Kco is widely used despite being negatively correlated with alveolar volume.
‡ See Fig. 12.4, page 371.
§ See Fig. 14.6, page 428.

This transformation has the further advantage that, if, as in the above example, the value for m is effectively constant between subjects then the result for each subject is defined by the parameter c. The proportional difference between two subjects or groups of subjects is then expressed by

$$100(c_1 - c_2)\% \qquad (3.25)$$

Decimal age

Age is commonly expressed in years rounded off to the nearest whole number but this may not be accurate for children or for longitudinal studies involving measurements made annually or after an interval of a few years. The requisite accuracy is then obtained by expressing the age in decimal years. The latter is obtained by subtracting the decimal date of the assessment from that of the data of birth. Decimal dates for each day of the year are given in Table 3.12 or they can be computed using the equation given in Table 3.13.

Table 3.12 The date expressed as decimal years, e.g. 16 August 1993 is 1993.622

Day	Jan 1	Feb 2	Mar 3	Apr 4	May 5	Jun 6	Jul 7	Aug 8	Sep 9	Oct 10	Nov 11	Dec 12
1	000	085	162	247	329	414	496	581	666	748	833	915
2	003	088	164	249	332	416	499	584	668	751	836	918
3	005	090	167	252	334	419	501	586	671	753	838	921
4	008	093	170	255	337	422	504	589	674	756	841	923
5	011	096	173	258	340	425	507	592	677	759	844	926
6	014	099	175	260	342	427	510	595	679	762	847	929
7	016	101	178	263	345	430	512	597	682	764	849	932
8	019	104	181	266	348	433	515	600	685	767	852	934
9	022	107	184	268	351	436	518	603	688	770	855	937
10	025	110	186	271	353	438	521	605	690	773	858	940
11	027	112	189	274	356	441	523	608	693	775	860	942
12	030	115	192	277	359	444	526	611	696	778	863	945
13	033	118	195	279	362	447	529	614	699	781	866	948
14	036	121	197	282	364	449	532	616	701	784	868	951
15	038	123	200	285	367	452	534	619	704	786	871	953
16	041	126	203	288	370	455	537	622	707	789	874	956
17	044	129	205	290	373	458	540	625	710	792	877	959
18	047	132	208	293	375	460	542	627	712	795	879	962
19	049	134	211	296	378	463	545	630	715	797	882	964
20	052	137	214	299	381	466	548	633	718	800	885	967
21	055	140	216	301	384	468	551	636	721	803	888	970
22	058	142	219	304	386	471	553	638	723	805	890	973
23	060	145	222	307	389	474	556	641	726	808	893	975
24	063	148	225	310	392	477	559	644	729	811	896	978
25	066	151	227	312	395	479	562	647	731	814	899	981
26	068	153	230	315	397	482	564	649	734	816	901	984
27	071	156	233	318	400	485	567	652	737	819	904	986
28	074	159	236	321	403	488	570	655	740	822	907	989
29	077	159	238	323	405	490	573	658	742	825	910	992
30	079	—	241	326	408	493	575	660	745	827	912	995
31	082	—	244	—	411	—	578	663	—	830	—	997

Table 3.13 Calculation of decimal age. The number of days from 1 January 1900 to any specified date can be calculated exactly from the following relationship which was compiled by Rossiter

---

No. of days = Integer $(365.25Y + 30.6M + D - 0.25L - 305.8)$

where Integer (A) is the integer part of A {i.e. Integer $(5.7) = 5$; Integer $(-1.6) = -1$}
D = number of days in date
Y = Integer $(Z/12)$, where $Z = 12 \times$ Year + Month + 9
$M = Z - 12Y$
$L = (Y - 1) - 4 \times$ Integer $\{(Y - 1)/4\}$

Then, Age = {No. of days (today) − No. of days (birthday)}/365.25
Example: to calculate age on 6 July 1998 if born on 24 February 1924: For 24 February 1924:

$D = 24$
$Y =$ Integer $(299/12) = 24$
$M = 299 - 288 = 11$
$L = 23 - 4 \times$ Integer $(23/4) = 3$

No. of days (birthday)
= Integer $(365.25 \times 24 + 30.6 \times 11 + 24 - 3 \times 0.25 - 305.8) = 8820$

Similarly for 6 July 1998:
$D = 6$
$Y = 99$
$M = 4$
$L = 2$

No. of days (today) = 35981
Hence:

Age = $(35981 - 8820)/365.25 = 74.363$

Rounding off

Numerical results are often reported using more digits than is appropriate since the accuracy of the measurement is seldom better than 1%. Thus results should be rounded off to three meaningful digits. A valid convention is to round off downwards all terminal digits of five or less and to round upwards the terminal digits six to nine. The alternative of rounding upwards at five or over can introduce error if the process is repeated. For example if the number 10.45 is rounded off downwards to 10.4 and then to 10, it is still a good estimate of the original. However, if the rounding off is upwards 10.45 becomes 10.5 and then 11 which is a less good estimate of what was first reported.

Averaging ratios

Some lung function results are expressed as ratios or percentages having the form y/x or 100 y/x%. This method of presentation can be misleading in the circumstances discussed on page 60. In addition error can arise if the results are averaged incorrectly. Averaging the ratios e.g. $0.5(y_1/x_1 + y_2/x_2)$ is fine but taking the ratio of the averages, i.e. $0.5(y_1 + y_2)/0.5(x_1 + x_2)$ is not acceptable.

A multiple regression equation is used to describe a variable which is related to several others, for example, FEV_1 in adults is related to age and stature. Hence:

$$y = mx + nz + c \tag{3.26}$$

where x is stature in metres, and z is age in years. The relationship can be simplified if either x or z can be expressed in the form of a proportionality. Thus in the above example, Cole has shown that, in adults, a proportionality exists between FEV_1 and the square of the stature (x^2). On this account FEV_1 can be related to age independent of stature using the form

$$y/x^2 = m'z + c' \tag{3.27}$$

The proportionality can also be used to standardise FEV_1 or other index to a common stature which for men might be 1.72 m. Thus:

$$FEV\ st = FEV\ obs \times 1.72^2/stature^2 \tag{3.28}$$

In addition to age and stature the dependent variable (y) may be related to other characteristics of the subject; for example in the case of FEV_1 the gender, ethnic group, occupational exposure and whether or not the subject smokes can influence the observed level. The contributions of these independent variables can be analysed by introducing into the multiple regression equation some categorical or dummy variables to which are allocated the value 1 if they are present and 0 if they are absent for the subject in question. There may also be a need for additional terms to denote interaction between variables, for example between age and smoking. Thus:

$$FEV_1 = a + b(\text{stature}) + c(\text{age}) + d(\text{smoking}) + e(\text{age} \times \text{smoking})$$
$$+ f(\text{occupational exposure}) + \text{etc.} \tag{3.29}$$

Since in this instance the smoking variable has been defined as 1 for smokers and 0 for non-smokers the regression coefficient of FEV on age is c for non-smokers and $c + e$ for smokers.

An equation of this type is often used to describe the FEV_1 of subjects participating in an occupational respiratory survey. The values of the coefficient terms are obtained by multiple regression analysis using an appropriate computer software package (e.g. SPSS[x]). However, prior to the analysis the independent variables should be scrutinised to establish that they are truly independent and not intercorrelated, hence do not exhibit colinearity. For example, the amount smoked in pack years* and the total dust exposure over a life-time spent in a dusty industry are both correlated with age. The inclusion of two or all of these indices in the same multiple regression analysis can lead to a misleading result. The subject is considered further on page 492.

---

* One pack year describes a tobacco consumption of one pack (i.e. 20 cigarettes) per day for 1 year.

The spread of the individual values about a multiple regression equation is described by the residual standard deviation (RSD) or coefficient of variation. These and some other statistical terms are given in Table 3.14. Aspects of their use are considered subsequently (pages 58, 68, 457, 492 and 506).

Table 3.14 Some statistical terms

Standard deviation [SD]	Describes spread of data
Standard error [SE, i.e. SD ÷ ($\sqrt{n}$ or $\sqrt{n-1}$)]	Indicates reliability of a mean value
Residual standard deviation [RSD]	SD about a regression line
Standard error of the estimate [SEE]	as for RSD
Coefficient of variation [C of V, i.e. 100 (SD or RSD) ÷ mean]	Describes spread if proportional (p 68)
Correlation coefficient [r]	Indicates extent to which two variables provide essentially the same information (range 0–1)
R^2 [correlation coefficient^2] *also called* coefficient of determination	Indicates proportion of variability in one index which is explained by another (range 0–1 or 0–100)

Logistic regression analysis is a form of multiple regression analysis used to describe a categorical variable, i.e. one which is present or absent, for example chronic bronchitis (page 516). Again the independent variables should not exhibit colinearity. In addition some computer software packages for logistic regression analysis have limitations so should not be used uncritically. Thus at this stage if not earlier a statistician should be consulted.

Guide to references

The references (Chapter 18) are classified under subject headings of which the following are particularly relevant to the present chapter:

4: Lung Function Testing; General Considerations

Why assess lung function?
Criteria for tests
Technical aspects
Choice of and setting up the tests

Training technicians
Conduct of the assessment
Reporting the results

Introduction

The respiratory physiologist can help to solve many respiratory problems (Table 4.1), but he can do so only if he chooses the right equipment, has sufficient time and skill to make use of it, and if he obtains the trustful co-operation of the subjects he investigates. These are the topics discussed in this chapter.

A well-equipped laboratory with well-trained staff can identify the type or pattern of dysfunction presented by a patient and can assess its severity. This will help to make or confirm a diagnosis, establish a prognosis, or suggest treatment, such as bronchodilator or oxygen therapy, or physical training. Serial testing can be used to monitor the effects of treatment. On the other hand the functional defect may be shown to be much less than the patient's symptoms imply, suggesting that there are factors apart from his lungs which contribute materially to his disability.

Consent

Prior to the tests the subject, or in the case of young children the parent, should be given a simple factual description of why lung function is to be measured and what is entailed. Any unusual features should be pointed out. This is particularly important for research investigations and for these the approval of an ethical committee should have been obtained. The subject should be given an opportunity to ask questions. These should be answered and explicit consent for the procedure should be obtained.

Criteria for tests

Acceptability

The tests should be safe, simple and not unpleasant for the subject. A procedure which is difficult to carry out will have a high failure rate and may yield unreliable results. One which is unpleasant will discourage

Table 4.1 Some applications of lung function tests

Field of application	Subdivision	Item
Human biology and physiology	Physiology	Normal function Changes with exercise, posture, barometric pressure, pregnancy, etc.
	Physiological anthropometry	Relation to age, sex, size, ethnic group, customary activity Variation due to time of day, season, climate, geographical location
Clinical science	Diagnosis	Causes of wheeze, breathlessness, cyanosis, finger clubbing and aspects of respiratory failure Interpretation of abnormal chest X-ray
	Clinical assessment	Diseases of the lung, chest wall, heart and circulation Diseases of the central nervous system Accidents involving the trunk
	Medical treatment	Oxygen therapy, bronchodilator therapy, assisted ventilation
	Surgical treatment	Suitability for operation
	Anaesthetics	Suitability for and management during and after anaesthesia
	Research applications	Evaluation of remedies Relationship of deranged function to abnormal structure Assessment of prognosis
Community medicine	Epidemiology	Effects of smoking and air pollution Prevalence of respiratory impairment Identification of high-risk cases
	Rehabilitation	Capability for physical work
Occupational medicine	Health in industry	Pre-employment, periodic and exit examinations, effects of respiratory hazards, suitability for strenuous work Establishment of safe conditions
	Diagnosis and assessment of occupational pulmonary diseases	Asbestosis, beryllium disease, byssinosis, farmer's lung, pneumoconiosis of coal-workers and other occupational groups Lung disease in grain handlers, hard-metal workers, silo fillers, those exposed to proteolytic enzymes, toluene di-isocyanate, etc.
Medicine and the Law	Assessment of disability	Function of the lungs and the capacity for exercise

follow-up measurements and lead to a high refusal rate amongst other patients. These difficulties can often be avoided by choosing tests which are submaximal, non-invasive and of short duration. Procedures which are of low acceptability include measurement of the ventilatory response to carbon dioxide, and maximal exercise. For arterial cannulation and measurement of lung compliance the acceptability is greatly influenced by the operator. One who is skilful will achieve a 95% success rate and a good follow-up experience. The unskilled may both fail to intubate and frustrate future attempts.

Objectivity

The result of a test should ideally be independent of the motivation of the subject and the personality of the operator. However, the pattern of breathing, the ventilation minute volume and the extent of any maximal effort are partly under voluntary control. Tests which are affected by the subject's co-operation include the peak expiratory flow, the maximal voluntary ventilation, some multi-breath indices of lung gas distribution and the capacity for exercise. These tests should where possible be replaced by less variable alternatives, for example the ventilatory capacity can be estimated from the forced expiratory volume, which is relatively independent of the effort made by the subject (see Fig. 5.14, page 117). Measurements of ventilation minute volume and the arterial blood gas tensions made during submaximal exercise may be more representative of the function of the lungs than measurements made at rest because the performance of work occupies some of the subject's attention. Multi-breath indices of lung mixing which include an allowance for the ventilation minute volume should be used in preference to those which do not. The capacity for exercise may be replaced by a submaximal procedure. However, any test which includes a maximal inspiration or a full expiration will sometimes be performed inadequately and any instruction as to how a test should be performed will occasionally be deliberately misinterpreted. The best means of avoiding this type of error are a persuasive but firm and vigilant operator and careful scrutiny of the results for undue variability and for internal inconsistencies, for example between estimates of vital capacity or residual volume obtained by more than one method. The acceptable limits for variability due to the operator are discussed below.

Repeatability

The repeatability of a test is usually expressed in terms of the variation between measurements made at a single session and the variation between sessions. The former is a function of the intrinsic variability of the procedure after an allowance has been made for the extent to which the results improve with practice. The latter represents the additional variability due to factors which operate on the subject, observer or equipment over a longer period. Some of this variability can be eliminated by the careful calibration of the equipment, the standardisation of the results for temperature and barometric pressure and the control of such variables as posture, activity, recent smoking and time of day, especially between morning and afternoon and in relation to meals. However, when all these factors are taken into account observations made on different occasions always show some residual variability which cannot be eliminated.

The residual variability can best be analysed when it is approximately the same for all values of the quantity which is being measured. The distribution of deviation from the mean value is then symmetrical and takes the form of a normal or Gaussian distribution curve. This is the case for some spirometric indices including FEV_1. For other indices the distribution is related to the size of the index. The distribution can then usually be 'normalised' by an appropriate transformation. The simplest transformation is to take the logarithms of the measurements. This is appropriate when the variability is *proportional* to the magnitude of the index as is approximately the case for the exercise cardiac frequency. For the diffusing capacity of the alveolar capillary membrane and volume of blood in the alveolar capillaries the reciprocals of the indices should be used (i.e. $1/Dm$ and $1/Vc$) (Fig. 10.4, page 314). This reciprocal transformation can also be used for the airways resistance (Fig. 5.12, page 111). Other transformations are discussed by Oldham and by Armitage and Berry amongst others. For data which have been normalised the contributions, to the overall scatter in the results, of variability within and between sessions can be expressed in terms of the total variance, which is the square of the standard deviation of the measurement. For r determinations on each of s sessions the total variance can be expressed in terms of the variance within sessions (A) and that between sessions (B) as follows:

$$\text{Total variance} = A/rs + B/s \qquad (4.1)$$

The variability of an index is normally expressed in terms of its standard deviation which, in this context, is the standard error of a single measurement made on one occasion. When the distribution of the untransformed data is Gaussian, the standard deviation is used without modification. When the distribution is log normal (i.e. the variability of the untransformed data is proportional to the magnitude of the index), the standard deviation is expressed relative to the mean value as the coefficient of variation (see Table 3.14, page 64):

$$\text{Coefficient of variation} = \frac{\text{standard deviation}}{\text{mean value}} \times 100\% \qquad (4.2)$$

In addition to describing distributions which are proportional the coefficient of variation is also used for comparing the respective variabilities of different indices. In laboratories where high standards are maintained most tests in regular use have coefficients of variation in the range 4−8%. Some tests which are less reproducible are also employed when they yield information on an aspect of function that cannot be assessed in other ways. However, where two tests measure the same attribute of function, that which has the lower coefficient of variation is usually to be preferred. For example, amongst tests of ventilatory capacity, the forced expiratory volume is more reproducible than the forced inspiratory volume, the peak expiratory flow rate, the forced mid-expiratory flow and the airway resistance; it is therefore the appropriate test for many applications. By contrast, the diffusing capacity of the alveolar capillary membrane and the lung compliance are poorly reproducible but provide information which can only partly be obtained in other ways; in these instances improved techniques are required.

Discrimination

The tests of lung function should be appropriate to the circumstances for which they are required. For example, in the investigation of patients with interstitial lung disease, the tests should discriminate with respect to the function of the lung parenchyma. Therefore, if only a limited number of tests can be applied, the compliance and the transfer factor (diffusing capacity) of the lung should be given priority over tests of airway calibre. However, once the lung parenchyma has been investigated the ventilatory capacity will yield additional information on the state of the airways; for this reason, despite its poor discrimination in interstitial lung disease, the forced expiratory volume should be included amongst any additional tests which are carried out.

Sensitive tests are those which identify correctly a high proportion of subjects with the feature for which they are being assessed. There are then few false negative results. Specific tests are those which identify correctly persons who do not have this feature. There are then few false positive results. These and other terms are defined briefly in Table 4.2.

No single test of function is comprehensive so in order to achieve adequate discrimination, a battery of tests should usually be employed; the tests should be selected with a view to their providing information on different aspects of function. This requirement need not involve great expense or the use of bulky apparatus since within each subdivision of lung function, there are several tests from which to choose; when setting up a laboratory the initial selection can therefore be made with a view to the intensive use of a small number of items of equipment. Some of the subdivisions of lung function and the groups of tests from which a choice can be made are listed in Table 4.3.

Technical aspects

When a new laboratory is set up it is usually the intention of those in charge that the items of equipment which are purchased should be inexpensive, accurate and portable, and yet simple to maintain and operate; they should also yield immediate answers which are valid in all circumstances. These criteria constitute a counsel of perfection! In practice, the choice of equipment represents a compromise in terms of cost, complexity, portability and convenience of use, which must be superimposed upon the fundamental requirements that are outlined in this and subsequent chapters. However, not all items of equipment

Table 4.2 Criteria for tests

Aspect	Criterion	Expression
Acceptability	Safe, simple and not unpleasant for subject	Arbitrary
Reproducibility	Within and between sessions, between occasions, observers, laboratories, etc.	Standard deviation or coefficient of variation
Accuracy	Extent of any systematic error (estimate affected by reproducibility)	Amount or percentage
Validity	Relevance or discriminative power of the test; now replaced by sensitivity and specificity	
Sensitivity	Proportion of affected persons who are identified by the test	Percentage
Specificity	Proportion of unaffected persons who are correctly identified	Percentage
False positives	Subjects who are wrongly identified as having the condition	May be reported as percentage
False negatives	Subjects who have the condition but are not identified by the test	
Technical considerations	Time for the test, bulk of equipment, convenience in use, output (analogue or digital), time for intermediate analysis	Arbitrary

Table 4.3 Relationship of tests to aspects of lung function

Aspect	Subdivision	Index and/or procedure
Lung expansion	Compliance of the lung	Oesophageal intubation; measurement of pressure and volume
	Total lung capacity and subdivisions	Gas dilution methods with spirometry Whole-body plethysmography Radiography
Lung movement	Resistance of airways (also chest wall and lung tissue)	Whole-body plethysmography Methods using interruption of air flow, forced oscillation or oesophageal intubation; measurement of pressure and flow
	Ventilatory capacity	Maximal voluntary ventilation, forced expiratory volume, peak expiratory flow, transit times Indices derived from flow−volume curves breathing air and helium
	Response to bronchodilator drugs	Forced expiratory volume, airway resistance, forced expiratory flow
	Air-trapping and distribution of inspired gas	Forced expiratory volume/forced vital capacity (%) and related indices incl. RV/TLC, V_A'/V_A, V_d/V_t

Table 4.3 *Continued*

Aspect	Subdivision	Index and/or procedure
Lung movement *continued*	Air-trapping and distribution of inspired gas *continued*	Single- and multi-breath indices of uneven ventilation Closing volume and capacity Appearance of spirogram
Respiratory muscles	O_2 consumption	Spirometry
	Maximal force	Relation to lung volume
Lung parenchyma	Ventilation–perfusion ratios	Alveolar–arterial tension differences for oxygen, carbon dioxide and nitrogen. Intra-breath R Venous admixture Tests of regional and lobar function
	Transfer of gas	Transfer factor (diffusing capacity) and its subdivisions
	Other indices	Ventilation in relation to the uptake of oxygen and the change in arterial oxygen tension during exercise
	Haemodynamics	Pulmonary vascular pressures in relation to blood flow
Regulation of respiration	Effectiveness	Tensions of O_2 and CO_2 in arterial blood
	Control mechanisms	Ventilation in relation to uptake of oxygen, tidal volume and duration of inspiration Respiratory responses to hypoxaemia and hypercapnia Indices of respiratory drive
Limitation of exercise	Respiratory component	Exercise ventilation and related variables
	Cardiovascular component	Cardiac frequency and stroke volume Electrocardiogram Relationships to oxygen uptake, respiratory exchange ratio and blood lactic acid concentration

meet the currently recognised standards such as those of the European Respiratory Society, European Coal and Steel Community or American Thoracic Society. In addition the objectives of the laboratory should not be sacrificed to expediency. For example, where there is a prospect of making serial measurements over a period of years an instrument should be selected which is capable of regular calibration *in the laboratory* (page 50). For comparison with results from other laboratories, the indices which are obtained should be given in absolute and not in arbitrary units. The output of data should, where possible, be in the form in which it is to be used; for this reason the provision of a numerical value is generally to be preferred to a graphical record which must be measured, counted or integrated before it can be interpreted. Where two variables are to be compared, a twin co-ordinate chart recorder which provides an immediate graphical solution will shorten the time of analysis compared with a recorder with two independent channels. For complex indices which require manipulation of intermediate results, the output from the instruments should preferably feed on to magnetic tape or on-line into a computer.

The interpretation of the result of an assessment often depends upon a number of variables being measured at one time. This has led to the manufacture of composite apparatus comprising several items. The specification and performance of each item should be scrutinised since one or more of the items could have undesirable features, although standards of manufacture are, in general, high. For example, there might be no provision for making a three point calibration in the laboratory or for adequate hygiene. The intermediate stages in processing the results might not be accessible for scrutiny or the indices which are obtained could be unique to the equipment and not comparable with measurements made using other apparatus. The additional time spent in making a careful selection of components for the laboratory can lead to improved reproducibility, greater accuracy and better understanding of the limitations of the method.

Choice of equipment

The choice of equipment will be determined by the type of work which it is proposed to undertake and is considered in depth in subsequent chapters. A chest clinic should have at least one and preferably two low resistance spirometers for measurement of forced expiratory volume and vital capacity. Other lung function tests and facilities for analysis of arterial blood gases will not normally be available in the clinic; they must be available in any hospital treating patients with acute diseases. The lung function laboratory will usually be equipped to measure the subdivisions of total lung capacity including residual volume, the transfer factor (diffusing capacity) and the physiological response to progressive exercise. The laboratory can also perform the arterial blood gas analyses. Alternatively these can be undertaken in the department of clinical chemistry or in intensive therapy units. Additional lung function tests and facilities for scanning the lungs should be available in specialist centres. The times for each of the recommended procedures, the equipment and the indices which are obtained are given in Table 4.4. Some of the other options which are available are listed in Table 4.5 and for lung mechanics in Chapter 6.

Setting up the tests

Once the choices have been made and the equipment has arrived at the laboratory, the tests will be brought into use. Usually this is done by the operator trying out the procedures first on himself and then on visitors and selected patients. In this way the operator gains experience with the test; however, in order to demonstrate that the results are satisfactory the performance of both the equipment and the operator

Table 4.4 Equipment for routine assessment of lung function

Measurement	Equipment	Index
Forced expiratory volume and vital capacity or forced vital capacity (page 133); 5–15 min	Low resistance dry spirometer with electronic timing device or recorder. It should be fitted with means for calibration and should preferably be battery operated	Forced expiratory volume (FEV_1). Forced vital capacity (FVC). FEV%. Change after bronchodilator drugs (and, where appropriate, after exercise)
Total lung capacity and sub-divisions (page 150); 15 min	Closed-circuit spirometer with kymograph and katharometer for analysing He or body plethysmograph with ancillary equipment	Total lung capacity (TLC). Functional residual capacity (FRC). Residual volume (RV). RV/TLC (%)
Transfer factor (diffusing capacity) by single-breath method (including index of distribution) (pages 302 and 222); 15 min	Bag-in-box system with appropriate tap. Spirometer. Infrared analyser for CO. Equipment for measuring lung volumes	Transfer factor (diffusing capacity) for the lung (Tl_{CO}), K_{CO} (Tl/V_A). Lung mixing index (V_A'/V_A)
Ventilation and cardiac frequency during exercise (page 425); 20 min	Treadmill or cycle ergometer. Ventilation meter. Mixing chamber. Physical gas analysers for O_2 and CO_2. Electrocardiograph. Dedicated computer	Exercise ventilation ($\dot{V}_E$) and tidal volume (Vt) O_2 consumption ($\dot{n}_{O_2}$) Respiratory and cardiac frequencies. Dyspnoeic index. Response to breathing O_2
Anthropometry (page 54); 5–10 min	Stadiometer and weighing scales. Skin calipers*	Height and weight. Fat-free mass*

* If laboratory is to undertake exercise testing.

should be assessed objectively. The equipment should be calibrated under the conditions in which it is to be used (page 50) and the result recorded in a book kept for this purpose. The reproducibility of the equipment and operator together should next be determined (page 67). For many tests of function this may be done by the operator making the measurement on a group of subjects on each of 5 days, but other procedures are also appropriate. The order of testing both within and between days should be arranged in the form of a randomised block or Latin square. In this way any systematic variation which may occur from day to day or as a result of the time in a session when the measurement is performed can be determined. When several operators are to use the equipment the comparability of the results which they obtain should also be determined (page 133).

Once it is established that the calibration of the equipment is satisfactory and the measurement is reproducible the magnitude of the results should be considered. The results are likely to be correct when the accepted procedure for the test is adopted, but systematic errors sometimes occur. They are usually due to either the neglect of some apparently trivial aspect of the procedure or a defect in the equipment that is not readily amenable to calibration. Such errors may be detected

Table 4.5 Equipment for additional tests of lung function

Measurement	Equipment	Index
Peak expiratory flow (page 139): 3–5 min	Peak flow meter, e.g. Wright	Peak expiratory flow (PEF)
Flow–volume curve (page 142): 10 min	Spirometer and differentiator or pneumotachograph and integrator, with appropriate recorder	MEF 50% FVC and related indices. Transit time. Volume of iso-flow
Airway resistance (page 167): 15 min	Body plethysmograph. Pneumotachograph. Pressure transducers. Equipment for forced oscillations. Oscilloscope	Airway resistance (Raw). Thoracic gas volume (TGV). Flow–volume curve, hence $MEF_{60\%}$ of TLC
Lung distensibility (page 161): 20 min	Oesophageal balloon and equipment for measuring pressure. Spirometer with potentiometer and twin co-ordinate chart recorder	Static compliance (Cl). Recoil pressure
Distribution of inspired gas (page 214): 5–20 min	Spirometer, rapid analyser for He, A, N_2 or Xe^{133} and twin co-ordinate chart recorder	Closing volume and capacity. Single breath N_2 index. A/N_2 index
Ventilation–perfusion ratios (page 250): 60 min	Blood gas analysers	Blood gas tensions (Pa,o_2 and Pa,co_2) and pH. Venous admixture ($\dot{Q}va/\dot{Q}t$ and $\dot{Q}s/\dot{Q}t$) at rest and on exercise
	Respiratory mass spectrometer	Intrabreath R

Test	Equipment	Measurement
Subdivisions of transfer factor (page 313): 15 min	As for Tl with additional paramagnetic meter for O_2 or gas chromatograph	Diffusing capacity of alveolar capillary membrane (Dm). Volume of blood in the alveolar capillaries (Vc)
Respiratory control (page 373): 10 min	Rebreathing bag, gas meter and analyser for CO_2. Interrupter and related equipment	Response of ventilation to CO_2. Respiratory drive
Regional and lobar function (pages 229 and 225): 15–60 min	For details see text	
Pulmonary circulation (page 239):	Rapid analyser for CO_2. Swan Ganz catheter. Pressure transducer. Densitometer or other appropriate equipment	Tension of CO_2 in mixed venous blood ($P\bar{v},co_2$). Pulmonary arterial pressure (P_{PA}) and cardiac output ($\dot{Q}t$) at rest and on exercise
Respiratory muscle function (page 577): 10–30 min	Pressure transducer and recorder Double lumen oesophageal tube Electromyograph	Maximal inspiratory and expiratory pressures. Transdiaphragmatic pressure (Pdi). Electromyogram. Respiratory muscle fatigue
Chest wall expansion	Magnetometers. Impediance pneumograph	
Sleep apnoea (page 350): 12 h	Oximeter. Jerkin plethysmograph. Electroencephalograph	Nocturnal hypoxaemia etc.

by the operator performing a biological calibration in which the test is applied to a group of subjects with apparently normal lungs. The results should be comparable with those published in the literature (Chapter 15). To ensure that this level of performance is maintained a routine should be established for the regular repetition of the calibration. The equipment is now ready for use.

Training the technician

The assessment of lung function and the physiological response to exercise require both technical expertise and ability to coax the subjects to perform respiratory gymnastics. Subjects usually respond best to an unassuming and friendly but firm approach. Some prospective technicians achieve this spontaneously and others during training but some never do. Such persons should be identified at the pre-employment interview. The candidate should have a background in biology, physiology or physics at an appropriate level. The training should be based on a recognised programme and lead to the award of a qualifying or higher certificate. Training on the job is seldom adequate though many technicians start in this way, combining practical work with a part-time course at a technical college or polytechnic. The theoretical part of the course should cover respiratory, cardiovascular and exercise physiology, respiratory pathophysiology, instrument and measurement technology and simple statistics. The practical course should be based on a specialist centre, and the course for the higher certificate should include a research project. The project should contribute to, but be assessed separately from, the final examination paper. Competence acquired during such a course should be reinforced by attendance at refresher courses and scientific meetings; in the UK these are organised by the Association of Respiratory Technicians and Physiologists. In addition the technicians should participate in review sessions with clinicians on the contribution of the lung function assessments to the clinical management of patients (pages 81 and 515).

Conduct of the assessment

This should normally bring together all the information which will be needed for compiling the report and identifying any inconsistencies with other aspects of the case.

For this purpose and in order to establish what tests are appropriate and safe to perform, the subject should complete a brief questionnaire on respiratory and cardiovascular symptoms based on the MRC Questionnaire (page 517) including questions on smoking and present medication. The blood pressure and, if appropriate, the electrocardiogram should be recorded and read by a trained observer, the haemoglobin concentration noted and the chest radiograph scrutinised by a competent person who will usually be a physician. The radiograph is useful because as well as indicating any thoracic pathology it provides a measure of thoracic gas volume with which that obtained by other methods can be compared.

The subject should ideally attend the laboratory in a relaxed post-absorbtive state having not smoked or consumed alcohol on the day of the test and not taken strenuous exercise within the preceding hour. Neglect of these precautions could affect particularly the results of the measurement of transfer factor (page 300) and physiological response to exercise (page 429). In addition if the response to a bronchodilator drug is to be assessed in a patient on bronchodilator therapy, he or she should preferably not have taken any β-adrenergic or anticholinergic drug within the preceding 4 h. If this condition is not met the time and dose of any therapy should be recorded.

The measurements should be preceded by a description of what is envisaged and why the tests are being undertaken. Explicit consent should be obtained (page 65). The assessment will normally start with the measurement of stature using a stadiometer (page 50). Before starting any lung function tests the subject should remove *loose* false teeth and loosen tight clothing, including surgical corsets and, sometimes, the brassière. The first test is dynamic spirometry and if the subject has not performed this previously, the technician should demonstrate the procedure or arrange that the subject watches whilst another subject is assessed. For this purpose it is an advantage if all tests except the compliance and physiological response to exercise are performed in one room. The measurement of FEV_1 and related variables is described on page 133. Next, if appropriate, an inhalation of salbutamol is administered by a standard method (page 640) and the lung volumes and transfer factor measured whilst the drug is exerting its effect; in the case of salbutamol this takes up to 45 min. However, if it is not intended to administer a bronchodilator some laboratories start with closed circuit spirometry for measurement of subdivision of total lung capacity then follow it with dynamic spirometry. This order facilitates the elimination from the lungs of helium which might otherwise affect the measurement of transfer factor. In any event, time must be allowed for clearance of test gases between tests and for this purpose it is sometimes convenient for one operator to alternate the tests between two patients. In patients given a bronchodilator drug the dynamic spirometry should then be repeated and if appropriate the compliance or plethysmography performed. The exercise should follow after the other tests. If the patient has symptoms suggestive of angina or a history of ischaemic heart disease the exercise should be preceded by recording a 12 lead electrocardiogram. This should be read by a trained observer. In addition the skinfold thicknesses and body mass should be recorded for calculation of fat-free mass (page 50). At the end of the exercise test the subject's degree of breathlessness and other symptoms should be recorded (page 387). After completing the measurements the subject should be thanked for participating and supplied with precise information as to when the results will be available, to whom they will be sent and how he or she can have access to them. The practice of commenting on the results as they come up on the printer can be helpful if they lead to the subject improving his or her performance but may cause misapprehensions which are difficult to correct subsequently.

Reporting the results

An assessment of lung function is not complete until the result has been compiled and reported on. A specimen report sheet (dimensions of original 28 cm by 20 cm (A4)) is given in Table 4.6. It includes spaces for personal details about the subject, anthropometric measurements, the clinical and radiographic information which should be to hand when the report is prepared, the results, the reference values, any previous result which may be relevant and the comment. The anthropometric measurements and the clinical information will usually be obtained at the time of assessment and the chest radiograph inspected at the time of preparing the comment. Reference values appropriate for most circumstances are given in Chapter 15.

The results and the reference values can be written onto the report sheet by the technicians who made the measurements; alternatively the data can be processed and printed automatically. In this event the print-out should be initialled by the technician as evidence of its accuracy. The report will normally be prepared by a physician or clinical physiologist who will also check (or enter) the clinical information. The report can be written by hand then photocopied. It may take into account any interpretation given by a computer programme. The latter should not be accepted uncritically since the programmes are, as yet, limited in scope and cannot take into account all the relevant indices and circumstance. This subject needs further development.

The reporter bases his comments on the list of results, provided he can trust their accuracy. His trust should be founded on familiarity with the equipment, an adequate laboratory routine and a procedure for finding faults which should involve both the technician who made the measurements and the reporter. The scrutiny should establish that the instruments were free from drift, the initial calibrations were satisfactory and not materially different from those made after the measurements, the mechanical equipment was functioning satisfactorily and the subject was able to comply with the instructions of the operator. The nature and, so far as possible, the cause of any difficulty in this respect should be noted. The instrumental displays and the intermediate results should also be of acceptable quality and should usually be inspected before the report is written. Some examples are given in Fig. 4.1.

In addition the reporter should preferably discuss the assessment with the technician; this can lead to improved quality control and may contribute additional information which the patient sometimes communicates to the technician but neglects to tell the physician.

The comment should be based on all the individual results; each

Table 4.6 Example of lung function report sheet

Name and Address No.		Result	Reference value	Previous result
	FEV_1 (before) (l)			
	(after)* (l & change, %)			
	FVC (before) (l)			
	(after)* (l & change, %)			
	FEV% (before) (% of FVC)			
	PEF (before (ls^{-1})			
Date	(after)* $(ls^{-1}$ & change, %)			
Birth Age Sex	$MEF_{50\% \ FVC}$ (ls^{-1})			
Occupation	$MEF_{25\% \ FVC}$ (ls^{-1})			
Referred by	Raw on insp. $(kPa\,l^{-1}s)$			
Clinical diagnosis/problem	at lung volume of (l)			
	sG_{AW} $(kPa^{-1}s^{-1})$			
B.P. (systemic) E.C.G.	TLC (pleth)			
Bronchitis grade† Wheeze grade† Breathless† grade	TLC (He dilution)			
Smoking	VC (two stage) (l)			
X-ray	IVC (l)			
	FRC (l)			
	RV (l)			
Ht (m) Wt (kg)	RV% (RV/TLC) (%)			
Hb $(g\,dl^{-1})$ FFM (kg) % fat	C static exp. $(l\,kPa^{-1})$			
Comment	insp. $(l\,kPa^{-1})$			
	Recoil pr.(max) (kPa)			
	at TLC-20% VC (kPa)			
	Tl $(mmol\,min^{-1}\,kPa^{-1})$			
	K_{CO} (Tl/V_A)			
	V_A'/V_A (%)			
	S_{CO_2} rebr. $(l\,min^{-1}\,kPa^{-1})$			
	Ergometer settings			
	$\dot{n}_{O_2}$ (exercise) $(mmol\,min^{-1})$			
	$\dot{V}_E$, breathing air $(l\,min^{-1})$			
	RER —			
.	$\dot{V}_E$, breathing O_2 $(l\,min^{-1})$			
	Vt_{30} (l)			
	f_C (treadmill/bike) (min^{-1})			
	Sa, o_2 rest (%) exercise‡ (%)			

* 45 min after inhalation of salbutamol (200 μg).
† From Questionnaire of respiratory symptoms.
‡ Can be replaced by blood gas tensions if arterial blood is sampled.

will be compared with the reference value which may be a previous result for that subject or one obtained from tables. For the principal indices the result under scrutiny can conveniently be allocated to one of four categories: normal, or slightly, moderately or grossly abnormal. In children before puberty the result can be expressed as a percentile (page 458). For some applications borderline abnormality linked to one standard deviation (1 SD) from the reference value can indicate a physiologically meaningful difference from the mean for the average subject. One SD for the forced expiratory volume in adult males is 0.5l and for the transfer factor $1.7 \, \mathrm{mmol \, min^{-1} \, kPa^{-1}}$ ($5 \, \mathrm{ml \, min^{-1} \, mmHg^{-1}}$). Using this criterion 16% of genuinely normal results will be considered suspect (cf. page 510) and some instances where a result for an index has fallen from an above-average to a below-average level will still be missed. Any arbitrary level has its disadvantages!

If abnormality is suspected or established the next step is to discover its nature. This will entail recognition of a characteristic pattern of

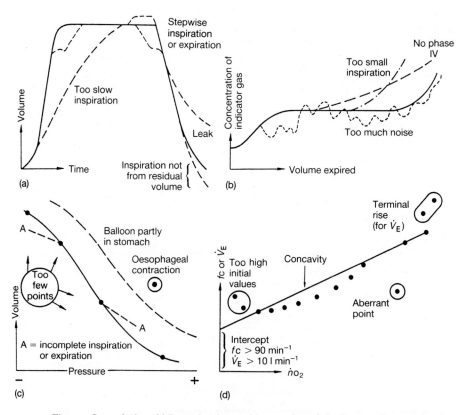

Fig. 4.1 Some faults which can be detected by scrutiny of the intermediate results; in most instances they constitute reasons for rejecting the measurement but it may be sufficient to exclude one or more points. *Top left*: transfer factor by the breathholding method. *Top right*: closing volume. *Bottom left*: static lung compliance. *Bottom right*: progressive exercise test.

abnormality such as one of the syndromes of abnormal function described in Chapter 16 or of physiological adaptation described in Chapter 15. For the report to be conclusive the pattern should be consistent with all the physiological results, the clinical features, the appearance of the chest radiograph and other information about the subject. Inconsistencies within or between any of these classes of information should lead to reappraisal of the findings with a view to achieving a comprehensive interpretation or deciding how the inconsistency should be resolved.

Guide to references

The references (Chapter 18) are classified under subject headings of which the following are particularly relevant to the present chapter:

5: Structure, Expansion and Movement of the Lung

Anatomy of the lung

The thoracic cavity is formed by the chest wall and the diaphragm. The cavity is subdivided by the mediastinum and heart which extends out into the left thoracic space. On this account the left lung is somewhat smaller than the right lung, the respective weights in healthy, young adult males being approximately 500 g and 600 g. The shape is nearly pyramidal with a height of approximately 20 cm and a density when fully inflated of about $0.2\,kg\,dm^{-3}$. The right lung is subdivided into superior, middle and inferior lobes which are each supplied by a division of the right main bronchus. The bronchus to the right inferior lobe is a nearly linear continuation of the trachea. The left lung is subdivided into the superior and inferior lobes and the lingula; the latter is supplied by the lingular or lower division of the left superior lobe bronchus and is analogous to the middle lobe of the right lung. The lobes are divided into segments; these are listed in Table 5.1. Within each segment the bronchus subdivides and gives off between 10 and 25 branches, of which the diameters range from about 1 cm downwards; the path length from the carina is in the range 8−23 cm.

Table 5.1 Nomenclature of bronchopulmonary anatomy

Right lung		Left lung	
Bronchi	Segments	Bronchi	Segments
Superior lobe	Apical (1)	Superior lobe	Apical (1)
	Posterior (2)		Posterior (2)
	Anterior (3)		Anterior (3)
Middle lobe	Lateral (4)		Superior (4)(lingula)
	Medial (5)		Inferior (5)(lingula)
Inferior lobe	Apical (6)	Inferior lobe	Apical (6)
	Medial basal (7)		Medial basal (7)
	Anterior basal (8)		Anterior basal (8)
	Lateral basal (9)		Lateral basal (9)
	Posterior basal (10)		Posterior basal (10)

The *pattern of branching* is described in terms of models of which two are in common use. In Weibel's model the right and left main bronchi constitute generation one and the generation number is increased at each dichotomy. This is useful for describing the larger airways, for example in relation to bronchoscopy. The model breaks down when describing the peripheral airways because these are allocated to different generations depending on their distance from the carina; this obscures the relationship of branch number to diameter. In addition if a common path length is assumed the model overestimates the number of terminal units and predicts incorrectly that the total cross-sectional area of the respiratory tract increases progressively with distance from the carina resembling the contour of a trumpet. These errors are avoided by ordering the airways from the periphery as is done in the procedure of Horsfield and colleagues (Fig. 5.1). Their model correctly describes the distribution of airway cross-sectional area as onion-shaped with a maximum some 12 cm from the carina. The average numbers and dimensions of airways in the different orders are given in Fig. 5.2.

The intrapulmonary airways are of endothelial origin and are fully differentiated by the 16th week of gestation. The proximal airways (i.e. bronchi) have cartilage in their walls, mucous glands beneath the basement membrane and columnar epithelium. The distal subdivisions are bronchioles and differ from the bronchi in having no cartilage or mucous glands and being lined by cubical rather than columnar epithelium. Both types of cell are ciliated and are interspersed with goblet cells. The goblet cells end distally at the level of the terminal bronchiole, which is also the last subdivision of the bronchial tree in which the lumen is surrounded by a continuous layer of smooth muscle. The terminal bronchioles have an internal diameter in the range 0.30–1.0 mm; their total number in the two lungs is of the order of 25×10^3.

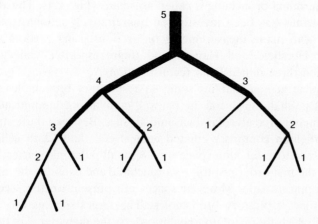

Fig. 5.1 Model of the bronchial tree showing asymmetrical branching. The ordering starts at the periphery. Where two branches meet the parent branch is one order higher than the higher-ordered daughter branch. (Source: Horsfield K, Cumming C. *J Appl Physiol.* 1968; **68**: 373–383.)

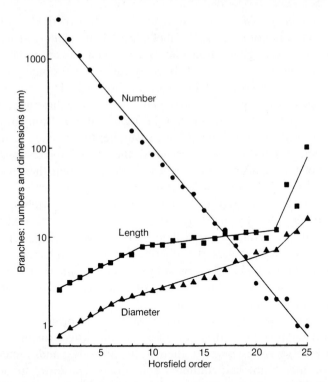

Fig. 5.2 Number, mean diameter, and mean length of branches in each Horsfield order of a cast of the human bronchial tree. Straight lines represent the regression equations. The ordering starts three bifurcations up from the terminal bronchioles ($n \approx 25\,000$). (Source: Horsfield K. *APS Handbook of Physiology. The Respiratory System III.* 75–88, 1986.)

Clusters of between three and five terminal bronchioles constitute the secondary lobules. Some of these units are surrounded by fibrous septa which render them visible to the naked eye. The portion of lung distal to one terminal bronchiole is called an *acinus* (Fig. 5.3). The structure of the acinus has been investigated quantitatively amongst others by Weibel who made measurements on sections using random samples and by Horsfield and Hansen and their respective colleages who attempted three-dimensional reconstructions.

A typical acinus contains some 14 respiratory bronchioles each of which has shallow alveoli in its wall and also communicates with approximately 100 alveolar ducts and air sacs. Between these structures the epithelium comprises ciliated cubical cells and Clara cells which have a secretory function (page 97). A small pulmonary artery usually adjoins the first order respiratory bronchiole and confines the air spaces to the opposite side. More air spaces are present on the second and third order respiratory bronchioles. The largest spaces are alveolar ducts of which there are up to eight orders; the diameter is in the range 0.6–2 mm. Air sacs are smaller and have few distinctive features.

Each *alveolar duct* is lined by flattened epithelial cells and is supported by a spring-like spiral fibre of collagen, elastin and smooth muscle

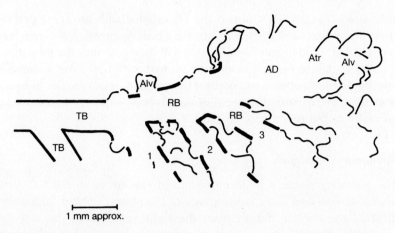

1 mm approx.

Fig. 5.3 The normal anatomy of the acinus or respiratory portion of the bronchiolar tree showing the terminal bronchioles (TB), three orders of respiratory bronchioles (RB1, 2 and 3), an alveolar duct (AD), an atrium (Atr) and alveoli (Alv). The acinus is approximately spherical and of average diameter 6 mm. (Source: Reid L. *Thorax* 1958; **13**: 110.)

cells. The alveoli emerge from between the turns of the spiral, usually five to eight per turn; they are roughly hexagonal in shape except for the terminal alveolus which is spherical. There are between 10 and 30 alveoli per duct and this unit constitutes a primary lobule. The vessels run between the alveolar duct systems and surround the alveoli.

The alveoli communicate with each other through the pores of Kohn which are discrete holes in the walls between alveoli, often with a cuboidal type II alveolar cell forming part of the aperture. These cells are considered further on page 76. Accessory communications between some bronchioles and their adjacent alveoli have been described by Lambert and there are also communications between alveolar ducts and between respiratory bronchioles; their diameter is up to 200 μm. These communications permit collateral ventilation between adjacent portions of lung tissue. Larger communications occur in the lungs of some other mammals, for example dogs, in which there is less inter-lobular connective tissue than in man.

Alveoli continue to develop after birth and increase in number throughout the period of growth. Depending on its size, the adult lung contains between 200 and 600×10^6 alveoli with an average diameter of about 0.25 mm; together with other air spaces they have a total surface area of about 70–80 m^2. The alveoli are lined by type I alveolar cells (epithelial cells) whose thickness away from the nuclei is in the range 0.04–0.07 μm. The cells lie on a basement membrane (Fig. 5.9, page 98); for two alveoli which are adjacent the basement membranes enclose the components of the interalveolar septum, including reticulin fibres, elastic fibres, the histiocytes (macrophages) and capillaries with their lining of endothelial cells. The epithelial cells are in close apposition and have minimal gaps between them; the mean pore size is 0.5 nm. By contrast the endothelial cells are separated by clefts and pores of diameter 12−15 nm which open when the capillary is distended; fluid containing albumen will then pass into the interstitial space. On this account, whereas the occurrence of alveolar oedema is rare, interstitial oedema will occur if the capillary intravascular pressure is increased. The total thickness of the alveolar capillary membrane is normally in the range 0.15−0.5 μm.

Pulmonary circulation

The pulmonary artery is developed from the artery to the left sixth branchial arch and is the main source of blood for the lung. It conveys most of the cardiac output from the right ventricle to the alveolar capillaries. The pulmonary artery divides into right and left pulmonary arteries and these in turn subdivide to provide up to eight generations of elastic-walled vessels of diameter more than 2 mm. The distal branches of diameters 2 mm down to 0.3 mm, are small muscular pulmonary arteries which run beside the airways supplying the paren-chyma of the lung. Other vessels enter the periphery of the lung units where they provide a collateral circulation. The arteries end as terminal arterioles which supply the individual acini; these vessels have thin walls, a diameter of less than 150 μm, and a surrounding perivascular space. Accumulation of fluid in the space can interfere with blood flow (page 190). The arterioles deliver blood to the capillary networks which lie in the septa between the alveoli; these networks, in turn, drain into the pulmonary venules which lie in the periphery of the lobules. The venules unite to form veins which run in the septa and join to form the main pulmonary veins that end in the left atrium.

Pulmonary arterioles do not anastomose with each other but they may communicate with the pulmonary veins through anastomotic channels bypassing the alveolar capillaries; the significance of the channels is not known. Blood which has not traversed the alveolar capillaries may also enter the pulmonary veins or the left atrium from the bronchial arteries and veins, the lower oesophageal veins and occasionally by anomalous drainage from the coronary sinus or the azygos veins.

Blood can enter the left ventricle from the coronary circulation through the Thebesian veins; however, the amount is normally less than 0.4% of cardiac output and the total quantity of blood which bypasses the alveolar capillaries is usually small (see Fig. 7.7, page 191). This physiological shunt is increased in a number of lung diseases including pulmonary fibrosis, bronchiectasis and bronchial carcinoma; in these conditions the bronchial arteries can be dilated and the fingers exhibit 'clubbing'. The oesophageal veins become enlarged when there is portal hypertension.

Bronchial arteries arise from the thoracic aorta and their arterioles provide nutrients to the visceral pleura, pulmonary arteries and conduct-ing airways down to and including the respiratory bronchioles. The primary lobules are supplied by branches of the pulmonary artery. The bronchial veins anastomose with the pulmonary veins. The bronchial arterioles communicate with the pulmonary arterioles in newborn infants but not in later life except when the pulmonary arteriolar flow is reduced by lung disease; oxygenated bronchiolar blood can then flow into the pulmonary circulation.

Pulmonary lymphatics drain the connective tissue spaces of the lung down to the level of the primary lobules including the interlobular, sub-pleural, peribronchial and perivascular spaces. They run proximally from the level of the alveolar ducts into the lymph nodes which adjoin the respiratory bronchioles; the latter, in turn, drain into nodes which lie along the course of the bronchi and at the hilum of the lung. From there drainage occurs into the cervical, para-aortic, subdiaphragmatic, and anterior mediastinal nodes. Flow of lymph also occurs both in the plexuses of lymphatics which lie beneath the pleura and in the lymphatics which accompany the pulmonary veins. Flow is directional due to the presence of valves. No lymphatics have been observed in the walls of atria or alveoli. For the right and left lung respectively the lymph drains into the thoracic duct and the right lymphatic duct; these vessels enter the systemic veins at the junctions of the subclavian and internal jugular veins.

The *autonomic nerve supply* to the lung is from the vagi and the fibres of the cervical and the upper six thoracic ganglia of the sympathetic nervous system. The post-ganglionic sympathetic fibres enter the pulmonary plexus; this forms a sheath round the bronchi and the bronchioles in which are embedded the parasympathetic ganglia. The ganglia provide a parasympathetic cholinergic motor innervation to the bronchial smooth muscle, the secretory epithelium and the bronchial glands. The plexus provides a sympathetic adrenergic motor innervation which supplies the bronchial the pulmonary blood vessels and submucosal glands but not the bronchial smooth muscle. The latter deficiency is compensated for by a high density of adrenoceptors especially β_2 receptors (page 198). An additional autonomic nerve supply to the lung is provided by the peptidergic or non-adrenergic non-cholinergic system (NANC). The mediators include vasoactive intestinal peptide and substance P which respectively relax and constrict bronchial smooth muscle. The role of the system has been investigated by Richardson amongst others. The sensory nerves arise from receptors in the upper respiratory tract, the lung and the pulmonary vascular bed; some are listed in Table 5.2.

The role of the receptors in the upper airways is mainly protective. The pulmonary receptors contribute to the pattern of breathing in a wide range of circumstances of which some are discussed subsequently. In addition, nodes of epithelioid cells resembling those in the carotid body (page 340), occur in the glomus pulmonale; this is located near the bifurcation of the pulmonary artery. Other types of receptor have also been described; many have still to be investigated in detail.

Table 5.2 Features of some respiratory receptors (after Widdicombe)

Name/site	Type and location	Nerve supply	Stimuli	Responses
Nose	Little information	Trigeminal	Dusts, vapours irritants	Sneeze, apnoea, bronchodilatation Secretion of mucus
Nasopharynx	Myelinated and non-myelinated	Glosso-pharyngeal	Pressure, etc.	Sniff and aspiration reflexes
Pharynx	Little information		Pressure, etc.	Swallowing reflex
Larynx	Free endings: (a) superficial (b) deep	Laryngeal (superior and recurrent)	Dusts, vapours, irritants	Swallowing (via epiglottis). Cough and expiratory effort (via vocal cords). Laryngeal and bronchoconstriction. Secretion of mucus
Lung irritant receptors	Superficial and deep, rapidly adapting near carina and main bronchi	Vagus (small myelinated)	Dusts, irritants, deep respiration, decreased lung compliance, microemboli, etc.	Cough, raised BP, laryngeal and bronchial constriction, secretion of mucus, hyperpnoea
Stretch receptors (in airways)	Complex, slowly adapting. In muscular membranous posterior wall of trachea and main bronchi	Vagus (large myelinated)	Stretch, inspiration, decreased lung compliance, hyperthermia, low Pa_{CO_2}	Inspiration often shortened, expiration often prolonged, vocal chords abducted (reflex weak in man)
Deflation receptors	As above		Deflation	Inspiration
J receptors (pulmonary c fibre receptors)	Juxtacapillary, also walls of bronchi (? and trachea)	Vagus (non-mylelinated)	Irritants, chemical mediators, interstitial oedema, microemboli	Apnoea, tachypnoea, tracheal and weak bronchial constriction, bradycardia, etc.

Functional anatomy of the chest cage

Relation to movement of the lung

Expansion of the chest cage takes place as a result of upward and outward movement of the ribs and downward movement of the diaphragm; it is effected by the contraction of the intercostal muscles and the muscle of the diaphragm. During vigorous breathing the action of these muscles is supplemented by that of accessory muscles which act upon the chest cage from other parts of the skeleton; the latter muscles include the sternocleidomastoids, the scaleni, the pectoralis major and minor and the latissimus dorsi. The expansion of the thoracic cavity lowers the pressure at the pleural surface of the lung relative to that in

the surrounding atmosphere; air then enters and expands the lung. The
expansion is not uniform throughout the lung. During spontaneous
breathing when the inspiration begins from functional residual capacity,
the expansion is predominantly at the lung bases but when the inspiration
follows a full expiration, the expansion is greater at the apex than at
the base. The movement is affected by the operation of gravitational
force and elastic, resistive and inertial forces in the lung; these factors
are discussed in subsequent pages.

During the expiratory phase of the respiratory cycle, the inspiratory
muscles relax and the intrapleural pressure becomes less negative with
respect to atmospheric pressure. The elastic recoil of the lung tissue
then compresses the alveolar gas and raises its pressure above that at
the mouth. This change reverses the direction of gas flow. The process
occurs passively without much assistance from the respiratory or accessory muscles of respiration but, even during quiet expiration, some
intercostal muscles contract to a small extent. During vigorous breathing
expiration is assisted by contraction of the abdominal muscles; the
contraction raises the intra-abdominal pressure and this forces the
diaphragm upwards. Compression by the thorax can contribute when
expiration is from near to total lung capacity or when the elbows are
used to reduce the size of the rib cage. These changes increase the
intrapleural pressure which rises towards and then exceeds atmospheric
pressure. The rise in pressure initially increases the rate of expiration
but its continuation may hinder expiration by compressing the airways.
The process is discussed on page 116.

Ribs

Posteriorly the ribs articulate with the thoracic vertebrae. Anteriorly
the upper six ribs articulate with the sternum, whilst the 7th to 10th
ribs are joined to the costal cartilages; the 11th and 12th ribs have no
anterior connections other than the soft tissue in the wall of the
abdomen. The first ribs on both sides of the body move together about
a transverse axis through the costovertebral joints; rotation about this
axis increases the antero-posterior diameter of the thoracic inlet and
raises the sternum. This movement is effected by the contraction of the
scaleni and the sternocleidomastoid muscles.

The 2nd to 6th ribs move about two axes which lie respectively in
the transverse and antero-posterior planes of the body. However,
Jordanoglou has shown that a single axis of rotation can describe both
movements. The axis is common to both sides of the thorax and passes
through the necks of the ribs; movement about this axis increases the
antero-posterior diameter of the thorax and raises the sternum. It has
been likened to the movement of the handle of a farmyard pump. In
females, due to greater mobility of the upper ribs, this movement is
relatively larger than in males. The second axis of rotation of the ribs is
separate for each side of the thorax and is through the angles of the
ribs and the costosternal joints; rotation about this axis causes an

outward and upward movement of the middle part of the ribs and an increase in the transverse diameter of the thorax. This movement has been likened to that of the handle of a bucket.

The 7th to 10th ribs exhibit the bucket-handle motion since rotation about their antero-posterior axes causes widening of the thorax. However, they do not exhibit the pump-handle movement. Instead, a rotatory movement in the transverse plane depresses the sternum and reduces the antero-posterior diameter of the chest.

Intercostal muscles

The internal and the external intercostal muscles form two incomplete layers between each rib and the one below. The function of the muscles during respiration has been deduced with the aid of electrodes placed either on the surface of the thorax or in the muscle. Bipolar needle electrodes are commonly used because there is then no artifact due to spread of electrical activity from other tissues.

Most fibres of the external intercostal muscles (intercostales externi) are in the posterior regions of the intercostal spaces. At the back of the thorax the fibres pass obliquely downwards and laterally, and at the side of the thorax downwards, forwards and medially from each rib to the one below. They contract during inspiration and relax during expiration. During quiet breathing the time of relaxation coincides with the start of expiration but during vigorous breathing the time of relaxation is delayed; this has the effect of smoothing the transition between inspiration and expiration. Most of the fibres of the internal intercostal muscles (intercostales interna) are in the anterior regions of the intercostal spaces; the fibres pass obliquely downwards and backwards. The function of the fibres is determined by the incline of the structures to which they are attached. The interchondral or parasternal fibres lie between the costal cartilages whose slope is upwards; the direction of these fibres resembles that of the external intercostal muscles and, like them, they contract during inspiration and have an inspiratory function. The associated electrical activity (EMG) can be used to monitor inspiration. The interosseous fibres lie between the ribs where they slope downwards and forwards. When the lung is moderately inflated these fibres contract during expiration and have an expiratory function. They also contract during speech.

Paralysis of the intercostal muscles causes loss of rigidity of the chest wall and reduces the lateral bucket-handle movement of the ribs. The intercostal spaces then become flaccid, and exhibit paradoxical movement, inwards during the inspiratory phase and outwards during the expiratory phase of the respiratory cycle.

Diaphragm

The muscles of the diaphragm arise from round the floor of the thoracic cavity, including the arcuate ligaments and crura, lower six ribs and the xyphoid process of the sternum. Medial and lateral arcuate ligaments bridge over the psoas major and quadratus lumborum muscles from insertions respectively over the body and transverse process of the first lumbar vertebra and the twelve rib. A median arcuate ligament bridges over the aorta. From its origins the muscle fibres of the diaphragm pass upwards to converge on the central tendon which mostly lies beneath and is attached to the percardium. The tendon is penetrated by the inferior vena cava and the diaphragmatic muscles by the oesophagus. In the absence of muscular contraction the position of the diaphragm is determined by the pressure difference between peritoneum and pleura and hence that between stomach and thoracic oesophagus; the latter is designated ΔPdi. Its measurement can contribute to investigation of diaphragmatic weakness (page 577). The maximal pressure is usually measured in the oesophagus with respect to atmospheric and can be achieved by sniffing (page 578). When the airway is closed the maximal pressure is developed during inspiration from near to residual volume (Fig. 5.4).

The diaphragm resembles other skeletal muscles in containing both fast twitch and slow twitch fibres. The fibres exhibit fatigue and respond to strength and endurance training (page 645). Fatigue can be demonstrated by serial measurements of ΔPdi,max and by electromyography which shows a shift in the EMG frequency spectrum towards lower frequencies. The costal and crural fibres of the diaphragm receive their

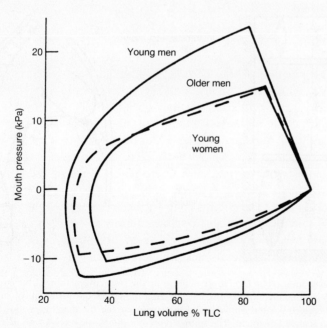

Fig. 5.4 Maximal volume–pressure loops showing the forces which can be developed by the respiratory muscles, including the accessory muscles, at different lung volumes. The data were for groups of subjects breathing with maximal effort into and out of air-tight containers of capacity 1.5–200 l. (Source: Cook CD, Mead J, Orzalesi MM. *J Appl Physiol* 1964; **19**: 1016–1022.)

innervation via the phrenic nerve from respectively the upper and lower cervical segments of the spinal cord. When all the fibres of the diaphragm contract together the central tendon is pulled downwards. The movement resembles that of a piston with a rolling seal: it leads to an increase in depth of the thoracic cavity and an increase in pressure in the abdomen including that part which is enclosed within the lower ribs. The increased abdominal pressure acts on the visceral surface of the ribs to displace them outwards. Upward and outward movement of the ribs and eversion of the lower margin of the thorax also follows contraction of the costal fibres of the diaphragm in isolation. This movement is a consequence of the position which the fibres normally occupy and does not occur when the fibres are horizontal; it therefore does not occur when the diaphragm is flat, as in some cases of emphysema. In these circumstances a contraction of the muscle of the diaphragm reduces the transverse and possibly the posterio-anterior diameters of the lower margin of the thorax. In supine obese subjects a similar response occurs. Isolated contraction of the posterior crural fibres of the diaphragm is believed to displace the rib cage downwards but not to influence the thoracic diameter. The subject is reviewed by De Troyer (Fig. 5.5).

The diaphragm contracts during inspiration and is relaxed throughout the greater part of expiration. During quiet breathing it is the principal muscle of inspiration; then its tidal excursion is on average 1.5 cm.

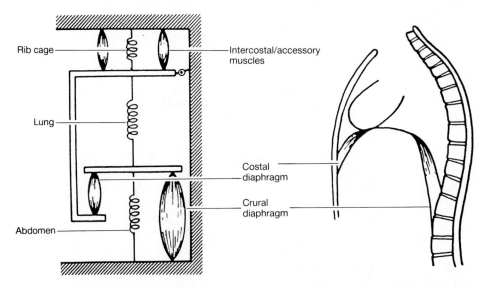

Fig. 5.5 Diagram used by De Troyer to illustrate the respective actions of the costal and crural fibres of the diaphragm. The hatched area represents the vertebral column, the inverted L-shaped bar the rib cage, and the transverse bar the diaphragm; this is assumed to remain horizontal. The springs represent the elastic recoil of rib cage, lungs and diaphragm. Both parts of the muscle of the diaphragm depress the central tendon. The costal fibres elevate the rib cage and evert the lower costal margin. The crural fibres depress the rib cage through the mediation of lung elasticity. (Source: *APS Handbook of Physiology. Respiration* III(i) p. 451. Adapted from Macklem PT, Macklem DM, De Troyer A. *J Appl Physiol* 1983; **55**: 547–557.)

During deep breathing Wade has shown that the excursion relative to the insertion of the diaphragm can be as much as 10 cm. This movement is responsible for about 75% of the volume of gas which is inhaled; the remaining 25% is attributable to movement of the ribs. Thus total paralysis of the diaphragm greatly reduces the ability to ventilate the lung but respiration can be maintained without it. Unilateral paralysis in subjects with normal lungs causes a reduction in the ventilatory capacity of about 20%; the decline is greater when the work of breathing is increased by disease of the lung or thoracic cage. The paralysed half of the diaphragm moves paradoxically by rising in the thorax during inspiration and falling during expiration; the movement reflects the differences in pressure between the thorax and the abdomen during the two phases of the respiratory cycle. Unilateral paralysis of the diaphragm may be diagnosed on X-ray screening of the chest by asking the subject to sniff. The consequences of diaphragmatic weakness and a strategy for assessing diaphragmatic function are considered respectively on pages 577 and 578.

Abdominal muscles

The abdominal muscles support and protect the abdominal contents and contribute to movement of the trunk. They also influence respiration both because the fibres arise from or are inserted into the lower ribs or costal cartilages and because contraction raises the intra-abdominal pressure. The main action on respiration is expiratory. Thus the rectus abdominus muscles occupy the medial half of the anterior abdominal wall; their contraction reduces the anterio-posterior and transverse diameters of the thorax. In conjunction with other abdominal muscles they raise the intra-abdominal pressure and displace in a cranial direction the central tendon of the diaphragm. The abdominal muscles are inactive during quiet breathing. They become active during phonation and during exercise when the ventilation exceeds approximately $40\,l\,min^{-1}$. Initially contraction occurs towards the end of expiration, but during maximal breathing it occurs throughout expiration. It also occurs during coughing and sneezing.

As well as causing expiration the abdominal muscles appear to have a subsidiary role of stabilising the rib cage or even causing some degree of chest expansion. Thus in the dog De Troyer found that isolated stimulation of the external oblique muscle expanded the lower ribs. Stimulation of the internal oblique and transversus abdominus muscles did not influence the position of the ribs. In man on account of the different configuration of the thorax the action of the abdominal muscles on the rib cage is believed to be restrictive with the possible exception of some fibres in the transversus abdominus which could have a stabilising effect.

During inspiration the abdominal muscles contribute to the function of the diaphragm by raising the intra-abdominal pressure. This causes cranial displacement of the central tendon, lengthening of the muscle fibres of the diaphragm, and an increase in their force of contraction in the direction of everting the lower costal margin. This synergistic action of the abdominal muscles has been demonstrated on changing from a supine to an upright posture, during exercise, voluntary hyperventilation and when the chemical drive to ventilation is increased.

Lung expansion

Introduction

When a normal subject inhales maximally after a forced expiration the volume of gas in the lung increases approximately four-fold. For the expansion to be uniform this would require an increase in linear dimensions of the lung by a factor of 4^{-3} or 1.6 which nearly obtains in practice. However, regional differences in expansion occur on account of the pyramidal shape of the lung and the operation of gravitational force. Most expansion takes place in the alveolar ducts and alveoli, which Storey and Staub have shown to enlarge to an equal extent. Thus expansion maintains constant branching angles between airways (isotropic expansion). It is made possible by both the structure of the lung tissue and the surface-tension properties of the material which lines the alveoli.

The framework of the lung is made up of bundles of elastic and collagen fibres which extend from the large airways to the alveoli and pleura. During development collagen appears first in the primitive airways and blood vessels and immature elastin in what will become the mouths of alveoli. Subsequently collagen contributes to the alveolar basement membranes. Both types of fibre increase in number after birth with the elastin contributing approximately 12% of dry lung weight by about 6 months. The proportion of collagen continues to increase throughout the period of growth. However, the two types of fibre are frequently in apposition and together they form the scaffolding of the lung. This has been described by Weibel as resembling crumpled wire netting but whereas the constituent fibres are relatively indistensible they can move with respect to each other so the bundles of fibres lengthen and uncurl and alter their relative positions like the threads of a nylon stocking when it is put on. The network of fibres extends into the walls of the larger airways and blood vessels so these structures also expand but to a lesser extend than the lung parenchyma. Here, during a breath which starts from residual volume, the coils of the spiral fibres of the alveolar ducts expand longitudinally and by so doing widen the mouths of the alveoli which lie between them. The accordion-like expansion is followed by stretching of the alveolar septa, loss of undulations in their walls (also called crumpling), opening up of pleats in the septa and recruitment of previously collapsed alveoli. These processes increase the area of alveolar surface. The increase facilitates the passage of gas across the alveolar capillary membrane. It is accompanied by a narrowing and elongation of those alveolar capillaries which lie in the central parts of the alveolar septa though not those which lie near the junctions of septa. The changes reduce the volume of alveolar capillary blood with which the exchange of gas takes place. The changes are illustrated in Fig. 5.6.

During normal expiration the changes in shape and dimensions are reversed. Deflation of the lung can also occur from contraction of muscle fibres present in the bundles which form the alveolar ducts and related structures. This pneumoconstriction does not necessarily affect the larger airways.

In the absence of constriction the network of bundles confers stability on the lung because a reduction in volume of a small part leads to a local increase in tension within the network around it; the resulting traction tends to restore the part to its original size. This interdependence was described by Mead, Takishima and Leith.

Elastic recoil of lung tissue; role of lung surfactant

During inspiration the respiratory muscles stretch the elastic and collagen tissues network of the lung and overcome the force of surface tension at the air to tissue interface. The work which is done is not dissipated as heat; instead it is stored in the structures which have been stretched and there exerts a retractive force which is the *elastic recoil of the lung tissue*. About half of this is due to stretching of lung tissue and half due to surface tension. The energy is used during expiration to restore the

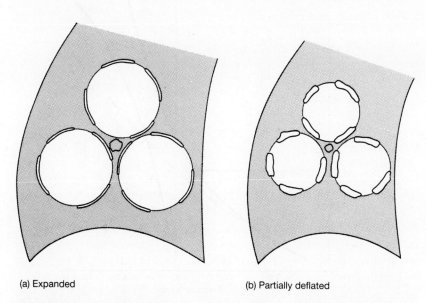

(a) Expanded   (b) Partially deflated

Fig. 5.6 Diagram illustrating the effect of lung expansion upon the size of the alveolar capillaries. When the lung is expanded (a) the capillaries in the alveolar walls are attenuated and the volume of blood which they contain is less than when the lung is partially deflated (b); by contrast the alveolar corner vessels and the extra-alveolar vessels in the interstitial spaces are increased in size due to traction from the surrounding structures.

lung to its initial volume. The elastic and the collagen tissue and the surface film may therefore be said to impose an elastic hindrance to inspiration. Where there is hysteresis they may also impose a viscous resistance (see below and page 165).

The force which must be applied to expand the lung varies with its volume. This is illustrated in Fig. 5.7 which shows the relationship between the applied pressure and the volume which this pressure is able to support under equilibrium conditions. The slope of the relationship between pressure (Pst) and volume (V) describes the distensibility of the lung. The slope at functional residual capacity is called the *compliance of the lung* (page 100); it is a chord measurement to a curvilinear function and has a different slope when measured on inspiration and on expiration. The resulting elipse is illustrated in Fig. 5.8. The figure is due to Radford who demonstrated that the area of the elipse (and hence the hysteresis) decreased when the lung was filled with saline. The reduction was evidence for the operation of surface forces which were inactivated when the gas-to-tissue interface was eliminated by the saline. At about the time when Radford made this observation, Pattle demonstrated that fluid expelled from lung tissue had an extremely low surface tension. Clements and his colleagues further found that the surface tension of a film of extract was less when the material was condensed into a small area than when it was expanded.

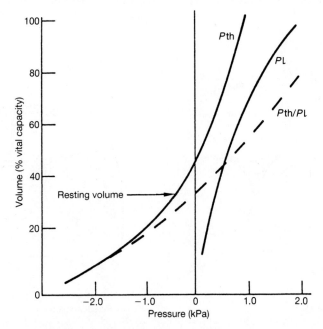

Fig. 5.7 Static volume−pressure curves for the thoracic cage (*P*th) and the lung (*Pl*) separately and in combination. They were obtained from measurements of pressure in the pharynx and in the oesophagus during relaxation against a closed mouthpiece after inspiration from a spirometer. The relationship can also be obtained during relaxation whilst breathing from a pressurised container. (Source: Knowles JH, Hong SK, Rahn H. *J Appl Physiol* 1959; **14**: 525−530.)

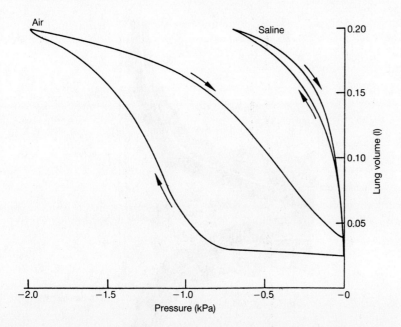

Fig. 5.8 Volume−pressure diagram for isolated cat lung. The directions of the arrows indicate inflation and deflation; their slopes reflect the lung compliance. The compliance is increased when the surface forces are eliminated by filling the lung with saline. (Source: Radford EP, Jr. In JW Remington, ed. *Tissue Elasticity*. Washington: A.P.S., 1957, 177−189.)

This important property of the surface layer has the effect of stabilising the lung during expiration; the mechanism is described below. The action is due to the presence of a lipopolysaccharide, dipalmitoyl lecithin; this is formed in the mitochondria of cuboidal granular pneumonocytes (type II alveolar cells) present in the alveolar walls. The surfactant is stored as lamellar bodies prior to being secreted onto the epithelium of the alveoli and alveolar ducts where it forms a monomolecular layer. The layer extends into the respiratory bronchioles. It is relatively smooth due to it bridging over irregularities in the epithelial surface which are filled with liquid hypophase, (Fig. 5.9); this contains apoproteins, alveolar macrophages and tubular myelin, comprising concertina-like packets of dipalmitoyl lecithin: the latter is in a form which can be reinserted into the surface layer.

Patency of airways

For the lung to function effectively the alveolar gas must be in communication with the environment, hence all classes of airways should be open. Four factors contribute to the patency of airways; in the bronchi cartilage provides some support and in the alveolar septa the blood vessels exert an erectile effect. The smaller airways are supported by the bundles of fibres, including elastic fibres, which permeate the lung. The fibres are inserted into and exert traction on the walls of airways; their function resembles that of the guy lines which hold apart

97

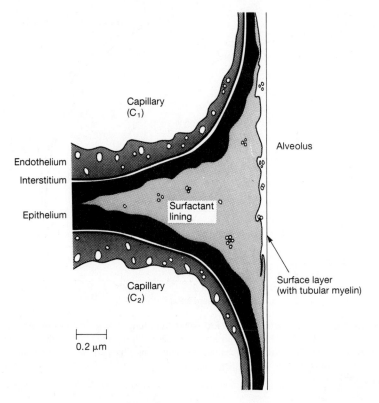

Fig. 5.9 Line drawing of a photomicrograph showing the surfactant lining of part of an alveolus at the junction between two alveolar capillaries (C_1 and C_2). The lining layer contains tubular myelin and is indicated by an arrow; the lining bridges over amorphous fluid (hypophase) in the trough between the capillaries. The alveolar capillary membrane comprising endothelium, interstitium, epithelium and surface layer is thickened in consequence. (Source: Weibel ER. *APS Handbook of Physiology Respiratory System* III(i), 100, 1986.)

the walls of a tent. The fibrous network also contains collagen fibres which restrain the lung as it expands and prevent rupture. The fourth factor relates to the surface tension of the fluid lining the alveoli. This exerts a force which tends to shrink or even close them, and thus to dilate the remaining intrathoracic structures.

LaPlace observed that the pressure in a bubble was related directly to the surface tension and inversely to the radius of curvature. Hence LaPlace's Law:

$$P = 2T/r$$

where P is the pressure within an air bubble surrounded by liquid, r is the radius of the bubble and T is the surface tension at the air to liquid interface. For a cylindrical air space the coefficient term is reduced from two to one whilst for a soap bubble which has two surfaces, it is doubled to four. Within the lung not all the air spaces are the same size. If LaPlace's Law applied the smaller ones would empty into the larger, and all air spaces would be at risk of collapse as their volume

diminishes during expiration. It is the modification of surface tension   *Lung expansion*
by surfactant that prevents such undesirable events.

Closure of air-filled structures

Normal closure. During normal breathing the alveoli are in communication with the environment due to the operation of the mechanisms
described above. However, closure of air-filled structures occurs during
forced or sustained expiration. The closure is due to the progressive
reduction throughout expiration of traction from guy lines and to
compression of the lung by a positive high intrapleural pressure. Yet
the lung still contains air. The air remains trapped after intubation of a
bronchus and this led Hughes and colleagues to suggest that the site of
closure is in the terminal bronchi. The distribution of the trapped gas is
influenced by the lung being subject to gravitational force which leads
to airways at the base of the lung closing first (page 180). At the point
of maximal closure the volume of gas remaining in the lung is the
residual volume (page 105), and the lung volume above residual at
which closure is first detectable is the closing volume (page 219).
Premature closure increases the residual volume; the commonest cause
is the loss of lung elasticity (increase of compliance) which occurs with
increasing age (page 487) and with emphysema (page 535). Premature
closure also occurs secondary to narrowing of the airways from other
causes, including contraction of bronchial muscles and thickening of
airway walls. A delay in airways closure during expiration has the
converse effect of reducing the residual volume. This occurs when the
quantity of collagen in lung tissue is increased by diffuse interstitial
fibrosis or one of its antecedent conditions.
    Closure of airways takes place as the lung volume approaches residual
volume. The walls of the airways are then in apposition and surface
tension forces tend to hold them together. The suction needed to effect
reopening in man is approximately 0.4 kPa; during inspiration this
pressure is achieved by the over-expansion increasing the elastic recoil
from regions not subject to closure during the preceding expiration.
The lung volume at reopening is usually below that at the end of a
normal expiration (functional residual capacity page 104). Macklem
has suggested that reopening occurs mainly from the central end. At
bronchial bifurcations this could lead to one branch opening before the
other or to the formation of a bubble or miniscus of fluid which could
then move up and down an airway causing a variable obstruction. The
closure of airways is the main factor causing hysteresis in the static
volume−pressure curve; this is shown for a cat lung in Fig. 5.8. Here
the inspiratory curve exhibits a critical opening pressure of approximately
0.8 kPa. At near to full inflation both inspiratory and expiratory curves
flatten off as they approach a volume asymptote which in the figure is
just in excess of 0.2 l. This maximal volume is determined by the
collagen component of the fibrous stroma of the isolated lung.

Abnormal closure. Peripheral air spaces begin to develop during intra-uterine life but they are effectively indistensible until the lung starts to produce surfactant at about the 24th week of gestation. This process is delayed in babies with respiratory distress syndrome (page 621, cf. page 448). The presence of surfactant enables the airspaces to fill with air during the first few breaths after birth. Subsequently they do not collapse unless either the production of surfactant is reduced or conditions predisposing to collapse supervene. Production of surfactant is interfered with if the lung parenchyma is damaged by breathing oxygen-enriched air (page 630), by severe shock and by diversion of pulmonary blood flow through an extra-corporeal circulation. These and related types of adult respiratory distress syndrome are described on page 569. Collapse of alveoli can also occur following absorption of gas distal to an obstructed airway. It is therefore a feature of bronchial carcinoma, and inhaled foreign body. It can occur during anaesthesia if the lung is ventilated at a low lung volume and in air-force pilots if they are exposed to high 'g' (or centrifugal) forces. Following the closure, the pressure in the obstructed region is reduced by the continued uptake of gas into the blood and this process is facilitated by the presence of a soluble anaesthetic gas or 100% oxygen. The end result is either atelectasis or re-expansion, the latter tending to occur at near to total lung capacity, when the lung retractive force is approaching its maximum. In the isolated lung, collapse of airspaces can also be produced by degassing *in vaccuo*. The subsequent re-expansion is associated with alveoli popping open haphazardly and not in a regular sequence. During expiration similar instability does not occur except when production of surfactant is diminished. The instability is due to the surface tension of the fluid lining of the alveoli; this is opposed by a retractive force exerted by the stroma of the lung (Fig. 5.10). Factors promoting instability include a small lung volume, diminished production of surfactant and excess fluid in the alveoli reducing the radius of the air spaces.

Compliance of the lung

The elasticity of the lung is essential for its proper function; it is depicted by the static volume−pressure curve (Fig. 5.7) which can be described mathematically. The most convenient model is a mono-exponential equation. This has been shown by Colbatch to fit the upper half of the expiratory curves of normal subjects and most patients. The relationship, shown in Fig. 6.16, page 164, has the form:

$$V = A - Be^{-kP\text{st}} \tag{5.1}$$

where A is the derived asymptote on the volume axis in excess of total lung capacity and B is the volume decrement below A at which trans-pulmonary pressure is zero. The exponent k is a shape factor which, in conjunction with the lung volume, describes the slope of the volume−pressure curve per litre of volume, (i.e. $k = \mathrm{d}V/\mathrm{d}P\text{st}\,(A - V)^{-1}$), and

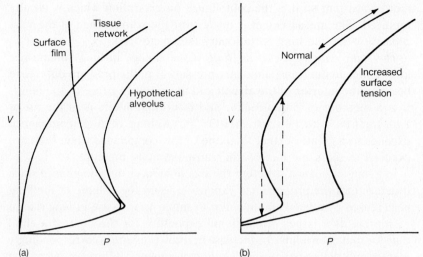

Lung expansion

(a)   (b)

Fig. 5.10 Diagram illustrating the volume−pressure characteristic of a hypothetical alveolus. It is the sum of two components due respectively to the tissue network of the lung and to the surface film (a). For the tissue network and for the surface film when the alveolus is not expanded beyond a hemisphere, the volume is directly related to the pressure; for the surface film at larger alveolar volumes (i.e. beyond the inflection in the curve) the volume increases abruptly unless the pressure is greatly reduced or the film is supported.

When the curves are combined to yield the alveolar curve (b) the kinked portion between the interrupted lines represents a region of instability. The alveolus during its initial inflation will follow the curve up to the point of inflection when the volume will increase abruptly to the new level indicated by the right-hand vertical arrow. During deflation it will follow the curve down to the left-hand vertical arrow when the volume will suddenly decrease. During normal tidal breathing the alveolus will move within the limits indicated by the double-headed arrow where the relationship is stable.

When the surface tension is increased a higher pressure is required in order to expand the alveolus; in addition the alveolus is now unstable over the range of pressures to which it is normally exposed. For both these reasons a rise in the surface tension is likely to be associated with atelectasis. (Source: Mead J. *Physiol Rev* 1961; **41**: 281−330.)

is analogous to the specific compliance (see below). The derivation neglects the quantity of lung tissue which also contributes to the total volume of the lung. In healthy adults k is of the order of $12 \pm 1.5\,\mathrm{Pa}^{-1}$ ($0.12 \pm 0.015\,\mathrm{cmH_2O^{-1}}$); it is increased with emphysema and reduced with stiff lungs.

The volume−pressure curve can also be defined in terms of the static recoil pressure at total lung capacity and the static compliance, where the latter is the slope of the central linear part of the curve; this may be approximated by a straight line:

$$Cl,st = \Delta V/\Delta Pst \qquad (5.2)$$

where Cl,st is static lung compliance, V is volume (litres BTPS) and Pst is static recoil pressure (kPa). On account of hysteresis the slope is influenced by whether the volume−pressure curve is obtained starting from full inspiration or from residual volume. The former curve is the more consistent so it is the compliance on expiration which is usually reported. The measurement is made over the whole range of the vital capacity when the lung is stationary (see page 162).

The static compliance of the lung is the change in lung volume per unit change in the transpulmonary pressure (i.e. the pressure difference between the interior of the alveoli and the pleural surface of the lung). It is a measure of distensibility, and in normal adults is in the range $1.0-3.9 \, l \, kPa^{-1}$ $(0.1-0.39 \, l \, cmH_2O^{-1})^*$. A lung of high compliance expands to a greater extent than one of low compliance when both are exposed to the same increase in transpulmonary pressure.

In a lung of normal structure the size influences the compliance since it determines the proportional expansion when the volume of the lung is increased by a fixed amount. For example an increase in lung size of $1 \, l$ represents a larger proportional expansion for the lung of a child than for that of an adult; the increase in recoil pressure is correspondingly greater and the compliance is less in consequence. However, when the change in lung volume is expressed in dimensionless units (e.g. as a fraction of the total lung capacity) the relationship of recoil pressure to lung volume is found to be independent of lung size; this has the effect that the compliance per litre of lung volume, which is the *specific compliance*, is effectively constant. The specific compliance (sC) is usually reported for expiration at functional residual capacity (page 162); it then has a value in normal subjects of 0.8 (range $0.3-1.4$) kPa^{-1} (0.08, range $0.03-0.14 \, cmH_2O^{-1}$).

Some factors which influence the static lung compliance are listed in Table 5.3. A lower compliance is usually associated with a small inspiratory capacity and subdivisions. Additional changes occur when the reduction is due to pathological changes in structure. The recoil pressure is then usually increased as is the work of breathing. The latter change is to some extent compensated for by a change in the pattern of breathing. The tidal volume is usually reduced and the respiratory frequency increased especially during exercise (page 432). If the person requires assisted ventilation, for example in relation to anaesthesia for a surgical operation, the force required to inflate the lung is increased. A high compliance is uncommon but it contributes to the clinical and physiological abnormalities of emphysema and, to a lesser extent, of old age, (pages 535 and 489 respectively).

Compliance may also be estimated during tidal breathing from measurements of lung volume and oesophageal pressure made at the ends of inspiration and expiration when the lung is *apparently* stationary. The index so obtained is called the *dynamic compliance* (Cdyn). In

---

* The ranges have been derived using Tables 15.18 and 15.22 (pages 496–7 and 511). For indices that are described by regression relationships the ranges extend by two standard deviations, or in the case of the compliance 1 SD, on either side of the expected values for the ages 20–25 years and 70 years, the heights in men of 1.6–1.8 m and in women 1.5–1.7 m also, for FRC, the weights in men of 50–90 kg and in women 45–85 kg. The appropriateness of representing the results in this way is discussed in chapter 15.

Table 5.3 Factors which affect static lung compliance

Aspect	Compliance low	Compliance high
Alveolar volume*	Small person Feeble respiratory muscles (page 577) Airway closure	Large person Some athletes Some asthmatics
Lung surfactant	Respiratory distress syndrome	—

Fibrous stroma	Disorders of lung
	   parenchyma (page 558)
		Age
		Emphysema
		Semicarbazide (breaks
		   cross-linkages)

Visceral pleural	Secondary to TB, asbestos exposure, haemothorax	—
Tone in muscle of alveolar ducts	Histamine Serotonin Hypoxia	Bronchodilator drugs reverse these effects
Pulmonary blood volume	Mitral stenosis Left ventricular failure Polycythaemia (?)	Isocapnoeic hypoxia Pulmonary stenosis Haemorrhage (?)

* Specific lung compliance usually normal; the principal exception is airway closure
if the alveolar volume is measured by plethysmography.

subjects with healthy lungs the two indices are similar but the dynamic
compliance is reduced by obstruction in the small airways. The reduction
is due to the pressure swing which is recorded being influenced by the
movement of gas within the lung (page 182). In these circumstances
the relationship of the dynamic compliance to the respiratory frequency is
an index of airflow resistance. Its measurement is considered on page 165.

Compliance of the chest wall

The position of the rib cage and the diaphragm is the resultant of a
number of factors; these include the forces which are exerted by the
muscles of respiration and the elastic recoil of the lung tissue and of
the thoracic cage; the last factor resembles the elastic recoil of the lung
in that it varies with the volume of the thorax over a wide range. The
relationship is illustrated in Fig. 5.7 where the slope of the left-hand
line is the compliance of the chest wall. In normal subjects the chest
wall compliance is in the range $1.0-3.61 kPa^{-1}$ ($0.1-0.35 l cmH_2O^{-1}$).
It is reduced when the mobility of the chest wall is impaired by
ankylosing spondylitis and other conditions which affect the integrity
of the skeleto-muscular apparatus of the thorax. The chest wall compliance is also reduced in the presence of obesity and by the skeletal
changes which accompany ageing.

The position of equilibrium of the chest wall varies with posture and,
when there is no pressure difference across it, differs from that when it

is exposed to the elastic recoil force of the lung. This may be seen at autopsy, when, on opening the thorax, there is a tendency for the chest cage to expand and for the lungs to deflate; similar changes occur following the induction of a pneumothorax. The difference is apparent in Fig. 5.7 which shows that the static pressure gradient across the thoracic cage is zero when the volume is approximately 45% of the vital capacity. At smaller volumes the elastic recoil of the thoracic cage exerts an inspiratory effect.

Subdivisions of the lung volume

Functional residual capacity. When the respiratory muscles are relaxed, the relationship between the lung volume and the applied static force is illustrated by the dashed line in Fig. 5.7. In the absence of muscular contraction the chest assumes an equilibrium position in which the tendency for the thoracic cage to expand is exactly balanced by the tendency for the lung to deflate. The equilibrium position is the functional residual capacity. During inspiration the chest is moved away from this position by the action of the respiratory muscles; it normally returns to it at the end of expiration. The *functional residual capacity* (FRC) can therefore be defined as the volume of gas in the chest at the end of a normal expiration when the elastic recoils of the lung and of the thoracic cage are equal and opposite. In an upright posture, the FRC of a healthy adult male is in the range 0.8−6.55 l. In females the range is 0.7−4.9 l (see footnote page 102). The recoil of the chest wall is influenced by posture which affects the component of force due to gravity and the extent to which compression of the abdominal contents raises the diaphragm; lying down also introduces a physical constraint from local pressure on the ribs. These factors together reduce the FRC by approximately 25% compared with standing up. Gravitational force can be decreased temporarily by use of a human centrifuge. This leads to ascent of the diaphragm which reduces the FRC by lowering the expiratory reserve volume (Fig. 5.11). The recoil of the lung is determined by lung elasticity and surface tension. The elasticity is reduced by emphysema and increased by interstitial fibrosis; converse changes occur in the lung compliance (the reciprocal of elasticity) and hence in FRC. The lung surface tension is increased in respiratory distress syndrome. It is also increased by shallow breathing; however, the associated reduction in FRC is then mainly due to temporary closure of airways. In addition the FRC is reduced when the tidal volume is increased by exercise or increased respiratory drive from hypercapnia or hypoxia.

Total lung capacity. The position of the chest wall at full inspiration determines the total lung capacity which is the resultant of a balance between on the one hand the elastic recoils of the lung and of the thoracic cage and on the other the inspiratory action of the respiratory

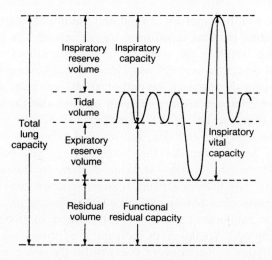

Fig. 5.11 Spirogram labelled to show the subdivision of the total lung capacity. The vital capacity is the volume expired on complete expiration after the deepest inspiration. However, in patients with lung disease, in order to avoid errors due to air-trapping (Fig. 6.12, page 155) the measurement is best made from residual volume when it is called the inspiratory vital capacity. It may also be obtained as the sum of measurements made on separate breaths of the inspiratory capacity and the expiratory reserve volume when it is called the two stage vital capacity.

muscles. The latter action is determined by both the strength of the muscles and the extent of the reflex inhibition to inspiration. Thus the *total lung capacity* (TLC) is the volume of gas in the thorax at the end of a full inspiration when the sum of the elastic recoils of the lung and thoracic cage is equal and opposite to the inspiratory force developed by the respiratory muscles. In healthy adult males, depending on their size, the TLC is in the range 3.6–9.4 l; in healthy females the range is 3.0–7.3 l (see footnote page 102). The total lung capacity is affected by all the factors which influence the static lung compliance (Table 5.3, page 103), the compliance of the chest wall and the strength of the respiratory muscles. This can affect the vital capacity and is discussed under this heading below. In addition enlargement may occur with acute isocapnoeic hypoxia and when the calibre of the lung airways is reduced fairly suddenly as during an acute attack of asthma. One possible mechanism is release of reflex inhibition to inspiration. However, the transpulmonary pressure at full inflation should then be increased, which does not seem to be the case.

Residual volume. The volume of gas in the lung at the end of a forced expiration is similarly determined by a balance of forces, including the strength of the accessory muscles of expiration, the inherent incompressibility of the thoracic cage, and the traction exerted on airways by the fibrous stroma of the lung, (page 94). In children and young adults the elastic recoil of the lung is relatively high so the airways mostly remain patent throughout expiration; the residual volume is then determined by the muscle strength and chest wall rigidity. With increasing age the chest wall becomes more rigid and the muscle strength diminishes. In addition the lung recoil pressure declines and on this account airway closure becomes the main factor limiting full expiration; the mechanism is described on page 99. Thus *residual volume* (RV) is the volume of gas in the chest at the end of a full expiratory effort when the combined effects of closure of small airways and the elasticity of the thoracic cage prevent further expiration. In healthy adult males, depending on their age and size, the residual volume is in the range 0.5–3.5 l; in healthy females the range is 0.4–3.0 l (see footnote page 102). The residual volume is reduced when the traction which is exerted by the guy lines is for any reason increased; this occurs, for example, in pulmonary fibrosis. The residual volume is increased when the traction is diminished; this occurs for example in emphysema and with increasing age. Weakness of the expiratory muscles has a similar effect. In addition constriction of the airways by reflex action, drugs or disease causes an increase in residual volume by trapping air at the end of expiration; the conditions in which this occurs are associated with a rise in the airways resistance and are discussed, under this heading, later.

Vital capacity and its subdivisions. Other subdivision of the lung volume are illustrated in Fig. 5.11. They include the tidal volume, which is the respiratory excursion per breath and the inspiratory and the expiratory reserve volumes of the lung. The sum of these subdivisions is also the extent to which the total lung capacity exceeds the residual volume and is called the *vital capacity*; its size is the resultant of all the factors which affect these two variables. In healthy males, depending on their age and size, the vital capacity is in the range 2.0–6.6 l; in healthy females, the range is 1.4–5.6 l (see footnote page 102). The vital capacity is reduced if the lung compliance is low, the respiratory muscles are weak or the residual volume is enlarged relative to the total lung capacity as occurs in emphysema and with narrowing of lung airways. The inspiratory capacity and hence the vital capacity are increased as a result of activities which strengthen the accessory muscles of respiration including deep sea diving, swimming and rowing. The average change in VC appears to be in the range 2–7%; it can be more in some individuals. The vital capacity is relatively independent of posture, but it is reduced by about 7% when the subject lies down; the change is due to displacement of gas by blood which enters the thorax from the legs and abdomen (see page 295). In contrast to the vital capacity, the inspiratory and the expiratory reserve volumes respectively increase and decrease on lying down because of the changes in functional residual capacity mentioned above. The tidal volume at rest is normally about 0.5 l. During exercise it increases linearly with the ventilatory requirement of the subject (see Fig. 15.30, page 509) up to a limiting value, which is about 50% of the vital capacity. Factors which influence the relationship of the breathing frequency to the tidal volume are discussed in Chapter 11.

Introduction

At any moment the degree of inflation of the lung is determined by a balance of forces between the respiratory muscles, gravitational force, and the elasticity of the lung and chest wall. Movement occurs when the equilibrium is disturbed; the rate of movement is then influenced by the strength of the applied force and the elasticity, resistance to movement and inertia of the thoracic cage, the lung tissue and the gas contained in the lung. As a first approximation the elastance (i.e. the reciprocal of compliance, C), is related to volume, the resistance (R) to velocity of airflow and the inertia (I) to the acceleration. The pressure difference across the lung can be described in terms of these variables:

$$P = 1/C\ V + R\ dV/dt + I\ d^2V/dt^2 \qquad (5.3)$$

Inertia

The force which must be applied to overcome the inertia of the respiratory system is a function of mass and acceleration, particularly that of the gaseous compartment.

The force can be represented as follows:

$$F = A\Delta P = n\ \rho,l,A\ (dv/dt) \qquad (5.4)$$

where ΔP is the pressure difference between the two ends of a gas column of cross-sectional area A; ρ, l and dv/dt are respectively the density, length and acceleration of the column of gas and n is a constant which is nearly unity. The inertance of the system can be represented as:

$$I = n\ \rho,l/A$$

where I is the inertance and all the other terms are as described above. The pressure drop across an inertance is greatest when the flow rate increases rapidly such as can occur when the frequency of breathing rises. The work done in accelerating the lung is stored as kinetic energy. However, during normal breathing inertial forces are of negligible magnitude; they can be material when a high frequency oscillation is applied for purposes of assisting ventilation or for investigating the mechanical characteristics of the lung (pages 647 and 169).

Resistance

The force required to overcome the resistance to movement of the lung and thorax is relatively large; thus the associated energy expenditure can represent a significant fraction of the maximal uptake of oxygen. For this reason the frictional resistance of the lungs and chest wall can limit exercise. It also, in part, determines the maximal rate at which air can move into and out of the lung.

The *total thoracic resistance* is the sum of components attributable to the rib cage, the diaphragm, the abdominal wall and contents, the lung tissue and the gas in the lung airways. As with electrical resistances in series, these are additive in their effect, so may be represented in the following form:

$$Ptotal = Pth + Pti + Paw \qquad (5.5)$$

where P is the force required to overcome the frictional resistance and th, ti and aw refer respectively to the thoracic rib cage and diaphragm, the lung tissue and the lung airways. For the thoracic cage the force is a simple function of the velocity of linear movement. The velocity cannot be measured directly, but can be described approximately in terms of the rate of air flow. Then as a first approximation:

$$Pth = Rth \times \dot{v}^{n1} \qquad (5.6)$$

where Rth is the resistance of the thoracic cage, in kPa (or cmH_2O) l^{-1} s and $\dot{v}$ is the velocity of movement of the thoracic cage expressed as flow rate of air in ls^{-1}. In most instances the value of the exponent $n1$ lies between 1.0 and 1.1.

Lung tissue resistance (Rti) and airway resistance (Raw) together make up the total pulmonary resistance:

$$Rl = Rti + Raw \qquad (5.7)$$

where Rl is the pulmonary flow resistance in kPa (or cmH_2O) l^{-1}s; it is therefore the pressure difference which must be applied between the pleural surface of the lung and the lips in order to secure a velocity of flow of $1 ls^{-1}$. This quantity can be derived from the slope of the initial part of the isovolume flow-pressure curve which is illustrated in Fig. 5.14 (page 117).

The *tissue resistance* normally represents approximately 10% of total pulmonary resistance (Table 5.4). The proportion is increased when the airway resistance is reduced by an increase in lung size as occurs at total lung capacity. The tissue resistance itself is increased in pulmonary fibrosis and other conditions where the quantity of interstitial lung tissue is increased (page 558). However, Gibson and Pride have pointed out that the increase can be simulated by a lung in which some lung units were indistensible whilst others were normal. The estimation of tissue resistance is relatively inaccurate because it is obtained by subtracting airway resistance from total pulmonary resistance (page 172).

The *airway resistance* is the principal component of the total pulmonary resistance and contributes about as much as the chest wall to the total thoracic resistance (Table 5.4). However, the force required to overcome these two resistances does not bear the same relationship to flow in each case. In the chest wall the relationship is nearly linear (equation 5.6), but in the airways it is complex because the flow of air is *laminar* in some regions but *turbulent* in others. In the periphery of the lung

Table 5.4 Average values for the total thoracic resistance and its components at a flow rate of $0.5\,\mathrm{l\,s^{-1}}$ in healthy young men. The values in women are higher

	Resistance SI units $(\mathrm{kPa\,l^{-1}\,s})$	Tradit. units $(\mathrm{cmH_2O\,l^{-1}\,s})$	Methods used to measure the different components
Mouth			
	0.05*	0.5*	
Larynx			
	0.05	0.5	
2–3 mm airways			
	0.02	0.2	Plethysmograph / Interrupter / Oesophageal balloon / Forced oscillation
Alveoli			
	0.02	0.2	
Lung tissue			
Chest wall	0.12	1.2	
Total	0.26	2.6	

* During gentle panting with the mouth wide open; higher values are obtained during normal breathing. The data are due to Pride.

the airways are of small diameter but there are many of them, so the total cross-sectional area is large. On this account the air moves relatively slowly in a stream-lined or laminar manner: gas molecules travel parallel to the long axis of the airway with those at the centre moving faster than at the periphery. The force which is required to overcome the frictional resistance is proportional to the mean forward velocity of flow (i.e. $Paw = Raw\ \dot{v}$) and the wave profile is parabolic (Fig. 7.3, page 185).

Compared with the peripheral airways the central airways are of larger diameter but there are fewer of them so the total cross-sectional area is smaller. Thus for a given volume flow rate the linear flow velocity is higher and the pattern of flow is often turbulent with gas molecules travelling transversely across the airway as well as longitudinally. Thus the wave profile is square and the frictional resistance is increased being proportional to the square of the mean forward velocity (i.e. $Paw = Raw\ \dot{v}^2$). The transition from laminar to turbulent flow is determined by the Reynolds number. This is described by the following relationship:

$$\text{Reynolds number} = \dot{v}D\rho \div \eta A \qquad (5.8)$$

where, in appropriate units, $\dot{v}$ is the bulk flow rate of gas at a cross-sectional area A, D is the corresponding airway diameter and ρ and η are the gas density and viscosity. Reynolds numbers of less than 100 and more than 10 000 are associated respectively with completely laminar and fully turbulent flow, with other values intermediate. In the trachea during quiet breathing the Reynolds number is about 1500 so the flow is partly turbulent. With an increasing minute ventilation it becomes progressively more turbulent and is completely turbulent during maximal ventilation. In the bronchi the gas stream becomes turbulent at flow rates of approximately $5 \, ls^{-1}$ but in the bronchioles at all levels of ventilation it is nearly laminar except at bifurcations where there are local eddies; these dissipate energy. In addition, because the total cross-sectional area of the larger airways is less than that of the smaller ones, changes in forward velocity and hence in kinetic energy occur as the gas molecules pass from one to the other.

The effect which is described as convective acceleration summates with that due to friction. It can be described by Bernoulli's theorem. The latter states that neglecting frictional losses the sum of the lateral pressure at the airway wall and the gas kinetic energy is independent of the cross-sectional area. Hence if the flow velocity profile is flat:

$$P_1 + \frac{1}{2}\rho \, (\bar{v}_1)^2 = P_2 + \frac{1}{2}\rho \, (\bar{v}_2)^2 + D/\dot{v} \qquad (5.9)$$

where the subscripts 1 and 2 refer to two sites of different cross-sectional area and D is the rate of energy dissipation in the region between them. This relationship which is due to Pedley, can be used to define the force which is required to overcome the resistance to air flow. Ainsworth and Eveleigh showed that the force can be described by an exponential equation similar to 5.6 above:

$$Paw = Raw \times \dot{v}^z \qquad (5.10)$$

where Paw is the force required to overcome the resistance to air flow and Raw is the lung airway resistance in kPa (or $cmH_2O)l^{-1}$; it is therefore the pressure difference which must be applied between the alveoli and the lips in order to secure a rate of flow through the airways of $1 \, ls^{-1}$. Depending on the degree of turbulence, the factor z varies between 1.0 and 1.9. The airway resistance can also be described by a quadratic equation which in effect provides separate terms for the laminar and turbulent components. Thus:

$$Paw = k_1\dot{v} + k_2\dot{v}^2 \qquad (5.11)$$

This approach is due to Rohrer.

The degree of turbulence and hence the airway resistance increase during maximal ventilation. In addition airway resistance can vary widely because it is greatly influenced by airway diameter. The relationship is described by Poiseuille's equation. This states that, for a simple tube, the resistance is related inversely to the fourth power of the radius; since in the bronchi the radius varies with lung size the airway resistance varies throughout the respiratory cycle. The resistance is lower at large lung volumes when the airways are expanded; it rises during expiration as the airways diminish in size and becomes infinite at residual volume when the airways close for reasons which are discussed on page 99. The relationship of the airway resistance to the lung volume of a normal subject is illustrated in Fig. 5.12. The resistance is increased when the airway diameter is reduced by disease (Table 5.6).

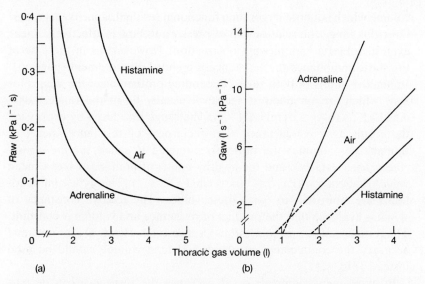

Fig. 5.12 *Left* Relationship between airway resistance (*Raw*) and thoracic gas volume for
a normal subject showing the effects of inhaling aerosols of histamine and then
adrenaline which respectively increase and decrease the resistance. *Right* The resistance
varies inversely with the volume of gas in the thorax at the time of measurement; thus
the relationship between airway conductance (*Gaw*, i.e. Raw^{-1}) and thoracic gas volume
is effectively linear. However, the conductance is not zero at zero lung volume, so the
practice of expressing conductance per l of lung volume (i.e. specific conductance) leads
to error; the conductance at a specified volume should be used instead. The data were
obtained by McDermott and her colleagues (unpublished).

The airway resistance is also influenced by the density and the
viscosity of the respired gas which affect respectively the turbulent and
laminar components of the resistance. Changes in gas density occur under
conditions of altered barometric pressure, (e.g. Fig. 5.17, page 125,
also page 471). Changes can also be introduced experimentally in
order to identify the components of the resistance. This is done by
administering gases of different density and viscosity, for example
helium or sulphur hexafluoride in oxygen (Table 5.5). The procedures
are described on page 143.

The airways resistance is usually measured during inspiration; it is
averaged over the range of flow rates from 0 to $0.5 \, \mathrm{l\,s}^{-1}$ at a lung

Table 5.5 Density and viscosity at 20°C of gas mixtures containing 80% nitrogen, helium
or sulphur hexafluoride with 20% oxygen

	Density (ρ, $\mathrm{kg\,m}^{-3}$)	Viscosity (η, $\mathrm{kg\,m}^{-1}\,\mathrm{s}^{-1}$) $\times 10^{-9}$	Kinematic viscosity (υ, $\mathrm{m}^2\,\mathrm{s}^{-1}$) $\times 10^{-9}$
N_2/O_2	1.286	1.792	1.393
He/O_2	0.429	1.952	4.550
SF_6/O_2	5.567	1.602	0.288

Note: in the lung the values are somewhat different due to the effects of temperature,
CO_2 and water vapour.

volume which is a little larger than functional residual capacity (page 104). Over this range the relationship of pressure to flow is effectively linear even in subjects with airways obstruction. However, as in the case of the static compliance the resistance is a chord measurement (page 96). In healthy adults of both sexes, depending on their size, the values for *Raw* which are obtained at sea level usually lie in the range $0.05-0.2\,kPa\,l^{-1}\,s$ ($0.5-2.0\,cmH_2O\,l^{-1}\,s$). The range is reduced by expressing the result as a conductance (i.e. reciprocal of resistance) per l of thoracic gas volume: the index so obtained is called *specific airway conductance* (sGaw), and for healthy adults of both sexes has a mean value of about $2.3\,kPa^{-1}\,s^{-1}$ ($0.23\,cmH_2O^{-1}\,s^{-1}$). The 95% confidence limits are from half to twice these values. The relative constancy of sGaw is evidence that the product of resistance and volume is constant. The term specific resistance (sRaw) is also used. However, for maximal accuracy the conductance at a specified lung volume should be used instead (Fig. 5.12).

In experimental animals or at necropsy the resistance can be partitioned between airways of different size by use of retrograde catheters to obtain the intra-luminal pressure: in this way it has been shown that during normal quiet respiration a large part of the total resistance is contributed by the nose, glottis and larynx (Table 5.4). For measurement of lung airway resistance these components may be reduced by panting (see page 168). Within the lung Macklem and his colleagues have shown that the resistance is mainly in the larger airways (diameter 3–8 mm). Obstruction in the periphery of the bronchial tree, such as occurs with bronchiolitis or loss of lung elasticity, needs to be intense before it exerts a material effect upon the overall resistance (see Table 5.4, page 109). Evidence for moderate obstruction to the peripheral airways may be obtained in the ways listed on page 527. These methods do not distinguish between the principal causes of a raised peripheral resistance; however, on theoretical grounds this should be possible in terms of the upstream resistance (*Rus*) which is described on page 172. *Rus* should be increased in the presence of inflammation of small airways or raised bronchomotor tone but normal if the small airway narrowing reflects loss of lung elasticity. Unfortunately these expectations have not been demonstrated in practice.

Factors which influence airway resistance. An increase in the airway resistance can be either extra- or intra-thoracic and, if the latter, extra-pulmonary or intra-pulmonary. In all these situations obstruction may be due to the accumulation of material within the lumen (endomural obstruction), to encroachment on the lumen by thickening of the epithelial or subepithelial tissue or to external compression by glands or by other space-occupying lesions. The intra-thoracic airways are subject to a number of other factors including variation in brochomotor tone. In addition, those airways which lie outside the lung are subject to compression if the intra-thoracic pressure rises above atmospheric. The airways which are intra-pulmonary are narrowed when the traction

Table 5.6 Types of generalized abnormality of airway calibre

Endo-mural obstruction	Viscid mucus: polyp or foreign body in large airway
Mural encroachment on lumen	Sub-epithelial inflammation or oedema: mucus gland hyperplasia: stricture in large airway
Bronchomotor tone increased	Asthma, wheezy bronchitis, exposure to cotton dust, histamine and other causes of bronchoconstriction
Extra-mural traction on intrapulmonary airways	*Reduced* at small lung volumes,* in the elderly and with emphysema *Increased* at large lung volumes* and with interstitial fibrosis
Mural deformability	*Reduced* with asthma and bronchitis *Increased* after bronchodilator drugs and with cylindrical bronchiectasis
Extra-mural compression of the lumen	*Static* with neoplasm or enlarged gland *Transient* with interstitial oedema *Dynamic* with coughing or during forced expiration

* Irrespective of cause and of lung compliance.

which is exerted on their walls by the recoil of the lung tissue is, for any reason, reduced. This is the case in emphysema. The traction is increased in interstitial fibrosis; it is also increased by the subject breathing at nearer to total lung capacity. This can occur in emphysema. It sometimes also occurs following a rise in bronchomotor tone, for example during an attack of asthma when the increase in thoracic gas volume has the effect of partly reversing the reduction in airway calibre which occurs. In all these circumstances the extent to which the forces which are applied deform the walls of the airways is determined by their rigidity; this is influenced by the thickness of the sub-epithelial layer and the prevailing bronchomotor tone. Thus the overall airway resistance is the resultant of a large number of processes which operate at several levels within the airways; these are summarised in Table 5.6. They have been described using mathematical models of varying complexity by a number of workers including Pedley and Van de Woestijne and their respective collaborators. As a basis for such a model the latter authors have described the resistance at a given airways generation (g) as follows:

$$Raw\ (g) = f[\dot{v},\ Ng, \phi(Ptm(g)] \qquad (5.12)$$

where f is a function of the density and viscosity of the gas, $\dot{v}$ is the gas velocity and Ng is the number of airways in generation g. ϕ describes the relationship of the diameter of the airway to $Ptm(g)$ which is the transmural pressure. This quantity ($Ptm(g)$) is the distending pressure for airways of the generation g. It is less than the static recoil pressure of the lung (Pst) by an amount which reflects the resistance of the upper airways between the alveoli and generation $g(Raw,\ alv \rightarrow g)$, thus during expiration:

$$Ptm(g) = Pst - [Raw,\ alv \rightarrow g] \times \dot{v} \qquad (5.13)$$

113

Through this relationship the characteristics of the upstream airways contribute to the apparent resistance of those which are nearer the mouth. Thus whilst the measured airway resistance reflects mainly that of the larger airways, its dependence on the resistance of the more peripheral airways leads to changes in the latter being more readily detectable than might otherwise be expected.

These relationships have important consequences for the interpretation of changes in airway resistance such as may occur following the administration of bronchoactive drugs. In particular the measurements should be made at the same velocity of air flow and the same value of Pst, i.e. at the same absolute lung volume. However, changes may occur to either or both the diameter and the distensibility of the airways (ϕ) and it is not easy to distinguish between them. In these circumstances it is desirable that the value of ϕ should also be investigated; this may be done by measuring the airway resistance at several lung volumes and obtaining the relationship of Raw to Pst.

Consequences of an alteration in airway resistance. The airway resistance influences directly the maximal minute ventilation. It also influences it indirectly by reducing both vital capacity and tidal volume since the factors which determine the calibre of the airways also influence the volume of the lung at which closure of the small airways occurs (see also page 97). As a result subjects with a high airway resistance have a residual volume which is large relative to the size of their lungs; thus not only is the maximal rate of air flow diminished but the maximal tidal volume is also less. Reduction of airflow is especially marked during forced expiratory effort since the factors which reduce the calibre of airways often increase their susceptibility to dynamic compression (page 112). In the converse situation, subjects who have a low airway resistance tend to have a small residual volume; when the cause is interstitial fibrosis the associated increase in recoil pressure, and hence in airway calibre then leads to the ventilatory capacity being larger than might be expected from the vital capacity (page 561). However, an additional factor is the lung tissue volume which also contributes to the anatomical size of the lung.

When airway narrowing occurs it does not affect all airways equally, those regions where the airways are most affected incur the greatest reduction in ventilation. In this way, a high airway resistance causes very uneven distribution of inspired air and this change in turn reduces the effectiveness of the lung as an organ of gas exchange. This aspect is considered in Chapter 7.

Maximal flow rates

Flow rates which are effort dependent

During inspiration the maximal rate of airflow varies directly with the applied pressure and hence the inspiratory effort. During expiration the peak expiratory flow rate is also effort dependent up to a limit which is determined by the maximal wave velocity (page 119). Thus these maximal flow rates are influenced by the force which can be applied by the respiratory muscles and are amenable to physical training. The force is expended in overcoming the resistance and inertia of the chest wall, the lung and the contained air (page 107). The force varies with the lung volume; this is illustrated for static conditions, in Fig. 5.4. The force under dynamic conditions is somewhat less because muscle power declines as the muscles shorten. The lung volume also influences both the airway resistance and the maximal wave velocity. The highest flows occur when the peak is achieved at near to total lung capacity. This is shown in Fig. 5.13a. Fig. 5.13b shows more typical relationships of maximal flow to lung volume (maximal flow−volume curves). In most circumstances the inspiratory limb of the curve is of fairly uniform shape. The expiratory limb comprises the effort-dependent part especially the peak expiratory flow and the effort-independent part which is described subsequently.

The peak expiratory flow is achieved with very little displacement of air. Thus an important component is air which is expelled from the airways themselves by compression of their walls. The displacement is influenced by the compliance of the airways and other variables; these are indicated in the following equation due to Van de Woestijne and Clement which describes the rate of change with respect to time of the volume of the conducting airways:

$$dVaw/dt = f(Caw, \dot{v}, Cl, dPpl/dt) \qquad (5.14)$$

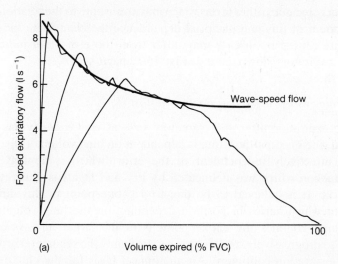

(a)   Volume expired (% FVC)

Fig. 5.13a Three maximal flow−volume curves in which the peaks were attained at different lung volumes relative to forced vital capacity (FVC), superimposed on the maximal flow curve defined by wave-speed theory. The highest peak was achieved with the shortest rise time and the greatest effort. Other effects of the degree of effort are shown in Fig. 6.3, page 137. (Source: Pedersen O.F. Personal communication.)

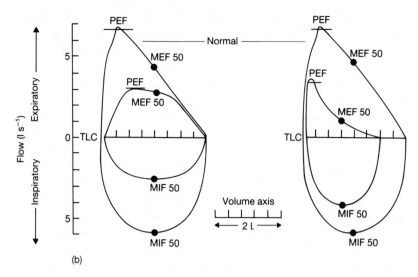

(b)

Fig. 5.13b Maximal flow–volume curves for a healthy subject (outer curves), a patient with moderate obstruction to the intrapulmonary airways (inner right hand curve) and with obstruction to the extra-thoracic airways (inner left hand curve). PEF is peak expiratory flow. MEF_{50} and MIF_{50} are the forced expiratory and inspiratory flow at the lung volume (RV + 50% VC). On expiration at lung volumes less than 80% TLC the flow rates are relatively independent of the expiratory effort which is exerted (see Fig. 5.14).

where the left hand term is the rate of change of airway volume. *Caw* and *Cl* are the compliance of the airways and of the lung, which are normally quite similar, and d*P*pl/d*t* is the rate of change with respect to time of the pleural pressure. *f* and *v̇* are defined in equation 5.12 above which, since the peak flow rate is also determined by the airway resistance, includes other terms which may contribute to the relationship. On account of this multifactorial dependence the changes in the peak flow rate caused by disease may differ from those of other indices of forced expiratory flow (see e.g. Fig. 16.1, page 519).

Flow rates which are independent of effort

During expiration after approximately 30% of vital capacity has been expired, the maximal flow rate is dependent on lung volume (Fig. 5.13) but is effectively independent of the effort which is applied. This phenomenon which was delineated by Fry and Hyatt is illustrated in Fig. 5.14. It is believed to be due to a choke point or flow-limiting segment which varies in position depending on the lung volume. At large lung volumes the choke point is in the larger airways and it moves to progressively smaller airways (probably the segmental bronchi) as the expiration continues. An anatomical basis for the choke point could be the airway narrowing which is visible at bronchoscopy during a forced expiration. However, whilst such narrowing might account for a choke point in small bronchi and bronchioles it appears not to explain the occurrence of a flow-limiting segment in large airways. The

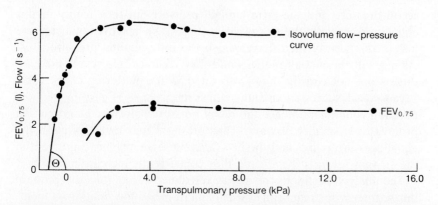

Fig. 5.14 The effect of variation in the force applied to the lung on the expiratory flow rate of normal subjects. The lower line shows the relationship of the $FEV_{0.75}$ to the maximal oesophageal pressure recorded during the expiration. The upper line is an isovolume flow–pressure curve: it shows the relationship of flow to pressure at the arbitrarily chosen volume of 50% of vital capacity above residual volume. The reciprocals of the initial slopes of these lines (Θ) describe total lung resistance (*Raw* + *Rti*). The data were obtained from a series of vital capacity manoeuvres performed with varying effort; flow was recorded with a pneumotachograph, pressure with an intraoesophageal balloon and lung volume with a body plethysmograph. The latter cannot be replaced by a spirometer, since the relevant volume is that of the lung when it is compressed during expiration and not total lung capacity minus the exhaled gas volume measured at atmospheric pressure. For interpretation see text. (Sources: 1. McKerrow CB, McDermott M. Unpublished. 2. Ingram RH, Jr, Schilder DP. *J Appl Physiol* 1966; **21**: 1821–1826.)

way in which the choke point operates has been approached through analysis of the mechanical forces acting on the lung and by application of wave mechanics.

Equal pressure point theory. The mechanical model of airway closure is due to Mead and Pride and their respective collaborators. It has given rise to the equal pressure point theory. This starts with the proposition that during active expiration the rise in intra-pleural pressure is to some extent transmitted through the lung parenchyma to the walls of the airways; the airways are compressed and may close in consequence. Whether they do or not is determined by the respective strengths of the compression and the opposing forces which are principally the elastic recoil of the lung tissue and the intra-luminal pressure. The compliance of the airway is an additional factor. The elastic recoil varies directly with lung volume. The intra-luminal pressure relative to atmosphere is highest in the alveoli and falls progressively along the length of the airway due to convective acceleration and to frictional losses in the airways. A relationship linking some of the variables is given in equation 5.13 (page 113).

When only moderate expiratory effort is applied the airways remain patent and the flow rate varies with the applied pressure. According to equal pressure point theory, with more marked effort the peribronchial pressure can temporarily become equal to or exceed the sum of the recoil pressure and the intra-luminal pressure. In the vicinity of this equal pressure point the airway closes (Fig. 5.15). The frictional pressure loss in this airway then decreases so the intra-luminal pressure rises. As a result the airway reopens and flow resumes. However, the conditions are not exactly those associated with a fluttering check valve because each successive opening allows the passage of gas; this reduces the lung volume and hence the recoil pressure. Closure then occurs in progressively smaller airways. Thus during a maximal expiration the equal pressure points and the flow-limiting segments move upsteam in the airways towards the alveoli; they concurrently increase in number.

The analysis partitions the airway resistance during forced expiration into segments upstream and downstream from the flow limiting segment. Thus:

$$Raw = \frac{Palv}{\dot{V}_{max}} = \frac{Pst + Ppl}{\dot{V}_{max}} = Rus + Rds \qquad (5.15)$$

where Pst and Ppl are the static recoil pressure and the pleural pressure; Rus and Rds are respectively the airflow resistances upstream and downstream of the equal pressure point.

The upstream resistance influences the maximal flow rate in the manner described. The downstream segment is subject to compression

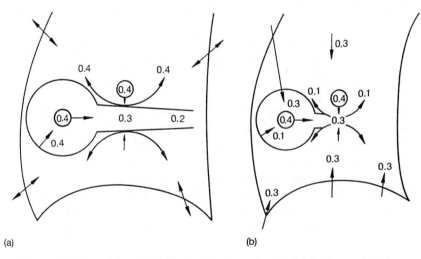

(a)   (b)

Fig. 5.15 Diagram (after Pride) illustrating airway closure. (a) Passive expiration (pleural pressure assumed to be zero). Expiration is effected by the elastic recoil pressure of the lung (0.4 kPa). The thin-walled portion of the airway is held open by both the recoil pressure acting on its wall and the intraluminal pressure; i.e. that transmitted from the alveolus. Both forces act against the alveolar pressure (0.4 kPa) and the elastic forces of the airway (not shown in the diagram). (b) Active expiration. The rise in intrapleural pressure caused by contraction of the accessory muscles (+0.3 kPa) initially assists expiration. It also tends to collapse the airway especially as the opposing force, due to the traction of the lung tissue and the intraluminal pressure, decreases progressively as the lung gets smaller. The site of closure is located where the pressure within the airway (0.3 kPa) plus that required to deform the wall of the airway (here 0.1 kPa) are equal to the outside pressure (here 0.4 kPa).

which is proportional to the expiratory effort but does not limit the maximal flow rate. These features resemble those in a river containing a waterfall or weir. Below the weir the river can be very lively but the quantity of water which flows is determined by the conditions at and above the weir and not below it. The equal pressure point mechanism could operate in small airways (diameter < 2 mm) towards the end of a forced expiration; however, it has not been possible to validate this. The theory has now largely been replaced by one based on fluid mechanics.

Wave mechanics theory. This was proposed by Dawson and Elliott and has been summarised amongst others by Wilson, Rodarte, Butler and Hyatt. According to this hypothesis flow limitation is due to interaction between wave velocity which is the maximal speed at which a pulse wave of gas can be transmitted along the airway and two other features of the airway; these are the compliance of the airway wall and the convective acceleration of the contained gas. The latter is discussed on page 110. It has the effect that as air is expired the linear flow rate increases progressively as gas passes from small to large airways (page 109). The driving pressure is the intra-luminal pressure. In the airways this pressure is less than alveolar pressure because energy is used to overcome flow resistance and to accelerate the gas. The intra-luminal pressure along the length of the airway then declines as does the transmural pressure which is the force tending to keep the airways open.

The loss of intra-luminal pressure due to frictional forces reduces the total cross-sectional area of larger airways. At a constant volume flow the convective acceleration then rises and this reduces even more the intra-luminal pressure; flow will not be maintained unless intra-luminal pressure rises. In a compliant airway such an increase could be dissipated by the airway distending: the airway would then act as a choke point independent of any increase in pressure outside the airway as would be required by equal pressure point theory. At small lung volumes this situation is believed to contribute to flow limitation at the bronchiolar level.

At larger lung volumes the cross-sectional area of the smaller airways is greater due to traction from 'guy lines'. Hence the pressure drop along the bronchioles is small so flow limitation does not occur at this level. Instead the choke point operates at the level of the bronchi which are less compliant but have a small total cross-sectional area. These factors are associated with a high linear flow velocity. The theory postulates that at the choke point the velocity approaches the limiting flow rate which is the pulse wave velocity. For any airway the pulse wave velocity is determined by the gas density and the rigidity of the vessel wall:

$$\dot{v}\text{pw} = \left(\frac{A dP}{\rho dA}\right)^{1/2} \qquad (5.16)$$

where $\dot{v}$pw is pulse wave velocity, A is total cross-sectional area and ρ is gas density and P is intra-luminal pressure. Hence the differential term is the slope of the pressure–area curve for the airway. The maximal volume flow rate is the product of pulse wave velocity and cross-sectional area:

$$\dot{v}\text{max} = \dot{v}\text{pw}A = A\left(\frac{AdP}{\rho dA}\right)^{1/2} \tag{5.17}$$

The general equation has also been derived for the lung using as a starting point the following equation for intra-luminal pressure.

$$P = \text{Pel} - \Delta\text{Pfr} - \frac{1}{2}\rho\dot{v}^2/A^2 \tag{5.18}$$

where Pel is the elastic recoil pressure (equal to alveolar pressure), ΔPfr is the pressure drop associated with frictional resistance, $\dot{v}$ is the volume flow rate of gas and the other items are as defined above. v/A is linear flow velocity and the right hand term which is due to Bernoulli is the pressure drop associated with convective acceleration. In large airways the component for frictional resistance is found to be small relative to that for convective acceleration; if the term is omitted, linear velocity (vl) substituted for $\dot{v}/A$ and the equation differentiated with respect to P:

$$dP = \rho(\dot{v}l^2/A^3)\, dA \tag{5.19}$$

then on rearrangement:

$$vl = A(A/\rho\,(dA/dP)^{1/2}) \tag{5.20}$$

This equation, which is similar to that for pulse wave velocity (5.17), describes the relationship of linear velocity to airway cross-sectional area and indirectly to intra-luminal pressure. The latter two attributes are inter-related and are a function of airway generation. Thus:

$$A = f(P.g) \tag{5.21}$$

where g describes the position along the airways. This equation is due to Fry; it differs from equal pressure point theory in relating the airway calibre to the intra-luminal pressure and not the transmural pressure. The equation can be used jointly with the Bernoulli equation to identify choke points where the linear velocity is maximal and equal to pulse wave velocity. According to wave velocity theory this circumstance should be met where the slope of the relationship of area to pressure is the same for both the Fry and the Bernoulli relationships. The former is given in equation 5.21; the latter by a version of equation 5.18 which makes the assumption that convective acceleration is the only cause for a change in lateral wall pressure with area. Equation 5.18 then becomes:

$$P = P\text{A} - \frac{1}{2}\rho\,\dot{v}^2/A^2 \tag{5.22}$$

where PA is alveolar pressure. Using this approach Hyatt and colleagues obtained pressure area curves for the first three airway generations and

120

flow volume curves in intact excised human lungs. They found near identity between observed values for $\dot{V}$max at large lung volumes and those predicted by wave velocity theory. The agreement did not extend to small lung volumes where other mechanisms may operate. Downstream from the choke point the airway is compressed but high linear velocities can occur. Pedersen has made similar observations in man (Fig. 5.13a, page 115).

Practical implications of flow limitation

The existence of flow-limiting mechanisms (at all but maximal lung volumes) have the effect that beyond a threshold level of effort the maximal expiratory flow reflects the intrinsic mechanical properties of the lung and only to a limited extent the expiratory effort. This has been used to validate the appropriateness of expiratory flow—volume curves for investigating the properties of different orders of airways. However, the limiting flow rate is critically dependent on lung volume and, therefore, when flow rates obtained on two occasions in the same individual are compared the measurements should relate to the same lung volume (page 145).

Relevance for coughing. The upstream migration of the choke point throughout expiration can contribute to the effectiveness of coughing by clearing progressively smaller airways as the cough continues. Thus between two successive coughs the lung volume diminishes and the choke point moves upstream; in doing so it loosens and the high flow velocity expels secretions from a more upstream segment of the airways. Since the downstream secretions are likely to have been removed by the earlier part of the cough there is now a clear path for the expulsion of secretions from the smaller airways. Premature collapse of airways such as occurs in emphysema and probably in bronchiectasis interferes with this mechanism and limits the cleansing action to the larger airways. It also leads to the development of high intra-pleural pressure which Langlands amongst others has shown to contribute to cough syncope.

Indices of maximal flow (ventilatory capacity)

Ventilatory capacity is the term used to describe maximal ability to move gas rapidly in and out of the lung. It includes both maximal breathing and single forced inspirations and expirations. The ventilatory capacity integrates the characteristics of the whole respiratory apparatus, including the lung, thoracic cage and respiratory muscles with their control mechanisms. Ventilatory capacity is one of the factors which determines exercise capacity (Chapter 12) and it is a good guide to prognosis of both chronic lung diseases and ischaemic heart disease (page 600). Tests of ventilatory capacity usually constitute the first stage in the assessment of lung function. This section describes some of the indices which can be used. The methods of measurement and the circumstances when the measurements might be used are given in Chapter 6.

Maximal breathing capacity (MBC) is the maximal volume of air which the subject can breathe in and out per min. When the manoeuvre is performed by voluntary hyperventilation, the index is called the *maximal voluntary ventilation* (MVV). The measurement is usually made over 15 s. For a longer period, e.g. 4 min, the term sustained MVV is used. Sometimes maximal exercise ventilation and maximal ventilation in response to inhaled carbon dioxide are also reported (page 134). The maximal voluntary ventilation in adults, depending on their age and size is in the range $47-2531\,min^{-1}$ in males and $55-1391\,min^{-1}$ in females (see footnote page 102). The measurement of maximal ventilation is discussed in Chapter 6; it is often used to assess training of the respiratory muscles.

Single-breath indices of ventilatory capacity relate to expiration and inspiration separately; they include instantaneous flow rates at defined points in the respiratory cycle, and flow rates averaged with respect to time or volume.

Indices derived from volume–time curves

The use of average flow rate over a timed interval was pioneered by Tiffeneau and by Gaensler. These workers measured the volume of gas expired during the first second of a forced expiration following a full inspiration. The index is called *forced expiratory volume* qualified by the time interval (e.g. forced expiratory volume 1 s or FEV_1 and similarly for inspiration the *forced inspiratory volume* 1 s or FIV_1). The FEV_1 is very reproducible and the most widely used of all lung function indices. Its magnitude in healthy adult males, depending on their age and size, is in the range $1.2-5.71$. In females the range is $0.8-4.21$. Other time intervals for example $FEV_{0.75}$ have also been used; they relate to the FEV_1 in a constant manner (e.g. Table 6.3, page 136).

$FEV_{0.75}$ was originally proposed by Kennedy for estimation of indirect maximal breathing capacity in patients with lung disease and was for a time used for assessing the ventilatory function of children. It has been replaced by FEV_1.

Comroe and Fowler suggested the use of the average flow rate over the middle half of the forced vital capacity; this index is called the *maximal mid-expiratory flow rate* (MMEF) (see Fig. 6.4, page 138). The maximal mid-expiratory flow is also called the *forced expiratory flow rate* (FEF) for the appropriate segment of the forced vital capacity (i.e. $FEF_{25-75\%\ FVC}$). The MMEF is used for detecting the early stages of airflow limitation. In healthy adult males it is in the range $0.2-7.41s^{-1}$. The corresponding range for females is $0.2-6.41s^{-1}$. The average flow rate late in expiration between expiration of 75% and 85% of vital capacity (designated forced late expiratory flow rate, $FEF_{75-85\%\ FVC}$), is believed to reflect the calibre of small airways. The $MEF_{25\%\ FVC}$ which is described below, provides similar information

122

more directly. Additional indices which may be derived from the maximal expiratory volume–time curve include the *mean transit time* (MTT) with its coefficient of variation and an *index of skewness* of the distribution of transit times, but the latter has a poor reproducibility. These indices are defined and illustrated in Fig. 6.5 (page 141). They differ from the $MEF_{25\%\ FVC}$ and similar indices in being derived from the whole of the forced expiration, and in being independent of the volume expired.

Mean transit time is highly correlated with FEV_1/FVC. The moment ratio and the coefficient of variation of transit times both reflect the proportion of lung units which empty late in expiration. These indices were proposed by Fish, Menkes, Neuburger and colleagues and modified by Miller and Pincock amongst others for detecting a minor degree of airway narrowing in respiratory surveys; their usefulness compared with other indices has still to be established (page 141). Some additional indices and abbreviations are listed in Table 2.2 (page 13).

The *peak expiratory flow* (PEF) is the maximum that can be sustained for a defined period, usually 10 ms (Fig. 5.13). The peak flow reflects mainly the calibre of the bronchi and larger bronchioles which are subject to reflex bronchoconstriction (Table 5.2 page 88); for this reason the index is widely used in the management of patients with variable airflow limitation. However, PEF is not independent of expiratory effort (page 114) and on this account is unsuitable for some debilitated patients. In healthy adult males, depending on their age and size, it is in the range $6-15\,l\,s^{-1}$; in females the range is $2.8-10.1\,l\,s^{-1}$. Higher values may be attained during coughing.

Indices derived from flow–volume curves

Peak expiratory flow is usually measured using a peak flow meter. It can also be obtained from the maximal expiratory flow–volume curve. A related but less widely used alternative is the maximal flow rate when 75% of the forced vital capacity remains to be expired ($MEF_{75\%\ FVC}$). This and other indices from the flow volume curve were formerly expressed as the forced expiratory flow rate at a point defined by the proportion of forced vital capacity exhaled from the lung hence $FEF_{25\%\ FVC}$ is the equal to $MEF_{75\%\ FVC}$. The latter terminology is preferable. The flow–volume curve is mainly used to obtain the flow rates at the points on the curve where 50% or 25% of the vital capacity remain to be exhaled ($MEF_{50\%\ FVC}$ and $MEF_{25\%\ FVC}$ respectively, or $\dot{V}max_{50\%}$ etc.; see Fig. 5.13 also the footnote to Table 2.2, page 14). For this purpose the curve can be delineated either from total lung capacity when it is a maximal expiratory flow–volume curve or from the end of a normal inspiration when it is a partial expiratory flow–volume curve. The former procedure was developed by Hyatt. The latter has the advantage that the flow rate is not modified by the breathing manoeuvre (page 142) but the disadvantage that the measurement requires the use of a body plethysmograph. The forced expiratory flow rates $MEF_{50\% \; FVC}$ and $MEF_{25\% \; FVC}$ are widely measured on respiratory surveys because they are believed to reflect the flow characteristics of airways of diameter respectively greater than and less than approximately 3 mm. However, the measurements are less reproducible than FEV_1 and the reference values have a wider dispersion. The indices have not made much contribution to clinical practice. Of greater use are the shape of the expiratory flow−volume curve and the maximal inspiratory flow rate; the latter is obtained from the maximal inspiratory flow−volume curve (Fig. 5.13b). The principal index is the $MIF_{50\% \; FVC}$. The average flow for the expiration of 1 l of gas starting 200 ml after the beginning of a forced expiration (i.e. $FEF_{200-1200}$) was formerly also used as an index.

Density dependence

The density of the respired gas can be changed by altering the ambient pressure as in a pressure chamber, or by flushing the lungs with a gas mixture comprising helium or sulphur hexafluoride in 20% oxygen (Table 5.5, page 111). Changing the density alters the extent to which the flow in large airways is turbulent; it does not affect laminar flow (page 111). The effects upon maximal breathing capacity are illustrated in Fig. 5.16 and upon the flow−volume curve in Fig. 5.17. The difference from breathing air is mainly confined to flow rates at large lung volumes: flow rates at small lung volume are entirely laminar and are not altered. There is also no change in vital capacity. The proportion of vital capacity over which the flow is independent of gas density between breathing air and a helium mixture is called the *volume of iso-flow* (*V-isov̇*); it indicates the lung volume during expiration at which the

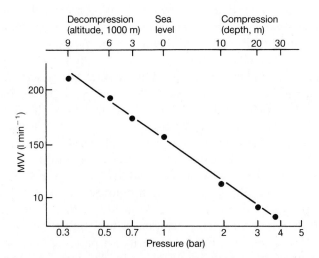

Fig. 5.16 The effect upon the maximal voluntary ventilation (MVV) in normal subjects of changes in the density and the kinematic viscosity of the respired gas caused by alterations in the ambient pressure in an altitude chamber. (Source: Miles S. *J Physiol (Lond)* 1957; **137**: 85P.)

forced expiratory flow rate is no longer limited by turbulence. The index is correlated with $MEF_{25\% \; FVC}$: it has rather poor reproducibility and is mainly of research interest. The change in $MEF_{50\% \; FVC}$ between breathing air and helium/oxygen is also used as an index.

Standardisation for vital capacity. Ventilatory capacity is greatly influenced by the size of the lung which for many purposes is represented by *forced vital capacity*. Forced vital capacity (FVC) is the maximal volume of air which can be expelled from the lung by forced expiration following a full inspiration. FVC enters into the derivation of maximal mid-expiratory flow (MMEF, page 140), maximal expiratory flow ($MEF_{50\% \; FVC}$ and $_{25\% \; FVC}$) and the volume of iso-flow (V-iso$\dot{v}$). It is also used to standardise the forced expiratory volume for lung size. For this purpose FEV_1 is reported as a percentage of forced vital capacity, then:

$$FEV_1\% = (FEV_1/FVC) \times 100$$

$FEV_1\%$ is used as a guide to airway calibre (page 517) and has the advantage for statistical analyses that unlike FEV_1 it is independent of FVC and nearly independent of body size and stature. However, forced vital capacity is an uncertain guide to total lung capacity because the other component, which is residual volume, can vary independently. For example changes in respiratory muscle strength influence vital capacity more than residual volume whilst the reverse is the case for changes in bronchomotor tone. Hence the use of FVC to correct

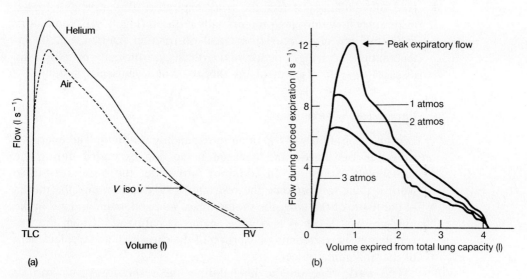

Fig. 5.17 Flow–volume curves in healthy subjects showing the effects of changes in gas density. The density affects the degree of turbulence and hence the flow rates at large lung volumes. (a) Breathing air and a helium/oxygen mixture (F_I, He = 0.8); the volume of isoflow (V-iso$\dot{v}$) is the point where the two curves meet. (b) Breathing under hyperbaric conditions in compression chamber. Some abnormal curves are shown in Fig. 16.1 (page 517).

ventilatory capacity for changes in lung size is inevitably approximate and can be misleading. For this reason the indices $FEV_1\%$, $FEF_{25\%-75\%}$, $MEF_{50\%\ FVC}$ and $MEF_{25\%\ FVC}$ should not be used to assess bronchial lability including the response to a bronchodilator drug. If these indices are to be used the allowance for lung size should be made in terms of alveolar volume measured by whole body plethysmography. Usually FEV_1 or PEF will be used instead (page 145).

Ventilatory capacity in disease of the lung

When the lungs are diseased the ventilatory capacity is affected mainly by changes in the effective cross-sectional area of airways and in the lung volume: more or less persistent reductions in cross-sectional area and hence an increased frictional pressure drop occurs from compression, active bronchoconstriction, thickening of the airway wall and accumulation of secretions. Dynamic compression is a consequence of loss of lung elasticity. All the conditions give rise to an obstructive type of ventilatory defect; this affects expiration more than inspiration (Fig. 5.13) and has distinct features depending on the site and mechanism of the obstruction. A restrictive type of ventilatory defect associated with restriction to lung expansion results in reduction of total lung capacity. The airway cross-sectional area and hence the forced expiratory flow rates are well preserved relative to the lung volume.

Extra-pulmonary airways respond differently from intra-thoracic airways because they are not held open by the elastic retractive force of the lung tissue. This has the effect that in the presence of an obstructive type of ventilatory defect the peak expiratory flow rate and forced inspiratory flow rates are preferentially reduced (Fig. 5.13). Ventilatory limitation can also occur from local obstruction (caused e.g. by inflammation, scarring, cricothyroid arthritis, acromegaly or neoplastic disease) or from diseases of the thorax or neuromuscular system.

Energy cost of breathing

During inspiration work is done in expanding the lung. The energy is stored in the elastic and collagen tissue and expended during the subsequent expiration. In addition, throughout the respiratory cycle work is done to overcome the resistance to movement and the inertia of the tissue of the lung, the thoracic cage and abdomen, and gas in the lung airways. Work is also done against gravity and, at high rates of ventilation, in overcoming distortion of the chest wall and displacement of the abdominal viscera.

The work done on the lung during one respiratory cycle can be obtained from the area which is enclosed by the curve relating the intrapleural pressure to the lung volume. The area which is pressure times volume has the dimensions of work which is a force multiplied by displacement, as shown by the following equation:

$$Fl = Fl^{-2}l^3 = FA^{-1}V = PV \qquad (5.23)$$

where F is force, l is distance, Fl^{-2} is force per unit area which is pressure (P) and l^3 is volume (V). A volume−pressure curve for an ideal lung is shown in Fig. 5.18 where the static compliance over a small range of volumes above functional residual capacity is represented by the slope of the diagonal ABC. Also shown is the corresponding static recoil relationship for the chest wall, which at functional residual capacity, is of equal magnitude but of opposite sign to that for the lung. The two relationships intersect at FRC which is indicated by the point A. During inspiration the work which is done by the inspiratory muscles in overcoming the elastic recoil of the lungs and chest wall is represented by the triangle ACD; it includes a component from the chest wall which assists lung expansion at small lung volumes but at larger volume opposes it. These are represented by the areas AE0 and EGD. The energy is stored in the stretched tissues. Additional inspiratory work is done in overcoming the resistance and inertia of the lung and thorax. The resistive components are illustrated in the diagram. During expiration the energy which is stored in the distended lung is used in part to overcome the forces which resist expiration, including the resistance of the airways and the lung tissue. This work is represented by the area C Exp.AC. Some of the stored energy is also used to overcome the resistance of the chest wall and the remainder is dissipated as heat.

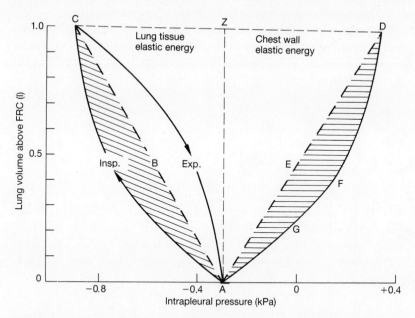

Fig. 5.18 Diagram after Campbell illustrating the relationship of the lung volume above functional residual capacity to the intrapleural pressure during quiet breathing. The slopes of the lines AC and AD represent the static compliance respectively of the lung and of the chest wall. These data can be obtained in the manner indicated in the caption to Fig. 5.7. The hatched areas represent work done during inspiration in overcoming resistance of the airways (oblique hatching) and chest wall (horizontal hatching). The use of the diagram to calculate the total work done by the inspiratory muscles is described in the text.

The total work done on the lung by the inspiratory muscles is represented by the area A Insp.CZA. This quantity has been measured during the inhalation of gas containing carbon dioxide when it has been shown by Milic-Emili and others to be a linear function of the hypercapnoeic drive to respiration. However, the work done on the lung is only part of the total performed during inspiration, which also includes the other components listed above. These quantities, which are represented by the area A Insp.C DFA, cannot easily be measured except when the force is applied externally to a subject in whom the respiratory muscles are paralysed; the results do not then apply to spontaneous breathing.

The energy for respiratory work is provided by the metabolic activity of the respiratory muscles; this has been investigated in animal models and to a lesser extent in man. The fraction of cardiac output which is used for external respiration goes mainly to the diaphragm except when expiration is obstructed: in this event more blood flow goes to the expiratory muscles. The diaphragmatic blood flow varies with the rate of respiratory work and is normally in the range $0.08-0.33\ ml\,g^{-1}$ min^{-1}. Higher flow rates are observed if inspiration is obstructed. The diaphragmatic blood flow is well preserved during conditions of low cardiac output including shock when the flow may exceed 20% of cardiac output. The blood flow sustains the aerobic oxidation of carbohydrate and free fatty acids. Rapid glycolysis seldom occurs except when the diaphragm is driven by phrenic nerve stimulation.

The oxygen consumed by the respiratory muscles is normally only a small proportion of total oxygen consumption so is difficult to measure accurately in man. The respiratory component is estimated from the

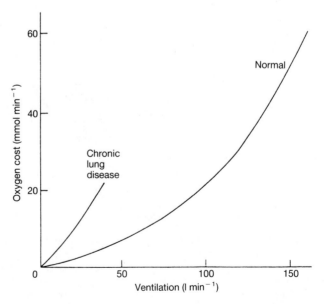

Fig. 5.19 The approximate oxygen cost of breathing in a healthy man and in a patient with severe lung disease.

increase in total consumption above resting which occurs when the ventilation is increased by voluntary hyperventilation, use of an external dead space, or addition of carbon dioxide to the respired gas. The procedure is described on page 377. The oxygen cost of breathing varies with the level of ventilation. During quiet breathing the consumption per litre of ventilation is in the range $10-90\,\mu\text{mol}\,l^{-1}$ ($0.25-2.0\,\text{ml}\,l^{-1}$); this is on average approximately 2% of the total consumption of oxygen by a resting subject. When the ventilation minute volume is $40\,l\,\text{min}^{-1}$, as occurs during moderate exercise, the oxygen cost is about twice as great, whilst at high rates of ventilation, the oxygen cost of breathing increases disproportionately (see Fig. 5.19). A situation can then arise when a further increase in ventilation requires the consumption of more additional oxygen than enters the pulmonary capillary blood as a result of the extra ventilation. This can occur during maximal exercise (page 392) or at rest if the work of breathing is greatly increased by obstruction of the airways. The energy cost of breathing is also high in patients with pulmonary fibrosis and in obese subjects in whom there is increased resistance to movement of the thoracic cage and abdomen. In all these conditions an increase in the work of breathing is an important cause of the onset of respiratory failure (see Chapter 16). The subject has been reviewed by Otis and by Roussos.

Guide to references

The references (Chapter 18) are classified under subject headings of which the following are particularly relevant to the present chapter:

6: Assessment of Bellows and Mechanical Attributes of the Lung

Measurement of ventilatory capacity and related indices	Lung compliance and resistance
Assessing bronchodilatation	Tissue resistance
Lung volumes	Total respiratory impedance
Use of whole body plethysmograph	Bronchial hyperreactivity

Introduction

The tests recommended for routine assessment of lung function are listed in Table 4.3 (page 70) and additional regularly used tests are given in Table 4.4 (page 73). Some features of the methods are summarised in Table 6.1. Those for ventilatory capacity yield numerous indices and some of these are characterised in Table 6.2. The equipment (Chapter 3), and the methods of measurement, should conform to internationally recognised standards such as those of the European

Table 6.1 Qualitative appraisal of assessment procedures

Aspects of lung function and method or apparatus	Technical aspects					Use	Page
	1*	2*	3*	4*	5*		
Lung volumes							
Closed circuit spirometry	B	A_2	A_2	C	C	Routine	150
Plethysmography	C	B	A_2	D	B	Specialist centre	157
Forced rebreathing	B	B	B	A	A	Surveys	154
Radiography	C	C	A_2	D	C	Research	155
Ventilatory capacity							
Bellows spirometer	A	A–C	A	A	A	Clinic	135
Rolling seal spirometer	B	B	A	B–C	B	Laboratory	135
Peak flow meter	A	B	A	A	A	Clinic	139
Pneumotachography	B	B	A	B	A	Laboratory	135
Resistance to flow							
Plethysmography	C	B	A_2	D	B	Specialist centre	156
Oesophageal balloon, etc.	C	C	C	C	C	Research	160
Airway interrupter	B	C	B	A	A	Surveys	173
Forced oscillation	C	C	C	C	B	Research	169
Lung elasticity							
Oesophageal balloon, etc.	C	C	C	C	C	Specialist centre	160

* 1 = complexity, 2 = calibration, 3 = reproducibility, 4 = portability, 5 = running cost.
Scale A–D where an A procedure is simple, readily calibrated, reproducible, portable and cheap to carry out.

Table 6.2 Some indices of ventilatory capacity

Index	Comment	Reproducibility*	Page†
Maximal voluntary ventilation (MVV)	Overall test, effort dependent, can assess endurance	xx	134
Forced expiratory volume (FEV$_1$) } Forced vital capacity (FVC) }	Overall test, first choice in most circumstances including for assessing bronchodilatation	xxx	135
Forced expiratory time (FET)	Guide to expiratory narrowing of airways	x	140
Inspiratory vital capacity (IVC)	Used in Tiffeneau index (FEV$_1$/IVC)	xxx	139
Peak expiratory flow (PEF)	Reflects large airway calibre, used to assess bronchodilatation; influenced by expiratory effort	xx	139
Indices from flow–volumes curve			
MEF$_{50\%\ FVC}$	As for MMEF	xx	142
MEF$_{25\%\ FVC}$	May reflect small airway calibre; FEF$_{75-85\%}$ is also used	x	142
MEF$_{75\%\ FVC}$	PEF yields similar information	xx	143
MEF$_{60\%\ TLC}$	Is independent of dynamic compression	xx	156
MIF$_{50\%\ FVC}$	Reduced by upper airway obstruction and respiratory muscle weakness. Is effort dependent. Has low acceptability	x	144
Maximal mid-expiratory flow MMEF (FEF$_{25-75\%}$)	Detects mild airflow limitation	xx	140
Transit times Mean (MTT), SD (SDTT) Index of skewness (IOS), Moment ratio	Usefulness unproven	xx	141

* Rating   xxx ≈ 2–3%;   xx ≈ 4–6%;   x > 8%, see page 67.
† Reference values are given in Chapter 15.

Coal and Steel Community (ECSC) and the American Thoracic Society. The ECSC 1992 update, which has been endorsed by the European Respiratory Society, can be read in conjunction with the present account. Reference values are given in Chapter 15.

Measurement of ventilatory capacity

What is being measured?

Ventilatory capacity is the maximal ability to move gas rapidly into or out of the lung. The measurement is of volume flow rate (rate of air flow). During forced expiration the outcome is determined mainly by the calibre of large airways, the size of the lung and the integrity of the respiratory system. During maximal voluntary ventilation the respiratory muscles provide the force that generates maximal inspiratory and peak expiratory flow rates. They contribute only slightly to FEV_1 and not at all to $MEF_{50\%\ FVC}$ and $MEF_{25\%\ FVC}$. Flow rates towards the end of a forced expiration ($MEF_{25\%\ FVC}$ $MEF_{75-85\%}$) may reflect the calibre of small airways; these do not make a material contribution to ventilatory capacity. The underlying physiology is discussed in Chapter 5 and the change in disease in Chapter 16.

Applications

These are summarised in Table 6.2.

Equipment

The equipment should meet the technical specifications given on pages 23–33. It should be calibrated at the start of each measurement session (page 50) and cleaned in the recommended manner (page 54).

Conditions of measurement

The measurement should normally be made during normal working hours but the error at other times seldom exceeds 2.5%. However, the lung volume is slightly reduced after a big meal. The bronchomotor tone can be increased by exposure to cold air or cigarette smoke and the ventilatory capacity exhibits diurnal and seasonal variation.

Serial measurements should preferably be made in a post-absorptive state at a specific time of day and season of the year. The ambient temperature should be within the range 16–25°C. In addition the same trained observer and apparatus should be used whenever possible. Alternatively if several observers are used, they should be calibrated against each other by measuring the ventilatory capacity of a group of subjects presented to each of them in random order. The observers should be in different rooms and not be audible to each other.

Subjects should be instructed to loosen any clothing which might restrict the movement of the chest or upper abdomen; dentures should not be taken out unless they are loose.

If the subject is new to the procedure this should be demonstrated by the operator; this aspect is discussed further on page 76. The measurement is performed with the subject in an upright position, usually seated but standing is acceptable. A nose clip is permissible but is not recommended except for children, negroes, subjects who produce variable results and those, including some Australian aboriginals, who play musical instruments through the nose.

Reporting the results

The volumes and flow rates are reported at body temperature and pressure, saturated with water vapour. For this purpose the apparatus temperature should be recorded and an appropriate correction made (page 18).

Reference values

These are given in Chapter 15.

Maximal breathing capacity (MBC)

Definition. MBC is the maximal volume of air which the subject can expire in 1 min when breathing as deeply and rapidly as possible. The measurement is usually that of maximal voluntary ventilation (MVV) over a period of 15 s. When recorded for a longer period (e.g. 4 min) it is called sustained MVV. The measurement of MBC can also be made during maximal exercise (VEmax ex), or maximal CO_2 ventilation while rebreathing into a bag. Such conditions should be specified. The measurement of MVV is described in this section.

Equipment. This is usually a rolling seal spirometer or pneumotachograph with an acceptably low flow resistance (page 23). Alternatively, use may be made of a bellows spirometer or a water spirometer with large cross-sectional area (page 24). Normally the subject rebreathes into the apparatus after any valves and absorber for carbon dioxide have been removed. However, if a pneumotachograph is used carbon dioxide at a fractional concentration of 0.05 may be added to the inspired gas to reduce the associated hypocapnia. The error from using an apparatus having a high flow resistance is illustrated in Fig. 6.1.

Procedures. The conditions of measurement are given above. The observer urges the subject to achieve the greatest possible depth and frequency of breathing and the result is influenced by the rapport which builds up between them. Thus both observer and subject can find the test tiring. The frequency of breathing should be reported (Table 2.2, page 14) and should preferably exceed 80 per min.

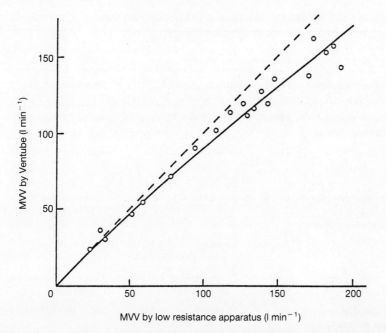

Fig. 6.1 Comparison of maximal voluntary ventilation (MVV) of 20 subjects obtained using a Ventube and a low-resistance apparatus. The back pressures at a flow rate of 80 l min^{-1} were respectively approximately 0.1 and 0.03 kPa. The line of identity is indicated by the interrupted line and the observed relationship by the circles and the continuous line. (Source: Thiruvengadam KV, McKerrow CB. *Dis Chest* 1962; **41**: 138.)

Estimation from FEV. In most circumstances maximal breathing capacity is highly correlated with forced expiratory volume over 0.75 or 1 s (correlation coefficient in the range 0.75−0.95). This has led to the use of FEV$_1$ to predict maximal ventilation in a variety of circumstances including exercise. Some relationships are given in Table 6.3.

Forced expiratory volume and vital capacity (FEV$_1$, FVC)

Definition. FEV$_1$ is the maximal volume of air which the subject can exhale in the first second of a forced expiration following a full inspiration. Other time intervals for example 0.5 or 3.0 s are also used. Forced vital capacity is the volume expired when the forced expiration is continued until no more air can be expelled from the lungs. In patients with airflow limitation FVC can be less than other indices of vital capacity including inspiratory vital capacity, slow expiratory vital capacity (performed in a relaxed manner) and two stage vital capacity (i.e. the sum of inspiratory capacity and expiratory reserve volume obtained by closed circuit spirometry). The difference is due to dynamic compression of airways and associated air trapping (page 126).

Equipment. This can be a bellows or a rolling seal spirometer, or a pneumotachograph or a rotating vane anemometer with an integrator. The apparatus should meet the technical specification given on page 23 and should be used in accordance with the manufacturer's

Table 6.3 Inter-relations between indices of ventilatory capacity

Variable to be predicted	Predictor	Relationship*	Source
Maximal voluntary ventilation	FEV_1	$MVV = 34.7\ FEV_1^{0.985}$ (C of V 18%, R^2 0.73)	McKerrow (1955)
Indirect maximal breathing capacity	$FEV_{0.75}$	$IMBC = 40 \times FEV_{0.75}$	Kennedy (1953)
$FEV_{0.75}$	FEV_1	$FEV_{0.75} = 0.92\ FEV_1$ -0.07 (95% limits $\pm 8\%$)	McKerrow *et al.* (1960)
Maximal exercise ventilation in respiratory patients	FEV_1	$\dot{V}E\ max\ ex = 35\ FEV_1$	Gandevia and Hugh-Jones (1957)
		$\dot{V}E\ max\ ex = 18.9\ FEV_1$ $+ 19.7\ (r = 0.82)$	Spiro *et al.* (1975)
		$\dot{V}E\ max\ ex = 33.1\ FEV_1 0.73$ (C of V 18%)	Cotes *et al.* 1982, see page 441
Maximal exercise tidal volume	VC	$Vt\ max\ ex = 0.65\ VC$ $-0.64\ (SD\ 0.21)$	Jones and Rebuck (1979)

* Volumes are expressed in litres and ventilation in $l\,min^{-1}$.
Abbreviations are given on pages 13 and 64.

instructions. For example, when using a Vitalograph the pen should start at the zero point on the graph paper and the readings should be made using the scale appropriate to each index. Calibration is described on page 50.

Procedure. The conditions of measurement and role of the operator are given on page 54. The subject takes the fullest possible inspiration through the mouth, then immediately puts the mouth round the mouth piece and exhales forcibly. The operator should ensure that the inspiration is unhurried and continued up to total lung capacity, the mouth piece is inserted without loss of gas or obstruction by the lips or teeth and the forced expiration is continued to completion without a pause and without loss of air around the mouth piece. Maximal encouragement is given during both inspiration and expiration (Fig. 6.2). Some common faults are given in Table 6.4. They include failure to take a full inspiration, hesitation early in expiration and pursing the lips as if blowing into a trumpet. These faults should be corrected by dialogue with the subject. In addition, in some patients the completion of the expiration may provoke coughing which in turn may lead to reflex bronchoconstriction. This difficulty can be avoided by the operator instructing the subject to stop breathing out after the first second has been recorded. When this is done the forced vital capacity must be measured separately. Subjects performing the test for the first time should make two or more practice blows to develop a correct technique. Thereafter three technically satisfactory blows are recorded.

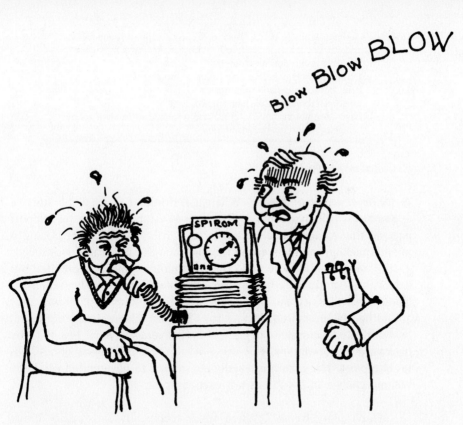

Fig. 6.2 Measurement of FEV_1 showing effort required of both the subject and the operator. Submaximal effort can lead to spuriously high values being recorded (Fig. 6.3).

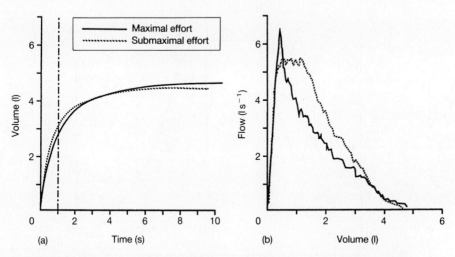

Fig. 6.3 Error in dynamic spirometry caused by submaximal effort in a healthy subject. The FEV_1, indicated by interrupted vertical line (a), is spuriously high (3.28 l compared with 2.81 l) due to there being less dynamic compression. Concurrently the apex of the flow–volume curve (b) is flattened and displaced to the right and the peak expiratory flow is submaximal ($5.4 l s^{-1}$ compared with $6.2 l s^{-1}$). Larger differences are observed in many patients with airflow limitation (page 126). Some mechanisms are discussed on pages 112–121.

Table 6.4 Common faults in performance of a forced expiratory manoeuvre

Previous inspiration not complete
Expiration begins before connecting to mouthpiece
Leak between lips and mouthpiece
Lips pursed or teeth partially closed
Expiration not maximally forced and sustained to residual volume
Coughing or premature inspiration

Calculation of results

(a) Start and end of breath. When a spirometer is used the start of
expiration is usually defined by backward extrapolation of the steepest
part of the volume time curve to zero volume (Fig. 6.4). Using a
pneumotachograph the starting time is when the flow rate first exceeds
0.5ls^{-1}. Results by these and other methods are highly correlated but
exhibit systematic differences. For example in many early studies including that of Kory and colleagues (1961), the starting point was after
200 ml had been expired. Values for FEV_1 by this method were found
by Smith and Gaensler (1975) to be on average 179 ml less than by
backward extrapolation. For other methods a difference of 2.5% is
fairly typical. The breath is usually considered to have ended when the
volume change in 0.5 s does not exceed 25 ml.

(b) Which blow is best? When three technically satisfactory blows
have been obtained the FEV_1 and FVC are usually taken as the
highest recorded values; they need not have come from the same

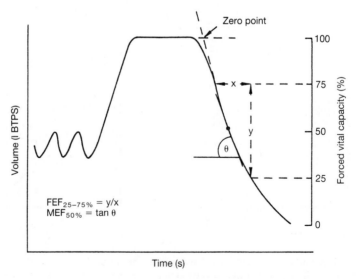

Fig. 6.4 Forced expiratory spirogram with volume axis adjusted to BTPS. The diagram
shows the derivation of the maximal or forced mid-expiratory flow (MMEF or $FEF_{25-75\%}$)
and $MEF_{50\%}$ $_{FVC}$, also the backward extrapolation method for locating the start of
forced expiration (i.e. $t=0$). The extrapolated volume should not exceed 0.1 l or 5% of
FVC whichever is greater.

forced expiration. However, as a check on the stability of the results the highest FVC should not normally exceed the next highest value by more than 5% or 0.1 l whichever is greater. In addition in order to avoid error due to submaximal effort (Fig. 6.3) the flow volume curve should preferably be recorded concurrently and be of acceptable quality (page 142).

(c) Standardisation for vital capacity. The dependance of FEV_1 on vital capacity may be eliminated by expressing the result as a ratio. Usually this is the percentage $FEV_1 \times 100/FVC$, also called FEV% or FEV_1/FVC. The ratio is independent of FVC but has the disadvantage that in the presence of airflow limitation the denominator is reduced by dynamic compression. This source of error is avoided by using instead either inspiratory vital capacity, slow expiratory (relaxed) vital capacity or two stage vital capacity. The index first proposed by Tiffeneau (1948) was $FEV_1 \times 100/IVC$. This format is recommended by the European Coal and Steel Community (see also page 517).

Comment. FEV_1 is independent of expiratory effort once a moderate effort has been made (Fig. 5.14, page 117). However, both FEV_1 and FVC are very dependent on the size of the preceding inspiration. FVC is also dependent on the expiratory effort. Measurements of FEV_1 and FVC are the most widely used of all lung function tests and have numerous applications; these are summarised in Table 4.1 (page 66). A low value for FEV_1% usually reflects airflow obstruction (page 517); it can also be due to an increased vital capacity (page 472). The assessment of responsiveness to bronchodilator drugs is given on page 145 and the estimation of maximal breathing capacity on page 134.

Peak expiratory flow (PEF)

Definition. PEF is the maximal flow rate which can be developed by forced expiratory effort following a full inspiration. The flow should represent an appreciable movement of gas and not a pulse wave. To this end the measurement should be made over a timed period of between 10 and 90 ms.

Equipment. In the clinic or for respiratory surveys PEF is measured using a peak flow meter (e.g. Wright, page 27). Before use the instrument should be inspected to establish that nothing is loose, the ratchet does not slip and the filter is clean. In the laboratory PEF can be measured using an appropriate spirometer or pneumotachograph (Table 3.2, page 24). The procedure for calibration is described on page 50.

Procedure. This is similar to that for measurement of FEV_1 and FVC which can be obtained concurrently if an appropriate spirometer or pneumotachograph is used. When only PEF is measured care should be taken that there is no delay between inspiration and expiration and that the flow is generated from the chest and not by the muscle of the cheeks; the subject should discontinue the expiration once the peak flow rate has been registered by the equipment.

Comment. Peak expiratory flow is correlated with ventilatory capacity and with other indices of forced expiratory flow at large lung volumes including $MEF_{75\% \; FVC}$ (page 143).

Peak expiratory flow reflects mainly the calibre of the bronchi; it is used for assessing bronchodilatation (page 145) and circadian variation in cases of suspected asthma (page 553). The flow rate is also dependent on the depth of the preceding inspiration, the strength of the muscles of expiration and the expiratory effort.

Other indices from volume–time curves

Maximal mid-expiratory flow (MMEF or $FEF_{25-75\%}$). This index is the flow rate over the middle half of the forced vital capacity: its derivation is illustrated in Fig. 6.4. In the presence of a normal FEV_1 a reduced MMEF is evidence for mild airflow limitation. However, when the FEV_1 is also reduced the MMEF does not provide much additional information. The index is recommended as a screening test for mild airflow limitation, but not for the clinical management of patients (see e.g. page 132).

Forced inspiratory volume (FIV_1). This index is the inspiratory equivalent of the FEV_1. It is measured by forced inspiration following a slow complete expiration, sterile apparatus must be used (see page 54). The index is effort dependent and the manoeuvre can be disagreeable so the measurement is seldom made except when there may be obstruction to extra-thoracic airways. In this condition better discrimination is obtained by using instead the $MIF_{50\% \; IVC}$.

Forced late-expiratory flow rate ($FEF_{75-85\%}$). This index is the average flow rate during exhalation of 10% of forced vital capacity starting after 75% of FVC has been expired. The index can be measured using equipment (e.g. Vitalograph recording to 12 s) which does not meet the technical specification for instantaneous flow rates. $MEF_{25\% \; FVC}$ yields similar information (page 143). The reproducibility of both indices is poor (Table 6.2, page 132).

Forced expiratory time (FET). This index is the time taken to expire a specified portion of the forced vital capacity, e.g. 99% (hence $FET_{99\%}$). It has a poor reproducibility which limits its usefulness as a quantitative index. $FET_{100\%}$ has the advantages of simplicity and of being measurable in a patient's home. An FET in excess of 4 s is evidence for some degree of airflow limitation.

Mean transit time (MTT) and its derivatives. MTT is the mean time taken for gas molecules to leave the lung during the expiration of the forced vital capacity. It is obtained by moment analysis which entails measuring the volumes expired in successive time intervals or the times for successive volume increments during the expiration. The volume–time curve which is measured should be that which has the shortest MTT from amongst curves which meet the criteria of acceptability given on page 136. Either the whole curve is used or the end of the expiration is omitted. The cut-off point can be defined by time, with truncation at 6 s but this can lead to a spuriously normal result in patients with airflow limitation. Alternatively truncation can be by volume at the point when a given percentage of FVC has been expired. Seventy-five per cent, 90% and 99% have been suggested but there is as yet no consensus as to which should be employed. The analysis yields three moments of which the first is the mean transit time. The subsequent moments are used to derive the standard deviation of transit time (SDTT), the moment ratio (MR) and an index of skewness (Fig. 6.5). SDTT can be expressed as a coefficient of variation (SDTT × 100/MTT, %). However, the moment ratio yields similar information.

MTT is highly correlated with $FEV_1\%$ which is more easily obtained. The standard deviation of transit times and related indices provide a numerical description of the latter part of the forced expiration. The indices might be expected to detect mild airflow obstruction at a time

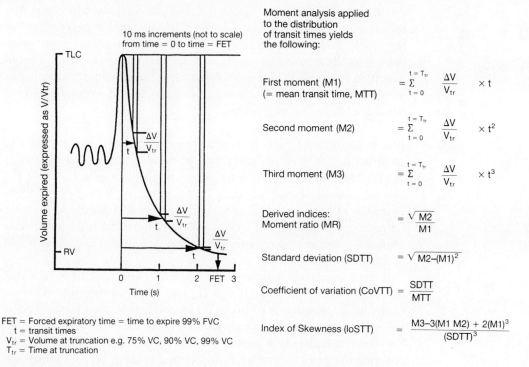

Moment analysis applied to the distribution of transit times yields the following:

First moment (M1) (= mean transit time, MTT)
$$= \sum_{t=0}^{t=T_{tr}} \frac{\Delta V}{V_{tr}} \times t$$

Second moment (M2)
$$= \sum_{t=0}^{t=T_{tr}} \frac{\Delta V}{V_{tr}} \times t^2$$

Third moment (M3)
$$= \sum_{t=0}^{t=T_{tr}} \frac{\Delta V}{V_{tr}} \times t^3$$

Derived indices:
Moment ratio (MR)
$$= \sqrt{\frac{M2}{M1}}$$

Standard deviation (SDTT)
$$= \sqrt{M2-(M1)^2}$$

Coefficient of variation (CoVTT)
$$= \frac{SDTT}{MTT}$$

Index of Skewness (IoSTT)
$$= \frac{M3-3(M1\ M2) + 2(M1)^3}{(SDTT)^3}$$

FET = Forced expiratory time = time to expire 99% FVC
t = transit times
V_{tr} = Volume at truncation e.g. 75% VC, 90% VC, 99% VC
T_{tr} = Time at truncation

Fig. 6.5 Derivation of transit time indices. (Source: Chinn DJ, Cotes JE. *Bull Eur Physiopathol Respir* 1986; **22**: 461–466.)

when the FEV_1 and $MEF_{50\%~FVC}$ are still relatively normal. However, the methodology is not yet fully standardised and the practical usefulness of the indices has still to be established.

Indices from expiratory flow−volume curves

Introduction. The characteristics of the airways from the trachea down to the level of the larger bronchioles mainly determine flow rates early in expiration when the lung volume is relatively large whilst the smaller airways determine flow later in expiration when the lung volume is reduced. Thus separation of the influence of large and small airways can be effected by measuring maximal flow rates at different lung volumes; the volumes are defined in terms of vital capacity (e.g. Fig. 5.13b, page 116) or total lung capacity. Plotting expiratory flow−volume curves has the theoretical advantage that flow rates defined in this way are independent of expiratory effort once about 30% of vital capacity has been expired (page 116).

A partial flow−volume curve starting from end-inspiration during tidal breathing is independent of effort after expiration of a small volume of gas from the central airways; in addition the airway calibre is then unaffected by reflex bronchodilatation and some effects of hystereris caused by prior inhalation to total lung capacity (page 199). However, when flow is related to the proportion of vital capacity remaining in the lung no allowance is made for compression of intra-thoracic gas by the rise in intra-thoracic pressure which accompanies forced expiration. True measurements of volume can be obtained in the whole body plethysmograph and its use is recommended when physiologically meaningful results are required. When assessing broncho-dilatation (page 146) the flow−volume curve is also subject to erroneous interpretation if changes in flow rates are compared without regard to possible changes in lung volume.

Practical aspects of flow−volume spirometry. The information used to construct a flow−volume curve can be obtained during measurement of FEV_1 and FVC by spirometry or by using a pneumotachograph; the former method should be used if the effect of 80% helium, 20% oxygen is to be assessed (Fig. 6.6). The equipment should be suitable for measuring high rates of airflow and meet the other technical specifi-cations for dynamic spirometry (page 24). At least three curves should be recorded.

The curves can be registered and analysed on-line using an oscilloscope or other suitable recorder (page 31) and a microprocessor. Alterna-tively the information is recorded on magnetic tape then transcribed at reduced speed onto a relatively slow recorder after the test expiration has been completed. Sub-maximal effort can distort the result by reducing the peak expiratory flow rate and causing less dynamic com-pression; the latter in turn is associated with relatively high values for $MEF_{50\%~FVC}$ and $MFF_{25\%~FVC}$. Criteria for acceptable curves include

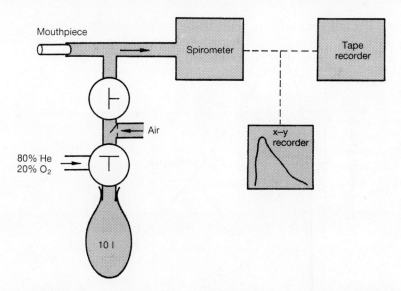

Fig. 6.6 Apparatus for recording the flow–volume curve breathing air and a helium/
oxygen mixture (e.g. Fig. 5.17, page 125). The test breaths are preceded by the subject
inhaling from the bag three full breaths of the appropriate gas and expiring to air. The
curves are best recorded on magnetic tape for subsequent reconstruction; they should
also be displayed on an oscilloscope or an $X–Y$ recorder having a time for full scale
response on the flow-rate axis of not more than 0.3 s.

that the FVC should meet the requirements for an acceptable measurement (page 139), the peak expiratory flow rates should not differ by
more than 10%, and the three curves should be of similar shape. This
should be established by inspection. The indices are in each case the
highest observed value and need not all come from the same curve; the
choice is made either from the numerical results or the three curves are
superimposed at total lung capacity and the outline is used for the
derivation. The flow rates are reported at given percentages of
the largest FVC. Derivation of the indices from the curve having the
highest value for FEV_1 plus FVC, as was formerly recommended by
the American Thoracic Society, can lead to error if the PEF is submaximal and is no longer acceptable. Commonly used indices are the
maximal flow rate when 50% and 25% of forced vital capacity remain
to be expired; these are designated $MEF_{50\% \ FVC}$ and $MEF_{25\% \ FVC}$
(Fig. 6.7). $MEF_{75\% \ FVC}$ is sometimes also used; it is highly correlated
with the peak expiratory flow rate. The terminology is discussed on
page 123.

Flow–volume spirometry performed whilst breathing gases of
different density can be used to assess the extent of turbulent flow in
the airways. In this case the test expirations are preceded by the
subject taking three vital capacity breaths of 80% helium in oxygen.
The test is performed as for breathing air. The result is reported as the
percentage changes in PEF and $MEF_{50\% \ FVC}$ and as the lung volume at
which the curves for air and helium first coincide; the latter point is
designated volume of isoflow (V-iso $\dot{v}$) and is reported as a percentage

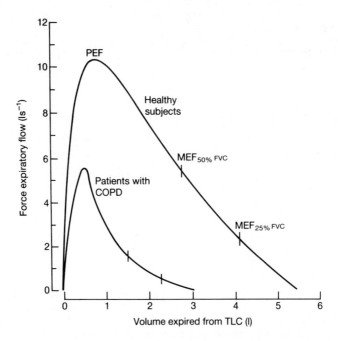

Fig. 6.7 Idealised flow—volume curve showing the principal indices. In practice the indices are the highest recorded from three technically satisfactory blows and need not all come from the same curve.

of forced vital capacity (Fig. 5.17, page 125). Alternatively if the lung volume is determined by plethysmography the volume is reported as a percentage of total lung capacity.

Comment. Flow—volume indices are often included amongst the results of dynamic spirometry. However, $MEF_{50\% \ FVC}$ is not as reproducible as FEV_1 with which it is correlated and the reference values have wider confidence limits: in isolation the index does not contribute additional information. In this it differs from the $MEF_{25\% \ FVC}$ which can provide evidence of narrowing of small airways in groups of subjects. The *V*-iso $\dot{v}$ is a research tool and is at present of limited usefulness. However, the role of flow—volume spirometry may need to be revised when more experience has been obtained of composite flow—volume indices such as have been proposed by Quanjer and colleagues. Partial flow—volume curves obtained by plethysmography can yield important physiological information but the method is unsuitable for routine assessments.

Inspiratory flow—volume curves. The inspiratory flow—volume curve is nearly symmetrical (Fig. 5.13b, page 116) and its characteristics are adequately described by the forced inspiratory flow rate ($MIF_{50\% \ IVC}$). This is obtained in a similar manner to FIV_1. The $MIF_{50\% \ IVC}$ can replace FIV_1 for assessing possible obstruction to extra-pulmonary airways (page 140) and weakness of the respiratory muscles. It may also have a place in assessing the ventilatory response to exercise.

Assessing bronchodilatation

The extent to which airflow limitation can be reversed by bronchodilator drugs is usually assessed by spirometry. The response can also be assessed in terms of a change in airways resistance measured using whole body plethysmography (page 167) or in exercise capacity (page 433). The drugs which can be used are described on page 639. The underlying pharmacology is considered on page 198, and bronchial hyper-reactivity on pages 174 and 555.

Administering the drug

The drug is usually administered from a pressurised inhaler which delivers a pre-determined dose. The subject should shake the dispenser, exhale to residual volume, insert the nozzle into the open mouth then activate the mechanism whilst at the same time making a full inspiration to total lung capacity at a moderate rate. The inhaler is then withdrawn, the mouth closed and the breath held for as long as is practicable. The procedure is repeated once after a delay of about 1 min. Many patients coming for assessment will have had inhalers prescribed but approximately 30% are likely to use them incorrectly. The assessment provides an opportunity to check the patient's technique and to provide retraining. Use of a placebo inhalant can be a help.

Measuring the response

The acute reversible bronchoconstriction caused by asthma or by inhaled particles is mainly in the trachea and bronchi so the tests used for assessment should be sensitive to airflow resistance at this site. They should also meet the other criteria for suitability given on page 69. Forced expiratory volume (FEV_1) is usually the index chosen. Peak expiratory flow (PEF) is also widely used particularly for serial monitoring (e.g. peak flow chart Fig. 17.6, page 644). The PEF reflects the calibre of large airways but is effort dependent and can be less reproducible than FEV_1. It is also affected by dynamic compression which can be facilitated by the bronchodilatation increasing the compliance of the airway wall; this can give rise to error if the peak flow rate is used for assessment. Greater accuracy can be obtained by expressing the response in terms of airflow resistance measured by whole body plethysmography. If the measurement is made during gentle panting it is relatively independent of dynamic compression but is sensitive to the reduction in functional residual capacity which can accompany bronchodilatation (page 106). The effect of the volume change can be allowed for by expressing the response in terms of specific conductance but this index is only moderately independent of lung volume (Fig. 5.12, page 111). Instead the measurement should be made at several lung volumes and the result at a standard volume obtained by interpolation (page 112). The response of large airways should not be assessed using

$FEV_1\%$ or maximal mid-expiratory flow (MMEF): for these indices the effect of the increase in FVC which accompanies bronchodilatation can nullify that due to an increased airway calibre; the bronchodilator response can then be missed or underestimated (Fig. 6.8). Indices of forced expiratory flow at small lung volumes are also inappropriate because they do not reflect the calibre of larger airways. The ways in which different indices change in response to a change in bronchomotor tone are illustrated in Fig. 6.9.

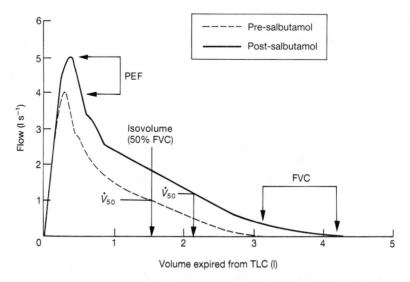

Fig. 6.8 Flow−volume curves before and after inhalation of a bronchodilator aerosol in a patient with airflow limitation which was partly reversible. The response was detected by the PEF, FEV_1 and isovolume $\dot{V}_{50}$ but not $MEF_{50\%\ FVC}$. The Tiffeneau index was more informative in this respect than $FEV_1\%$. The numerical results are given in Table 6.5.

Table 6.5 Effects of salbutamol upon the lung function of the patient with airflow limitation whose maximal expiratory flow−volume curves are given in Fig. 6.8 (male, age 69 years, height 1.84 m, body mass 60 kg).

Index	Before	After	% change*	Reference value
FEV_1 (l)	1.64	2.20	29	3.10
FVC (l)	3.24	4.34	29	4.43
$FEV_1\%$	50.6	50.7	0	66.1
IVC (l)	3.70	4.32	15	4.43
Tiffeneau index	44.3	50.9	16	66.1
PEF (ls^{-1})	4.1	5.1	22	8.9
$MEF_{50\%\ FVC}$ (ls^{-1})	1.0†	1.2	18	3.0
TLC (l)	7.98	7.99	0	7.44
RV (l)	4.28	3.67	−15	2.68
Tl ($mmol\,min^{-1}\,kPa^{-1}$)	9.81	9.84	0	9.5

* expressed as $100 \times \Delta x/\bar{x}$
† Flow at isovolume $1.9\,ls^{-1}$; change in flow at isovolume 62%.

Constriction of small airways occurs with bronchiolitis such as accompanies subacute asthma, most forms of chronic bronchitis, chronic smoking and inhalation of cotton dust or asbestos fibres. The degree of reversibility should be assessed using indices which are sensitive to changes at this site. Again FEV_1 is the first choice because of its reproducibility and sensitivity to narrowing of all classes of airway. $FEV_1\%$ and MMEF should not be used for the reason given above and PEF can be insensitive to narrowing at this site. Forced expiratory flows at small lung volumes are in general, suitable but not when the flows are reported at given percentages of vital capacity (see preceding paragraph). The error can usually be avoided by measuring thoracic gas volume using plethysmography and reporting the change in flow rate at a given lung volume.

Strategy

The procedure for assessing bronchodilatation depends on the objective and the time available for assessment. A casual assessment in a patient

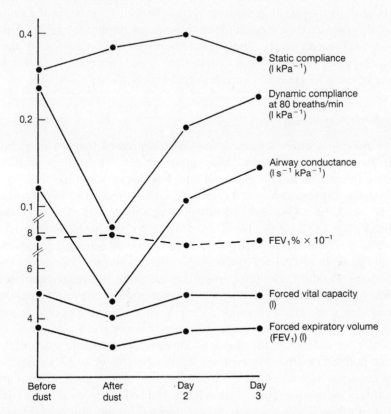

Fig. 6.9 Effect of mild bronchial obstruction caused by inhalation of cotton dust upon the lung function of a healthy subject studied by McDermott and colleagues. In order to illustrate the relative magnitudes of the changes the data are plotted on a semi-log scale.

147

is usually performed at a single session. In this event a positive response is evidence for bronchial lability but a negative response does not exclude this possibility. Greater certainty is achieved by first making baseline measurements over a few days then assessing the response to the drug at more than one time of day. When this is done the time between treatments should be at least 4 h. Serial measurements are essential when the response is not immediate, when the drug can cause euphoria and when the administration is prophylactic. For example, to assess the benefit from steroid drugs the assessment might be performed twice daily for three periods of 7–14 days with the drug administered during the second period only. In the case of prednisone the dose might be 40 mg daily for up to 14 days (page 642). A similar protocol would be suitable for assessing the prophylactic use of sodium cromoglycate (SCG). Alternatively the tests might assess the ability of SCG to prevent bronchoconstriction in response to provocation with a specific antigen; this is considered on page 643. The extent of bronchodilatation is also used to compare the effectiveness of alternative bronchoactive drugs. For this purpose groups of subjects are studied: their airway calibre and bronchomotor tone should be similar at the start of each period of treatment. The response should include the magnitude and the duration of bronchodilatation. Freedman and Hill proposed that this be done by adjusting the dose so that both drugs produce the same initial response, then recording the subsequent amplitude and duration by serial measurements. The measurements should be continued until the response has returned to its control level; this end point should take account of circadian variation (page 555).

Reporting the result

For individual subjects most studies have suggested that the bronchodilator response is related to the result of the test before administration hence the change is a proportional one. For this reason it has traditionally been expressed as the percentage change from the initial value (i.e. $100 . \Delta x / x_1$). Oldham and others have shown that the use of the initial value can lead to bias. This is avoided if the mean level is used instead (i.e. $100 . \Delta x / \bar{x}$, page 59). The proportional model is consistent with the Weber–Fechner psychophysical law relating a stimulus to the resulting sensation. The law implies that the subjective relief associated with bronchodilatation is related to the proportional and not the absolute change in lung function. Thus the proportional model indicates the likely clinical improvement. An improvement greater than 12% is usually an indication for therapy. However, Tweeddale and others have pointed out that the reproducibility of a change of FEV_1 reflects the accuracy with which the FEV_1 can be measured. This is an absolute quantity, independent of the mean level. Hence the presence or absence of a bronchodilator response is best decided by the absolute change. Both approaches have merit. They can be combined by reporting the percentage change in circumstances where the absolute change in FEV_1

exceeds the critical level which Tweeddale and colleagues estimated to be 190 ml. Where this difference is not attained the existence of bronchodilatation is unproven. Adjustment of the response for body size can be achieved by expressing the change as a percentage of the reference value. This has been recommended by Quanjer and colleagues. However, where the patient has some irreversible airflow obstruction the reference value is not a realistic target. A more relevant value is then the maximum observed in remission or the maximum achieved during intensive therapy.

For studies comparing the properties of different drugs the response can be assessed in terms of its peak amplitude, its duration and the area under the response–time curve. Alternatively the curve can be described by an equation which models the biological action of the drug. The response is then described by the coefficients (parameters) of the individual terms as suggested by Oldham and Hughes.

Lung volume

The ventilatory capacity and the ability to exchange gas with the blood are greatly influenced by the volume of the lung. The measurement of lung volume starts with spirometry. This gives the readily accessible subdivisions of total lung capacity but not residual volume. The second stage is the measurement of functional residual capacity from which residual volume can be obtained by subtracting expiratory reserve volume. The FRC is obtained by a closed or open circuit gas dilution method, whole body plethysmography or three-dimensional chest radiography.

Open circuit gas dilution method

Principle. The nitrogen present in the alveolar gas is flushed out of the lung by the subject breathing oxygen; the expired gas is collected and the quantity of nitrogen is determined by analysis. The change in alveolar nitrogen concentration over the period of washout is also measured and these two quantities are used to calculate the lung volume at the start of washout. Allowance is made for nitrogen which enters the lung from the pulmonary capillary blood and lung tissue as soon as the concentration in the alveolar gas becomes less than that in the body. This technique has the advantage of also providing information on the effectiveness of gas mixing in the lung (page 223); it has the disadvantages of requiring both very accurate gas analysis and a standard allowance for nitrogen excretion, which is an average for a number of subjects and does not necessarily apply to individuals. The method is not recommended for routine measurements except where lung-gas mixing is of special interest.

Practical details. The subject should preferably be in a seated upright position, wearing a nose clip and breathing through a mouthpiece and valve box. Oxygen which is nitrogen-free is supplied through a demand system. Usually the expired gas is collected in a Douglas bag or Tissot spirometer but the volume can also be obtained using a pneumotachograph and integrator. The subject makes a full expiration and a sample of alveolar gas is collected for measurement of the initial nitrogen concentration (page 33). The subject is then connected to the oxygen supply at the end of a normal expiration and breathes oxygen for 7 min or until the alveolar nitrogen level has fallen to a fractional concentration of 0.02. At this point a second alveolar sample is obtained and analysed for nitrogen. The analysis is usually done by measuring the fractional concentrations of oxygen and carbon dioxide, then obtaining the nitrogen by difference (cf. Table 3.5, page 34). Alternatively the nitrogen concentration is measured directly using a nitrogen meter or respiratory mass spectrometer. The gas collected during the period of washout is then analysed for nitrogen; the required accuracy is of the order of 0.01% which for an FRC of 3l will result in a measurement error of ±60 ml (±2%). The FRC is calculated as follows:

$$FRC = \frac{(V_E + V_{DS})(F_{E,N_2} - F_{I,N_2})}{F_{A_1,N_2} - F_{A_2,N_2}} - 0.275l \text{ BTPS} \qquad (6.1)$$

where V_E and V_{DS} in l BTPS are the volumes of the gas expired during the period of breathing oxygen and the deadspace of the collecting system, F_{I,N_2} and F_{E,N_2} are the fractional concentrations of nitrogen in the oxygen and in the mixed expired gas and F_{A_1,N_2} and F_{A_2,N_2} refer to the concentrations in the alveolar gas before and at the end of the period of breathing oxygen. The volume of 0.275l is a correction expressed in terms of alveolar gas during breathing air, for the nitrogen that entered the alveoli from the blood during the period of breathing oxygen.

Closed circuit gas dilution method

Principle. The subject rebreathes from a closed circuit spirometer containing some helium or other indicator gas made up in 21% oxygen with the remainder gas nitrogen. During rebreathing the indicator mixes with the alveolar gas hence the spirometer concentration falls whilst the alveolar concentration rises until the two are equal. The dilution of the indicator reflects the ratio of the volume of the spirometer to that of the spirometer plus alveolar gas so if the spirometer volume is known the alveolar volume can be calculated. Helium is commonly used as the indicator because the appropriate analyser (katharometer) is accurate, robust and cheap. The overall accuracy of the method is approximately 2% except in subjects with grossly impaired lung mixing. For such individuals the residual volume is likely to be underestimated compared with the plethysmographic method or by radiography; error can be minimised in the manner described below. This method is recommended for routine use.

Equipment. The method requires a katharometer or other appropriate analyser (see Table 3.5, page 34) and a 9 l spirometer. This is arranged to record on a kymograph and is fitted with a soda-lime canister for absorbing carbon dioxide. The canister should be mounted vertically to ensure uniform distribution of the granules and changed after every 20 determinations or when the CO_2 concentration in the circuit rises above 0.5%. A fan with an output of not less than $180 \, l \, min^{-1}$ (Fig. 6.10) secures both the mixing of the gases and a steady flow through the katharometer; the pressure in the mouthpiece should be atmospheric when the fan is running. When setting up the apparatus the operator should calibrate the spirometer by the method outlined in Table 3.8 on page 52, and then test for leaks by running the kymograph for 20 min with the pump switched on, the mouthpiece occluded and a 1 kg weight placed on the bell. Should outward leakage of gas occur, the source should be traced by the application of soap solution particularly to the shaft of the pump and rim of the soda-lime canister. The linearity of the katharometer should also be confirmed. This is best done by serial dilution of a gas mixture containing helium; the initial concentration should register nearly full-scale deflection on the analyser. The dilution is carried out by one of the methods illustrated in Fig. 3.8 (page 49) and the precautions to be taken when using a katharometer

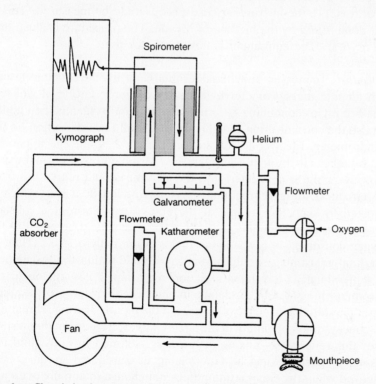

Fig. 6.10 Closed circuit apparatus for the measurement of total lung capacity and its subdivisions. The apparatus may be combined with that for measurement of the transfer factor (see Fig. 10.1, page 305).

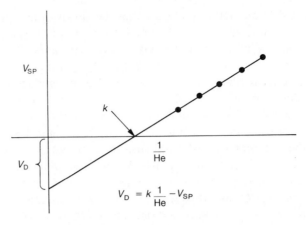

$$V_D = k \frac{1}{He} - V_{SP}$$

Fig. 6.11 Procedure for measuring the deadspace of the closed circuit apparatus. Starting with the apparatus full of air and the spirometer bell depressed, helium is added until almost full-scale deflection is registered on the katharometer. The gas in the apparatus is then diluted progressively with air in increments of 0.5 l. During dilution the volume of gas in the spirometer (V_{SP}) is plotted against the reciprocal of the concentration of helium ($1/He$). The relationship should be linear. The deadspace of the apparatus (V_D) is numerically equal to the intercept on the Y axis when $1/He$ is zero.

are considered on page 304. Once the spirometer and helium katharometer have been calibrated the volume of gas in the closed circuit apparatus, i.e. the instrument deadspace, should be measured. This is best done *in situ* by the method of Meade. The procedure is illustrated in Fig. 6.11. The equipment is now ready for use.

Procedure. To measure functional residual capacity, the circuit is flushed with air and the spirometer bell set at an appropriate level which is usually 2 l. Gas containing 80% helium and 20% oxygen is then added to raise the concentration of helium to near full-scale deflection on the katharometer. Meanwhile the subject is seated beside the apparatus and breathes air through a mouthpiece. At the end of a normal expiration he or she is connected into the spirometer and rebreathes from the circuit. During rebreathing oxygen is added at a rate which is adjusted to keep the volume at the end of expiration at a constant level; this can be done automatically. The rate should be equal to the oxygen consumption of the subject; this is normally $0.2-0.25 \, l \, min^{-1}$. The final adjustment should normally be made within the first minute of rebreathing as any later variation may impair gas mixing in the spirometer lung system. A change in end-expiratory level of the spirometer may also be evidence of leakage at the mouth. During rebreathing the concentration of helium in the circuit falls at a steady but diminishing rate; this reflects gas mixing in the lung, solution in body fluid and passage into the stomach. Gas mixing is considered to have been achieved when the concentration does not change materially over 30 s. This point is reached within 5 min in healthy subjects and up to 20 min in patients with emphysema.

Subsequently additional air may need to be introduced into the spirometer. The subject is asked to make a forced expiration to residual volume and then, after a few tidal breaths, a full inspiration to total lung capacity. This manoeuvre is then repeated twice without the tidal breaths. In each case the operator urges the subject to maximal effort. When this instruction is obeyed the movement of the spirometer bell, as recorded on the kymograph, will be seen to move to the new position exponentially and not abruptly. The volume of gas at BTPS which can be expired by the subject from the resting respiratory level is the expiratory reserve volume. The volume of gas inspired from the resting level is the inspiratory capacity; it is the sum of tidal volume and inspiratory reserve volume (Fig. 5.11, page 105). These volumes together make up the two stage vital capacity. The inspiratory vital capacity is also recorded.

The functional residual capacity is given by:

$$FRC = V(He_1 - He_2)/He_2 \text{ l BTPS} \tag{6.2}$$

where FRC is functional residual capacity and V is volume of gas in the circuit (both in l BTPS) and He_1 and He_2 are initial and final concentrations of helium. The latter is the concentration at the end of rebreathing except when no plateau has been reached. If this is due to an inadequate oxygen flow rate the correct concentration can sometimes be estimated from the graph relating helium concentration to time by backward extrapolation of the curve to zero time. However, the procedure is not always reliable. Equation 6.2 neglects any displacement of the volume axis which may arise from the subject being switched into the breathing circuit at a volume other than FRC or from a change in resting respiratory level during rebreathing. The displacement can readily be allowed for. In addition a correction is needed because the gas in the spirometer is at ambient temperature and pressure (ATPS). For a spirometer temperature of $t°C$, a barometric pressure of P_B and a water-vapour pressure at $t°C$ of $P_{H_2O}(t)$, the functional residual capacity may be calculated as follows:

$$FRC = \left(\frac{He_1}{He_2} (V_1 + DS) - (V_2 + DS) \right) \times \frac{310}{273 + t}$$
$$\times \frac{P_B - P_{H_2O}(t)}{P_B - P_{H_2O}(37)} \text{ l BTPS} \tag{6.3}$$

where V_1 and V_2 are the volume of gas in the spirometer at switch in and at equilibrium and DS is the deadspace of the closed circuit apparatus. The total lung capacity and its other subdivisions are then obtained in the manner shown in Fig. 5.11 (page 105).

Alternative gas dilution methods. During respiratory surveys there may be insufficient time or laboratory space for the closed circuit measurement of lung volume. However, if the subjects have relatively normal lungs, the lung volumes can be estimated using single breath or forced rebreathing techniques. The single breath measurement is usually made in conjunction with either a single breath test of lung mixing for example the single breath nitrogen test, or the single breath measurement of transfer factor; the procedures are described respectively on pages 214 and 310. These methods underestimate the lung volume in subjects with airflow limitation, the underestimation being less in the case of the transfer measurement which entails breath holding than the mixing test which does not. Van Ganse and colleagues have suggested that the underestimation can be allowed for empirically but the correction is inevitably approximate. Greater accuracy can be secured by the forced rebreathing technique.

Forced rebreathing technique. In the version of Wilmore as modified by Sterk and colleagues the subject exhales to residual volume and is then connected to a bag-in-bottle system which is completely filled with 6–8 l of 100% oxygen. The subject inhales slowly to total lung capacity, exhales slowly to residual volume then takes eight deep breaths each of duration 2 s. During rebreathing the flow rate is monitored with a heated pneumotachograph, volume is measured with a spirometer and nitrogen concentration at the mouth using a nitrogen analyser or respiratory mass spectrometer. The residual volume is calculated per breath for the last three breaths and the value at breath number 7.5 obtained by interpolation. Residual volume is given by:

$$RVn = V_B F_{B,N_2}/(F_{A,N_2} - F_{B,N_2}) + V_I - VCmax \qquad (6.4)$$

where RVn is residual volume at breath n, F_{B,N_2} and F_{A,N_2} are fractional concentrations of nitrogen respectively in the bag (measured during inspiration) and alveolar gas when breathing air. V_B, V_I and VCmax are respectively the volume of oxygen, inspired volume and vital capacity, all at body temperature saturated with water vapour. F_{A,N_2} is obtained from mean expired nitrogen concentration (area under the expired concentration volume curve divided by expired volume) corrected for anatomical deadspace (i.e. $F_{E,N_2}.Vt/(Vt - Vad)$ where F_{E,N_2} is mean expired nitrogen concentration, Vt is tidal volume and Vad is anatomical deadspace). The within subject coefficient of variation is reported as 7.7%. The method requires practice. It is suitable for healthy subjects and for use in respiratory surveys but not for patients with impaired lung mixing.

Air trapping. In a normal subject after a full inspiration the respiration returns immediately to its previous pattern; however, in a patient with narrowing of the lung airways the resting respiratory level may remain elevated for several breaths. This phenomenon, which is illustrated in Fig. 6.12, is due to the trapping of gas behind small airways which were opened during the forced inspiration and then closed prematurely during the subsequent expiration. The closure may be due to a diminution in the elastic recoil of the lung tissue or to surface forces acting on the airways.

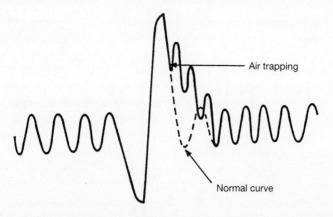

Air trapping

Normal curve

Fig. 6.12 Spirogram illustrating air trapping during measurement of the total lung capacity by the closed circuit method. After a full inspiration the spirogram returns gradually over a series of breaths to its previous level. In this it differs from the spirogram for a healthy subject where the return is immediate. Trace reads from left to right with inspiration upwards.

Radiographic method for total lung capacity

Principle

The thoracic cavity is subdivided into a number of horizontal slices whose width and depth are obtained by measurement of postero-anterior and left lateral chest radiographs. The radiographs are taken at full inspiration. The volume of each slice is calculated from the thickness of the slice and the appropriate width and depth measurements; the latter are corrected for magnification due to the film being a finite distance from the centre of the thorax. The slice volumes are summed to give a total cavity volume from which lung volume is obtained by subtracting the volume of the heart and other structures.

Practical details

The basic method is that of Barnhard and colleagues and is performed manually. The slices are considered to be elliptical cylinders for which the volume is given by:

$$\text{slice vol.} = 0.25\pi \times \text{width} \times \text{depth} \times \text{thickness} \qquad (6.5)$$

Five slices are used and their limits are given in Fig. 6.13. The heart is considered as a whole ellipsoid; the appropriate dimensions and equation for calculating its volume are given on page 250. The space beneath the dome of each half of the diaphragm (Vsd) is treated as one-eighth of an ellipsoid. Its volume is given by:

$$V\text{sd} = 0.13\pi \times \text{width} \times \text{depth} \times \text{height} \qquad (6.6)$$

where the width and depth are taken from line vi in Fig. 6.13 (i.e. r_1 and r_3) and the height is the vertical distance from the line to the appropriate cardio-phrenic angle i.e. r_2(R) and r_2(L).

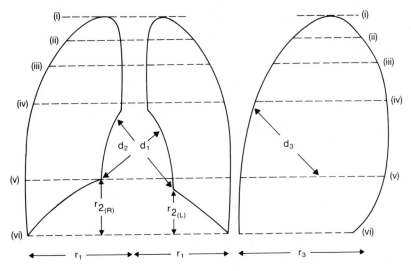

Fig. 6.13 Measurements used for calculation of radiographic lung volume by the method of Barnhard. The distances (i–ii) and (ii–iii) are each 2.5 cm. (v) is at the upper border of diaphragm and vi between the two costophrenic angles. (iv) is midway between (iii and v). d2 and d3 are respectively at right angles to and parallel with d1 which terminates at the junction of the right atrium with the left border of the heart; within these constraints all three are maximal intra-cardiac dimensions. (Source: O'Shea J, Lapp NL, Russakoff AD *et al. Thorax* 1970; **25**: 544–549.)

In more sophisticated versions of the method the radiographs are marked by hand then scanned and the coordinates of successive points fed into a computer. The method of Pierce and colleagues uses 200 slices and their area is taken as one-third way between an elipse and the enclosing rectangle. As well as the heart and sub-diaphragmatic regions the thoracic structures include the arch of the aorta and the vertebral column. The contribution to the slice cross-sectional area of each of these structures is considered to be elliptical. The method has an average accuracy of ±0.2l, when compared with plethysmography.

Whole body plethysmography

Introduction

The whole body plethysmograph is an air-tight box made of transparent plastic in which the subject sits. It can provide instantaneous values for the volume of gas in the thorax and intra-alveolar pressure. The method was developed for measurement of airway resistance by Comroe, Botelho and DuBois and used subsequently for measurement of lung volumes and construction of flow–volume curves based on thoracic gas volume. Curves obtained in this way are free from the effects of compression of intrathoracic gas, which can distort flow–volume curves based on the volume of air expired (see page 142). The plethysmograph lung volume differs from that measured by gas dilution by including any non-ventilated spaces, for example large emphysematous bullae. It

156

also includes intestinal gas; however, the error on this account is small. The method is accurate but technically demanding. It is an essential tool for the study of lung mechanics and can monitor uptake of a soluble gas for measurement of cardiac output (page 246).

The plethysmograph can be either of constant volume when the measurement is of pressure change or of constant pressure when the measurement is of volume change. These two quantities are reciprocally related through Boyle's Law which is described below.

The *constant volume plethysmograph* is also called a pressure plethysmograph. It is used for measurement of airways resistance and thoracic gas volume. The system has a high frequency response and can also be used to record gas uptake over fractions of the cardiac cycle (page 246) and hence cardiac output. The *constant pressure plethysmograph* which is also called a volume displacement plethysmograph, was designed by Mead; here the volume change is monitored using a spirometer or obtained by integration of the signal from a large pneumotachograph in the wall of the box. The spirometer should preferably have a high frequency response and the connection should have a large diameter so as not to introduce a resistance artefact. Electronic compensation for phase lag in the system is provided by a signal proportional to the box pressure. The volume displacement plethysmograph is used for delineation of flow−volume curves and also for measuring thoracic gas volume.

The principal source of error is from the air in the plethysmograph changing in humidity or in temperature during the procedure. The error can be minimised in one of the ways given below. Error can also arise if the amount of carbon dioxide which is evolved differs from the amount of oxygen which is absorbed; the effect of this is usually small. In addition in patients with airflow obstruction the transmision of alveolar pressure to the mouth can be impaired. This can lead to material overestimation of thoracic gas volume and underestimation of airway resistance.

Plethysmograph method for lung volume

Boyle's law states that if a given mass of gas is compressed at constant temperature, the product of pressure (P) and volume (V) is constant. This relationship can be applied to the lung when the subject is enclosed in a whole body plethysmograph. The equipment is illustrated in Fig. 6.14. An important feature is a shutter which can be actuated by remote control to stop the airflow. The pressure and the volume of gas in the lung are varied by the subject making inspiratory and expiratory efforts against the shutter with the glottis open. In these circumstances the following relationship applies:

$$PV = (P + \Delta P)(V - \Delta V) \qquad (6.7)$$

where P is alveolar pressure and ΔP is the change in pressure during panting against the shutter; V is the thoracic gas volume and ΔV is the

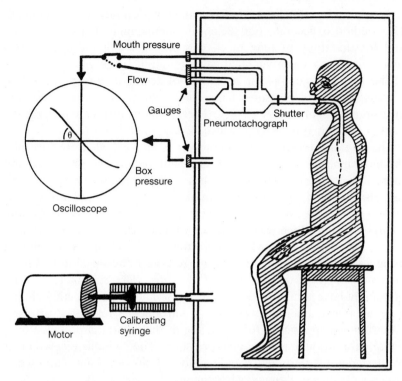

Fig. 6.14 Body plethysmograph (constant volume) and ancillary equipment for measuring the thoracic gas volume and airway resistance. The volume of the plethysmograph is about 700 l and full-scale deflection on the oscilloscope is obtained with a change in volume of 70 ml, equivalent to a change in pressure of 10 Pa (0.1 cmH$_2$O). Tan θ is the pressure in the mouth during panting against the closed shutter expressed as a fraction of the pressure in the box. For calculation of thoracic gas volume tan θ is compared with the ratio of the signal due to movement of the calibrating syringe to the pressure in the box. For measurement of airway resistance tan θ is compared with the ratio of the signal from the pneumotachograph during gentle panting with the mouth open to the pressure in the box.

change in volume due to compression of the chest by the respiratory muscles when the airway is obstructed. When the terms within the brackets are multiplied, the product $\Delta P. \ \Delta V$ is small relative to the other terms, so may be neglected. The error this introduces is equal to ΔV. The relationship then simplifies to:

$$V = P \ \Delta V / \Delta P \qquad (6.8)$$

Because water vapour condenses when compressed, its pressure remains constant and it does not influence the result. Hence the alveolar pressure (P) is effectively the barometric pressure less the pressure of water vapour in the lung (i.e. $P_B - P_{H_2O}$ at 37°C). The change in the alveolar pressure during panting against the shutter (i.e. ΔP cmH$_2$O), is measured with a pressure transducer; this is arranged to record the pressure in the mouth which, when the movement of air is stopped by the shutter, is equal to that in the alveoli. The change in the volume of the lung (ΔV) is measured indirectly from the change in the pressure of the air in the plethysmograph. The conversion of pressure change to volume change is calibrated by injecting a known volume (about 50 ml) of air into the plethysmograph and recording the ensuing rise in pressure within the box.

In practice, when the subject enters the plethysmograph the temperature of the air rises; it causes a rise in the pressure in the box which is released by opening a port to atmosphere. The subject breathes quietly through the pneumotachograph until, at the end of a normal expiration, the operator actuates the shutter to block off the mouthpiece and at the same time closes the port which permits the equalisation of pressure between the box and atmosphere. The subject pants against the shutter with the cheeks supported by the hands to minimise any change in volume of the buccal cavity. The mouth pressure and the box pressure are displayed on the two axes of the oscilloscope in the manner illustrated in Fig. 6.14 and the angle θ is recorded. Then provided the two manometers have similar calibrations:

$$\tan \theta = \Delta P / \Delta P\text{box} \qquad (6.9)$$

where $\Delta P\text{box}$ is the change in pressure in the plethysmograph. If the calibrations differ a calibration factor will be required.

The relationship of the pressure in the plethysmograph to the volume of air which it contains is next determined separately by noting the change in pressure which occurs when a measured volume of air is displaced into and out of the box by a calibrated syringe of capacity 50 ml (0.05 l); this is illustrated in Fig. 6.14. The calibration is usually performed when the plethysmograph is empty but it should be noted that the procedure then introduces a small error due to the assumption that the changes in the box are isothermal (i.e. obey Boyle's law) when they are in fact adiabatic. This error is avoided if the subject remains in the box during the calibration. In either event the box pressure with respect to atmospheric pressure and the syringe volume are displayed respectively on the horizontal and the vertical axes of the oscilloscope, and the coefficient of proportionality, which is the tangent of the angle to the horizontal, is obtained. This coefficient (S_1) is the change in the volume of the air in the box per unit deflection on the pressure recorder (i.e. $\Delta V / \Delta P\text{box}$). In the absence of a subject it applies to the empty plethysmograph but may be adjusted to the smaller volume of air due to the presence of a subject in the box by means of the following relationship:

$$S_2 = S_1(V\text{box} - W/1.07)/V\text{box} \qquad (6.10)$$

where S_1 and S_2 are the initial and corrected coefficients of proportionality, $V\text{box}$ is the volume of the plethysmograph in litres, W is the body weight of the subject in kilograms and the factor 1.07 is the average density of the human body. From these data the thoracic gas volume (V) is calculated as follows:

$$V = (P\text{B} - P_{H_2O} \text{ at } 37°C) \, S_2/\tan \theta \times \text{BTPS correction} \qquad (6.11)$$

The measurement of the thoracic gas volume requires only about 10 min of the subject's time and is readily performed when the airway resistance is recorded (see page 167). The residual volume and the total lung capacity can then be obtained by spirometry performed immediately after the period of panting. To this end the expiratory reserve volume and inspiratory capacity are measured and respectively subtracted from and added to the thoracic gas volume. For subjects with normal lungs the residual volume is numerically equal to that recorded by the closed circuit helium dilution method. However, in the presence of airway obstruction a larger volume may be obtained by plethysmography because the method registers gas in non-ventilated parts of the lung, and the mouth pressure which is recorded may be lower than of that in the alveoli (page 183).

Oesophageal pressure

Introduction

Measurement of compliance and recoil pressure require knowledge of the pressure difference across the lung between the alveoli, where the pressure is effectively atmospheric, and the pleural space. The lung has a density of approximately $0.2\,g\,ml^{-1}$; consequently the pressure in the pleural space is less negative at the base of the lung than at the apex. When the subject is seated the pressure gradient between these points is approximately $0.5\,kPa$ ($5\,cmH_2O$). An average pressure may be obtained by inducing a small artificial pneumothorax then measuring the pressure directly. However, the induction may itself affect the pressure and on ethical grounds it is only justifiable if the pleura is to be canulated for medical reasons. The pleural pressure is transmitted to the oesophagus so in favourable circumstances oesophageal pressure can be used instead. Ideally the site of measurement should be at the level of the middle of the lung. Difficulty arises when the tone of the oesophageal wall is increased, or there is peristalsis, or the oesophagus is compressed by the heart or affected by pulsations transmitted from it. Oesophageal peristalsis occurs during swallowing and in proximity to the times of meals and the cardiac artefact is increased by a supine posture; accordingly a time remote from meals and an upright posture are recommended.

Procedure. Oesophageal pressure relative to mouth pressure is measured using a differential pressure transducer of small internal volume (Chapter 3). The transducer is connected to an air-filled polythylene tube of internal diameter 1–1.5 mm which is passed through the nose or mouth. To obtain a representative pressure the end of the tube is surrounded by a flexible Latex rubber balloon. The optimal balloon dimensions are: length 10 cm, diameter 1 cm, and wall thickness 0.06 mm. It should be tapered at its upper end to fit closely round the tube which should be perforated near to this point. On distension to a

volume of 6 ml there should be no measurable back pressure. The
balloon should contain 0.4 ml of air. This is injected from a syringe
before or after the balloon is inserted. The pressure which is measured
is that at the site of the air bubble, usually the upper end of the
balloon. As an alternative to a balloon the tube can be filled with
water. The system then has a more rapid frequency response but is
liable to error due to hydrostatic forces and to the pressure being
measured at only a single point. In addition, the presence of water in
the oesophagus may provoke peristalsis.

To insert the balloon into the oesophagus the operator first establishes
which of the subject's nostrils is widest by asking him to sniff through
each in turn; then if a local anaesthetic is to be used, inquiry is made
into previous drug sensitivity. The dose is 1 ml of 3% lignocaine
hydrochloride solution (Xylocaine) administered through a spray fitted
with a long nozzle; the spray is directed to both the front and back of
the nasopharynx and 5 min are allowed for the anaesthetic to exert its
effect. However, anaesthesia is seldom necessary. To make the insertion
the operator faces the subject who sits with the neck slightly flexed.
The operator lubricates the balloon with a tasteless lubricant (e.g.
K-Y, Johnson and Johnson), and passes it gently into the nose whilst
the subject makes a series of swallowing manoeuvres. Swallowing is
assisted by having the subject suck up water from a glass through a
flexible drinking straw which is held between the lips. The tube should
now descend into the oesophagus. This should be checked by seeing
that the tube has passed over the back of the tongue and is not coiled
in the nasopharynx as sometimes occurs when a very flexible tube is
employed. Swallowing is continued until the balloon comes to lie in the
stomach, where its presence is confirmed by the response to sniffing
which should cause a rise in the pressure in the tube. The tube is now
withdrawn 10 cm or more into the oesophagus where sniffing causes a
fall rather than a rise in the pressure. The balloon is too high if at
constant lung volume the recorded pressure is affected by the subject
performing a forced expiratory or inspiratory manoeuvre against a
closed mouthpiece or moving the neck, or by the observer pressing on
the suprasternal notch. Placement is satisfactory when a respiratory
rhythm is obtained which is not obscured by pressure fluctuations
transmitted from the heart. The main source of error is tonic contraction
of the oesophageal muscle. This is particularly liable to occur at near
to total lung capacity and is best overcome by waiting. Peristaltic
contractions have a duration of between 2 and 5 s and occur especially
in the lower part of the oesophagus; they may be identified by monitoring the pressure on an oscilloscope. Contractions due to the procedure
usually disappear within a few minutes. Those due to hunger may be
alleviated by a cup of tea.

Lung compliance

The compliance of the lung is the change in volume in l BTPS per unit change in pressure gradient between the pleura and the alveoli. It can be measured during breath-holding or a very slow expiration, when it is static compliance (page 96), or during regular breathing, when it is dynamic compliance. The latter index is influenced by the airway resistance (page 165). The change in volume is measured with a spiro-meter or by integration of the output from a pneumotachograph. The change in pleural pressure is measured indirectly from the oesophagus (see above). The alternative proposed by Bevan of using the supra-sternal notch as a null point indicator proved not to be successful.

Static compliance

Outline. Static compliance is obtained from consecutive measurements of oesophageal pressure and mouth pressure at a number of lung volumes throughout inspiration and expiration, starting from residual volume. The test breath is preceded by one or two full inspirations to total lung capacity; these prevent closure of some airways which might otherwise influence the result. The volume steps are made by closing the airways with a shutter for periods of about 1 s at intervals of approximately 500 ml; during interruption the subject should not breathe but relax against the shutter. Provided that the glottis is open when the flow of gas is interrupted, equalisation of pressure occurs between the alveoli and the mouth; this is usually complete within 0.4 s. However, particularly at near to total lung capacity a time of 2 or 3 s may be required for the elastic recoil of the lung to accommodate to the change of volume.

Practical details. Pressure and volume are plotted in the form of a volume–pressure diagram such as that illustrated in Fig. 5.7 (page 96). The compliance is the slope of the middle linear part of the tracing; it is usually measured over 1 l starting from functional residual capacity. The pressure difference across the lung is obtained by using a differential manometer to subtract mouth pressure from oesophageal pressure. The conditions are static so the recording equipment can have a relatively slow response time, for example a water manometer of small bore and recording spirometer. However, the procedure is simplified by using a differential electromanometer, and a twin coordi-nate chart recorder, in which the volume and the pressure are displayed on two axes at right angles. The record can be analysed directly provided there are no artefacts due to cardiac systole. These are best avoided by synchronising the periods of recording to follow the R wave of the ECG. Alternatively, the pressure fluctuations due to cardiac systole can be identified by the oesophageal pressure being recorded against time during periods when the airway is occluded by the shutter (see Fig. 6.15). Compliance (slope) is measured for inspiration and expiration separately but the latter is usually reported because it is not as affected by hysteresis (page 99). The pressure–volume diagram is

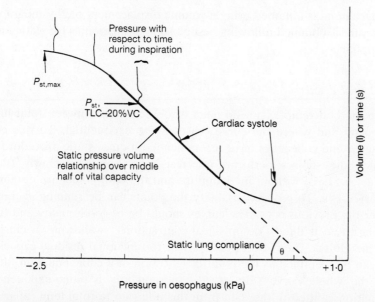

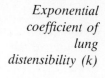

Fig. 6.15 Method for measuring static lung compliance using an interrupter and $X-Y$ recorder developed by Hart, McKerrow and Reynolds. The shutter which interrupts the subject's airflow during slow inspiration or expiration is actuated for alternate periods of 1 s. After each interruption there is an interval of 0.4 s before the pen makes contact with the recorder paper; during the next 0.6 s pressure is recorded on the X axis. On the Y axis volume is recorded at the instant when the pen touches the paper; the time is recorded for the remainder of each interruption. The static lung compliance is the slope of the line joining the starting points of the tracings, except when these are deflected by pressure fluctuations due to cardiac systole. The fluctuations may be detected by inspection of the record and an appropriate allowance made. Pst is the elastic recoil pressure of the lung.

also used to obtain the elastic recoil of the lung. This can be reported for inspiration and expiration separately at a lung volume 1 l or 20% below total lung capacity; alternatively the lung volume can be reported at a standard transpulmonary pressure, for example 0.5 kPa. The maximal recoil pressure at total lung capacity is also reported; it has the disadvantage of being rather variable, except when measured with the subject relaxing against the closed shutter. During the procedure the additional measurement of the rate of airflow immediately prior to interruption permits the calculation of pulmonary resistance and hence the relationship of pulmonary conductance to lung recoil pressure (page 112).

Exponential coefficient of lung distensibility (k)

Outline

The index (k) is the exponent in the equation used to describe the shape of the upper part of the static volume–pressure curve (equation 5.1, page 100). The volume is expressed as percentage of total lung capacity and is obtained using a volume displacement plethysmograph. Pressure is obtained following oesophageal intubation as for static lung compliance.

Practical details

The method requires 30−40 pairs of observations between total lung capacity and where the curve ceases to be exponential. To this end Gugger and colleagues have recommended a quasi-static procedure in which the subject performs the test expiration very slowly (flow rate $< 0.21s^{-1}$) without interruptions and the data points are obtained every 0.25 s. To reduce variability the points can be running averages over the previous 0.5 s. The curves should be of good quality and free from artefacts due to oesophageal contractions, swallowing or closure of the glottis. The cut-off point is near to functional residual capacity. It can be identified as the point of inflection of a cubic equation fitted to the whole curve (Fig. 6.16). Subsequently a mono-exponential equation is fitted to the data from this point up to total lung capacity. The residual variance above the curve expressed as a percentage of the total variance for volume over the range used should not exceed 10%.

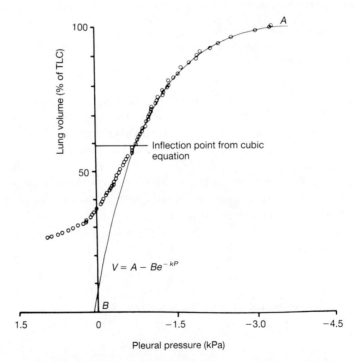

Fig. 6.16 Quasi-static PV curve from a normal subject in the units % TLC and kPa. Data points are those actually collected. The continuous line is an exponential curve fitted to the data above the inflection point. $k = 0.120$. (Source: Gugger M, Wraith PK, Sudlow MF. *Clin Sci* 1990; **78**: 365−369.)

Comment

The procedure is technically demanding. In additional falsely low values for k are obtained if airways close during the test expiration. The main use is for study of early emphysema. Some evidence is provided by Osborne and colleagues.

Dynamic compliance

Outline

Dynamic compliance differs from the static compliance in that the measurement is made during tidal breathing. Under these circumstances the relationship between lung volume and pressure is not a single line as in Fig. 5.7 (page 96) but takes the form of an ellipse (see Fig. 5.18, page 127). The linear relationship represents the force which is required to overcome surface tension and the elastic recoil of the lung tissue; the curvilinearity is due to the additional force which is needed under dynamic conditions to overcome the resistance to movement of both lung tissue and gas in the airways. At respiratory frequencies of the order of 90 per min the inertia of the gas in the lungs also contributes to the curvilinearity. The resistive component of the applied force is assumed to be zero when the lung is stationary at the time of the change from inspiration to expiration and again at the end of expiration, i.e. the points A and C in Fig. 5.18. The pressure swing, between the two points of zero flow, is accurately mirrored by the pressure swing in the oesophagus, provided there is little or no airways obstruction to cause internal movement of air within the lung (page 182). The dynamic compliance is the slope of the line ABC in the diagram.

Practical details

To make the measurement, the pressure is measured by a trans-ducer having a high frequency response and a range of $0-5.0\,kPa$ $(0-50\,cmH_2O)$; the volume is measured with either a spirometer, which is modified by the connection of a potentiometer to the axle of the pulley wheel, or a pneumotachograph fitted with electronic inte-gration, or a plethysmograph. The pressure and volume channels should be in phase and the dynamic responses of the volume and pressure transducers should be similar. The pressure and volume are displayed synchronously on the two axes of an oscilloscope or X−Y recorder. For convenience of measurement the oscilloscope beam is automatically brightened or a mark is made on the pressure trace at times when the flow is zero. The slope of the line through the points of zero flow on the diagram can be estimated approximately by eye with the aid of a protractor. For greater accuracy the component of pressure which is applied to overcome the lung resistance is eliminated by electronic means. During very quiet breathing (i.e. in the absence of turbulence)

165

this is done using the proportional relationship which exists between the velocity of airflow and the resistive pressure. The pressure record on the oscilloscope is backed off by an amount proportional to the velocity of airflow, which, in turn, is obtained from the output of the pneumotachograph before integration. In this way the short axis of the volume−pressure ellipse (Insp-B-Exp. in the diagram) is narrowed down to a straight line. Alternatively the dynamic compliance can be obtained during the measurement of the pulmonary resistance by the pressure−flow method (page 171).

The measurement of dynamic compliance is normally made during slow quiet breathing when the resistive component of the pressure swing is minimal. The resistive component can be increased by performing the measurement at imposed breathing frequencies up to 60 per min. In the presence of airway obstruction the dynamic compliance falls as the frequency is increased. This *frequency dependence of compliance* can provide evidence for narrowing of small lung airways. To avoid technical artefacts the tidal volume and the resting respiratory level must be kept constant. To obtain the change with frequency the dynamic compliance at each frequency is expressed as a percentage of the static compliance.

Lung resistance

Introduction

The total lung resistance (Rl), which is the driving pressure divided by the flow rate, is equivalent to the pressure difference between the pleural surface of the lung and the mouth when the flow rate at the lips is $1 ls^{-1}$. It is the sum of the airway resistance (Raw) and the tissue resistance (Rti) for which the corresponding driving pressures are the pressure gradients between the alveoli and the mouth and between the pleura and the alveoli. Thus:

$$Rl = Raw + Rti \qquad (5.7)$$

The indices are calculated from measurements of velocity of air flow at the lips ($\dot{v}$) and pleural or alveolar pressure relative to pressure at the mouth (Ppl and PA respectively). For laminar flow, such as occurs when velocity is less than $0.5 ls^{-1}$, the relationship can be written in the form:

$$Ppl/\dot{v} = PA/\dot{v} + (Ppl - PA)/\dot{v} \qquad (6.12)$$

Velocity is measured with a pneumotachograph (page 27). Pressure at the pleural surface of the lung is measured in the oesophagus; alveolar pressure is measured either at the mouth after interruption of the air stream or by application of Boyle's law using a body plethysmograph. These techniques form the basis for three distinct methods of estimating the lung resistance. The relationships between them are indicated in Table 5.4 (page 109). In addition, the total thoracic resistance which includes the resistance of the chest wall (see equation 5.5, page 108), may be obtained by the method of forced oscillation, in which the pressure at the mouth is measured during the imposition of small cyclical fluctuations in lung volume; these are produced by a sine-wave pump or a loudspeaker diaphragm which is arranged to oscillate at the resonant frequency of the thorax.

Lung resistance is usually reported in the units of resistance (i.e. kPa or $cmH_2Ol^{-1}s$). However, the reciprocal of the resistance, which is the conductance (G), is often preferable because it is almost linearly related to the thoracic gas volume (page 110) and transpulmonary pressure. The conductance is often expressed per litre of the thoracic gas volume when it is called specific conductance (sG). The term specific resistance sRaw is also used.

Plethysmography is the best way of measuring airway resistance because it is accurate, acceptable to most subjects and in addition yields thoracic gas volume; the latter is necessary for interpreting resistance measurements. Knowledge of thoracic gas volume also has other uses (see for example page 537). Total thoracic resistance measured by forced oscillation can monitor rapid changes in airway calibre — for example those due to bronchodilatation or bronchial provocation. The technique does not require the active co-operation of the subject so is suitable for young children and during anaesthesia. However, the method is technically demanding, and it is subject to error caused by the mouth and pharynx absorbing some of the imposed oscillation. There is no concurrent estimate of thoracic gas volume. This is also a defect of the classical pressure—flow method of measuring pulmonary resistance, a method which involves oesophageal intubation; however, both methods can be applied in the absence of a plethysmograph. The interrupter method is a less sensitive guide to airways obstruction than the other methods, but has the advantage, for surveys, that it is readily portable.

Plethysmographic method

Outline. This method requires a body plethysmograph (see page 156), pneumotachograph and pressure recorder and a mouthpiece fitted with a shutter which can be operated by remote control. These items of equipment are also used for the estimation of the thoracic gas volume; they are illustrated in Fig. 6.14, which shows a constant volume plethysmograph. The method using a constant pressure plethysmograph is essentially similar. When the subject is seated in the constant volume plethysmograph the pressure within it fluctuates through the respiratory cycle. This is because the driving pressure required to force the alveolar air through the airways affects the alveolar volume. On inspiration the volume increases and on expiration it decreases; these changes respectively compress and expand the air in the plethysmograph. The greater the airway resistance the greater are the pressure swings in both the chest and the plethysmograph. With suitable calibration the alveolar pressures can be obtained from the box pressures. The calibration factor is the relationship between the two pressures. It is determined in the absence of air flow so is not subject to the errors which affect the measurement of alveolar pressure by the interrupter method. It therefore provides a true measure of the airway resistance which is usually obtained during panting. This pattern of breathing is adopted to minimise heating and cooling of the respired gas during breathing through the pneumotachograph. Alternatively the need for panting can be reduced by the provision of air which has been heated to 37°C and saturated with water vapour. The measurement may then be made during quiet breathing. This procedure is more acceptable for the subject, but is associated with material loss of sensitivity in detecting changes in airway resistance because the resistance of the larynx is relatively larger and more variable in these circumstances than during panting. The airway resistance should be related to the lung volume or the transpulmonary pressure at the time of measurement (see Fig. 5.12 and page 111); the volume is also measured in the plethysmograph (page 157).

Practical details. The pressure transducers should be capable of measuring accurately variations of the order of 10^{-3} kPa. They should be in phase and the frequency responses should be at least 10 Hz (page 24). Calibrations should be performed in relation to each batch of measurements and the appropriate calibration factor should be used in the calculation. The relationship of alveolar pressure to box pressure is obtained whilst the subject performs gentle panting movements against the closed shutter. In these circumstances, because of the absence of flow, the pressure is nearly uniform throughout the respiratory tract, so can be measured at the mouth. This pressure and the pressure which is measured simultaneously in the box are displayed on the axes of a cathode-ray oscilloscope or twin co-ordinate chart recorder; the slope of the resulting diagram (tan θ in Fig. 6.14) is the ratio of the change in alveolar pressure to the change in box pressure ($\Delta Pa/\Delta Pbox$). The measurement of box pressure is repeated with the shutter open whilst the subject pants gently and shallowly through the pneumotachograph at flow rates of between 0 and $0.5 ls^{-1}$. The pressure and the output from the pneumotachograph are displayed as before and the slope of the relationship is again determined ($\dot{v}/\Delta Pbox$). The airway resistance (*Raw*) is obtained from the ratio of the two slopes in the following manner:

$$Raw = \frac{\Delta Pa}{\Delta Pbox} \times \frac{\Delta Pbox}{\dot{v}} \text{ kPa (or cmH}_2\text{O)l}^{-1}\text{s} \qquad (6.13)$$

The airway resistance is usually measured at a flow rate of $0.5 ls^{-1}$ but a flow rate of $1 ls^{-1}$ is sometimes adopted. During inspiration the resistances at the two flow rates are, in practice, similar; during expiration the resistance is higher at the higher flow rate because the air flow is partly turbulent and the lung volume is changing. An allowance can be made for the latter factor when the relationship of airway resistance to lung volume is known. However, the airway resistance during expiration is also affected by the rise in intrapleural pressure (see page 112); the effect of this factor is minimised by the subject performing the panting manoeuvre as gently and shallowly as possible; the frequency of panting should be less than $1\,Hz$ and the expiratory flow rate should not exceed $0.5\,\mathrm{l\,s^{-1}}$. A satisfactory result is then obtained in the majority of subjects, even though they have no previous experience of the method. In a small number the result during expiration can be difficult to interpret, because the relationship of flow to pressure ($\dot{V}/\Delta P\mathrm{box}$) is not linear, but exhibits expiratory looping. This phenomenon is usually associated with airway obstruction.

Forced oscillation method

Outline. When the thorax is subjected to forced oscillation from a pump connected to the mouth a back pressure is developed. This is a function of both the amplitude of the oscillation and the total impedance of the respiratory system; the latter has three components, resistance, compliance and inertance. The component due to compliance is a function of the change in volume of the thorax: this is inversely related to the frequency of the oscillation which is imposed. The component due to inertance is a function of the acceleration of the thorax: this is directly proportional to the frequency. Thus when the frequency of the imposed oscillation is changed these two components of the total impedance are affected in opposite ways: thus there is a frequency at which they are of equal magnitude and effectively neutralise each other. At this resonant frequency, which is normally about $9\,Hz$, the impedance of the lungs and thorax is almost entirely due to the resistive component. The measurement which is usually made is of input impedance at the mouth in which both the forced oscillation and the volume change relate to the mouth. In transfer impedance the two relate to different sites with usually the pressure directed at the chest and the volume change measured from the mouth. The reverse is the case for the transfer impedance at the mouth (Fig. 6.17). This is the sum of the airway, lung tissue and chest wall resistances. Use may be made of the resonant frequency for measurement of the total thoracic resistance. The method was developed by DuBois and colleagues, then modified by Grimby, Mead and others. The subject has been reviewed by Peslin and by a working group of the Commission of European Communities Biomedical Advisory Committee.

Practical details. The measurement of input impedance at the mouth is made with the subject seated and the head in a vertical position; flexion of the neck should be avoided. The subject breathes through a pneumotachograph which is connected to a sine-wave pump. Alternatively a loudspeaker can be used but has the disadvantage that standing waves can develop in the speaker chamber. The frequency of oscillation

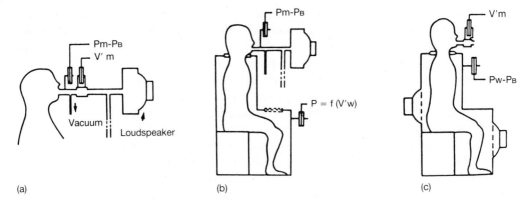

(a)

(b)

(c)

Fig. 6.17 Alternative approaches to measuring respiratory mechanical impedance. (a) pressure input at the mouth and flow measured at the mouth (input impedance at the mouth); (b) pressure input at the mouth and flow measured at the chest (transfer impedance at the mouth); (c) pressure input at the chest and flow measured at the mouth (transfer impedance at the chest); Pm, Pw, P_B: mouth, body surface and barometric pressures, respectively; $V'm$, $V'w$: flows at the mouth and at the chest, respectively. (Source: Peslin R. *Bull Eur Physiopathol Respir* 1986; **22**: 621–631.)

should cover the range 4–32 Hz. The amplitude of oscillation is usually 40 ml for adults and less for children. The pneumotachograph is continuously flushed with air (flow rate $\approx$ 12 l min^{-1}) to minimise accumulation of expired gas. The applied pressure is measured at the lips using a suitable transducer (page 29). The pressure and the flow are displayed on the X and Y axes of an oscilloscope where convenient scales per cm of screen are respectively 0.16 kPa (1.6 cmH$_2$O) and 0.4 l s^{-1}. During the application of the forced oscillations the signal on the screen takes the form of an oblique loop; in normal subjects this reduces to a straight line at the resonant frequency. However, in patients with airways obstruction, because the compliance is frequency dependent, the resonant frequency can be very high and exceed the maximal frequency of the equipment. In these circumstances the looping can be reduced by subtracting from the pressure axis a signal which is proportional to either the integral or to the differential of the flow rate; these signals, which are proportional to the changes in volume and in acceleration of the imposed forced oscillation, relate respectively to the compliance and inertance components of the overall impedance. If the subject were not breathing spontaneously, the thoracic resistance would be the slope of the linear relationship which is obtained. In practice the subject is breathing and this leads to variability in resistance between breaths. The variability can be reduced by averaging the pressures and flows (but not the resulting resistances) over a series of breaths.

Comment. The method depends on the transducers for pressure and flow having a negligible impedance and similar phase and amplitude characteristics. In addition an appropriate allowance should be made for the proportion of oscillatory flow which is taken up in the cheeks and upper airways. The proportion is increased in the presence of intrathoracic airways obstruction. The resistance is underestimated in consequence. The error can be reduced by cupping the cheeks in the hands or by applying a compensatory oscillation externally. Alternatively the error can be eliminated by applying the oscillation to the trunk via a partial body plethysmograph which does not include the head, as suggested by Mead. The resulting transfer impedance at the chest has the further advantage that only the flow is measured at the mouth; the flow meter can then be open to the atmosphere and have a less demanding specification than when the applied pressure and the flow are both measured at the mouth. The methodology for transfer impedance offers scope for further development.

Pressure—flow method

Outline. The pressure—flow method for measuring the total lung resistance requires the intubation of the oesophagus and, if compliance is measured concurrently, it takes about 40 min of the subject's time. For these reasons it has been superseded by other methods except when measurement of the tissue resistance, or the resistance upstream of the equal pressure points (page 172) is required.

To make the measurement the velocity of airflow and oesophageal pressure in excess of mouth pressure are displayed as a pressure—flow diagram on a cathode ray oscilloscope (see Fig. 6.16). The slope of the long axis of the diagram is the relationship of air flow velocity to total applied pressure; this is a first approximation to the desired relationship which is between air flow velocity and *resistive* pressure. The latter is obtained by subtracting from the total pressure the component due to elastic recoil of the lung; this pressure is the product of the change in volume and the lung elastance.

Correction for compliance component of pressure. The correction is made using the relationship of lung volume to pressure obtained concurrently with the flow—pressure curve. An example is given in Fig. 5.18. Here the resistive pressures at the points I and E are represented by the lengths Inspn-B and B-Expn. The total lung resistance at the points I and E is obtained by dividing the resistive pressures by the corresponding rates of air flow. The division can be performed electronically since above functional residual capacity the force which is required to overcome the elastic recoil of the lung is nearly proportional to its volume: the volume is obtained by electrical integration of the output of the pneumotachograph. A component which is proportional to this volume is now subtracted from the pressure axis of the pressure—flow diagram (Fig. 6.18). This manoeuvre converts total pressure into resistive pressure; the slope of the long axis of the new diagram so obtained is the total lung conductance. The correction to the pressure axis is adjusted to minimise the area enclosed by the pressure—flow

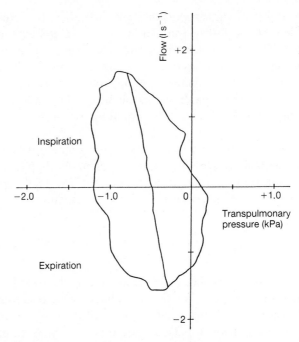

Fig. 6.18 Pressure−flow diagram during quiet breathing. The diagonal line was obtained by the method of Mead and Whittenberger which is described in the text. (Source: *J Appl Physiol* 1953; **5**: 779.)

loop; in this circumstance the magnitude of the correction (i.e. the potentiometer setting) is a measure of the dynamic lung compliance (cf. page 165). The loop will reduce to a straight line as in Fig. 6.14 when both the air flow is entirely laminar (range of flow rates 0.5− $1.0 l s^{-1}$) and the tidal excursion is small. The resistance is then unaffected by variations in lung volume during the procedure. However, it is affected by the average volume, which should also be reported (see Fig. 5.12, page 111).

Tissue resistance. Lung tissue resistance (Rti) is obtained as the difference between total lung resistance (Rl), which is measured by the pressure−flow method and the airway resistance (Raw), which is measured by the plethysmograph method:

$$Rti = Rl - Raw \qquad (5.7)$$

On account of breath-to-breath variations it is essential that both resistances are measured during the same respiratory manoeuvre. Tissue resistance is normally small relative to airways resistance so the procedure is not particularly exact except when the tissue resistance is increased.

Upstream resistance. The concept of upstream resistance arises from equal pressure point theory, which is now superseded by a theory based on wave mechanics. It is of theoretical interest but appears not to be of practical use. Upstream resistance is the resistance of peripheral airways under conditions of maximal flow, at which time the driving force is the static elastic recoil of the lung. At any lung volume it is given by the relationship:

$$Rus = Pst \div \dot{v}max \qquad (6.14)$$

where Rus is the resistance of airways upstream of the equal pressure point, Pst is the static or elastic recoil pressure of the lung at the lung volume specified, and $\dot{v}max$ is the maximal rate of air flow at that volume. The lung volume is measured by plethysmography. The appropriate values for pressure and flow are obtained from separate determinations of the relationships between recoil pressure and lung volume (Fig. 5.7, page 96), and between maximal flow rate and volume (Fig. 5.13b, page 116); the relationship between νmax and Pst (Fig. 5.14, page 117) is linear over a wide range of lung volumes. The slope (θ) is the upstream conductance and the intercept on the pressure axis is a measure of bronchial collapsibility.

Interrupter method

Outline. For this method of measuring airway resistance the alveolar pressure is measured at the mouth during interruption of the flow of gas by a shutter. When the shutter is closed the pressure equalises throughout the respiratory tract, so the pressure in the mouth rises to the level of that in the alveoli immediately prior to interruption. When the rate of air flow before the interruption is also known the airway resistance can be calculated. The measurement is usually made during a series of interruptions whilst the subject breathes through a resistance; this is adjusted to have a relationship of pressure to flow similar to that of the lung airways.

Practical details. The flow of gas down the airways is assumed to be partly turbulent to the extent that the pressure is proportional to the flow raised to the power of 1.6. Then, by analogy with equation 5.10 on page 110:

$$Paw = Raw \times \dot{v}^{1.6} \qquad (5.10)$$

where Paw is the pressure difference between the alveoli and the mouth, $\dot{v}$ is volume flow rate of gas and Raw is airway resistance. The method was proposed by Ainsworth and Eveleigh and developed by Clements. Interruption is effected by a rotating shutter which occludes and opens the airway for alternate periods of 0.05 s. This occlusion is too brief to give rise to sensation so the subject is able to breathe through the apparatus at an apparently steady rate of flow. The pressure in the mouthpiece when the shutter is open (P_1) is a measure of the rate of air flow through the apparatus. The pressure when it is closed (P_2) is that required to overcome the resistances of both the lung airways and the apparatus. The airway resistance (*R*aw) is then given by the following relationship:

$$Raw = \frac{P_2 - P_1}{P_1} \times Rc \text{ kPa (or cmH}_2\text{O) l}^{-1}\text{s} \qquad (6.15)$$

where *R*c is the resistance coefficient of the apparatus. The airway resistance is usually recorded at rates of gas flow of 0.5 and 1.0ls^{-1}.

Comment. In practice, the interrupter method yields a result which more nearly resembles the total lung resistance than the airway component. This is because, during the period of equalisation of pressure after interruption, the pressure in the alveoli changes. In addition, when the airway resistance is high, the pressure which is measured at the mouth is not representative of that in the alveoli. This is due to movement of gas within the lung (Pendelluft effect, see Fig. 8.7, page 226). Amongst the useful features of the method are that it is quick and simple for the subject, does not involve large or complex apparatus or tedious calculations and is appropriate for making serial measurements.

Assessing bronchial hyperreactivity

Background. The responsiveness of bronchial smooth muscle to agents which cause bronchoconstriction varies both between individuals and within the same individual at different times. An increased response can be specific to one substance, for example, an agent which causes occupational asthma (page 549), or non-specific when any constrictor stimulus can elicit an exaggerated response. This non-specific bronchial hyperreactivity is a feature of some abnormal conditions of the lung (page 555); it also occurs in approximately 5% of healthy persons who are then at increased risk of developing air flow limitations in response to inhaled irritant substances. The procedure for assessment is described below. The converse procedure for assessing the response to bronchodilator drugs is given on page 145, and that for challenge using a specific allergen on page 555.

Outline. Non-specific bronchial hyperreactivity is assessed using an aerosol of histamine or methacholine in progressively increasing doses. An inhalation of cold air or exercise can also be used as the provoking agent but the response is then usually assessed qualitatively. The bronchoconstrictor response to provocation is monitored in terms of the resulting change in ventilatory capacity or specific airway conductance. The use of ventilatory capacity, either forced expiratory volume or peak expiratory flow rate, is the more convenient and often more reproducible but has the disadvantage of entailing full inspiration to total lung capacity; this causes reflex bronchodilatation which can partly inhibit the bronchoconstrictor response (page 198). The error can be avoided by assessing the response at near to functional residual capacity in a whole body plethysmograph. Airway resistance and thoracic gas volume are measured and the response is reported in terms of the specific conductance. In laboratory studies the stimulus and response are used to construct a dose–response curve and the reactivity is reported as the dose which causes a predetermined degree of bronchial narrowing for example a 20% reduction in FEV_1 (Fig. 6.19): this is designated provocation concentration 20% or PC_{20, FEV_1}. When specific airway conductance is used the end point can be a 35% change ($PC_{35, sGaw}$). The former index is the more reproducible and is more widely available but the end point appears to reflect a greater degree of bronchoconstriction.

Practical details. Uncontrolled provocation can lead to severe broncho-constriction so a recognised protocol should be adopted and carried out under medical supervision. The subject should preferably be asymptomatic, have no material airflow limitation and not be taking medication at the time of testing. The histamine provocation test is performed by alternating measurements of forced expiratory volume

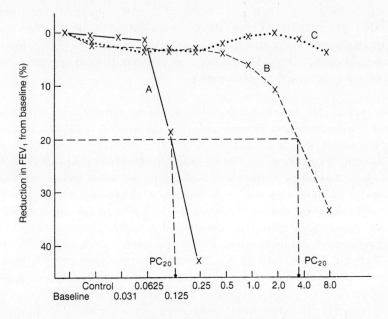

Fig. 6.19 Testing for bronchial hyperreactivity in subjects suspected of having asthma. The FEV_1 was normal between attacks. Subjects inhaled saline and then graded doses of histamine solution from a Wright nebuliser for 2 min with 3 min intervals between. During these times measurements of forced expiratory volume were made every 0.5 min. Subject A showed marked hyperreactivity; subject B was moderately reactive; subject C did not react to histamine in the dosage used. The small reduction in FEV_1 occurring after the control inhalation of saline was probably physiological; a larger reduction would have been an indication for postponing the histamine challenge as the result could not have been interpreted satisfactorily. (Source: Keaney NP, King B in Cotes JE, Steel J. *Work-Related Lung Disorders*. Oxford: Blackwell Scientific Publications, 1987, 357.)

or specific conductance with inhalations of dilute solutions of histamine. The inhalations are either for 2 min from a Wright nebuliser, or five vital capacity breaths from a demand nebuliser (e.g. De Vilbiss) or five tidal breaths from a dosimeter. The FEV_1 is measured 90 s after the inhalation is completed. Using a Wright nebuliser with a flow rate of air or O_2 of 8 l min^{-1} and solution volume of 5 ml the initial histamine concentration is 0.03 mg ml^{-1}; the concentration is doubled for each subsequent inhalation up to a maximum of 32 mg ml^{-1}. If there has been any airflow limitation it is reversed with salbutamol or other β stimulant drug. The PC_{20, FEV_1} is obtained by interpolation of the semi-log plot of FEV_1 on histamine concentration (Fig. 6.19). Alternatively the cumulative dose of histamine may be so plotted when the index is designated PD_{20, FEV_1}. However, some subjects fail to respond so do not provide a quantitative score. This can be a disadvantage for respiratory surveys. The difficulty has been overcome by O'Connor and colleagues who used instead the slope of the relationship of the percentage reduction of FEV_1 on the final cumulative dose of the drug used for the challenge. The non-responders then have a score of zero.

The methacholine test is performed similarly to that for histamine using doses in the range 0.01 – 25 mg ml^{-1}; it is equally effective and yields a quantitatively similar, though not identical result. The two test substances are equally effective but compared with methacholine, histamine is possibly safer as the induced bronchoconstriction appears to be more easily reversed by salbutamol.

Comment. The full procedure for assessing non-specific bronchial hyperreactivity is not disagreeable for the subject and has a good reproducibility ($\pm$ one dilution level) but takes up to an hour to complete. It can be shortened by omitting the lower doses in subjects who have no history of atopy and by stopping the test at an intermediate dose, for example 8 mg ml^{-1} of histamine. Alternatively, for respiratory surveys, this dose can be used as a single challenge for subjects who, from answers to questions, are considered unlikely to react. In addition, the procedure can be shortened by limiting the reduction of FEV_1 to 10% but the reproducibility of the index is then impaired. A lesser degree of airway obstruction can also be detected by monitoring the conductance ($PC_{35, sGaw}$) instead of the ventilatory capacity (PC_{20, FEV_1}). The choice of procedure will be influenced by the particular application. Difficulty may arise if results are to be compared between laboratories since there is a high probability that different methods will have been used. Some work on standardisation has been undertaken but more is needed if this difficulty is to be resolved.

Exercise-induced airflow limitation

Exercise-induced airflow limitation, also called exercise-induced asthma (EIA), is assessed by measurement of FEV_1 before and 6 min after moderately heavy exercise. Either running, cycling or stepping exercise of duration 6 min may be used; swimming is unsuitable as it provides a less powerful constrictor stimulus than other forms of exercise. A reduction in FEV_1 in excess of 10% which is reversed by subsequent inhalation of salbutamol aerosol is positive evidence for EIA. The bronchoconstriction is due to constrictor stimuli acting on airways which are either unduly responsive or have a raised bronchomotor tone prior to stimulation (Fig. 16.6, page 549). The bronchomotor tone is further increased if the exercise entails breathing cold air as this initiates reflex bronchoconstriction via receptors in the large airways supplied by branches of the vagi. A positive response is followed by a refractory period lasting up to 4 h. The response is blocked by the prior administration of disodium cromoglycate. The test is suitable for children and for physically active adults. It is not suitable for persons with a reduced FEV_1 or those who have recently taken a bronchodilator drug.

Cold air provocation test

This test is usually performed at rest and does not entail pharmacologically active substances so is particularly suitable for elderly subjects. The provoking agent is air which is cooled to $-10°C$ by passage through a coil surrounded by a refrigerated sheath or a bucket of ice and salt. The subject performs the manoeuvre for measurement of FEV_1 then breathes the air through the mouth for 6 to 10 min taking deep rapid breaths; hypocapnia is avoided by using a mouth piece with a large deadspace or by providing 2% carbon dioxide as the respired gas. Other aspects of the procedure are as for exercise induced airflow limitation including the contra-indication, the end point, the refractory period and the effect of cromoglycate.

Guide to references

The references (Chapter 18) are classified under subject headings of which the following are particularly relevant to the present chapter:

7: Distribution of Ventilation and Perfusion

Introduction

Gas exchange between the body and its environment takes place in the parenchyma of the lung where only the alveolar and capillary membranes separate air from systemic venous blood. The alveoli are ventilated during each respiratory cycle by that part of the tidal volume which traverses the anatomical deadspace (page 191); in adults at rest the volume of this alveolar component of the tidal volume is about 0.4 l; it can vary between 0.3 and 6.0 l, depending on the depth of the breath and the dimensions of the airways. The gas is added to that present in the lung (which is functional residual capacity); under quiet resting conditions this has an average volume in adults of about 2.5 l. Thus the dilution factor is normally about 1.2 (i.e. $(2.5 + 0.4) \div 2.5$). The pulmonary capillaries receive 50 to 150 ml of mixed venous blood during each cardiac cycle. An approximately equal volume of blood is in contact with the alveolar gas (page 194). It is nearly completely replaced with each systole. The flow of blood is pulsatile; its distribution is influenced by gravitational force. The distribution is also regulated by constriction of smooth muscle in the walls of small pulmonary arteries and by events taking place in adjoining lung tissue. The distribution of ventilation is similarly determined by a combination of factors of which gravitational force is possibly the most important. Other factors which contribute to uneven ventilation are the shape of the thoracic cavity, the orientation of the respiratory muscles and uneven distribution of lung resistance and compliance. The intervention of active regulatory mechanisms usually ensures that for the great majority of alveoli the ventilation is appropriate for the perfusion; however, even in normal lungs some gas is wasted in ventilating those alveoli, which on account of inadequate perfusion contribute little to gas exchange. Similarly some blood is imperfectly oxygenated because it perfuses alveoli which are poorly ventilated.

These topics are considered in the present chapter. The diffusive characteristics of the lung and gas exchange in individual alveoli are considered in Chapter 9.

The pleural space

The lung is free to move within the thoracic cavity except at the hilium where it is attached to the mediastinum. Elsewhere the structures are separated by a layer of fluid between the visceral and parietal pleura. This pleural fluid resembles interstitial fluid in being formed by ultra-filtration from serum. The fluid contains relatively little protein (concentration in the range 1–2%) so reabsorbtion occurs because its osmotic pressure is less than that of plasma. Reabsorbtion is into lymphatics in the parietal pleura and is accompanied by some protein. The volume of pleural fluid is small (probably less than 10 ml) because on average the capillary osmotic pressure only slightly exceeds the relevant mechanical forces; these are (1) the capillary hydrostatic pressure, (2) the recoil pressures of the lung and chest wall which are subatmospheric throughout most of the respiratory cycle (e.g. Fig. 6.18, page 172), (3) gravitational force which provides a gradient of pressure in the vertical plane and (4) any traction or support from the hilum of the lung. The result is a relatively dry pleural space. In any posture the pressure gradient is more negative at the top than at the bottom of the lung. Under static conditions it is less for the lung than for pleural fluid due to the respective densities being in the ratio 0.22:1.0. However, under dynamic conditions pleural fluid is in motion, and this leads to the vertical pressure gradient being the same in pleural liquid and at the pleural surface of the lung. The movement of fluid is probably influenced by anatomical factors and is not solely due to gravity. The earlier evidence has been reviewed by Agostoni. Recent advances have been made amongst others by Lai-Fook and colleagues. The pleurae are porous to gases but the space does not contain air. This is because the sum of the tissue gas tensions is considerably less than atmospheric, so any gas in the pleural space is reabsorbed (see page 18).

Mechanical factors which affect distribution of inspired gas

Gravitational force

Effect of pleural surface pressure on lung expansion. Due to the operation of gravitational force, the pressure with respect to atmosphere at the pleural surface of the lung is more negative at the top than the bottom of the lung. In an upright posture the gradient down the lung (distance approximately 0.3 m) is about 0.75 kPa (7.5 cmH$_2$O). The consequences for regional distribution of inspired gas have been investigated using inert gases labelled with radioactive tracers, particularly by Milic-Emili and West and their respective colleagues; some of the techniques are described in Chapter 8. The simplest of these entails the inhalation by the subject of a small quantity of radioactive xenon. Its distribution in the lung is recorded by scintillation counters placed outside the chest. In this and other ways it has been shown that during slow inspiration from residual volume, the first gas to be inhaled goes to the upper part of the lung; in the middle range of inspiration the air is distributed between the regions. As inspiration continues, a larger proportion goes to the lower region until, at near to total lung capacity, the apex is almost fully inflated and the last air to be inhaled goes mainly to the bases. The lung bases are also the recipients of most of the tidal volume during normal breathing. The regional distribution of the respired gas is greatly influenced by the slope of the volume—pressure curve and by the point on the curve where inspiration begins. The probable mechanism is illustrated in Fig. 7.1. In addition for a given vertical pressure gradient a lung of high compliance will exhibit larger regional differences in ventilation than a lung of low compliance. The perfusion of the lung is distributed similarly (page 187).

During expiration the emptying of the different lung regions occurs

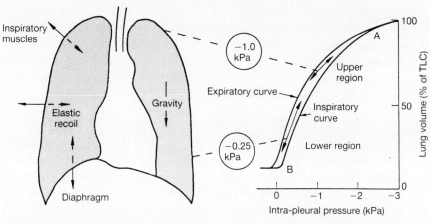

Fig. 7.1 Diagram after Milic—Emili and West showing the effect of pleural surface pressure on regional distribution of ventilation. The lung has superimposed on it the forces which are applied during inspiration; these are opposed by the elastic recoil of lung tissue which varies with volume. The relationship of volume to pressure is shown on the right hand side of the diagram (cf. Fig. 5.8, page 97); it is assumed to be the same for upper and lower regions. The vertical gradient of pleural surface pressure leads to the alveoli of the upper region being more expanded (i.e. they lie higher up on the volume axis) than those of the lower region; their volume at functional residual capacity is, therefore, relatively greater; their potential for further expansion is limited so these alveoli lie on a relatively flat part of the volume—pressure curve. A further change in pressure then leads to a smaller volume change than in the lower region which is on the steeper part of the curve. This difference in expansion ratios is more marked at near to total lung capacity when the upper region, because it is then on the horizontal part of the curve (A in the diagram), does not expand at all. By contrast, at near to residual volume, when the upper region (intra-pleural pressure −0.4 kPa) has a large expansion ratio, the lower region (intra-pleural pressure +0.35 kPa) is on the flat part of the curve where there is no expansion (B in the diagram).

in the reverse order from inspiration with the bases tending to empty before the apices, hence *first in is last out*. The regional differences are less clear than during inspiration, especially at large lung volumes. The more uniform emptying is contributed to by the absence of hysteresis during expiration and by a paradoxical increase in tone of the muscle of the diaphragm which tends to reduce the gradient of pleural pressure. However, the regional differences become more pronounced at near to residual volume due to the closure of airways which serve the lung bases. The lung volume at which closure becomes detectable by current methods is called the *closing capacity*. It is the resultant of all the factors which determine the calibre of the intrapulmonary airways (page 112). The measurement is discussed and described on page 219.

The vertical gradient in lung expansion is reflected in the alveolar diameter which is normally greater in the upper than in the lower regions, especially at small lung volumes. The difference disappears at total lung capacity when all alveoli are fully expanded. Below total lung capacity the alveolar size is related to the pressure tending to expand the lung, which may be represented in the form:

$$P = W \div A \tag{7.1}$$

where P is the gravitational pressure at any horizontal plane across the lung, A is the cross-sectional area of the plane and W is the weight of the lung below it. This relationship points to the mechanical stresses on the lung being less at the lung bases than in the upper lobes and the apices of the lower lobes; it is probably no coincidence that these places are also the commonest sites of emphysema. The association has been analysed by West.

Uneven distribution of compliance and resistance

Lung units with a high compliance tend to have a high expansion ratio, and vice versa; such variation contributes to spatial inequality of ventilation. Differences in lung resistance give rise to temporal inequality in which lung units fill and empty sequentially. Alveoli served by airways which are wide and short tend to fill quickly and hence early in inspiration whereas those which are served by relatively long and narrow airways take longer to fill and so on average fill later in inspiration. Similar differences obtain on expiration when the alveoli served by the wider airways empty sooner than those served by the narrower ones, hence *first in is first out* (cf. regional inequality above).

A lung composed of units of equal compliance but unequal airway resistance may be expected to exhibit temporal inequality of ventilation. Whether or not there is also spatial inequality will depend on the duration of inspiration. If it is prolonged then, for a given change in pleural surface pressure, all alveoli will achieve the same expansion ratio but if it is brief the lung units having a high resistance will expand less than the lower resistance units. The behaviour of the lung in these terms has been investigated theoretically and from experiments on models by, amongst others, Otis and McKerrow. They consider the lung as a series of parallel units each consisting of a tube of resistance R leading into a container having a compliance C. When such a system is ventilated using a pump which delivers a sine wave, the extent to which the pressure applied to the lung is out of phase with the rate of air flow can be expressed in degrees as the phase angle θ (Fig. 7.2). By analogy with electrical alternating current theory:

$$\tan \theta = \frac{1}{2\pi fCR} \qquad (7.2)$$

where f is respiratory frequency. The product of the compliance and the resistance is the 'time constant of the lung' which is the time after the sudden application of a pressure gradient across the lung for the flow to arrive at within $1/e$ or 36.8% of its equilibrium value. For the model the time constant is larger when either the resistance or the compliance is increased. In practise an increase in resistance is the more relevant; it is associated with a reduced rate of airflow. According to the model the phase angle is small when pressure and flow are nearly in phase. When two compartments have different phase angles due to differences in resistance, gas can be flowing out of one at a time when it is flowing into the other and vice versa. This 'Pendelluft' phenomenon has been demonstrated in the lung (Fig. 8.7, page 226). It reduces the effective tidal volume; it also reduces the accuracy of measurements of resistance and compliance for the whole lung, especially when the measurements are made at high frequencies of breathing. In such circumstances, the dynamic compliance of the model is less than and the airway resistance is greater than that given by summation of the

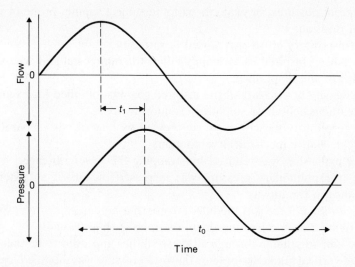

Fig. 7.2 Diagram illustrating the derivation of the phase angle from the pneumotachograph record of air flow and the pressure applied across the lung between the pleural surface and the mouth. The phase angle is the segment of the respiratory cycle between peak flow and peak pressure (t_1) expressed as a fraction of the complete cycle (t_0), when the latter is 360°. Then $\theta = t_1/t_0 \times 360°$.

resistance and compliance of the component units. Similarly in man, when the airway resistance is increased, the dynamic compliance is lower than the static compliance (see pages 102 and 165). There are also both temporal and spatial inequality of ventilation which are most marked at high frequencies of breathing. The time constant is short when the resistance and compliance are reduced. This combination can occur in diffuse interstitial fibrosis; it is associated with a reduced ability to expand the lung but the proportion of vital capacity which can be expired in 1 s (i.e. the $FEV_1\%$) is usually increased and the peak expiratory flow may be within normal limits (page 561). A reduction in compliance has relatively little effect upon those indices of inequality of distribution of gas which assess temporal rather than spatial inequality. On this account the inequality is sometimes overlooked.

Uneven contraction of respiratory muscles

In any posture except the lateral decumbent the vertical gradient of pleural surface pressure and the wide range of regional time constants explain most of the observed variations in regional lung gas distribution. However, a number of discrepancies have been identified, many of them by Milic Emili, Macklem and colleagues at McGill and Paiva and colleagues in Brussels. Their observations were often made initially using single breath techniques in which either the nitrogen present in the lung was diluted by a single breath of oxygen or the test breath was tagged using a bolus of radioactive xenon (^{133}Xe) or other isotope (page 229). The discrepancies arose in a number of circumstances, and their diversity illustrates the ingenuity and persistence of respiratory physiologists! The circumstances included:

1 different postures for example with the subject supine, prone or in a lateral position;
2 the inspiratory effort was varied in intensity;
3 the subject inspired using mainly either the intercostal and accessory muscles or the diaphragm;
4 the density or viscosity of the inspired gas was modified for example by breathing helium or sulphur hexafluoride;
5 the respiratory muscles were suppressed by anaesthesia or paralysis and replaced by mechanical ventilation;
6 lung expansion was reduced by strapping the lower rib cage;
7 the transpulmonary pressure was increased by use of an external resistance in the airway;
8 gravitational force was modified by use of a human centrifuge, space craft or aircraft accelerating or in a parabolic trajectory.

The unifying theme through all these studies appeared to be that the normal vertical gradient or pleural surface pressure was modified locally by predominant contraction of one or other group of respiratory muscles. In any posture forced inspiration from residual volume but not from functional residual capacity usually augmented the flow to the apex of the lung; this was due to increased contraction of the intercostal and accessory muscles. D'Angelo demonstrated that the redistribution was associated with local distortion of the rib cage. Accentuated contraction of the diaphragm increased the flow to the lung bases in all postures but particularly in the lateral decumbent position when its piston-like action is enhanced by the diaphragm forming much of the lateral boundary of the chest (cf. Fig. 5.5, page 92). The evidence has been reviewed by Engel.

Movement of gas by bulk flow and by diffusion in the gas phase

During inspiration the gas enters the lung by convection in which the molecules travel together by a process of bulk flow. The flow is mainly laminar (see page 108), so the gas passes along the airways with a parabolic profile, leaving along the walls of the airways a thin layer of the gas already present in the lung (Fig. 7.3). The distribution of the gas may be studied by the inhalation of an aerosol of inert particles. The particles should be of sufficiently small size that few of them become impacted on to the walls of the airways, but large enough not to be subject to Brownian movement and so be dispersed by diffusion. These requirements are met by particles of diameter 0.5 or 1 µm of sodium chloride coated with di-2-ethyl hexyl sebacate; the procedure is described on page 227. Using this material Muir and others have shown that for a tidal volume of 600 ml the aerosol penetrates the primary lobules to the level of the alveolar ducts but does not enter the alveoli: the latter movement occurs by diffusion in the gas phase. This process is almost instantaneous over distances of the order of one alveolar diameter, so is effective for regions of the lung which are

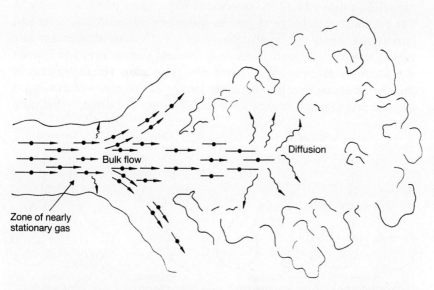

Fig. 7.3 Diagram after Muir showing laminar flow of gas molecules into an acinus during tidal breathing. Penetration down to the level of the alveolar ducts is by bulk flow. The ventilation of the alveoli and of the zone of nearly stationary gas takes place by diffusion (cf. Fig. 5.3, page 85).

185

ventilated. The rate of diffusion is similar for each of the gases normally present in the lung, but is faster for substances of low molecular weight, for example hydrogen or helium, and slower for substances of high molecular weight like sulphur hexafluoride. The effectiveness of gas distribution by diffusion is enhanced by breath holding and a slow respiratory frequency. This provides time for diffusion of gas to take place between adjacent lung units along both normal and collateral channels, which is of particular importance during breath-holding at small lung volumes, when many small airways are occluded.

During normal tidal breathing intrapulmonary mixing appears to be optimal at lung volumes just above those associated with airway closure. Any further increase in tidal volume improves the uniformity of distribution by convection (i.e. by bulk flow of gas). Thus, Crawford and colleagues found that gas mixing within the acinus was normally complete within five breaths. They used a tidal volume of 1 l and measured the difference in slope of the alveolar plateau between helium and sulphur hexafluoride during washout with successive breaths of oxygen. The slope was expressed relative to the average expired concentration of the indicator gas. For each gas the slope increased in successive breaths but the difference in slope between helium and SF_6 increased only over the first five breaths and remained constant thereafter. The results suggested that for a 1 l tidal volume the slope of the single breath washout curve for nitrogen was mainly due to local convection and diffusion jointly contributing to washout of nitrogen within acini or very small lung regions. The changes during subsequent breaths reflected sequential emptying of larger regional units containing gases at different concentrations. The latter effect was due to uneven expansion ratios caused by anatomical factors and possibly gravity; it was not much affected by diffusion. Mixing by diffusion is of increased importance when the local delivery of gas by bulk flow is for any reason impaired. Models illustrating some of the abnormalities which can occur are given in Fig. 7.4 (see also page 266). The integration of the contributions to intrapulmonary mixing of the many determinants of local and regional convection and diffusion has clarified what until

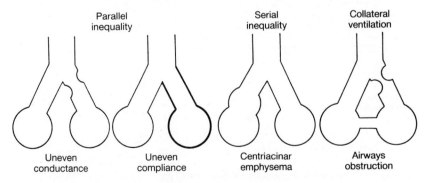

Fig. 7.4 Examples of uneven lung function. The effects of parallel and serial inequality can be described in terms of parallel and serial deadspaces; the latter can also be represented as stratified inhomogeneity.

recently has been a confusing and controversial aspect of lung function. The developments have also pointed to weaknesses in the traditional procedures for assessing lung mixing including the two compartmental analysis of multi-breath nitrogen washout curves (page 223) and single breath indices of lung mixing based on the nitrogen test of Fowler and Comroe (page 214). These and more recently developed tests are considered on page 218.

Effects of cardiac systole

Contraction of the heart redistributes blood both within the thorax and between the thorax and the main systemic circulation; it also generates a pulse wave which is transmitted to the lung tissue via the pulmonary circulation. These perturbations stir up the gases within the lung; the effect varies directly with the density of each gas and on this account differs from mixing by diffusive conductance in being greater for sulphur hexafluoride than for helium; it might be expected to be greater for carbon dioxide than for oxygen but any difference would be small. Cardiac systole also draws gas along the airways (cf. page 226). At rest the volume displaced is about 60 ml per heart beat. The changes lead to oscillations in the alveolar concentrations of oxygen and carbon dioxide in the expired gas (cardiogenic oscillations): the changes are illustrated in Fig. 8.3 (page 217). Fowler and Read found the amplitude of the oscillations to reflect the unevenness of distribution of ventilation–perfusion ratios within the lung.

Mechanical factors which affect distribution of pulmonary blood flow

The stroke volume of each ventricle is normally in the range 50–100 ml. It has a maximal value which in most circumstances reflects the capacity for exercise: the maximum is readily attainable, for example by lying down or performing moderate exercise. It is increased by physical training. A reduction in stroke volume occurs during tachycardia from any cause or if the venous return is reduced: this may result from a rise in alveolar pressure, venodilation, haemorrhage or pooling of blood in the legs. The latter can be reversed by counter pressure from an inflated anti-gravity (G) suit or by leg exercise. A volume of blood equal to the stroke volume is ejected into the pulmonary artery during each cardiac systole. The ejection raises the pulmonary arterial pressure, distends the blood vessels of the lung and displaces blood from the pulmonary arterioles into the pulmonary capillaries where the flow is to some extent pulsatile.

The pulmonary vascular bed can normally accept a volume of blood in excess of the stroke volume. On this account, whilst the majority of vessels contain circulating blood, some are empty and others contain blood which is stationary. The proportion in the first category is determined mainly by cardiac output; the distribution between the second and third categories is determined by a number of factors including gravity and the alveolar pressure. The distribution of blood has been investigated by a number of methods of which some are described in Chapter 8.

The operation of gravity upon the pulmonary circulation leads to the perfusion varying down the vertical axis of the lung; four zones may be identified, and are illustrated in Fig. 7.5. Their location is determined mainly by the perfusion gradient. This is the resultant of the pulmonary arterial and venous pressures, which are subject to the influence of gravity, and the pressure in the alveoli (alveolar pressure) which, in the absence of airflow obstruction is nearly uniform throughout the lung. For flow to occur the intravascular pressure or the traction exerted on the vessel walls must exceed the alveolar pressure which will otherwise compress and empty the alveolar capillaries. Compression can occur at the apex of the lung (zone one) when the subject is at rest

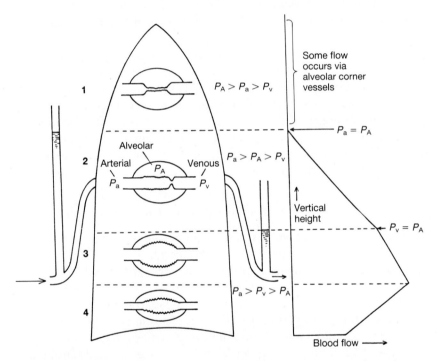

Fig. 7.5 Diagram showing the distribution of blood flow in the lung. In zone 1 the alveolar pressure (Pa) exceeds the pulmonary arterial pressure (Pa), so the alveolar septal vessels, but not the alveolar corner vessels, are collapsed. In zone 2 the arterial pressure exceeds the alveolar pressure, which in turn exceeds the venous pressure (Pv): hence the distal parts of the alveolar vessels are compressed, and flow is reduced. The intravascular pressure then builds up and flow is resumed intermittently. This is the principle of the Starling resistor. On account of gravity affecting the venous pressure the compression is greater and hence the flow is less at the top than at the bottom of this zone. Throughout zone 3 the driving pressure is the difference between the arterial and the venous pressures. The intravascular pressure increases down the zone and the flow increases accordingly. The intravascular pressure is highest in zone 4 where it contributes to a rise in the interstitial pressure; this is of little consequence except when the interstitial pressure is also increased from other causes (see discussion of zone 4 in text). (Source: West JB. *Ventilation/Blood Flow and Gas Exchange.* 3rd ed. Oxford: Blackwell Scientific Publications, 1977.)

in an upright posture. The compression affects the capillaries in the alveolar septa; it is due to the local pulmonary capillary pressure being less than the alveolar pressure and is relieved if the pulmonary arterial pressure is increased by exercise (see Fig. 11.2, page 327), hypoxic vasoconstriction, or a change in posture from upright to supine. The closure does not affect the alveolar corner vessels which are distended by inflation of the lung (cf. Fig. 5.6, page 95). These vessels provide a pathway for perfusion of superior parts of the lung. The mechanism has been demonstrated by Lamm and colleagues. In the upper part of the perfused region (zone 2) the pulmonary arterial pressure exceeds the alveolar pressure during systole but not during diastole. All these pressures exceed those in the pulmonary veins. In zone 2 the flow is intermittent or pulsatile and is determined by the arterial to alveolar pressure difference: Permutt and his colleagues have pointed out that the conditions of flow resemble a waterfall, though a dam or weir might be a better analogy. Similar conditions obtain in a Starling resistor (Fig. 7.5). In the main lower part of the perfused region (zone 3) the pulmonary venous pressure exceeds the alveolar pressure; the vessels are then distended with blood throughout their length and the flow is determined by the arterial to venous pressure gradient. By these means the blood flow increases almost linearly from the top to the bottom of the perfused region. The distribution of blood flow is also influenced by the degree of lung expansion, hence the blood flow per alveolus varies with the depth of inspiration (Fig. 7.6). Thus blood

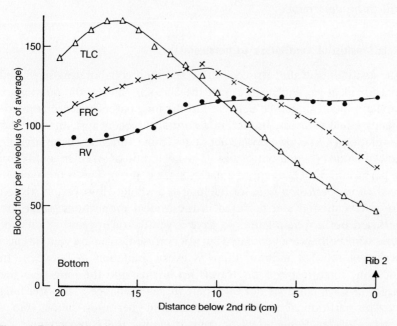

Fig. 7.6 Relationship of blood flow per alveolus to distance below the 2nd rib in seated subjects holding the breath at different lung volumes. Blood flow is expressed relative to the average; TLC, FRC and RV are defined in Table 2.2 (page 13). (Source: Hughes JBM, Glazier JB, Maloney JE, West JB. *Resp Physiol* 1968; **4**: 58–72.)

flow at the bases is reduced during forced expiration to residual volume. In addition the increase in hydrostatic pressure down the vertical axis leads to transudation of fluid into the interstitial tissue at the lung bases. The amount is normally small and the resulting increase in interstitial pressure is unimportant unless the pulmonary venous pressure and/or transudation of fluid are increased. The causes include left ventricular failure, mitral stenosis, an infusion of dextran, a fall in the pH of the blood and the effect of some drugs. In these circumstances the expansion of the lung parenchyma is reduced and the blood flow at the base of the lung (zone 4) is decreased.

Blood vessels can be subject to critical closure, which occurs when the pressure within the lumen is reduced below a critical level. The process operates for some systemic arterioles; it could do so for the lung but this has still to be proved. The mechanism has been elucidated by Burton and his associates. It depends partly on the property of smooth muscle that it relaxes and contracts slowly. Hence if the pressure within the lumen of an arteriole is suddenly reduced the muscle does not immediately relax to a comparable extent. Instead the excess tension summates with the elastic recoil of the wall of the vessel, to cause abrupt closure of the lumen. The pressure proximal to the point of closure then rises; when it exceeds the critical closing pressure the patency is restored. The mechanism of critical closure provides a means for maintaining the pressure in the pulmonary artery at a relatively constant level by permitting rapid adjustment of the number of arterioles which are perfused with blood; its possible role in the human lung has still to be determined.

Relationship of ventilation to perfusion

The analyses of Rahn, Briscoe, Riley and their collaborators suggested that for ideal gas exchange at rest the alveolar gas and the pulmonary capillary blood should be delivered to the lung parenchyma in approximately equal volumes. In fact, in a normal subject at rest, the alveolar ventilation ($\dot{V}\text{A}$) is on average about $4.5 \, \text{l} \, \text{min}^{-1}$ and the corresponding flow of blood ($\dot{Q}$) is about $5 \, \text{l} \, \text{min}^{-1}$, giving a ratio of alveolar ventilation to perfusion ($\dot{V}\text{A}/\dot{Q}$) of approximately $4.5/5.0$ or 0.9. This is the average *ventilation−perfusion ratio* for the lung as a whole. However, all alveoli are not ventilated and perfused in these ideal proportions; some are perfused but not ventilated, so have a ventilation−perfusion ratio of zero, whilst others are ventilated but not perfused, so have a ventilation−perfusion ratio of infinity; there is every gradation in between. In addition, some inspired gas travels no further into the lung than the larger airways, so does not take part in gas exchange. Thus the lung may be partitioned, in terms of ventilation−perfusion ratios, into a number of functional units or compartments; the compartments do not, in most cases, have discrete anatomical identities but they provide convenient points of reference for analysis of lung function. The five compartment model of Riley and others is illustrated in Fig. 7.7 and

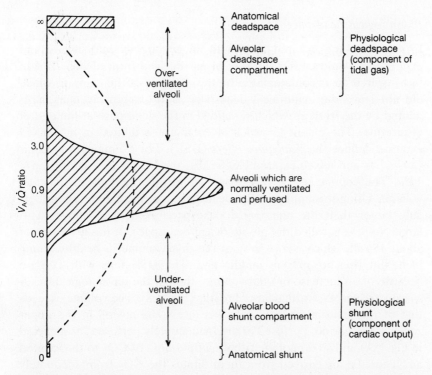

Fig. 7.7 Terminology for the five compartment model of lung ventilation–perfusion relationships of Riley and others. The term venous admixture effect can refer to the blood which perfuses the alveolar blood shunt compartment but more often it describes the physiological shunt. The shaded areas are for a normal subject. The interrupted line indicates a wide range of $\dot{V}_A/\dot{Q}$ ratios. The diagram is schematic. The gaseous composition of the compartments is indicated in Table 7.2 (page 207).

described below. The multi-compartment model of Farhi, Wagner and West is considered on page 196.

Anatomical deadspace

Anatomical deadspace is the volume of the airways from nasopharynx to terminal bronchioles in which no material exchange of O_2 and CO_2 occur. It is ventilated but not perfused, so has a ventilation–perfusion ratio of infinity and does not participate in gas exchange. The volume of the anatomical deadspace varies with the size of the lung, the tone of the bronchial musculature and the amount of traction exerted on the walls of the airways by the supporting tissue of the lung; these factors are themselves influenced by the degree of lung expansion and by bronchoactive drugs. The mean anatomical deadspace, normally re-ported at functional residual capacity, is about 150 ml in healthy young males and rather less in females. The anatomical deadspace varies with age and body size (page 310); the changes in disease are discussed in Chapter 16. The procedure for measurement is given on page 214.

Physiological deadspace

In an ideal lung inspired air would all go directly into alveoli and expired air would consist entirely of gas derived from alveoli. But in fact inspired air is contaminated by the remnant of the expirate which did not leave the anatomical deadspace, and expired alveolar gas is diluted by the fresh air which remained in the deadspace at the end of inspiration. The extent to which alveolar gas is diluted in the mixed expirate defines the *deadspace effect* (DSE). For example, if alveolar $CO_2 = 6\%$ and mixed expired $CO_2 = 4\%$, the DSE $= (6 - 4)/6 \times 100 = 33\%$. The volume of the deadspace would then be 33% of the tidal volume. Using this approach the deadspace, so calculated, is considerably larger than the anatomical deadspace as defined above. This larger volume is called the physiological deadspace. It has a volume of about 180 ml, which is 25–30% of the tidal volume in healthy young men, but rises to 40% in middle age. The DSE falls with exercise because of an increase in tidal volume, though the physiological deadspace also increases with deeper breaths (Fig. 7.8). The volume exceeds that of the anatomical deadspace because some alveoli in the upper zones are either not perfused or are inadequately perfused (as depicted in Fig. 7.5) and so do not contribute a full quota of CO_2 to the expired air. Thus the air derived from them dilutes the CO_2 from adequately perfused alveoli, and this excess of dilution ensures that the physiological deadspace is larger than the anatomical. The difference between these two deadspace volumes is the *alveolar deadspace*. When the lung is more completely perfused, for example during exercise, the alveolar deadspace shrinks. It is enlarged when pulmonary embolism or thrombosis obstructs one or more branches of the pulmonary artery, and also when narrowing of airways interferes with the distribution of

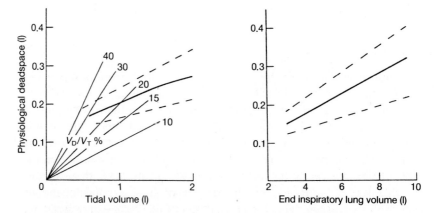

Fig. 7.8 Relationship of physiological deadspace to tidal volume and to end-inspiratory lung volume at rest and during exercise in healthy young adults. Higher values are observed in older subjects. The isopleths are for deadspace as a percentage of tidal volume (*Vd/Vt%*). (Sources: Asmussen E, Nielsen M. *Acta Physiol Scand* 1956; **38**: 1–21; Lifshay A, Fast CW, Glazier JB. *J Appl Physiol* 1971; **31**: 478–483.)

ventilation. The reason why airways obstruction has this effect is not immediately obvious, but is readily explained (see Chapter 16).

Physiological shunt

As explained above the over-ventilation of some alveoli relative to their blood supply increases the alveolar deadspace. Under-ventilation relative to the blood supply leads to the affected alveoli receiving insufficient oxygen to saturate the blood. This reduces the systemic arterial oxygen tension and content. The effect of underventilation in causing hypoxaemia resembles that of blood bypassing the lungs altogether, such as may occur in congenital heart disease and arterial anomalies of the lungs. The extent of underventilation can be categorised by the *venous admixture effect* (analogous to physiological deadspace) which describes the arterial saturation as though it were a mixture of blood exposed to ideal alveolar air (about 98% saturated) and mixed venous blood (about 75% saturated at rest). Thus if arterial saturation is found to be 90% the venous admixture effect would be $(98 - 90)/(98 - 75) \times 100 = 34.8\%$. (See also page 207.) The effect is derived from two sources, a true anatomical shunt through vessels which bypass the alveoli, and an alveolar blood shunt compartment from underventilated alveoli. The two together are the *physiological shunt*. The two components can usually be differentiated by inhalation of oxygen; this does not affect the blood traversing any anatomical shunt which completely bypasses the alveoli. It does, however, raise the alveolar oxygen tension in underventilated alveoli sufficient to eliminate the alveolar component of the hypoxaemia. Investigation of physiological shunting is described on page 253.

The physiological shunt in normal subjects is about 2% but it is increased in some congenital diseases of the heart and arteries and in circumstances when either airways obstruction or compliance are abnormal, provided the abnormalities are unevenly distributed, or are so severe as to cause respiratory failure. Localised obstruction of the airways at the base of the lungs (dependent obstruction) occurs at low lung volumes. The threshold volume for closure is designated *closing capacity* (page 182). Dependent obstruction is an important cause of hypoxaemia in elderly subjects on account of loss of lung elasticity (page 488) and in the obese due to lung volume being reduced by intrathoracic and abdominal fat (page 489); these causes of hypoxaemia are exacerbated by adopting a reclining posture which is associated with a reduced functional residual capacity compared with sitting up. Dependent obstruction also occurs if the volume of interstitial fluid in the lung is increased by an increase in pulmonary venous pressure (pages 603 and 605), a reduced plasma osmotic pressure secondary to protein deficiency or inflammation. An anatomical shunt due to abnormal pulmonary vessels can occur with bronchiectasis (page 545) and with portal cirrhosis (page 568). An extra-pulmonary shunt occurs in some forms of cyanotic congenital heart disease (page 602). In the

193

latter two conditions, the lung function is usually normal. Other differentiating features are discussed in Chapter 16.

Effective alveolar ventilation

On inspiration the alveoli receive per breath that proportion of the tidal volume (normally about 70%) which does not constitute the physiological deadspace. The ventilation per min is the alveolar ventilation:

$$\dot{V}_A = (V_T - V_D)f_R \, l \, min^{-1} \qquad (7.3)$$

where V_T and V_D are respective tidal volume and physiological deadspace (l BTPS), $\dot{V}_A$ is the alveolar ventilation (l BTPS^{-1}) and f_R is respiratory frequency per min.

Ideal alveolar air

The point of reference for analysis of lung $\dot{V}_A/\dot{Q}$ relationships is gas from alveoli which have a $\dot{V}_A/\dot{Q}$ close to the average for the whole lung. These alveoli contain gas of similar, but not of identical, composition. An average sample can be obtained during expiration after exhalation of gas in the anatomical deadspace (page 191). However, the sample is likely to be biased in favour of regions which have a relatively high ventilation–perfusion ratio. To overcome this difficulty Riley, Rossier and their respective colleagues proposed the use of an ideal alveolar air; its composition is that which would give rise to the observed respiratory exchange ratio if ventilation and perfusion were uniformly distributed. For its derivation the alveolar tension of carbon dioxide is assumed to be that of the arterial blood and the respiratory exchange ratio that of the mixed expired gas. The alveolar oxygen tension is then that which is consistent with these two values. It is calculated by using the alveolar air equation (page 252). Gas of this composition may not exist anywhere in the lung since the derivation assumes that all alveoli have the same ventilation–perfusion ratio, but for the analysis of the actual range of ventilation–perfusion ratios this is an advantage. The way in which the analysis is performed is described in Chapter 8.

Ideal alveolar air is the starting point for the graphical analysis of lung gas exchange by means of the oxygen–carbon dioxide diagram (Fig. 7.9). The diagram is derived from the dissociation curves for oxygen and carbon dioxide which are illustrated in Fig. 7.12; in its construction use is made of the premise that the rate at which carbon dioxide flows from blood to alveoli is exactly balanced by the rate at which ventilation carries it from the alveoli in the expirate; similarly the in-flow of oxygen in the inspirate is balanced by its uptake in the blood. The diagram describes the composition of alveolar gas in terms of the ventilation–perfusion and respiratory exchange ratios and the compositions of inspired gas and mixed venous blood; when values for any three of these variables are known or assumed the fourth can be

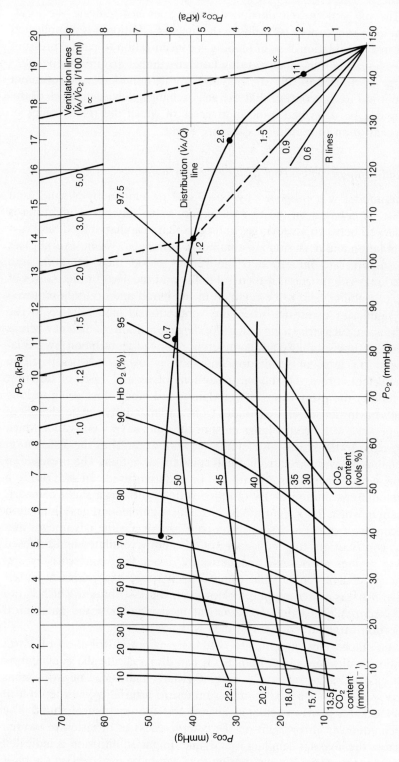

Fig. 7.9 O_2–CO_2 diagram of Rahn and Fenn. The grid of curved lines illustrates the normal relationships of the tensions of oxygen and carbon dioxide to the haemoglobin saturation and the content of carbon dioxide in blood. The lines for respiratory exchange ratio (R lines) radiate from a point (I) which describes the inspired gas (in this case air). Alveolar ventilation (units l/min per 100 ml of oxygen uptake) is represented by parallel lines of which that for infinite ventilation has an R value of infinity. The curved distribution line illustrates the combinations of oxygen and carbon dioxide tension associated with different ventilation–perfusion ratios: its limits are inspired gas ($\dot{V}_A/\dot{Q} = \infty$) and mixed venous blood ($\dot{V}_A/\dot{Q} = 0$). The dashed lines converge on a point on the distribution line where the $\dot{V}_A/\dot{Q}$ ratio is 1.2. For an alveolus having this ratio of ventilation to perfusion the alveolar ventilation would be expected to be 2.0 l/100 ml, the respiratory exchange ratio 0.9 and the tensions of oxygen and carbon dioxide respectively 13.9 and 5.2 kPa. The corresponding values for oxygen saturation and carbon dioxide content of blood can also be read off the diagram. (Source: Rahn H, Fenn WO. *A Graphical Analysis of the Respiratory Gas Exchange*. Washington DC: American Physiological Society, 1955.)

read off the diagram. Its use is described by Fenn and Rahn and by Farhi.

The oxygen–carbon dioxide diagram does not indicate the localisation or range of $\dot{V}A/\dot{Q}$ ratios in the lung; in addition it is complicated because the relationships of blood gas concentration to partial pressure for oxygen and carbon dioxide are both curvilinear and inter-dependent (page 278). Historically the diagram was a remarkable achievement and it led to the concept that the gas exchanging characteristics of the lung can be described using inert gases in which the relationships of concentration to partial pressure are linear.

Multi-compartment model of lung gas exchange

This model was proposed by Farhi and developed by Wagner and West. It is based on the two assumptions that gaseous equilibrium is achieved between alveolar gas and pulmonary capillary blood, and that ventilation and perfusion are continuous processes. When several gases in solution are infused into the venous blood their excretion into the lungs is a function of their solubility and the $\dot{V}A/\dot{Q}$ ratio. Gases of high solubility tend to be retained in the blood and are only removed in significant quantities when the ventilation is high relative to the perfusion; such gases have a high blood–gas partition coefficient whereas gases of low solubility are completely removed from blood by a relatively low level of ventilation and have a low blood–gas partition coefficient. From the relative retentions of several gases of different solubility the proportions of ventilation and blood flow going to lung units having any of 50 $\dot{V}A/\dot{Q}$ ratios from zero to infinity can be identified. In persons with healthy lungs most of the units have $\dot{V}A/\dot{Q}$ ratios which are close to the mean value of approximately 0.9. Thus the distribution is unimodal with a relatively small standard deviation. The presence of lung units which are overventilated or underperfused can give rise to a bimodal distribution of $\dot{V}A/\dot{Q}$ ratios with or without a shunt compartment in which the $\dot{V}A/\dot{Q}$ ratio is zero. This multiple inert gas elimination technique (MIGET) is described on page 255. It has the advantages that the contributions to gas exchange of differently ventilated and perfused lung regions are assessed concurrently rather than consecutively and the procedure, unlike that using oxygen (page 253), does not itself alter what is being measured. However, the distribution which is described relates to the mathematical model and not the anatomical location of any abnormality which is detected.

MIGET provides an estimate of the frequency distribution of $\dot{V}A/\dot{Q}$ ratios in different circumstances. It can also indicate the contribution to gas exchange of cardiac output (which influences mixed venous oxygen tension), hence the contribution to arterial oxygen tension of blood from poorly ventilated alveoli and the anatomical shunt. The technique can throw light on the completeness of diffusion of oxygen across the alveolar capillary membrane; impaired diffusion is indicated by a lower arterial oxygen tension than would be expected on the basis of ventilation–perfusion inequality alone (page 322). In normal subjects the method yields intuitively sensible distributions which change in the expected direction as a result of interventions (Fig. 7.14, page 209).

However, the model is possibly less representative of disease states because it neglects a number of factors which could reduce the effects on gas exchange of a wide range of $\dot{V}_A/\dot{Q}$ ratios. Thus the method does not take into account deadspace, collateral ventilation, cardiogenic mixing, and oscillations in gas exchange over the respiratory and cardiac cycles. It also overlooks the bronchial circulation which can contribute materially to gas exchange when there is pulmonary vascular occlusion. Some of these limitations are only of theoretical interest whilst others have been largely resolved. The method has illuminated many aspects of abnormal gas exchange including those associated with asthma, pulmonary embolism, cirrhosis of the liver and haemodialysis. These conditions are described in Chapter 16. MIGET is a useful if expensive tool for intervention studies. The subject has been reviewed by Farhi, Hlastala and Robertson, and Rodriguez-Roisin and Wagner.

Adjustment of ventilation and perfusion

Ventilation and perfusion are distributed mainly in response to the physical forces which are described above. These are imperfectly matched, and as a result there is a range of ventilation–perfusion ratios throughout the lung. The range is reduced by the operation of regulatory mechanisms.

Distribution of deadspace gas

After the completion of expiration, the deadspace of the lung contains gas from the alveoli which emptied last. In the presence of airways obstruction the gas comes from regions which were most affected by temporal inequality of ventilation so had a low ventilation–perfusion ratio. During the succeeding inspiration the gas passes into the alveoli which expand first; they are also those which tend to have a high ventilation–perfusion ratio. The sites include apical alveoli where the perfusion is minimal and perihilar alveoli where, for anatomical reasons, the expansion ratios are relatively high. Distribution of deadspace gas to these sites decrease the range of ventilation–perfusion ratios for the whole lung. This was pointed out by Farhi.

Distribution of inspired gas

Vertical gradient in lung expansion. The existence of a vertical pressure gradient in the pleural space leads to postural differences in distribution of ventilation. In an upright posture the lower lobes are better ventilated than the upper lobes. In a lateral posture, the inferior lung has rather better ventilation than that which is superior whereas in the supine position the ventilation per unit of lung volume is relatively uniform. These postural differences in the distribution of ventilation are similar to the differences in perfusion caused by gravity; consequently they tend to diminish $\dot{V}_A/\dot{Q}$ inhomogeneity.

Bronchial smooth muscle. The distribution of ventilation is partly regulated by the action of bronchial smooth muscle which is under the control of the autonomic nervous system. The parasympathetic component constricts primarily the larger airways which receive a rich cholinergic innervation from ganglia in the airway walls. The smaller airways are sparsely innervated and the constrictor response is less. Constriction is mediated by acetylcholine which is liberated from the nerve endings in response to vagal stimulation of the ganglia; it is potentiated by anticholinesterases and is inhibited by atropine. This drug increases the airways conductance of healthy subjects. The increase is usually more pronounced in patients with airways obstruction, particularly asthmatics indicating the presence of resting parasympathetic tone. The parasympathetic tone is augmented by propranolol which inhibits the bronchodilator action of catecholamines. Bronchoconstriction can also be caused by substance P which is a neurotransmitter for non-cholinergic excitatory nerves and by calcitonin gene-related peptide. The role of the latter substance is considered on page 203. The only bronchodilator innervation to the airways is provided by non-adrenergic non-cholinergic nerves. They extend from the larynx to the terminal bronchioles, and their stimulation in animals causes long-lasting dilatation, especially of the larger airways and can also activate mucous glands. The neurotransmitter substance appears to be vasoactive intestinal peptide (VIP) or the related substance, peptide histidine isoleucine. The role of this system in controlling normal airway tone is unclear. The subject is reviewed by Barnes. Sympathetic nerves appear not to supply the airway smooth muscles; instead they supply the mucous glands, the blood vessels and ganglia in the airway walls; through the latter connection an increase in sympathetic activity can inhibit bronchoconstriction caused by vagal activation. It also causes bronchodilatation by releasing adrenaline which acts on β receptors in the airway walls. This action unlike that of the vagi affects all classes of airways. The pharmacology of bronchodilation is considered on page 641.

Changes in bronchomotor tone occur in a number of circumstances; the reduction in tone associated with a raised carbon dioxide tension of intrabronchial gas directly reduces ventilation−perfusion imbalance. Other responses may also do this indirectly, but the majority of responses are directed to protecting the respiratory tract from inhaled noxious substances and their effect on ventilation−perfusion relationships is adverse not beneficial. They have been investigated by Nadel and by Widdicombe amongst others.

Deficiency of carbon dioxide in the intraluminal gas causes bronchoconstriction. This can affect all classes of airways as, for example, when it is achieved by voluntary hyperventilation. Alternatively it can occur locally in response to reduced delivery of CO_2 to part of the lung following occlusion of a pulmonary artery or reduction in local blood flow. These effects are reversed by the inhalation of CO_2 in a fractional concentration of 0.06; this concentration also partly reverses the bronchoconstrictor action of drugs including histamine and acetylcholine. The effect of hypocapnia is attenuated by atropine which is evidence that it is mediated in part via the vagi. There is also a local action of CO_2 on bronchial smooth muscle. The reaction provides a mechanism whereby the ventilation to a part of the lung is adjusted in response to local variation in blood flow; this was first suggested by Severinghaus and colleagues. The response to embolisation of a part of the pulmonary arterial tree is discussed on page 606.

Paradoxicallly a material increase in the intra-luminal concentration of carbon dioxide can also cause bronchoconstriction. This response is unaffected by atropine or isoprenaline so is believed to be a local reaction either of the bronchial muscle itself or an axon reflex arising from the larynx. Its role is unclear. This is also the case for the bronchoconstriction which occurs in response to hypoxia. The reflex is mediated via the carotid body and the vagi. It is inhibited by isoprenaline. A similar hypoxic bronchoconstriction can occur in patients with chronic lung disease; the constriction differs from that due to other aspects of the disease process in responding to oxygen enrichment of the inspired gas.

Bronchomotor tone is modulated by reflexes arising from receptors in the lungs. The reflexes are mediated via the vagi. Thus bronchomotor tone varies inversely with lung volume in response to the activation of stretch receptors in the walls of airways. The tone is increased by stimulation of receptors in the nasal mucosa which respond to cold, and by receptors in the larynx which respond both to many chemical substances and to mechanical stimulation. Bronchomotor tone is also increased by stimulation of nerve endings which lie beneath the epithelium of the airways. The receptors in the larger airways usually adapt quickly; they contribute to the cough reflex. The receptors in the smaller airways often adapt slowly and give rise to bronchoconstriction; they have been called irritant receptors by Widdicombe. A bronchoconstrictor response was first observed following inhalation of small dust particles by Dautrebande and DuBois, who noted that the response was independent of the composition of the dust; it was, however, related to the dose of dust (Fig. 7.10). A similar response has been observed following inhalation of tobacco smoke, sulphur dioxide and histamine aerosol. The deposition and clearance of aerosols is described on page 227.

Changes in airway resistance affect distribution of gas by convection and via anastomotic pathways. The distribution within the acinus is also influenced by the tone of muscle fibres which surround the openings to the alveolar ducts (see page 84). Constriction occurs in a number of circumstances (page 102) and can impair local distribution of gas by diffusion. The constriction also reduces the lung compliance. Systemic mechanisms have less effect on distribution because their action is

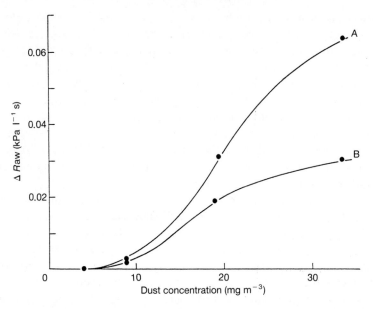

Fig. 7.10 Response of airway resistance (*R*aw) in healthy subjects to breathing inert dust for 4 h. Airway resistance was measured before exposure, immediately afterwards and 1 h later. The abscissa is mass concentration of respirable dust (particle diameter 1–7 μm) per cubic metre of inspired gas; the ordinate is change in airway resistance in subjects who inhaled dust adjusted for the change which occurred in control subjects over the same period. Each point is the mean of determinations on six subjects. The curves A and B show respectively the immediate changes and those at 1 h. (Source: McDermott M. *J Physiol* 1962; **162**: 53P.)

generalised. The carotid body contributes to the bronchoconstrictor response to hypoxia which is referred to above. The aortic baroreceptors can initiate bronchoconstriction in response to a fall in the systemic blood pressure. By contrast strenuous exercise can exert a bronchodilator effect; this is due at least in part to diminution of vagal tone. The converse phenomenon of post-exercise bronchoconstriction is discussed on page 176. The mechanism is indicated in Fig. 16.6, page 549.

Regulation of perfusion

In 1946 von Euler and Liljestrand showed that, in cats, ventilation of the lung with gas deficient in oxygen or containing carbon dioxide increased the pressure in the pulmonary artery. They attributed the rise to pulmonary vasoconstriction and suggested that local hypoxic vasoconstriction acted to reduce the perfusion to parts of the lung which were poorly ventilated. The response provided a mechanism for minimising hypoxaemia due to local hypoventilation. Subsequent work has confirmed this hypothesis and has shown that the mechanism operates in man. It appears not to operate for some mammals and birds which live at high altitude including the llama and bar-headed goose: these species unlike man are not subject to pulmonary hypertension in that environment.

200

The stimulus to vasoconstriction appears to be the oxygen tension of the pulmonary arterial vascular smooth muscle. This is determined by the oxygen tensions of the alveolar gas, the mixed venous blood and blood in the bronchial arteries which supply the vasa vasorum in the walls of the pulmonary arteries.

Hypoxic vasoconstriction is immediately reversed by breathing oxygen except when the condition is of long duration and associated with hypertrophy of smooth muscle in the walls of small pulmonary arteries (page 541). The response to breathing oxygen influences the relationship of pulmonary vascular pressure to blood flow; this exhibits a nearly parallel shift (Fig. 7.11). The mechanism is not known. The shift could be due to the opening of vessels via the Starling resistor mechanism illustrated in Fig. 7.5. However, Mitzner and Huang have an alternative explanation.

The action of hypoxia is mainly a direct one on the pre-alveolar and alveolar vessels since they respond after denervation and in the isolated lung; the post-alveolar vessels are not affected. There is also a neural component which is initiated by hypoxaemia stimulating the carotid body (page 340) and effected via the autonomic nervous system. The reflex is weaker in man than in some other mammals. It could contribute to the generalised pulmonary vasoconstriction which occurs at high altitude but not to the localised constriction which is a feature of many lung diseases. The response to hypoxia is maximal at tensions of oxygen in the range 2.7–13 kPa (20–100 mmHg); it is augmented by an increase in the concentration of hydrogen ions in blood perfusing

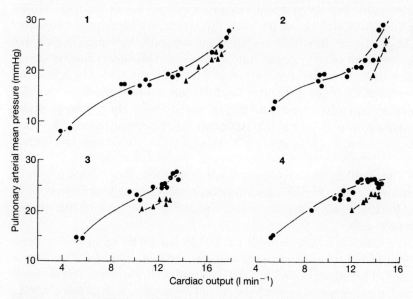

Fig. 7.11 Parallel shifts in the relationship of pulmonary arterial mean pressure to cardiac output in response to breathing oxygen instead of air during exercise (▲ and ● respectively). The subjects were four asymptomatic working coal miners with normal lung function and pulmonary arterial mean pressures. (Source: Field GB, Cotes JE. *Clin Sci* 1970; **38**: 461–477.)

the lung. The vasoconstriction is reversed by profound hypoxia and by some sympathomimetic drugs including aminophylline and isoprenaline.

In the fetus the presence of hypoxia of physiological origin is a principal cause of high pulmonary vascular tone (page 448). In the newborn hypoxia occurs as part of the syndrome of respiratory distress; it then leads to the circulation failing to adjust to the conditions of extra-uterine life (page 524). In people living at high altitude hypoxia is a cause of pulmonary hypertension and of fluid retention which can present as failure of the right ventricle (page 617). Howard and others have shown that the changes are partly due to a reduced renal blood flow. The latter conditions are also complications of hypoxaemia due to chronic lung disease (page 541). The hypoxaemia can be aggravated by the use of those bronchodilator drugs which have a vasodilator action on the pulmonary circulation (e.g. isoprenaline). However, alternative bronchodilator drugs which do not have this action are also available (page 641).

Pulmonary vasoconstriction is the result of interaction between actin and myosin filaments in the smooth muscle cells. In the relaxed state the myosin is present in an inactive form. It is activated as a result of phosphorylation by an enzyme (kinase) which in turn is activated through the mediation of calcium ions. The calcium ions are normally present mainly in the plasma and extracellular fluid and their entry into the cells is through calcium inflow channels which open in response to depolarisation of the cell membrane or to the attachment of mediator substances to adjacent receptors. Subsequent to the contraction the calcium ions are sequestered in the mitochondria and endoplasmic reticulum. The sequestered calcium ions can be re-used to initiate further contractions but the extent to which this happens is uncertain. The ions can also be excreted from the cells by routes which are independent of the calcium inflow channels. The energy for the movement of calcium ions within and out of the cells is provided by adenosine triphosphate (page 401). The local oxygen tension influences the pulmonary vasomotor tone over a range of tensions from hyperoxia where oxygen is a vasodilator to hypoxia where it is a vasoconstrictor. The same mechanisms probably operate throughout this continuum to regulate the delivery of ionised calcium to the contractile apparatus.

Theoretically the oxygen tension could affect the calcium inflow channels either directly or via mediator substances. Alternatively or in addition it could influence events within the cytoplasm of the smooth muscle cells.

The calcium inflow channels can be blocked by antagonist substances; these include the dihydropyridines nitrendipine, nifedipine and verapamil. They appear to act by taking up unpaired electrons. The channels can have their opening times prolonged by agonists such as BAY K 8644 which is an electron donor. The effect of these substances on the pulmonary vasculature is correlated with their redox properties. An oxygen radical is essentially an unpaired reactive electron source so it could modulate the calcium channels by this mechanism.

202

The action could involve the sulphydryl redox status which affects the synthesis or the constrictor leukotrienes C4 and D4 from glutathione; these substances appear to modulate the magnitude of the response to hypoxia. Alternatively or in addition it might involve the level of adenosine triphosphate *vis-à-vis* adenosine diphosphate (ATP/ADP + Pi, page 403); this affects the movement of calcium ions away from the sites of muscular contraction. Oxygen could also act in cytochrome P450 to which it can become attached; the cytochrome both contributes to the cellular metabolism and, in its oxidised form, is a source of superoxide anions. Thus there are a number of ways in which oxygen could influence the movement of calcium ions into, within and out of the smooth muscle cells and hence the tone of pulmonary vascular smooth muscle. Exactly how this is done has still to be established.

Oxygen might also affect the receptor-activated calcium channels by influencing the amount or the availability of the relevant substances; these include the vasoconstrictors angiotension II, histamine and prostaglandin F2α. However, whilst each of these substances can cause pulmonary vasoconstriction none of them is essential for hypoxic pulmonary vasoconstriction (HPV).

Opioid peptides can cause pulmonary vasoconstriction but whilst they act in this way in response to lung injury, the endogenous production is not increased during hypoxia. The site of production of the transmitter substances appears to be in the pulmonary vascular endothelium and this discovery has focused attention on endothelial-derived constricting and dilating factors. An example of the former is platelet activating factor (PAF) which includes amongst its actions the ability to dilate or, in higher concentrations, to constrict pulmonary blood vessels. The production of PAF is stimulated by hypoxia but whilst at least one PAF antagonist also inhibits hypoxic vasoconstriction, in the view of Barnes and colleagues, PAF is not the normal transmitter substance. Instead they suggest a role for endothelial-derived relaxing factor (EDRF) which is nitric oxide synthesised from L-arginine. EDRF is a potent pulmonary vasodilator which appears to inhibit HPV since the latter is enhanced by EDRF blockade.

Pulmonary vasodilatation can be caused through release of EDRF by acetylcholine, superoxide dismutase, bradykinin and substance P. Acetylcholine can also cause dilatation via release of prostacyclin in the pulmonary vasculature. Other substances including calcitonin gene-related peptide and vasoactive intestinal peptide (VIP) appear to act directly. One or more of these substances may contribute to pulmonary vasodilatation in patients with portal hypertension (page 558).

The inhalation of gas containing carbon dioxide causes pulmonary vasoconstriction in a number of species including man but the response is small compared with that to hypoxia. The vasoconstriction is probably due mainly to a local rise in the concentration of hydrogen ions since a fall in the blood pH has similar effect, whilst a rise in pH is associated with vasodilatation. For a given change in [H$^+$] the vasoconstrictor response to carbon dioxide is less than that to the infusion of acid. This has led some workers to conclude that apart from reducing the pH the CO_2 molecule has a vasodilator action.

Hypercapnic vasoconstriction can occur when there is no response to hypoxia and vice versa; thus the mechanisms are different. In practice that due to hypoxia is the more important and is the main cause for the local reduction in perfusion which occurs as a result of local under-ventilation of the lung in man. Read and others found that people differed in the intensity of their vasoconstrictor responses to hypoxia, whilst Grover and his colleagues, from study of cattle at altitude showed that the responsiveness was genetically determined. Responsive subjects are at greater risk of developing pulmonary hypertension than their less responsive contemporaries if they should travel to high altitude or acquire lung disease. The control of the pulmonary circulation is reviewed by Weir and colleagues including Archer and Reeves.

Effects of ventilation−perfusion inequality

The preceding sections have shown that the distribution of pulmonary ventilation and perfusion are subject to regulation by control mechanisms. These operate at the level of the acinus and primary lobule as well as for the lung as a whole and provide a means whereby ventilation and perfusion can be appropriately matched in the presence of factors which impose a local change in either of them. The mechanisms are imperfect and easily disturbed, particularly by circumstances which change the distribution of lung perfusion, for example an upright posture, haemorrhage or assisted ventilation involving positive end-expiratory pressure. These circumstances enlarge the perfusion zone one of West (page 188). A deranged distribution of either or both alveolar ventilation and pulmonary blood flow from any cause increases the range of the ventilation−perfusion ratios. Analysis of the contributory factors is difficult because the control system involves a large number of substances, many with multiple actions. There is also a high degree of interaction so the same stimulus can elicit widely differing responses depending on the levels of other variables. The responses can involve both blood vessels and airways as in the case of calcitonin gene-related neuropeptide, substance P, neurokinin A and bradykinin. These substances are both vasodilators and bronchoconstrictors and their release in response to immunological stimulation of the lung could contribute to the gross ventilation−perfusion imbalance seen in many disease states including asthma. The imbalance can sometimes be reduced by almitrine and the associated hypoxaemia can be alleviated by giving oxygen (page 621). The reason why hypoxaemia occurs and the consequences of ventilation−perfusion inequality are considered below.

Alveolar−arterial tension differences for oxygen and carbon dioxide

In a healthy lung gas exchange across the alveolar capillary membrane proceeds nearly to equilibrium in which the gas tensions are the same in the alveoli and the blood leaving the alveolar capillaries (page 270). Heterogeneity is introduced by ventilation and perfusion not being uniformly matched throughout the lung so there is a range of ventilation–perfusion ratios. This leads to differences in gas tension between acini. Small differences occur within regions and larger differences between regions, with the largest difference between the apex and base of the lung (e.g. Fig. 7.15, page 210).

Overall gas exchange is the resultant of gas from all the alveoli merging to form mixed alveolar gas and blood from all the capillaries merging to form pulmonary venous blood. However, these amalgamations cannot fully compensate for the underlying inequalities; instead gas exchange for the whole lung is less effective than that for the constituent parts. The first adverse factor is the *distribution effect* whereby the mixed alveolar gas, being composed mainly of gas from acini whose ventilation is excessive for their perfusion, has a low tension of carbon dioxide and a high tension of oxygen. Similarly the pulmonary venous blood, being composed mainly of blood from acini whose perfusion exceeds their ventilation, has a high tension of carbon dioxide and a low tension of oxygen. Thus a wide range of $\dot{V}A/\dot{Q}$ ratios leads inevitably to differences in gas tension between mixed alveolar gas and systemic arterial blood. The distribution effect is illustrated by a numerical example in Table 7.1 where the calculations are based on a model comprising two compartments in parallel (cf. Fig. 7.15, page 210). The $\dot{V}A/\dot{Q}$ inequality has the effect that for a given output of carbon dioxide the arterial oxygen saturation is lower and the alveolar ventilation higher than in a single compartment lung. For the model the respective values for arterial oxygen saturation are 95% and 98% and for alveolar ventilation $5 \, l \, min^{-1}$ and $4.4 \, l \, min^{-1}$. A second factor which increases the alveolar–arterial gas tension differences for the whole lung is the shape of the dissociation curve for oxygen (*dissociation curve effect*). The shape contributes to blood picking up oxygen in the lungs and unloading it in the systemic capillaries (see page 278). However, the blood is almost fully saturated at the alveolar oxygen tension of 15 kPa. Thus alveoli having an oxygen tension greater than this cannot raise the saturation further so their additional oxygen is not utilised. By contrast the oxygen content of blood from acini having a low $\dot{V}A/\dot{Q}$ ratio is inevitably reduced. When mixing occurs between blood from poorly ventilated and well-ventilated alveoli the quantity of oxygen in blood from alveoli with a high ventilation–perfusion ratio does not make up for the diminished quantity in the blood from poorly ventilated alveoli. The content of oxygen in the mixed blood is reduced in consequence.

In the presence of $\dot{V}A/\dot{Q}$ inequality the dissociation curve effect contributes to gas exchange for oxygen because the curve is asymptotic (i.e. has a flat top). It is relatively unimportant for carbon dioxide because for this gas the dissociation curve is essentially linear over the

Table 7.1 Consequences for gas exchange of $\dot{V}_A/\dot{Q}$ inequality: a numerical example based on a hypothetical two compartment model. Diffusion equilibrium across the alveolar capillary membrane and a linear CO_2 dissociation curve are assumed but are not essential to the outcome. The compartments are ventilated in the ratio 4:1 but are allocated equal blood flows. The a-A difference for O_2 (components are indicated by arrows) is due partly to the distribution effect (i.e. 15.2/13.0 kPa) and partly to the curvature of the dissociation curve (i.e. 13.0/11.3 kPa) (cf. Fig. 7.15)

		Compartment			A-a difference (kPa)
		C_1	C_2	Combined*	
Gas phase					
Ventilation	l min^{-1}	4	1	$\dot{V}_A$ 5	
O_2 tension	kPa (mmHg)	16.7 (125)	9.3 (70)	P_{A,O_2} 15.2 (114)	
CO_2 tension	kPa (mmHg)	4.5 (34)	6.7 (50)	P_{A,CO_2} 4.9 (37)	
N_2 tension	kPa (mmHg)	74 (554)	79 (593)	P_{A,N_2} 75 (562)	
Blood phase					
Blood flow	l min^{-1}	2.5	2.5	$\dot{Q}t$ 5	
O_2 tension	kPa (mmHg)	16.7 (125)	9.3 (70)	13.0 (97.5)†	
Saturation	%	98.5	92	Sa,O_2 95	
				Pao_2 11.3 (85)‡	3.9 (29)
CO_2 tension	kPa (mmHg)	4.5 (34)	6.7 (50)	P_{A,CO_2} 5.6 (42)	0.7 (5)
N_2 tension	kPa (mmHg)	74 (554)	79 (593)	Pa,N_2 76.5 (573)	1.5 (11)
$\dot{V}_A/\dot{Q}$	—	1.6	0.4	1.0	

* In gas phase C_1 contributes four parts and C_2 one part. In blood phase C_1 and C_2 contribute equally.
† Assuming linear dissociation curve.
‡ From dissociation curve.

physiological range (Fig. 7.12). The curve is also steeper so, under quiet resting conditions, the washout of carbon dioxide in the lung lowers the carbon dioxide tension of the blood by less than 1 kPa. For the lung as a whole the reduced tension of carbon dioxide in blood from well-ventilated alveoli tends to compensate for the increased tension in blood from alveoli which are poorly ventilated. Thus for carbon dioxide only the distribution effect contributes to alveolar—arterial tension differences whereas for oxygen both effects are important. These features are summarised in Table 7.2 and by a numerical example in Table 7.1.

For oxygen the two effects result in a tension difference for oxygen between mixed alveolar gas and systemic arterial blood (A-a Do_2) in healthy subjects of 0.7—2 kPa (see also Table 15.22, page 511). In patients in whom there is a wide range of ventilation—perfusion ratios the difference can be much greater (Fig. 7.13). The a-A differences for carbon dioxide are in general smaller. For both gases large A-a differences are mainly due to lung units which have a high $\dot{V}_A/\dot{Q}$ ratio. Such differences reflect uneven lung function but not the extent to which the gaseous composition of the blood is abnormal. For oxygen this is mainly determined by the amount and composition of blood which perfuses poorly ventilated alveoli and the blood shunt compartment.

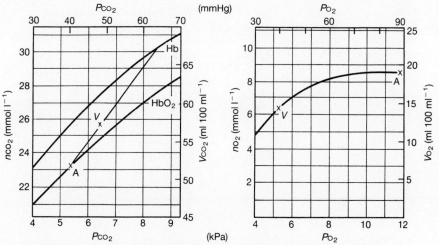

Fig. 7.12 Whole blood dissociation curves for carbon dioxide and oxygen over the physiological range in a healthy subject at rest. The points A and V are respectively for arterial and mixed venous blood. Between A and V the relationship for CO_2 is effectively linear but not that for O_2. (Sources: Christiansen J, Douglas CG, Haldane JS. *J Physiol* 1914; **48**: 244; Dill DB. *Handbook of Respiratory Data in Aviation*. Washington DC: Office of Scientific Research and Development, 1944.)

Table 7.2 Table summarising the levels of oxygen and carbon dioxide associated with the five compartment model of ventilation—perfusion relationships (Fig. 7.7). The dominant effects on mixed alveolar gas and pulmonary venous blood are indicated.* They are due solely to the distribution effect except in the case of oxygen in blood where the contribution of the dissociation curve is indicated by italics

Site	$\dot{V}_A/\dot{Q}$ ratio	Alveolar tension		Blood content	
		Oxygen	Carbon dioxide	Oxygen	Carbon dioxide
Anatomical shunt and non-ventilated alveoli	0	As mixed venous blood		As mixed venous blood	
Anatomic deadspace and non-perfused alveoli	∞	As inspired gas*		—	—
Underventilated or overperfused alveoli	0–0.9	Low	High	Low*	High*
Ideal alveoli	0.9	Normal	Normal	Normal	Normal
Overventilated or under-perfused alveoli	0.9–∞	High*	Low*	*Not raised*	Low
Principal consequences		$\dot{V}_A$ increased		Sa_{O_2} reduced	

Blood shunt compartment

Shunted blood is mixed venous blood; its composition can be derived from the following relationship:

$$\dot{n}_{O_2} = \dot{Q}t\,(Ca,_{O_2} - C\bar{v},_{O_2}) \qquad (7.4)$$

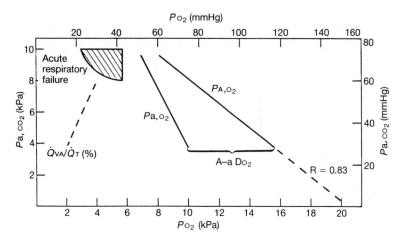

Fig. 7.13 O_2–CO_2 diagram for patients in respiratory failure. The lines describe the inter-relationships between alveolar and arterial blood gas tensions, and venous admixture effect for 487 patients with lung disease. The alveolar oxygen tensions (P_A, $_{O_2}$), calculated using the alveolar air equation (page 252), lie on the line for $R = 0.83$ (cf. Fig. 7.9). The diagram shows that patients with a *high* arterial tension of carbon dioxide can have a smaller alveolar–arterial oxygen tension difference (A-aDo_2) but a larger venous admixture ($\dot{Q}_{VA}/\dot{Q}_T$) than patients with a *low* tension of carbon dioxide; the difference reflects the level of alveolar ventilation and hence the alveolar oxygen tension. Thus the two indices of uneven distribution are not interchangeable. The shaded area indicates the arterial blood gas tensions before treatment with oxygen in 81 patients with acute respiratory failure. The lowest recorded A-a, o_2 was 2.5 kPa (19 mmHg) and the highest Pa,$_{CO_2}$ 11.7 kPa (88 mmHg). (Sources: Refsum HE, Kim BM. *Clin Sci* 1967; **33**: 569–576; McNicol MW, Campbell EJM. *Lancet* 1965; **1**: 336–338.)

where $\dot{n}o_2$ is oxygen uptake, $\dot{Q}t$ is cardiac output and the term within the bracket is the difference in oxygen content between arterial and mixed venous blood.

Cardiac output is the product of cardiac frequency (fc) and stroke volume (SV) whilst Cao_2 is a function of the oxygen dissociation curve (f), haemoglobin concentration [Hb] and arterial oxygen saturation (Sa,o_2). Then on substitution and re-arrangement:

$$C\bar{v},o_2 = f[Hb]\ Sa,o_2 - \dot{n}o_2/(fc.sv) \qquad (7.5)$$

The contribution of shunted blood to hypoxaemia is greatest when the mixed venous oxygen content is reduced. From the above equation this is likely to be the case when oxygen consumption is increased by exercise or cardiac output is low because of bradycardia, vascular obstruction or shock. The $C\bar{v},o_2$ is also reduced when oxygen transport is impaired by anaemia or an altered dissociation curve or when the oxygenation of blood perfusing better ventilated alveoli is reduced by pulmonary oedema or breathing an hypoxic gas mixture. The contributions of some of these factors in individual medical conditions has been unravelled using the multiple inert gas elimination technique (e.g. Fig. 7.14). Further results are given in Chapter 16. The measurement of the venous admixture and blood shunt are given in Chapter 8.

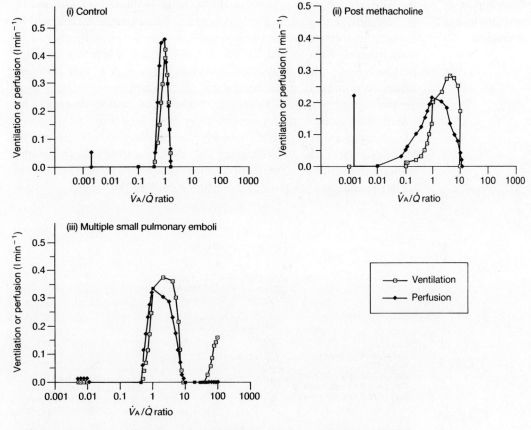

Fig. 7.14 Distributions of ventilation and perfusion obtained by the multiple inert gas elimination technique in two dogs showing: (i) a normal distribution; (ii) the change in distribution following induction of bronchoconstriction with metacholine; this reduced the ventilation to part of the lung and caused a compensatory reduction in perfusion. The dispersion of $\dot{V}_A/\dot{Q}$ ratios and the size of the blood shunt compartment were then increased; (iii) the effect of reducing the pulmonary blood flow with glass microspheres: this resulted in part of the lung being overventilated relative to the perfusion. The distribution of ventilation was then bimodal. The dispersion of perfusion was increased with some alveoli having very little ventilation (low $\dot{V}_A/\dot{Q}$ ratio). (Source: Reed JW, Guy H. Unpublished.)

Arterial–alveolar tension difference for nitrogen

Nitrogen in the body behaves mainly as an inert gas as it participates in metabolism to only a very limited extent. The tension of nitrogen in the blood is therefore determined mainly by pulmonary factors; these have been analysed by Klocke, Rahn and others. Within an alveolus the tension of nitrogen is determined by the dry gas pressure and the co-existing tensions of oxygen and carbon dioxide. The latter are influenced by the ventilation–perfusion ratio which therefore also influences the tension of nitrogen. Because of the dissociation curve effect, the volume of oxygen which is absorbed from an alveolus with a high $\dot{V}_A/\dot{Q}$ ratio is less than the volume of CO_2 excreted into it. In these circumstances the respiratory exchange ratio exceeds unity and the nitrogen which is present in the alveolus is diluted by addition of carbon dioxide to a greater extent than it is concentrated by removal of oxygen; the tension of nitrogen in such an alveolus is relatively low in consequence. By contrast, in an alveolus having a low ventilation–perfusion ratio the respiratory exchange ratio is low and nitrogen which is present is concentrated by the absorption of oxygen to a greater extent than it is diluted by addition of carbon dioxide. The nitrogen tension is therefore relatively high (see Fig. 7.15). Since nitrogen passes freely across the alveolar capillary membrane similar tensions exist in the blood leaving the alveolar capillaries. In healthy subjects the ventilation–perfusion ratios are affected by gravity and are higher in the superior than in the inferior parts of the lung (Fig. 7.15).

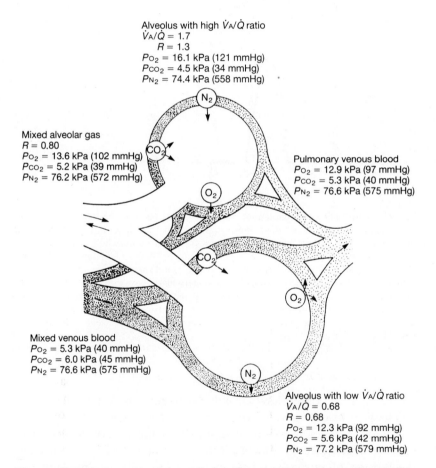

Alveolus with high $\dot{V}A/\dot{Q}$ ratio
$\dot{V}A/\dot{Q} = 1.7$
$R = 1.3$
$Po_2 = 16.1$ kPa (121 mmHg)
$Pco_2 = 4.5$ kPa (34 mmHg)
$PN_2 = 74.4$ kPa (558 mmHg)

Mixed alveolar gas
$R = 0.80$
$Po_2 = 13.6$ kPa (102 mmHg)
$Pco_2 = 5.2$ kPa (39 mmHg)
$PN_2 = 76.2$ kPa (572 mmHg)

Pulmonary venous blood
$Po_2 = 12.9$ kPa (97 mmHg)
$Pco_2 = 5.3$ kPa (40 mmHg)
$PN_2 = 76.6$ kPa (575 mmHg)

Mixed venous blood
$Po_2 = 5.3$ kPa (40 mmHg)
$Pco_2 = 6.0$ kPa (45 mmHg)
$PN_2 = 76.6$ kPa (575 mmHg)

Alveolus with low $\dot{V}A/\dot{Q}$ ratio
$\dot{V}A/\dot{Q} = 0.68$
$R = 0.68$
$Po_2 = 12.3$ kPa (92 mmHg)
$Pco_2 = 5.6$ kPa (42 mmHg)
$PN_2 = 77.2$ kPa (579 mmHg)

Fig. 7.15 Numerical example of the vertical gradient in lung gas exchange for a healthy subject studied by West. The reasons for the gradient are given in the text and illustrated in Figs 7.1 and 7.5. The upper alveolus has a relatively high $\dot{V}A/\dot{Q}$ ratio. Due to the dissociation curve effect the upper alveolus has a higher respiratory exchange ratio and lower nitrogen tension compared with the lower alveolus. Due to the distribution effect this inequality leads to a finite tension difference for nitrogen between mixed alveolar gas and pulmonary venous (i.e. mixed arterial blood). The corresponding tensions of oxygen and carbon dioxide are also given.

On this account, West has shown that, compared with mixed venous blood, the nitrogen tension in apical alveoli is low whilst that in basal alveoli is high. There is then a circulation of nitrogen from blood to alveoli in superior parts and from alveoli to blood in dependent parts, but the total quantity of nitrogen inhaled and exhaled per breath remains nearly constant. The tensions of nitrogen are identical in systemic arterial and mixed venous blood, hence any overall difference in nitrogen tension between blood and mixed alveolar gas cannot be due to an anatomical shunt, as is partly the case for oxygen. Instead Rahn and his colleagues have shown that it mainly reflects the presence of alveoli having a low ventilation−perfusion ratio. In this it complements the mixed alveolar to arterial tension difference for carbon dioxide which is mainly due to the presence of alveoli having a high ventilation− perfusion ratio (cf. page 205). For healthy subjects, in whom the proportion of low $\dot{V}A/\dot{Q}$ alveoli is small, the arterial alveolar tension difference for nitrogen is about 0.4 kPa (3 mmHg) (Fig. 7.15); in patients in whom the proportion is increased on account of lung disease the difference increases up to about 3 kPa (20 mmHg). The measurement of a-ADN$_2$ is described on page 261. It is mainly of historical interest since the multiple inert gas elimination technique provides more complete information.

Slope of the alveolar plateau

During a single expiration after exhalation of deadspace gas the tensions of oxygen, carbon dioxide and nitrogen measured at the mouth each attain a nearly constant level; this is the alveolar plateau or phase 3 for the gas in question. The term phase 3 is preferable because, as the expiration continues, the tension of oxygen falls progressively whilst those of carbon dioxide and nitrogen rise, e.g. Fig. 8.7 (page 226) and Fig. 8.3, (page 217). In healthy subjects phase 3 is nearly horizontal; most of the slope is due to gas exchange continuing during the expiration. The slope for carbon dioxide can then be described in terms of the volume and composition of inspired gas, the alveolar volume, the flow rate and composition of mixed venous blood and the time of expiration. The changes which take place have been used by Kim, Rahn and Farhi as a basis for measurement of cardiac output, Fig. 8.16 (page 245).

The slope of phase 3 is the resultant of all the factors which determine the regional distribution of ventilation and perfusion including gravitational force, the distribution of compliance and resistance and uneven contraction of respiratory muscles; these and other factors are discussed earlier in this chapter. In the presence of uneven lung function the slope is related to $\dot{V}A/\dot{Q}$ inequality because the alveoli which empty later in expiration usually have a lower ventilation−perfusion ratio than those which empty earlier. Since low $\dot{V}A/\dot{Q}$ ratios are associated with low respiratory exchange ratios (RER) and vice versa the slope of phase 3 for respiratory exchange ratio is affected by the uneven distribution of time constants within the lung. This is the basis for the

211

intra-breath R test which is described on page 259. Changes in time constants are usually a consequence of airways obstruction but can be due to uneven distribution of compliance (e.g. Fig. 8.19, page 182).

Guide to references

The references (Chapter 18) are classified under subject headings of which the following are particularly relevant to the present chapter:

8: Assessment of Distribution of Ventilation and of Blood Flow Through the Lung

Single breath and multibreath indices of uniformity of ventilation
Lobar analysis of lung function
Analysis by particle deposition characteristics
Use of radio-isotopes

Cardiac output and pulmonary blood flow
Inequality of ventilation–perfusion ratios including three compartment model, multiple inert gas elimination technique (MIGET) and intrabreath R

Types of assessment

The extent of uneven distribution of ventilation is usually assessed using a single breath procedure in which the subject inhales a test breath of oxygen; this dilutes the nitrogen already present in the lung and the extent of uneven distribution is inferred from changes in concentration of nitrogen at the mouth during the subsequent exhalation. Somewhat different information is obtained if instead of using nitrogen, which is the resident gas, the test is based on an inert gas which is foreign to the lung, for example a test breath or bolus of helium, argon or neon. A radioactive isotope of xenon, nitrogen or krypton can also be used in this way. Alternatively the radioactive gases can be used in conjunction with scintillation counters on the chest wall to monitor the distribution of ventilation on a regional basis. This technique has been used for investigating vertical gradients in lung function including those due to gravity. It can also locate regions of abnormal function. Localisation on an anatomical basis can be achieved by sampling gas from a bronchoscope with its tip placed in a lobar bronchus. Changes of distribution of ventilation with respect to time can be assessed by analysis of a series of breaths; this can be done with the subject breathing oxygen in open circuit or rebreathing a gas mixture containing helium from a closed circuit spirometer. These procedures are usually combined with measurement of functional residual capacity (page 149).

Distribution of perfusion can be assessed on a regional basis from the distribution of a radioactive marker such as human albumen labelled with technetium (^{99}Tc). The regional perfusion can then be compared with the regional ventilation obtained using for example radioactive krypton (^{81}Kr). For the whole lung the extent of uneven distribution of perfusion can be inferred from measurements which reflect the range of ventilation–perfusion ratios.

The distribution of ventilation with respect to perfusion can be obtained in terms of a five compartment model; this involves measuring the physiological deadspace and venous admixture effect by gasometric methods. The procedure entails analysis of arterial blood. The extent of ventilation–perfusion inequality can be assessed by using the intra-breath R single breath test, or by the multiple inert gas elimination technique of Wagner and West; the latter yields a numerical distribution of ventilation–perfusion ratios.

For epidemiological and occupational surveys the single breath nitrogen test is widely used because it is a simple and sensitive indicator of slight abnormalities of ventilation not reflected in the forced expiratory volume.

For in-depth studies of the mechanisms of hypoxaemia the multiple inert gas elimination technique is appropriate but available only at a few centres. The physiological deadspace and venous admixture effect can also be informative. For clinical investigation of suspected pulmonary embolism the assessment of regional function should be considered. The other tests are now mainly of research interest.

Indices of uniformity of ventilation

Single breath nitrogen tests

These procedures yield the anatomical deadspace (Fowler deadspace), the Fowler index of uneven ventilation, the slope of the alveolar plateau, the closing volume and an estimate of residual volume from which the closing capacity can be calculated. The methods were introduced by Ward Fowler following the development by Lilly of a rapid ultraviolet emission analyser for nitrogen. Other indicator gases can also be used to obtain these and additional indices; the latter are mentioned under alternative procedures below.

Apparatus. Volume is recorded by using a spirometer or from integration of the output of a pneumotachograph. Nitrogen concentration is measured with the ultraviolet emission analyser mentioned above. Alternatively the nitrogen concentration can be obtained using a respiratory mass spectrometer. The volume and gas concentration are displayed on an XY recorder; the components of the recording system should each have a minimal response time of 0.1 s and the records of volume and concentration should by synchronous. Oxygen is delivered from a demand valve, bag or spirometer. A convenient tap assembly is illustrated in Fig. 8.1. It should include a means of registering the flow rate during expiration, either an orifice resistance (diameter 4 mm) and pressure gauge, as recommended by Green and Travis, a pneumotachograph or a spirometer and differentiator. A flow signal is preferable as the orifice can influence the distribution in the lung of the test breath. The apparatus is arranged so that the subject is studied seated in an upright posture. A nose clip is worn.

Procedure for anatomical deadspace

The subject breathes normally through the mouthpiece to air, then at

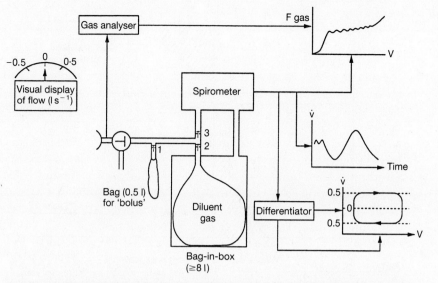

Fig. 8.1 Apparatus for single breath tests of uneven lung function. The valves 1 and 2 are adjusted so that the bag containing the test gas empties before the subject inhales from the bag-in-box (Donald, Christie box). The respiratory flow rates during inspiration and expiration should be in the range $0.3-0.5 \, l \, s^{-1}$ for 95% of the expiration. The display should be visible to the subject. The instruments should have response times of less than 0.1 s and the records of volume and of concentration should be synchronous; when two gases are to be analysed this is best done using a mass spectrometer and not separate analysers.

the end of an expiration is switched to the oxygen reservoir (this is labelled 'diluent gas' in Fig. 8.1). A single tidal breath of oxygen is inhaled and the subject then exhales normally. The time between the end of inspiration and the start of expiration should be standardised at 0.4–0.6 s. During expiration the nitrogen concentration is recorded. A schematic result is illustrated in Fig. 8.2; it has three parts. In phase 1 the nitrogen concentration is effectively zero. During this phase the gas which is sampled is oxygen from the mouth and airways down to the level of the terminal bronchioles. In phase 2 the nitrogen concentration rises rapidly. This phase represents the transition from sampling dead-space gas to sampling gas from alveoli (phase 3) in which the nitrogen already present has been diluted by the inhaled oxygen. The anatomic deadspace is taken as the volume expired up to the point when half the nitrogen in phase 2 has been expired. This can be defined graphically (Fig. 8.2).

The shape of phase 2 is influenced by the degree of turbulence (page 108) and the extent of diffusive mixing in the airways. The latter is increased by any delay between completing the inhalation of oxygen and starting to breathe out. To reduce variation on this account Norris suggested that the post-inspiratory pause should be standardised at 0.4–0.6 s. The anatomical deadspace varies with body size and lung volume so the tidal volume and functional residual capacity or thoracic gas volume should be recorded. The deadspace is, for practical purposes,

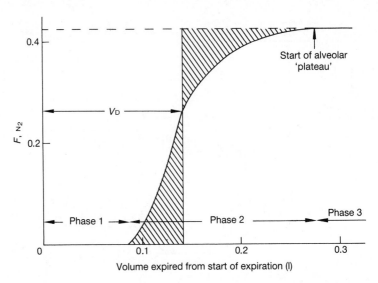

Fig. 8.2 Method for obtaining the anatomical deadspace following the inhalation of a single tidal breath of oxygen. The fractional concentration of nitrogen at the lips and the volume expired are recorded or replotted from separate records. The time between the end of inspiration and the start of expiration should be standardised at 0.4–0.6 s. The anatomical deadspace is obtained by dividing the rising part of the curve so that the two shaded areas are equal.

equal for all gases except those which are very soluble in an aqueous medium. Thus *modified procedures* have been developed using for example helium in oxygen ($F_{He} = 0.8$) or carbon dioxide in air as the indicator gas. The gases can be analysed using a respiratory mass spectrometer, or in the case of CO_2, a rapid infrared gas analyser.

Procedures for nitrogen indices of gas mixing within the lung

Vital capacity method. The subject breathes quietly through the mouthpiece to air, takes two deep breathes, then makes a full, relaxed expiration to residual volume. He signals that expiration is complete, the operator turns the tap connecting the mouthpiece to the oxygen reservoir and the subject makes a slow full inspiration to total lung capacity. He then immediately makes a slow full expiration to residual volume. During these manoeuvres the flow rate should not deviate outside the range $0.3-0.5 \mathrm{l s}^{-1}$. Alternatively if a constriction in the mouthpiece is used the pressure proximal to the constriction should not exceed 0.7 kPa (7 cmH$_2$O) The *Fowler nitrogen index* is the difference between the concentration of nitrogen in expired gas sampled at 750 ml and at 1250 ml after the start of expiration. The units are percentage of nitrogen in dry gas and the reference values, depending on the age and sex of the subject, are in the range 0.4–1.7% (Fig. 15.24, page 502). The merits and limitations of the index are discussed below. The *slope of the alveolar plateau* is depicted by the linear part of phase 3 (Fig. 8.3); this is usually taken from when 30% of vital capacity has

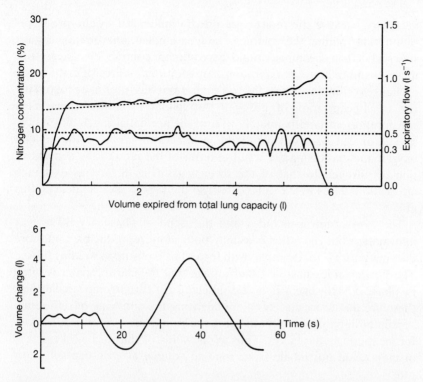

Fig. 8.3 Records obtained during the performance of the single breath nitrogen test by a normal subject. The upper figure shows nitrogen concentration and expiratory flow rate plotted against volume of gas expired and the lower figure the lung volume changes plotted against time. The flow rate is at the upper limit of what is acceptable (cf. Fig. 8.1). The inclined line represents the slope of phase 3 and the shorter vertical line the onset of phase 4 after allowing for cardiogenic oscillations. The latter are mainly confined to phase 3. (Source: El-Gamal FM. PhD Thesis, University of Newcastle upon Tyne 1986.)

been expired to the start of phase 4. The latter is defined under closing volume below. The position of the best fitting line can be determined by eye or a suitable computer programme can be used. However, errors in commercially available programmes have been reported so these should be checked carefully. The units are $\Delta[N_2]\% \, l^{-1}$. The measurement should be repeated until three technically satisfactory results have been obtained. For this purpose the inspired and expired volumes should agree to within 5%, the expired volume should be within 10% of vital capacity, the curve should not be interrupted by step changes and the flow rates should be within the prescribed limits. The mean result should be accepted. However, if the subject has difficulty with the procedure the mean of two, or even a single result, should be used, as repeated attempts (e.g. more than six) can be counterproductive. The interval between tests should be sufficient to wash out the additional oxygen from the lungs, this is 3–5 min in healthy subjects but up to 10 min in patients with poor lung mixing.

The procedure as described is that of a working group of the US National Heart and Lung Institute. The strict criteria were considered necessary because the indices are greatly influenced by the pre-inspiration lung volume, the volume of oxygen inhaled, uneven lung expansion such as can accompany rapid inspiration or contraction of accessory muscles and the rate of expiration. An additional source of error is gas exchange continuing during the test expiration; this leads to a progressive rise in concentration of nitrogen throughout expiration (page 211) which represents approximately 10% of the normal nitrogen difference. The error can be avoided by adding helium or argon to the inhaled oxygen and expressing the result in terms of the ratio of the concentration of nitrogen to that of the foreign gas (Fig. 8.4). Gas exchange affects both gases to the same extent so the ratio is independent of this effect.

The Fowler nitrogen index and the slope of phase 3 yield similar information but the latter is usually both more reproducible and more discriminatory — for example, with respect to exposure to welding fumes. The Fowler index has the disadvantage that the starting point is often in phase 2. However, it is less affected by cardiogenic oscillations; these are due to cardiac systole influencing the emptying of differently ventilated lung units. In both cases the procedure presents difficulties for inexperienced subjects. Thus in one study of shipyard workers 22% of men could not inhale from residual volume at an acceptably slow rate.

The numerical values for nitrogen slope $(\Delta[N_2]\% \, l^{-1})$ resemble those for the nitrogen index $(N_2 \%)$ despite the units being different. Both indices are increased by narrowing of small airways and by structural changes within the acinus altering the path length for diffusion. On this

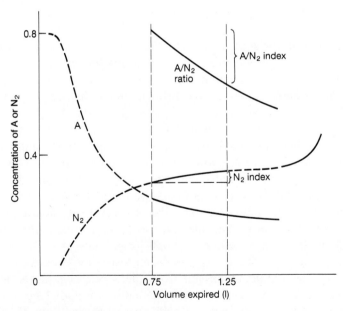

Fig. 8.4 Argon/nitrogen index of uneven ventilation. For this test the test inspirate is 80% argon, 20% oxygen. The gases are analysed using a mass spectrometer.

account Paiva and colleagues have suggested that the slope might be a guide to the presence of emphysema but this has still to be confirmed.

The sensitivity of the slope indices can be improved by starting the test inspiration from near to functional residual capacity. This modified method resembles that originally proposed by Fowler and is described below. It leads to fewer lapses on technical grounds than the vital capacity method but the latter has the advantage of also providing estimates of closing volume and capacity as well as fairly reproducible nitrogen slopes. Closing volume and capacity are described below.

Modified single breath methods. These methods are based on evidence by Paiva and others that, compared with the vital capacity method, more information can be obtained by beginning the test inspiration of oxygen from a lung volume between closing capacity and functional residual capacity; this is near to the mid-point of the expiratory reserve volume. The volume of the test breath is 1 l or 25% of the predicted vital capacity. The simplest modified procedure entails a test inspiration of 1 l of oxygen starting from functional residual capacity (FRC). The inspiration is preceded by two deep breaths to open any airways which may have been closed then three normal tidal breaths to re-establish the FRC. The inspiration and subsequent complete expiration are made slowly with minimal delay between them. The slope indices are calculated in the manner described above. Closing volume is not detected by this method. However, it can be obtained if the modified test inspiration is continued to total lung capacity. This procedure yields a more distinct phase 4 but higher values for closing volume and nitrogen slope compared with the vital capacity procedure. Information on the contribution of gaseous diffusion can be obtained if gases of different diffusivity are studied, for example, helium and sulphur hexafluoride (Table 5.5, page 111). Thus Paiva and colleagues have evidence that using a test inspirate of 0.5 l the difference between the slopes of phase 3 for helium and for sulphur hexafluoride may be a sensitive index of bronchiolitis. The respective relationships of the slopes to the volumes of the test inspirates may also be informative.

Closing volume and capacity

Single breath nitrogen method for CV and CC. The closing volume and capacity are usually obtained during the course of estimating the single breath nitrogen slope by the vital capacity method. They can also be obtained by the bolus method which is described subsequently. The nitrogen slope (phase 3) occupies most of expiration. It is followed by a fourth phase in which the nitrogen concentration rises above that in phase 3 (Fig. 8.3). This rise occurs towards the end of expiration, and in some subjects is followed by a sharp fall in concentration which is designated phase 5.

The closing volume is defined as the lung volume above residual volume at which closure of lung airways first occurs as indicated by the start of phase 4. The closing capacity is the lung volume at which closure first occurs expressed as a percentage of total lung capacity.

$$CC(\%) = 100 \ (CV + RV)/(VC + RV) \qquad (8.1)$$

where CC is closing capacity, CV is closing volume, RV is residual volume and VC is vital capacity. Thus the denominator is total lung capacity. In healthy subjects the presence of phase 4 is evidence of regional differences in lung filling and emptying. The explanation for this terminal rise in nitrogen slope is that during inspiration from residual volume the upper zones have a lower expansion ratio than the lower zones (Fig. 7.1, page 181). Hence at the end of the test inspiration, the oxygen concentration in the upper zone is lower and nitrogen concentration higher than in the bases. Both zones contribute gas to the subsequent expiration; however, towards the end of expiration some basal airways close. Thereafter the gas which is expired comes mainly from the upper zones. Since gas from this zone is relatively rich in nitrogen the recorded concentration rises.

The procedure for recording closing volume is that described for the single breath nitrogen slope by the vital capacity method. The onset of phase 4 is then the point at which the nitrogen concentration rises above the inclining phase 3; in its identification allowance needs to be made for the cardiogenic oscillations. Closing volume extends from this point to residual volume which should therefore be delineated correctly. This is particularly important in adolescents and young adults in whom closing volume may occur near the end of the vital capacity manoeuvre. For such subjects acceptance of the criterion that the expired volume should be at least 90% of vital capacity can lead to the closing volume being missed. A 99% criterion increases the yield. In addition a bolus of air can be administered at the start of the inspiration during which oxygen is inhaled. Manual compression of the thorax at the end of expiration can also be considered but this manoeuvre needs to be validated.

Closing capacity is defined by equation 8.1. It is calculated from closing volume, vital capacity and residual volume; the last is best obtained by an independent method, for example, closed circuit spirometry, whole body plethysmography or the nitrogen rebreathing method. These are described in Chapter 6 (pages 149–154). Alternatively for subjects with normal or moderately impaired gas mixing the alveolar volume can be calculated from information obtained during the single breath test. Then:

$$V_A = \frac{V_I, \ F_{A,N_2} - (V_{E,N_2}) \ (Vd/(V_E - Vd))}{F_{A,N_2} - (V_{E,N_2})/(V_E - Vd)} \ (l) \qquad (8.2)$$

where V_A, V_I, V_E and Vd are respectively the alveolar volume, the inspired and expired volume and the volume of the anatomical deadspace in lBTPS. F_{A,N_2} is the fractional alveolar concentration of nitrogen before the test breath and V_E, N_2 is the volume of nitrogen expired; this is given by the area under the single breath curve. The method can underestimate the alveolar volume when there is airways obstruction (cf. page 302).

Closing volume is usually reported as a percentage of vital capacity (CV%); in these units it is relatively large in early childhood, falls to a minimum of 10% on average in early adulthood, and then rises nearly linearly to an average of 30% in older subjects (Fig. 15.24, page 502). CV% is increased in most smokers and persons with airflow obstruction.

Bolus method for closing volume. The method differs from that described above in that a foreign indicator gas is used instead of nitrogen. Radioactive xenon (^{133}Xe) was first used for this purpose by Dollfuss but helium, argon or neon are preferable. The procedure is exactly as described except that the test inspiration from residual volume is a bolus of approximately 0.31 of the chosen gas followed by air; an appropriate analyser is used, for example a respiratory mass spectrometer or a critical orifice helium analyser. By this method the phase 3 usually exhibits marked cardiogenic oscillations but these disappear at the onset of phase 4 due to the closure of airways. The closing volume is apparent in all subjects including those in whom it is not detectable by the nitrogen method. However, compared with the nitrogen method the closing volume is invariably higher. It can also respond differently to acute airflow obstruction. This is due to the mechanism for producing a closing volume being different in the two situations. By the nitrogen method inequality is detected in terms of expansion ratios (page 180). By the bolus method the separation is anatomical with the test gas being inhaled mainly into the upper zones which normally fill earlier and empty later than the lower zones (page 180). Phase 3 obtained by the bolus method should not be used because it is greatly influenced by technical and other factors associated with the measurement.

Other methods for closing volume. A closing volume is demonstrable in the relationship of transpulmonary pressure to lung volume and of airflow resistance to thoracic gas volume. The volumes are larger than those seen by gas dilution methods.

Nitrogen slope and closing volume as epidemiological tools

The nitrogen slope arises mainly from local variations in ventilation and gaseous diffusion within and between acini (page 185), whereas the closing volume arises from regional differences in expansion ratios. Thus the two indices are complementary. In different circumstances both have been found useful in epidemiological surveys but there are snags. A proportion of subjects cannot perform the slow vital capacity which the unmodified nitrogen method requires and in some the closing volume is not detectable. Other methods of measuring closing volume often give different results. Closing volume is also strongly associated with smoking which can be assessed more directly by questionnaire. Thus closing volume appears to be of limited usefulness except in those who have never smoked, or where an environmental factor such as welding fumes interacts with smoking. The nitrogen slope may detect narrowing of small airways and, possibly, the early effects of emphysema but these abnormalities are usually considered to be indicated with greater certainty by the flow—volume curve and loss of transfer factor respectively. In addition, despite early promise, the nitrogen indices have not proved to be consistent predictors of a subsequent accelerated decline in forced expiratory volume. Thus the single breath nitrogen test using a vital capacity breath of oxygen is now seldom recommended for respiratory surveys; the evidence is reviewed by Viegi and colleagues. However, the prospects for modified single breath procedures such as those developed by the Brussels school (pages 219 and 669) are excellent and further work is indicated.

Multibreath indices of gas mixing

Lung volume index of uneven ventilation. This index is the ratio of the alveolar volume (i.e. total lung capacity minus anatomical deadspace) estimated by a single breath technique to that by a multibreath or plethysmographic method. It is therefore the ratio of the accessible or effective lung volume to the total lung volume; it is designated $V_A,\text{eff}/V_A$. In subjects with normal lung mixing the accessible and static volumes are nearly identical but with uneven total ventilation the accessible volume is reduced. This occurs when increasing age or disease processes affect the lung airways. The reference values of $V_A,\text{eff}/V_A$ are in the range $1.0-0.85$ (Table 15.22, page 511). A value below 0.85 is usually evidence for uneven ventilation but a value above 1.0 is due to technical error and is not diagnostic.

The index is obtained if the measurement of the transfer factor for carbon monoxide by the single breath method is combined with a separate estimate of alveolar volume (page 302). The $V_A,\text{eff}/V_A$ is correlated with forced expiratory volume as a percentage of vital capacity ($FEV_1\%$) and residual volume as a percentage of total lung capacity (RV%). The three indices can be combined in an empirical index of airflow obstruction (COI):

$$COI = 75 + 0.5 \, RV\% - 40 V_A,\text{eff}/V_A - 0.3 \, FEV_1\% \quad (8.3)$$

where COI is combined obstruction index. The index which was proposed by Cotes, can be used, with others, to provide a multi-dimensional description of lung function (page 69). Reference values are given on pages 496–7.

Closed circuit mixing index. The index is obtained during measurement of functional residual capacity by the closed circuit helium dilution method. It is the number of breaths completed by the subject up to the point when the concentration of helium in the circuit has fallen to within 10% of the equilibrium value. Depending on the tidal volume 15–30 breaths are normally required. The number is increased in the presence of uneven ventilation and is influenced by the ratio between tidal volume and alveolar volume. The result is also influenced by the volume and mixing characteristics of the closed circuit apparatus and the response time of the helium analyser. These features are difficult to standardise and therefore this index is not recommended.

Open circuit indices of gas mixing. The open circuit method for measuring functional residual capacity which is described on page 149, yields three classes of mixing indices. These relate to quiet resting conditions.

1 The *concentration of nitrogen in alveolar gas* after breathing oxygen for 7 min. The concentration is normally less than 1.5% at age 20, increasing to less than 2.5% at age 60. Higher values obtain when gas mixing in the lung is impaired by narrowing of lung airways. No allowance is made for the rate of ventilation which also affects the result.

2 The *lung clearance index* used by Becklake, Bouhuys and others. This is the volume of oxygen which must be breathed in order to lower the concentration of nitrogen in end tidal gas to 2%. The volume is expressed as a multiple of functional residual capacity. In healthy young adults the lung clearance index is in the range 5.0–9.0. Higher values obtain in older subjects and when the effectiveness of gas mixing is impaired.

3 Indices derived by *exponential analysis.* This model describes lung mixing in terms of one or more groups of alveoli all having the same expansion ratio. For such a group the nitrogen concentration falls rapidly at first and then more slowly as the nitrogen is washed out. The fall in concentration of nitrogen per breath is proportional to the concentration present and is linear when the log of the concentration is related to the number of breaths, provided the breaths are of equal volume. In healthy young adults the semilog plot is slightly curvilinear (Fig. 8.5); this is evidence for the presence of a range of expansion ratios. The range is widened by ageing or airway narrowing. For purposes of analysis the washout curve can be partitioned into two or more exponentials. Where two exponentials are fitted these represent two hypothetical chambers of different size and different expansion ratios which, if they were connected in parallel, would yield a washout curve similar to that which is observed for the intact subject. The analysis does not provide a unique description because the same washout curve could be described in more than one way. However, the procedure permits the construction of a model of lung expansion on which can be grafted similar descriptions of the perfusion and diffusion characteristics of the lung. The best account is still that of Gilson, Hugh-Jones, Oldham and Meade.

As an alternative to the nitrogen clearance curve, Cumming suggested using the decay curve (Fig. 8.6) in which, at any time, the volume of nitrogen remaining in the lung is related to the volume of oxygen which has been inhaled. Linear deviation from the relationship for an

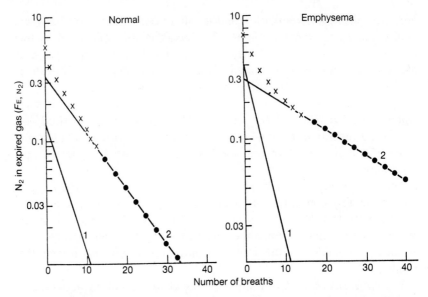

Fig. 8.5 Nitrogen washout curves obtained during breathing oxygen by a healthy subject and a patient with emphysema. The curves are subdivided into two components which represent alveoli which are well and poorly ventilated; these respectively have a high and low expansion ratio. To perform the analysis the slow mixing compartment of the lung is defined by the best fit for the tail of the curve where it is marked with dots. This is designated line 2. The fast mixing compartment is then defined by line 1 which is obtained by replotting the difference between the upper end of line 2 and the proximal part of the curve where it is marked with crosses. The rate of gas replacement in each compartment is described by the slope of the appropriate line; the rate for the poorly ventilated alveoli is slower in the patient with emphysema than in the healthy subject.

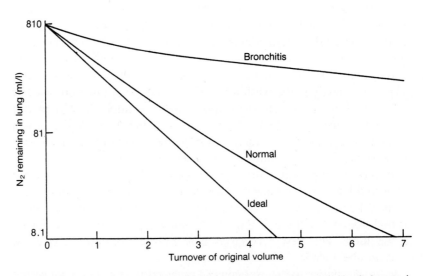

Fig. 8.6 Lung decay curves obtained by Cumming, showing the washout of nitrogen by breathing oxygen. The ordinate is the volume of nitrogen remaining in the lung expressed per litre of lung volume. The abscissa is the volume of oxygen inhaled, expressed per litre of lung volume. For interpretation see text.

ideal single chamber lung is then evidence for impaired mixing between
the inhaled gas and the alveolar gas within lung units (stratified
inhomogeneity) whilst curvilinearity is due to differences in time
constants between the units. Stratified inhomogeneity appears to be
the main cause of impaired mixing in patients with bronchitis.

A more sophisticated interpretation is possible if the washout is
controlled; this has been done by Crawford and colleagues who used a
1 l tidal volume inhaled at a constant flow rate (page 186).

Lobar analysis of lung function

The function of the right and left lungs can be studied separately by
bronchospirometry using a Carlens catheter. This has a double lumen
and inflatable cuffs to secure an airtight fit into the right and left main
bronchi. Ventilation, lung volume, gas exchange and pulmonary blood
flow can then be measured on each lung separately. From these and
other data the range of the ventilation—perfusion ratios and the surface
for gas exchange can be estimated. In unilateral lung disease useful
information can be obtained from measurements made with the subject
lying in the left or right lateral positions. The arterial oxygen tension
is often higher when the diseased lung is uppermost, whilst in this
position the increase in resting respiratory level compared with the
supine position is less than when the diseased lung is dependent.

However, this procedure has now largely been replaced by fibre
optic bronchoscopy and bronchial catheterisation using a tube of diameter 0.5−1.0 mm. The sampled gas is analysed using a respiratory
mass spectrometer (page 34). The techniques were pioneered by
Hugh-Jones and West and developed by Denison and colleagues amongst
others.

Lobar volume can be measured by gasometric methods which estimate
the ventilated volume accessible to the respired gas. The methods
include:

1 Washout of argon delivered to the lobe or segment from a locally
placed catheter; for this purpose a 20 ml bolus of argon is injected
during a slow inspiration from residual volume. The catheter is then
connected to the respiratory mass spectrometer and the local argon
concentration is analysed during the subsequent expiration. The accessible volume is calculated from the dilution of the argon.

2 A balloon catheter (e.g. Swan-Ganz 4F) is placed in the lobar or
segmental bronchus, the subject inhales a vital capacity breath of a gas
mixture containing argon in appropriate concentration and the balloon
is inflated. Subsequently the subject makes a full expiration into a
spirometer. The balloon is then deflated whilst expiratory effort is
continued; the additional volume expired and the local argon concentration during expiration are recorded and used to calculate the accessible
gas volume. The relationship of this volume to the total gas volume is
considered on page 534. The latter can be obtained by chest radiography
in subjects who have identifiable inter-lobar fissures on the lateral

view. If the fissures cannot be identified or if segmental volume is required, the relevant part can often be outlined using the radioactive gas krypton-81m (page 237). This is administered by the bolus method described above. The subsequent measurements and calculations are given by Pierce and colleagues. They are based on those for total lung capacity described on page 310.

Dynamic lobar volumes including flow volume curves can be obtained by spirometry performed with and without occlusion of the relevant airway; depending on circumstances the latter can be the lobar or segmental bronchus or the right or left main bronchus. The response of the occluded section can be obtained either directly or by subtraction from that for the intact lung.

Lobar ventilation−perfusion relationships can be obtained by lobar sampling using carbon dioxide as the indicator gas. An example is given in Fig. 8.7. Alternatively the lobar gas exchange can be studied in detail using a test gas mixture containing an inert gas (helium or argon), a very soluble gas (acetylene or freon-22) and carbon monoxide (e.g. $C^{18}O$) in air. These gases are used respectively to estimate the alveolar ventilation, blood flow and transfer factor all expressed per unit of alveolar volume. The method is described by Denison and colleagues. Some of the procedures are facilitated by use of a very long (30 m) sampling tube from the probe to the respiratory mass spectrometer. This delays the arrival of the sample without introducing significant disturbance. Thus two tubes of different lengths can be used in

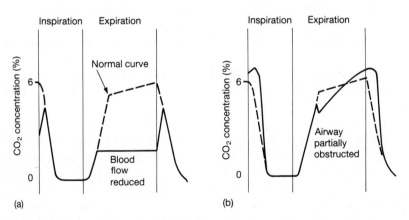

(a)   (b)

Fig. 8.7 Capnigram obtained by sampling from a lobar bronchus. The normal fluctuations during the respiratory cycle are shown by the interrupted line. When the lobar blood flow is reduced (left hand diagram) the alveolar concentration during expiration is diminished. At the start of inspiration the concentration rises briefly due to the entry into the lobe of deadspace gas which has come from normally perfused regions of the lung. When the airway is partly obstructed (right hand diagram) the concentration during expiration rises to an initial peak, declines and then rises again. The initial peak is due to the affected lobe continuing to inspire gas from adjacent lobes which are starting to expire (Pendelluft effect). The high alveolar plateau is due to the lobar ventilation being reduced and the continuation of the plateau into the subsequent inspiration is due to the affected lobe ventilating out of phase with the rest of the lung. (Source: Hugh-Jones P, West JB. *Bull Physiopathol Respir* 1967; **3**: 419−428.)

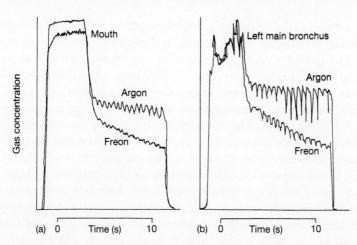

Fig. 8.8 Bronchial and oral concentrations of argon (A) and freon-22 ($CH_2F^{22}Cl$) in a normal subject lying on the left side. The subject inhaled the test gas from residual volume, held the breath then exhaled slowly. Sampling was concurrent via probes of different lengths. Compared with gas from both lungs sampled at the mouth, that from the left main bronchus contained more argon but no more freon-22; this was evidence for increased ventilation and perfusion of the dependent lung. (Source: Williams SJ, Pierce RJ, Davies NJH, Denison DM. *Br J Dis Chest* 1979; **73**: 97–112.)

conjunction with a single mass spectrometer to service several rooms or analyse consecutively two specimens of gas sampled concurrently (e.g. Fig. 8.8).

Analysis by particle deposition characteristics

Deposition and clearance of aerosols

Some of the small particles which enter the respiratory tract deposit on the respiratory epithelium and are then disposed of by ciliary action or in other ways. The process normally operates to protect the lung but can be used to delineate selectively structures having different deposition characteristics. Separation is achieved by using particles of different sizes. The size is expressed as aerodynamic diameter; this is the diameter of a sphere of unit density having the same terminal settling velocity as the relevant particle or fibre. Monodispersed particles (i.e. particles of uniform size ±10%) are used in the investigation of mucociliary clearance and the delivery and action of inhaled drugs, but this technique can also yield anatomical information such as the size of air spaces and it can indicate narrowing of small airways.

Particles of aerodynamic diameter 5 μm are used for delineating the bronchi including the bifurcations, where the particles accumulate by impaction, and the airway walls, where they deposit by sedimentation. Smaller particles in the range 2.0–0.5 μm are used to study the gas exchanging region of the lung. The 2.0 μm particles deposit by sedimentation in both bronchioles and alveoli whilst the 0.5 μm particles settle mainly in alveoli. The proportional deposition is greater for the larger particles. Both sizes can provide evidence of airway narrowing but the larger particles, which deposit in the bronchioles, are commonly used. The particles can be human albumen labelled with radioactive technetium (^{99}Tc); formerly the labelling was with iodine-131. The particles are produced using a spinning top generator, then diluted with air by passage through a nebuliser into a bag-in-box system (Fig. 8.1, page 215). The subject inhales the aerosol during tidal breathing: this should be controlled for volume, flow rate and pauses at times of zero flow since all these factors influence deposition. Scintillation counters placed outside the chest are used to assess when an adequate dose has been inhaled; their use is described under regional function below. The subject then rinses the mouth and oro-pharynx with water, and the distribution of radioactivity due to deposition is recorded immediately. Subsequently measurements can be made at 15 min intervals for 2 h and at longer intervals up to 24 h in order to monitor the clearance. For study of small airway function the relevant counting field is usually defined on a postero-anterior view as the outer third when the lung is subdivided vertically, or as the outer 50% by area when it is subdivided circumferentially. However, any two-dimensional approach leads to the lung periphery also contributing to the more central region which is used as a reference point. This is avoided if the periphery and central regions are defined in three dimensions. The peripheral deposition relative to that in the central region is expressed as a penetration index:

$$PI = \frac{\text{cps/pixel in periphery}}{\text{cps/pixel in central region}} \qquad (8.4)$$

where cps is the regional integrated count per second. The penetration index for particles can also be compared with that for a gas distributed uniformly throughout the lung; for example ^{81}Kr. The use of this gas is considered under regional function below. The variance of counts from different sites within the lung periphery provides an index of uneven distribution of penetration and hence of airway narrowing.

For studies of alveolar deposition the 0.5–1.0 μm particles can be of sodium chloride coated with di-2-ethylhexyl sebacate prepared in a modified La Mer-Sinclair generator, a process which involves volatilisation in nitrogen and heating with the sebacate vapour at 400°C. Alternatively triphenyl phosphate particles can be used. The concentration of particles in inhaled and exhaled air is determined using a Tyndallometer in which a light beam from a quartz halogen lamp illuminates the aerosol as it enters and leaves the mouth. The scatter of light at right angles to the beam is monitored using a photomultiplier.

The particles are inhaled from the bag-in-box during a single test inhalation made under controlled conditions of flow and volume; the subsequent expiration can be either immediate (e.g. Fig. 8.9) or after breath holding for up to 30 s. The accumulation of particles in the alveoli (and hence their removal from expired alveolar air) increases exponentially with time of breath holding so a half-time can be calculated

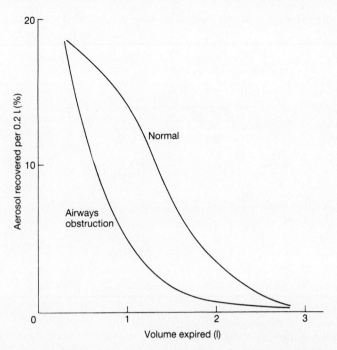

Fig. 8.9 Aerosol recovery curves for a healthy subject and a patient with airways obstruction showing the decline in concentration of aerosol particles (diameter 0.5 μm) during exhalation following a single test inhalation. The separation between the curves reflects the degree of airways obstruction. The procedure was that of Muir. (Source: Cotes JE, Houston K, Saunders MJ. *J Physiol (Lond)* 1971; **213**: 22P.)

if the test is repeated a number of times with different durations of breath holding; allowance must be made for deposition during expiration. In men of mean age 36 years Hankinson and colleagues found the mean half time to be 20 s (SD 4.4 s). The equivalent mean air space diameter was 0.55 mm. The half-time and mean airspace diameter were increased in the presence of conditions commonly associated with emphysema. The subject has been developed by, amongst others, Morrow, Albert, Newhouse, Lourenco, Pavia and their respective collaborators.

Use of radio-isotopes to study the lung

General principles

Substances which emit gamma radiation can be used to monitor most aspects of lung function. The particular application dictates the physical and chemical characteristics of the test substance which in turn influences which radioactive label is appropriate. Some gaseous isotopes are given in Table 8.1 and other substances in Table 8.2.

The use of radioactive substances depends on the ability of γ radiation to traverse the lung and chest wall and activate scintillation counters placed outside the chest. The activity is detected by a luminescent crystal and a camera which comprises a battery of photomultiplier

Table 8.1 Properties of some radioisotope gases used for studying the lung: the absorbtion is for a 2.5 cm thick layer of soft tissue

	Source	Half life	γ energy (KeV)	Absorption (%)	Example of use
Inert gas					
^{133}Xe	Nuclear reactor	5.3 days	80	45	Ventilation– perfusion* regional tomography§
^{127}Xe	Nuclear reactor	30 days	200	37	
^{85m}Kr	Nuclear reactor	4.4 days	150	40	
^{81m}Kr	^{81}Rb‡	13 s	190	38	
^{13}N+	Cyclotron	10 min	511	28	
Soluble gas					
$C^{15}O_2$+	Cyclotron	2 min	511	28	Perfusion
Reactive gas					
^{11}CO+	Cyclotron	20 min	511	28	Lung haemoglobin
Technetium					
^{99m}TC	99Mb¶	6.0 h	140	40	See Table 8.2

* Administered dissolved in saline.
‡ Obtainable from MRC Cyclotron Unit, Hammersmith Hospital, London.
§ Single photon emission computed tomography (SPECT).
¶ From nuclear reactor.
+ Positron emitter.

Table 8.2 Some radioisotope substances used to investigate the lung; the substances are administered intravenously except where indicated

Perfusion distribution	^{99m}Tc-HMPAO* (lipophilic aerosol)
	^{99m}Tc-albumin microspheres diameter $20-40\,\mu$m†
Ventilation distribution	^{99m}Tc-albumin (aerosol) diameter $1-2\,\mu$m
Pulmonary embolism	^{111}In-P256 (binds to fibrinogen receptors) or albumin microspheres
Alveolar capillary permeability	
Endothelium	^{113m}In-transferrin
Epithelium	^{99m}Tc-DTPA‡ (aerosol)
Trapped haemoglobin	^{11}CO (gas)§
Lung metabolism	^{18}F deoxyglucose§ (combines with glucose-6-phosphate)

* Hexamethyl pentanoic-amine oxine. $C^{15}O_2$ can also be used (Fig. 8.8).
† Combined with renal scans can assess AV shunts.
‡ Diethylenetriamine pentacetate.
§ Detected by positron emission tomography (PET).

tubes. Detection is broadly confined to one energy level: this is achieved using a pulse height analyser whose 'window' is set to reject all γ energies except the principle energy of the isotope in question. The width of the window is usually $\pm 20\%$ of the peak energy. The diameter of the camera should preferably be equal to that of the lungs so a 40.6 cm (16 inch) crystal is commonly used. The crystal is protected from low energy background and scattered radiation by a lead shield of which the thickness is determined by the energy of the relevant radiation. A thickness of 0.5 cm is appropriate for ^{133}Xe and more for higher energy radiation. The lead is perforated by holes which provide access to the camera. Usually the holes are parallel. A diverging collimeter can be used to enlarge the field which is scanned. For a standard source the amount of radioactivity is determined by the energy of the γ emission, the distance from the source to the detector (inverse square law) and the focusing provided by the lead collimator. In the thorax loss occurs from absorption of radiation by the tissue of the chest wall and to a lesser extent the lung. The absorption varies inversely with the γ emission energy (Table 8.1). For a low energy isotope (e.g. ^{133}Xe), the activity which is detected is mainly from the lung tissue immediately beneath the counters. The amount of lung tissue and the thickness of the chest wall varies down the lung so counts made at apex and base cannot be compared directly. However, this geometric factor is eliminated when the ratios of two counts are compared. For the ratio to be meaningful the tissue absorption should be the same for both signals. In this way valid regional comparisons can be made for ventilation/perfusion, ventilation/volume and perfusion/volume provided the same or similar isotopes are used for the component measurements. Error due to tissue absorption is increased if isotopes of different energy are used.

Error can also arise from isotope leaving the lung and entering the chest wall via the systemic circulation. This is likely to occur with soluble and partially soluble isotopes (e.g. respectively $C^{15}O_2$ and ^{133}Xe or ^{127}Xe) but not with insoluble isotopes or those having a very short half life (for example ^{81}Kr). Correction for the chest wall activity can be made in some circumstances. Recirculation of isotope can also occur into the lung.

Activity in the depth of the lung can be detected using counters on both sides of the chest, but for low energy isotopes the sensitivity is poor. It can be increased by using high energy isotopes particularly those which emit pairs of positrons; these are discharged in opposite directions and are detected by coincidence counting using banks of detectors on both sides of the chest. Coincidence counting provides a high signal-to-noise ratio and permits three-dimensional tomography with a spatial resolution of approximately 0.7 cm. Positron-emitting isotopes are produced in a cyclotron and, having a short half life (Table 8.1), can only be used on site.

Radioactive decay is a random phenomenon so the count rate per second is described in terms of the mean and standard deviation; the accuracy of estimation can be poor when counting times are short. Formerly counting was by rate meter but now detection is usually by γ camera (e.g. Anger's) which is interfaced with a computer having a visual display; the display is colour coded to highlight regions of contrasting activity and the output is also stored on disc for subsequent processing.

*Use of radio-
isotopes to study
the lung*

Lung ventilation and perfusion: outline of methods

The radio-isotope xenon-133 was introduced for study of regional lung function by Knipping in 1957 and the potential of the method was explored by Bates, West and their respective co-workers. Its introduction was closely followed by that of oxygen-15 which in the form $C^{15}O_2$ was used by West and Dollery to investigate regional pulmonary blood flow (Fig. 8.10). The blood gas partition coefficient of ^{133}Xe is approximately 0.13. This solubility is low enough to confine most of the inhaled gas to the lung, where the radioactivity depicts the distribution of ventilation. At the same time sufficient isotope can be dissolved in saline for intravenous injection with a view to studying lung perfusion. The use of the same isotope for both ventilation and perfusion scans avoids error due to differential tissue absorption (page 231). ^{133}Xe has the disadvantage of low energy, particularly for the Anger camera, and poor tissue penetration. These disadvantages are less for ^{127}Xe or ^{85m}Kr which can be used instead but these isotopes are expensive. In addition, for washout studies, all three isotopes have the limitation that their persistence in the body can cause error from circulation of isotope to the chest wall and recirculation to the lungs. The error can be avoided by using instead either technetium-labelled aerosol particles which do not enter the bloodsteam or a relatively insoluble gas such as ^{13}N, which has a blood–gas partition coefficient of only 0.013 (Fig. 8.12, page 235). The latter procedure depends on the laboratory having access to a cyclotron. Alternatively, use can be made of ^{81m}Kr which has too short a half life for material recirculation to occur. This gas has the further advantages of giving a low radiation dose and of being administered during normal breathing. Its use is recommended

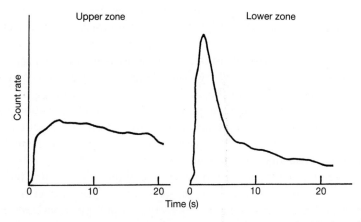

Fig. 8.10 Regional count rates for the upper and lower zones of a healthy lung during the inhalation of $C^{15}O_2$ followed by breath holding. The initial rise reflects the arrival of the isotope by ventilation bulk flow, the subsequent clearance reflects the blood flow per unit of tissue volume; this is greater for the lower than for the upper zone. An arrangement for counting is shown in Fig. 8.11. (Source: West JB, Dollery CT. *J Appl Physiol* 1960; **15**: 405–410.)

for clinical ventilation scans and for regional tomography. The scans can be compared directly with perfusion scans obtained using technetium-labelled microspheres or HMPAO (Table 8.2) because ^{81m}Kr and ^{99m}Tc have similar energy levels (Table 8.1) so the tissue absorption is the same for both isotopes. The comparison can contribute to investigation of pulmonary embolism. The diagnosis is likely if the perfusion scan shows a filling defect whilst the ventilation scan is normal. However, some reduction in ventilation normally occurs and more specific methods involving detection of constituents of a thrombus are now being developed (see Table 8.2 and page 230).

For clinical purposes technetium perfusion scans can also be compared with technetium ventilation scans or tomograms obtained using labelled aerosol particles of diameter $1-2\,\mu m$. In healthy subjects the distribution of aerosol closely resembles that of labelled gas: however, in the presence of airflow limitation the distribution of aerosol to poorly ventilated regions is less than that of labelled gas. The difference appears to be due to the gas being distributed partly by diffusion whilst the aerosol is distributed by convective ventilation (bulk flow of air) only. This has the effect that unevenness of ventilation is amplified and more readily apparent with the aerosol method. However, if the scan is part of an investigation of possible pulmonary embolism the amplification is a disadvantage because it can lead to the ventilation of poorly perfused regions of lung being underestimated (page 227). Both the aerosol and krypton methods can be applied to patients in bed or receiving intensive care; the procedures are suitable for serial monitoring of treatment as well as for diagnosis.

Other pulmonary applications of radioisotopes are given in Table 8.2.

Xenon-133

This section describes the use of ^{133}Xe. It also applies to ^{127}Xe or ^{85}Kr when these gases are used (but see page 231). ^{133}Xe, when inhaled, can be used to indicate regional ventilation and volume or, when dissolved in saline and injected intravenously, regional blood flow. When either of these procedures is followed by rebreathing in closed circuit from an anaesthetic bag or spirometer the scintillation count rate rises to a plateau which reflects the product of lung volume as seen by the counter and the geometric factor for ^{133}Xe; for this purpose the subject is switched into closed circuit at the end of the injection. The measurements which can be obtained are outlined in Fig. 8.11. Following intravenous injection, the peak activity reflects the arrival of ^{133}Xe with a distribution proportional to pulmonary blood flow; because of its low blood−gas partition coefficient about 87% of the isotope passes into the alveolar gas where it remains as long as the subject holds the breath. On resumption of breathing, the decline in radioactivity reflects the ventilation of perfused tissue. A slow clearance suggests a relatively low ventilation−perfusion ratio ($\dot{V}A/\dot{Q}$) within the field of counting.

The counting field comprises many overlapping lung units (at least 10^7) and this can affect the values for $\dot{V}A/\dot{Q}$ ratio obtained by dividing a measurement of regional ventilation by a separate measurement of regional perfusion. For example, a counting zone might consist of two compartments of equal volume and blood flow but unequal ventilation, with $\dot{V}A/\dot{Q}$ ratios of 1.0 and 0.01. Because they overlap in the counting field, the $\dot{V}A/\dot{Q}$ ratio from external counting would be 0.5 which, assuming a normal mixed venous blood composition, is equivalent to a P_{A,O_2} of 10.7 kPa (80 mmHg) or a venous admixture (or shunt) of 10%. But, in reality, the venous admixture would be almost 50% and the mean P_{A,O_2} 6.7 kPa (50 mmHg).

The lower right hand quadrant of Fig. 8.11 shows a wash-in of ^{133}Xe in closed circuit followed by a wash-out. The equilibration plateau is evidence that the ^{133}Xe concentration is the same in all alveoli. The local count rates then reflect the volume of alveolar gas in the counting fields. The *perfusion per unit volume* for any region is obtained by dividing the peak counts (during breath holding after intravenous injection) by the equilibrium count. Both measurements should be made at the same lung volume (e.g. total lung capacity), in order that the geometric factors in the chest wall and differences in detector sensitivity do not influence the result. Healthy subjects will reach equilibration after 1–2 min of rebreathing, or less if some vital capacity

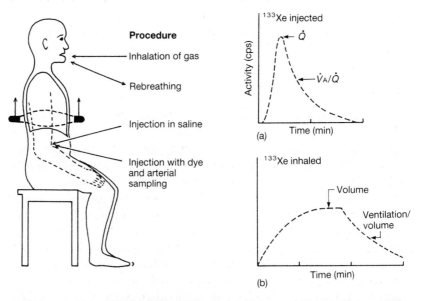

Fig. 8.11 Assessment of regional lung function using ^{133}Xe. (a) After injection the initial peak reflects the regional blood flow ($\dot{Q}$); the isotope then passes into the gas phase where the clearance during normal breathing reflects the ventilation of lung tissue which is perfused. A slow wash-out indicates a low ventilation–perfusion ratio ($\dot{V}A/\dot{Q}$).
(b) During re-breathing the plateau count rate when mixing is complete, reflects the volume of lung gas in the field of counting. The slopes of the wash-in and wash-out curves indicate the ventilation per unit volume.

breaths are taken at the start of rebreathing. Patients with airways obstruction may not reach full equilibrium in 20 min during which time isotope accumulates in the blood and chest wall.

The *ventilation per unit of lung volume* can be obtained from the initial slope or half-time $(t_{1/2})$ of the wash-in or wash-out of ^{133}Xe during regular breathing (Fig. 8.11). The wash-out curve cannot be interpreted beyond the $t_{1/2}$ on account of activity in the chest wall and from the recirculating blood (Fig. 8.12). Thus little information is lost by terminating the rebreathing after 4 min. The ventilation per unit of lung volume ($\dot{V}/V$) can also be obtained by the subject taking in a tidal breath of ^{133}Xe and then holding the breath. The index $\dot{V}/V$ is given by the ratios of the activity after the breath to the equilibrium level at the same lung volume. Alternatively, a bolus of ^{133}Xe can be injected close to the mouthpiece just before the start of an inspiration which is then continued up to full inflation. The distribution of the bolus is then that of gas inspired at end-expiratory volume, reflecting the early phase of inspiration. However, to the extent that ventilation is sequential, it is preferable to label the whole tidal breath. A bolus given at the beginning of inspiration after a maximal exhalation to residual volume is distributed preferentially to the lung apex; this is the basis for the measurement of closing volume (page 221). The distribution of ^{133}Xe after an inspiratory capacity breath in terms of either $\dot{V}/\dot{Q}$ or $\dot{V}/V$, reflects regional compliance, not regional ventilation and measures the regional inspiratory capacity; this is discussed below.

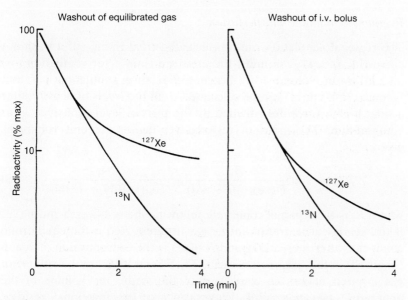

Fig. 8.12 Comparison of clearance of two radioactive gases of medium and low solubility (respectively ^{127}Xe and ^{13}N). The deviation of the ^{127}Xe curve to the right of that for ^{13}N is caused by ^{127}Xe in the chest wall and recirculating in the blood. The data are for the lower zone of a healthy subject. (Source: Rosenzweig DY, Hughes JMB, Jones T. *Respir Physiol* 1968; **8**: 86–97.)

Regional lung volume

The gas dilution principle is used to calculate the inspiratory capacity (ICr) or the vital capacity (VCr) of the region covered by the counter. The subject inhales radioactive gas from a spirometer to total lung capacity starting from functional residual capacity or from residual volume. At maximal inflation the activity over the chest and the xenon concentration in the spirometer are recorded, and related to the radio-activity at the same volume after equilibrium. For an inspiration from end expiration to total lung capacity (neglecting the regional dead space) it follows that:

$$Fi(xe).ICr = Fr(xe).TLCr \qquad (8.5)$$

where ICr and TLCr are the regional inspiratory capacity and total lung capacity, $Fi(xe)$ is the inspired concentration of ^{133}Xe, and $Fr(xe)$ is the regional concentration of xenon. The latter is represented by:

$$Fr(xe) = N_1.Feq(xe)/N_2 \qquad (8.6)$$

where N_1 and N_2 are the number of counts at total lung capacity for the single breath and equilibration manoeuvres respectively and $Feq(xe)$ is the spirometer concentration at the end of equilibration. Hence:

$$ICr/TLCr\% = 100.N_1.\ Feq(xe)/(N_2.Fi(xe)) \qquad (8.7)$$

The ratio FRCr/TLCr% may then be obtained by subtraction. Similar calculations may be made for VCr and RVr.

Regional ventilation and perfusion

The regional ventilation can be calculated from the $t_{1/2}$ of a wash-out curve (i.e. $0.693/t_{1/2}$ in min); the units are $1\,\text{min}^{-1}$ for ventilation ($\dot{V}$) and litres for volume (V), hence the relative ventilation per unit volume ($\dot{V}/V\ \text{min}^{-1}$) can be calculated from the levels of activity after a tidal breath (or bolus) divided by the plateau level of activity after equilibration. The index of regional ventilation per unit volume is given by:

$$\dot{V}/V\% = 100 \frac{R_1}{Fi(xe)\ (Vi - Vd)} \div \frac{Req}{Feq(xe)(Vi - FRC)} \qquad (8.8)$$

where R_1 is the regional count rate following the test breath and $Fi(xe)$ is the xenon concentration in the gas inspired, Req is the equilibrium count rate after rebreathing and $Feq(xe)$ is the concentration of xenon (in mCi/l) in the spirometer circuit. Vi, Vd and FRC are the volume of gas inspired under the conditions of the study, the volume of the apparatus and anatomical deadspaces and the functional residual capacity respectively. For the corresponding index of perfusion, the denominator in the first term is replaced by $xe(inj)$, the quantity of xenon injected in mCi. With gamma cameras and sets of counters which encompass the whole lung field a simpler and more usual form of normalisation expresses the regional counts (R_1 and Req) as a percentage of the total lung counts for each measurement. The terms FI(xe) (VI − Vd) and Feq(xe) (VI − FRC) are then omitted. The procedure is described by Bull and colleagues.

Krypton-81m

The isotope is generated on site by elutriation from an ion exchange resin column containing 81Rb (Table 8.1). The flow rate of air through the column is approximately 1 l min^{-1}; the isotope is delivered through a disposable face mask to the patient who will normally be breathing quietly, sitting in front of a gamma camera (Fig. 8.13). An image which represents the distribution of ventilation is obtained by accumulating over about 12 respiratory cycles a pre-set number of counts (e.g. 300 000). The image is affected by the volume of lung scanned by the counter (geometric factor). ^{81m}Kr has a half life of only 13 s (Table 8.1) so when it is breathed continuously the alveolar concentration never approaches the inspired concentration. Instead at the levels of ventilation found at rest the ratio of the alveolar to the inspired concentrations is linearly related to the ventilation per unit of lung volume. In equilibrium the ^{81m}Kr count rate reflects the balance between the arrival and removal of radioactivity, i.e.:

$$^{81m}\text{Kr} = \dot{V}\text{I}.C\text{I}/(\dot{V}\text{E}/V + \lambda) \qquad (8.9)$$

when $\dot{V}$I and CI are respectively inspired ventilation (l min^{-1}) and inspired radioactive concentration, representing regional isotope arrival; $\dot{V}$E/V is expired ventilation per unit volume (l min^{-1} l^{-1}) which, with

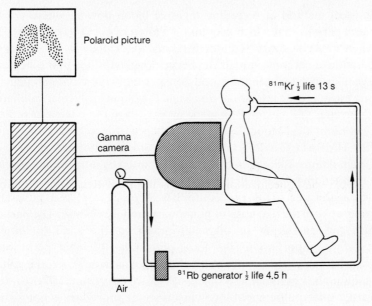

Fig. 8.13 Diagram of apparatus for ^{81m}Kr ventilation scan.

the radioactive decay constant λ, represents the removal processes. The normal values at rest for $\dot{V}E/V$ is $1-1.8\,\mathrm{min}^{-1}$ and for λ $3.2\,\mathrm{min}^{-1}$. Thus the denominator of the equation is determined mainly by the value for λ. However, since CI and λ are common to all parts of the lung the local ^{81m}Kr signal reflects the regional ventilation ($\dot{V}E/V$). When $\dot{V}E/V$ is greater than λ e.g. in hyperventilation, the advantage of the short half life is nullified and the ^{81m}Kr signal tends to reflect the local lung volume and not the ventilation. The inhalation of ^{81m}Kr gives a signal proportional to ventilation and not ventilation per unit volume, but an assessment of ventilation per unit volume can be made during the wash-out of ^{81m}Kr as $0.693/t_{1/2}$ — where $t_{1/2}$ is in min. A volume scan can be obtained by equilibrating with another radioactive gas of similar energy but longer half life, such as ^{127}Xe or ^{85m}Kr (Table 8.1).

The advantages of ^{81m}Kr are considerable, particularly in a clinical context. The radiation dose is low; the procedure is quick and very simple, and there is no interruption of normal breathing. In a single subject, using multiple views the distribution of ventilation can be recorded in a few minutes. Minute to minute changes in ventilation distribution can be monitored and the effects of physiotherapy, bronchodilator drugs, etc. observed. In addition a ^{81m}Kr ventilation scan is a companion to the more familiar ^{99m}Tc lung perfusion scan. The images for each scan look similar and a quick clinical assessment can be made. For example, there are many causes of perfusion defects on the ^{99m}Tc scan, but if the ^{81m}Kr ventilation scan is normal, pulmonary embolism is extremely likely.

Regional pulmonary blood flow

The ideal method of recording regional blood flow is, where circumstances permit, that which uses an inhalation of $C^{15}O_2$ (Fig. 8.10). The oxygen molecules rapidly enter the lung water pool as $H_2^{15}O$ via the mediation of carbonic anhydrase; hence the initial slope of the clearance curve is proportional to the blood flow per unit volume of parenchymal tissue including the interstitial tissue and the blood in alveolar capillaries. A delayed $C^{15}O_2$ clearance may be an early sign of oedema or reflect a reduction in local blood flow. In the absence of a cyclotron the aerosol ^{99m}Tc HMPAO (Table 8.2) can provide similar information.

The pulmonary circulation is usually explored by intravenous injection of technetium-99m-labelled human serum albumen microspheres or macroaggregates. This procedure has virtually replaced pulmonary angiography in the diagnosis of pulmonary embolic disease. The particles which are $20-50\,\mu m$ in diameter-impact in the small pulmonary vessels in proportion to the local perfusion. Regional perfusion is measured, not perfusion per unit volume, so, as with ^{81m}Kr, the volume of lung in the counting field influences the measurement. The particles obstruct some pulmonary blood vessels so the procedure is not without risk for patients with severe restriction of the pulmonary vascular bed.

In addition some particles enter the systemic circulation, through right to left intrapulmonary or intracardiac shunts. However, these emboli appear not to cause side effects. The size of the shunt can be estimated by scanning the kidneys to obtain the lung/kidney activity ratio. This correlates with the shunt measured by the oxygen method (page 253) but in absolute terms may exceed it because some channels allow the passage of 30 µm particles whilst at the same time being small enough to take part in gas exchange.

Radiation dose. The radiation exposure from most pulmonary isotopic procedures is low and mainly confined to the lungs. A typical ^{81m}Kr scan gives 0.2 mGy and a ^{133}Xe or ^{99m}Tc study 2–4 mGy. The annual permitted dose is 5 mGy.

Cardiac output and pulmonary blood flow

In most circumstances the outputs of the right and left ventricles are effectively equal so either quantity provides an estimate of cardiac output and pulmonary blood flow. The two quantities differ when cardiac output is changing or there is an intravascular shunt such as can occur with congenital heart disease. One must then consider which flow rate is being measured and if the procedure is valid. Most procedures entail measuring over a timed interval the dilution of a known amount of indicator material all of which must be accounted for. This application of the law of conservation of matter was proposed for measurement of cardiac output with oxygen as the indicator by Fick in 1870 and the Fick principle is the basis of all indicator dilution methods. The relationship has the form:

$$F.C\alpha.\text{out} = j + F.C\alpha.\text{in} \tag{8.10}$$

where F is flow rate, $C\alpha$ is the equilibrium concentration of indicator material entering or leaving the mixing chamber and j is the rate at which the indicator is added to or removed from the system. Hence for oxygen:

$$\dot{Q}\text{t} \,(1\,\text{min}^{-1}) = \frac{\dot{n}O_2}{44.6} \div (Ca,o_2 - C\bar{v},o_2) \tag{8.11}$$

where $\dot{Q}\text{t}$ is cardiac output and $\dot{n}o_2$ is oxygen consumption (mmol min^{-1}). When oxygen consumption is obtained in litres the conversion factor (44.6) is omitted. The term in the bracket is the difference in oxygen content between arterial and mixed venous blood expressed in litres STPD per litre; it is the volume of oxygen added to 1 l of blood in the lungs. Other gases which can be used include carbon dioxide, which like oxygen enters into reversible combination with blood, and the moderately soluble gases acetylene, nitrous oxide and freon-22. For acetylene a correction of approximately 10% is made for the quantity which dissolves in lung tissue. Highly soluble gases, for example diethyl ether, cannot be used because uptake occurs into the epithelium of the upper respiratory tract, and insoluble gases, such as helium or argon, are unsuitable because the quantity exchanged is too small to be measured accurately. The principle of mass balance also applies to substances administered by injection including indo-cyanine green dye and cold saline. For the latter substance the resulting temperature change provides a nearly unique signal in not being affected by recirculation of blood back to the lungs from the systemic circulation.

Cardiac output can also be measured by physical methods of which the most satisfactory is that of aortic blood flow velocity by the Doppler ultrasound technique with separate estimation of aortic diameter. Electrical bio-impedance, ballistocardigraphy and other techniques can be used but their accuracy is lower.

Direct Fick method for oxygen

This is the standard against which other methods are compared. It entails cannulation of a peripheral artery (page 37) and catheterisation of the right heart for placement of a catheter in a pulmonary artery. The placement is usually made by the flotation technique of Bradley which employs a double lumen catheter (Swan-Ganz) with an inflatable balloon at its end. When the balloon reaches the right atrium it is inflated and this leads to the catheter being carried by the flow of blood into a pulmonary artery. Collections of systemic arterial blood, mixed venous blood from the pulmonary artery and mixed expired gas for measurement of oxygen consumption (page 35) are made concur-rently under steady state conditions usually over a 2 min period. The calculation is given in equation 8.11.

Indirect Fick methods: rebreathing method using oxygen

A modified Fick method for oxygen has been developed by Cerretelli and others. It is non-invasive and valid for most subjects but not those with markedly uneven lung mixing, a material pulmonary vascular shunt or a right to left intravascular or intracardiac shunt. The contents of oxygen in arterial and pulmonary pre-capillary blood are calculated from the respective gas tensions using the dissociation curve and other relevant variables. These are given on page 280. The calculation of cardiac output is made in the manner described above. The arterial oxygen tension is estimated from that in end tidal gas sampled at the lips. The latter quantity (Pet,o_2) exceeds the tension in arterial blood (Pa,o_2) by an amount (a) which is approximately 1.6 kPa (12 mmHg) Hence:

$$Pa,o_2 = Pet,o_2 - a \qquad (8.12)$$

In the presence of a shunt this estimate of systemic arterial oxygen tension is no longer accurate. The pulmonary precapillary oxygen tension is estimated by rebreathing test gas from a bag. The gas mixture is usually carbon dioxide (fractional concentration 0.09) in nitrogen. The volume is equal to the functional residual capacity of the subject, the rebreathing time is 10 s and the subject rebreathes deeply and rapidly. The oxygen concentration at the lips is monitored using a respiratory mass spectrometer. During rebreathing the expired oxygen concentration falls and the bag concentration rises until the two come into equilibrium; the plateau is usually reached within 4 s and persists thereafter (Fig. 8.14). At this point the oxygen tension is equal to that of mixed venous blood, which falls to a very low level during strenuous exercise; therefore, it is dangerous to use this method at high levels of oxygen consumption and in subjects with arterial hypoxaemia or severe anaemia. It is also unsuitable for subjects with atherosclerosis. On account of these limitations the method is used mainly for young adults; in other circumstances the carbon dioxide method is preferable.

Rebreathing method using carbon dioxide

This method resembles that for oxygen so is invalidated by poor lung mixing and right to left cardiac or pulmonary vascular shunts. It also has the theoretical disadvantage that fluctuations in the quantity of carbon dioxide dissolved in lung tissue can influence the result. In practice the agreement with the direct Fick method is excellent and the method is widely used. The carbon dioxide output is obtained by collection and analysis of expired gas (page 36). The CO_2 tension in systemic arterial blood is obtained in one of three ways: (1) analysis of arterialised blood from an ear lobe (page 37); (2) calculation from that

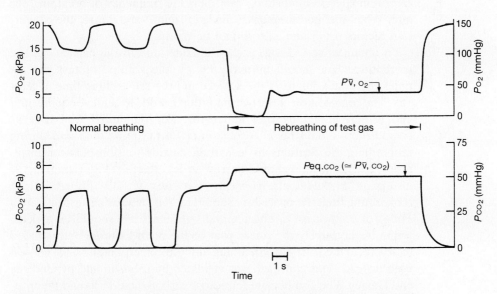

Fig. 8.14 Measurement of mixed venous gas tensions by rebreathing. The record, which was obtained using a mass spectrometer, shows sustained equilibria for both oxygen and carbon dioxide. The rebreathing bag initially contained carbon dioxide in the fractional concentration 0.08 with the remainder nitrogen. The plateau for oxygen is attained more readily following the addition of some oxygen to the gas mixture. For details see text. (Source: Cerretelli P, Cruz JC, Farhi LE, Rahn H. *Respir Physiol* 1966; **1**: 258–264.)

in mixed expired gas assuming a value for the physiological deadspace (page 192); (3) derivation from the mean alveolar or end tidal CO_2 tension during continuous analysis of expired gas at the lips; this is performed using a rapid infrared gas analyser or respiratory mass spectrometer. The tension of CO_2 in pulmonary pre-capillary blood (i.e. mixed venous blood, $P\bar{v},co_2$, Fig. 8.14) is obtained by rebreathing a gas mixture containing 30% O_2 and 9–13% CO_2. Some subjects experience discomfort during the rebreathing.

The blood gas tension difference $(P\bar{v},co_2 - Pa,co_2)$ is used to calculate the corresponding content difference $(C\bar{v},co_2 - Ca,co_2)$ which in turn is inserted into the Fick equation for cardiac output:

$$\dot{Q}t = \frac{\dot{n}co_2}{44.6} \div (C\bar{v},co_2 - Ca,co_2) \tag{8.13}$$

The terms and units are as for equation 8.11 but with carbon dioxide substituted for oxygen.

Practical details. The arterial carbon dioxide tension is obtained from the tension in end-tidal gas using the empirical relationship of N.L. Jones and colleagues:

$$Pa,co_2 = Pet,co_2 - 0.133 \left(0.004 \frac{\dot{n}co_2}{44.6} - 0.13f_R + 0.75 \right) \text{ kPa} \tag{8.14}$$

where Pa,co_2 and Pet,co_2 are respectively the tensions of carbon dioxide in arterial blood and end-tidal gas in kPa, $\dot{n}co_2$ is the output of carbon dioxide in mmol min^{-1} and f_R is the frequency of breathing per min. When the measurement is made in l min^{-1} and mmHg the conversion factors 0.133 and 44.6 should be omitted.

To obtain mixed venous carbon dioxide tension the capacity of the rebreathing bag should normally be 5 l, the volume of test gas 1.5 times the tidal volume of the subject and the rebreathing time at least 12 s. The composition of the test gas is that needed to achieve equilibrium and is determined by trial and error. For the initial trial the gas composition should be FI,O_2 0.3, FI,CO_2 0.11, FI,N_2 0.59 and during rebreathing the fluctuations in carbon dioxide tension between inspiration and expiration should narrow to less than 0.1 kPa (1 mmHg). If instead of a plateau the concentration rises or falls throughout the rebreathing then the procedure should be repeated using respectively a FI,CO_2 of 0.09 or 0.13. The interval between trials should be at least 3 min. Alternatively the linear part of the record can be extrapolated to 20 s from the start of rebreathing and the corresponding CO_2 tension used instead. This approach was validated by Denison and by Godfrey and Davies. The equilibrium tension of carbon dioxide should theoretically be equal to that in pulmonary precapillary blood and this is usually the case at rest. However, on exercise the equilibrium gas tension exceeds the blood tension by a small amount. This was formerly thought to be due to the chemical reaction between CO_2 and blood only reaching equilibrium after the blood has left the pulmonary capil-

242

laries (hence *downstream effect*) or to the surface of the pulmonary capillary endothelium carrying a negative charge. However, Scheid and Piiper have evidence that the difference is technical in origin.

It can be allowed for empirically using the equation of Jones and colleagues:

$$Pox,\bar{v},co_2 = Peq,co_2 - 0.133 \left(1.4 + 2.6 \frac{\dot{n}co_2}{44.6}\right) kPa \qquad (8.15)$$

where $Pox,\bar{v},co_2$ is the tension of carbon dioxide in oxygenated mixed venous blood, Peq,co_2 is the equilibrium tension of carbon dioxide and $\dot{n}co_2$ is output of carbon dioxide in mmol min^{-1}. The constant terms 0.133 and 44.6 are omitted when traditional units are used.

The conversion from the tension to the content of carbon dioxide in blood is best done using the following relationship:

$$Cco_2.blood = Cco_2.plasma \left(1 - \frac{0.0289[Hb]}{(3.352-0.456.So_2).(8.142-pH)}\right)$$
$$(8.16)$$

where $Cco_2.plasma = 2.226.s.plasma\ Pco_2.(1 + 10^{pH-pK'})$, Cco_2 is CO_2 content, So_2 is O_2 saturation, s is the plasma CO_2 solubility coefficient, and pK' is the apparent pK from the equations of Kelman. (Source: Douglas A, Jones NL, Reed JW. *J Appl Physiol* 1988; **65**: 473–477.) Alternatively the nomogram of McHardy (Fig. 8.15) can be used instead.

Single breath methods using carbon dioxide

By these methods the tensions of carbon dioxide in systemic arterial and mixed venous blood are obtained from an analysis of gas sampled at the lips during a single slow expiration. The resulting blood gas tension difference is converted to a content difference and used in the Fick equation as described above. The basic method, developed by Kim, Rahn and Farhi, is described in Fig. 8.16. It suffers from three limitations. First, the value for cardiac output is critically dependent on the shape of the Pco_2/Po_2 relationship; this should be for alveolar gas not deadspace gas or gas expired after closure of some airways (phase 4). The accuracy is improved by introducing a single rebreathing stage before the test expiration, starting the sampling after the expired carbon dioxide tension has risen to 4 kPa (30 mmHg) and having tight criteria for what is an acceptable amount of scatter about the line of best fit. These aspects were reviewed by Ohta and colleagues. Second, the respiratory exchange ratio is influenced by uneven lung function (page 211) which can therefore affect the result. Third, the lung volume falls during the slow expiration on account of uptake of oxygen; the carbon dioxide in the lung–bag system rises in consequence. More carbon dioxide then enters the blood and lung tissue but the transfer lags behind that of oxygen. The exchanges invalidate the basic assumption of gaseous equilibrium across the alveolar capillary membrane at

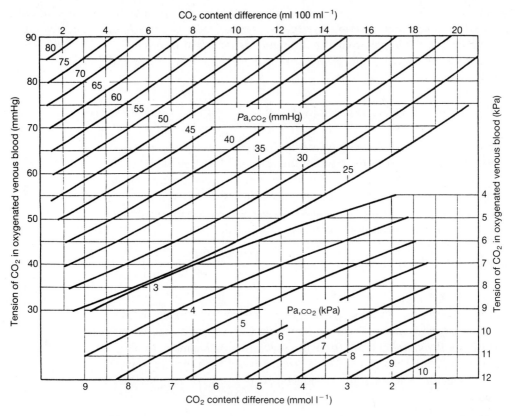

Fig. 8.15 Differences in content of carbon dioxide between venous and arterial blood ($C\bar{v},co_2 - Ca,co_2$) for a range of tensions of carbon dioxide in arterial and oxygenated venous blood. They are calculated for a saturation of oxygen in arterial blood (Sa,o_2) of 95% and a blood concentration of haemoglobin monomer of 9.2 mmol l^{-1} (15 g dl^{-1}). Where one or both of these quantities deviate materially from the assumed values, the true CO_2 content difference may be obtained by addition of a factor (f); in traditional units this is calculated as follows:

$$f = 0.015(\text{Hb} - 15)\,(P\bar{v},co_2 - Pa,co_2) - 0.064\,(95 - Sa,o_2)\ \text{ml dl}^{-1}$$

(e.g. Pa,co_2 and $P\bar{v},co_2$ respectively 40 and 55 mmHg, Hb 10 g dl^{-1}, Sa,o_2 100%. The factor is then -0.8 and the corrected difference 5.3 ml dl^{-1}). (Source: McHardy GJR. *Clin Sci* 1967; **32**: 299–309.)

the point of measurement; the result can be in error by up to 10% in consequence. The error can be avoided by use of the technique of Farhi and colleagues in which the subject rebreathes oxygen-enriched air. The alveolar carbon dioxide tension falls initially and then rises. The definitive measurements are made when the tension has returned to the level observed immediately before the start of rebreathing. The method has the further advantage over the standard rebreathing method that all the data required for the calculations are obtained during the test expiration. The measurement can therefore be repeated at intervals of no more than 40 s for following changes in cardiac output, for example, those at the start or end of exercise.

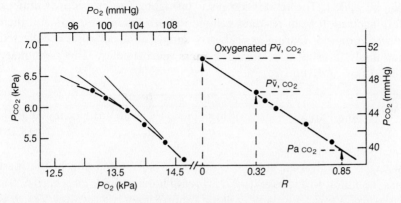

Fig. 8.16 Derivation of the tensions of carbon dioxide in arterial and mixed venous blood from analysis of expired gas for oxygen and carbon dioxide during a single expiration. The data are plotted in the form of an O_2–CO_2 diagram (cf. Fig. 7.9 (page 195) and the best curve is fitted. The slopes (S) at successive points on the curve are used to calculate values for respiratory exchange ratio (R) using the alveolar air equation (page 252) rearranged into the form:

$$S = [R + (1 - R) \, F_{I,CO_2}] \div [1 - (1 - R) \, F_{I,CO_2}]$$

P_{CO_2} is plotted against R, when a linear relationship is obtained. The P_{CO_2} of arterial blood is that associated with the steady state R (usually 0.85). The P_{CO_2} of mixed venous blood is that associated with an R of 0.32. This is because at $R = 0.32$ the CO_2 output relative to the oxygen uptake (0.32:1.0) is due solely to oxygen displacing CO_2 from combination with haemoglobin (Haldane effect, page 289); the P_{CO_2} remains constant and equal as between arterial and mixed venous blood. The P_{CO_2} of the oxygenated mixed venous blood is similarly defined by $R = 0$, when there are equal *contents* of carbon dioxide in arterial and mixed venous blood. (Source: Kim TS, Rahn H, Farhi LE. *J Appl Physiol* 1966; **21**: 1338–1344.)

Methods using inert gas

Single breath method. For acetylene, nitrous oxide and freon-22 which do not react with blood the Fick equation has the form:

$$\dot{Q} = \dot{n}TG/a(P_A - P\bar{v}) \; \mathrm{l \, min}^{-1} \qquad (8.17)$$

where $\dot{Q}$ is cardiac output ($\mathrm{l \, min}^{-1}$), $\dot{n}TG$ is the uptake of test gas ($\mathrm{mmol \, min}^{-1}$) and P_A and $P\bar{v}$ are respectively the tensions (kPa) in alveolar gas and mixed venous blood. The factor (s) is the solubility of the gas in blood at 37°C; this is given in Table 9.3 (page 272).

The tension in alveolar gas is usually obtained by analysis of a sample collected after exhalation of 750 ml to flush the deadspace (page 216). The tension in mixed venous blood is zero when the gases are inhaled for the first time. It rises after about 20 s on account of recirculation of blood containing gas absorbed during the previous passage through the lung; the rebreathing or breath holding must, therefore, be completed within this time. The measurement can be combined with that of transfer factor for carbon monoxide. In this event the test gas already contains carbon monoxide, helium or other insert insoluble gas and oxygen, the latter in a fractional concentration of 0.18 (page 304). For measurement of cardiac output 4% freon-22

245

can be added. The remainder gas is nitrogen. The procedure entails a full inspiration from residual volume, breath holding for $10\,s$ and then slow expiration. During expiration a sample of alveolar gas is collected for analysis using a respiratory mass spectrometer. The pulmonary blood flow is given by:

$$\dot{Q}c = \frac{V_A.P_B/(P_B - P_{H_2O})}{s\beta.t[V_A/(V_A + sti\,Vti)].\log\,e[V_A/(V_A + sti\,Vti).(F_{A,fr_0}/F_{A,fr_t})]}$$

(8.18)

where V_A is alveolar volume estimated from the dilution of the inert gas (equation 10.11, page 310), t is breath holding time, P_B is barometric pressure, Vti is lung tissue volume (approximately 11.5% of V_A), S is Bunsen solubility coefficient for freon respectively in blood (β) and lung tissue (ti) (page 272) and $F_{A,fr}$ is the alveolar concentration of freon-22. The concentration at time 0 is calculated from the inspired concentration and the initial and alveolar concentrations of the inert gas, that at time t is obtained from the alveolar gas sampled at the end of breath holding. The method which can also be used to estimate lung tissue volume is due to Cander, Johnson and colleagues who used acetylene; the intermediate calculations are as for the measurement of transfer factor (page 308). The reproducibility, expressed as the standard error of the estimate, was found by Kendrick and colleagues to be approximately $0.7\,l\,min^{-1}$ and the relationship to the direct Fick method was given by:

$$\dot{Q}\,\text{freon-22} = 1.37 + 0.77\dot{Q}\,\text{Fick} \pm 0.49 \qquad (8.19)$$

Plethysmograph method. The instantaneous flow rate can be obtained by the method of Lee and Dubois using a whole body plethysmograph. The measurement is made at rest or during cycle ergometry in a whole body plethysmograph. The subject first inhales a vital capacity breath of oxygen to raise the alveolar oxygen tension. This is followed by a vital capacity breath of 100% nitrous oxide then exhalation and breath holding for $15\,s$ at functional residual capacity. The subject subsequently breathes out. When a constant volume plethysmograph is used the uptake of nitrous oxide by blood causes a fall in pressure. This is converted to volume by use of the calibration factor for the box (page 159). The fall in pressure is modified by contractions of the heart, production of heat by the subject, and changes in volume due to the different rates of uptake and evolution of oxygen and carbon dioxide in the lung (R effect). The contribution of these factors is allowed for by subtracting the pressure changes observed when the subject inhales air in place of the test gas.

Using a constant pressure box the change in volume can be obtained using a pneumatic servo-system which adds gas at the rate needed to keep the pressure constant. The rate has a steady component which reflects changes in temperature and a variable component; the latter reflects uptake of nitrous oxide and the R effect. Both components exhibit a pronounced cardiac rhythm. This is evidence that blood flow through the pulmonary capillaries is pulsatile. The pulsation is imparted to gas exchange across the alveolar capillary membrane.

The concentration of nitrous oxide in gas expired during the breathing manoeuvre is obtained by analysis with an infrared gas analyser or respiratory mass spectrometer. The values before and after breath holding are used to calculate the mean alveolar concentration. The cardiac output is then calculated using a version of equation 8.10.

Indicator dilution methods

For this application of the Fick principle the cardiac output is determined from the dilution of an indicator substance which is injected rapidly into the superior vena cava or pulmonary artery. The dilution is measured at a site distal to where mixing with blood takes place; this is usually a systemic artery, but for material injected into the superior vena cava the pulmonary artery is sampled instead. The output from the analyser has three parts, an initial flat portion which represents the time for the indicator to reach the point of sampling, a period of rising concentration and a period of decline when the concentration is falling nearly exponentially towards the initial value; the decline may be interrupted by a secondary rise due to some of the indicator material traversing the lungs a second time. The effect on the dilution curve of recirculation of indicator material is eliminated by replotting the exponential portion of the curve on semi-log paper when the decline is effectively linear and can be extrapolated to zero. This line describes the relationship which would have obtained if no recirculation of indicator had taken place.

The cardiac output is calculated from the quantity of the indicator which is injected and the total area under the dilution curve expressed in log normal units. The method for obtaining the area is illustrated in Fig. 8.17. Indicators in current use include the dye indocyanine green, human albumen labelled with iodine-133 or Tc-99 and cold saline solution. Indocyanine green has an absorption band at 805 nm (8050 Å) where the spectral absorption of haemoglobin is independent of its saturation with oxygen. The concentration of dye is determined by spectrophotometry using an ear oximeter or cuvette through which arterial blood is drawn at a constant rate by a motor-driven syringe; the cuvette is not susceptible to movement artefact which can be an advantage for exercise studies. Indocyanine green has the advantage over Coumassie blue that the quantity of dye is small so the skin is not discoloured, excretion into the bile is rapid so measurements can be repeated at 2 min intervals, and the method is independent of the arterial oxygen saturation. In addition the procedure does not require a steady state or uniform ventilation and perfusion of the lung. It is the method of choice for investigation of patients with lung disease. Labelled albumen is detected using a scintillation counter. This can be applied to samples of blood collected serially every half second from an arterial

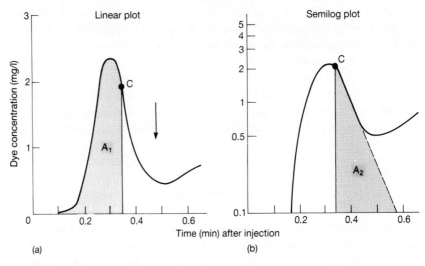

Fig. 8.17 Measurement of cardiac output by the indicator dilution method. Here the principle of the method is illustrated using indocyanine green as indicator. The detector was a cuvette through which blood from the brachial artery was drawn at a constant rate. Dye concentration was determined photo-electrically from absorption of light of wavelength 805 nm (8050 Å); calibration was by analysis of samples prepared by serial dilution of dye with the subject's blood. (a) Shows the changes in concentration following rapid injection of 3 mg of dye into the superior vena cava. The arrow marks the recirculation of dye through the systemic circulation. In (b) the data have been replotted on a semilog scale. The interrupted line is a linear extrapolation of the descending exponential portion of the curve before recirculation of dye has taken place. The area under the exponential part of the curve (A_2) is obtained from the following relationship:

$$\text{area } (A_2) = \frac{\text{concentration of dye at C}}{\text{slope of exponential}}$$

The remaining area (A_1) is obtained by planimetry. The total area is the product of time (min) and mean concentration of dye ($mg\,l^{-1}$); the cardiac output ($\dot{Q}t$) is obtained as follows:

$$\dot{Q}t = \frac{\text{dose of dye}}{A_1 + A_2}\,l\,min^{-1}$$

cannula; alternatively the counter can be placed over the precordium but measurements from this site are less reproducible. With the cold saline method the changes in temperature are recorded with a thermistor which is inserted through a needle into the pulmonary artery or a large systemic artery; measurements made at the periphery are less satisfactory due to dissipation of the thermal signal. The method has the advantage that there is no recirculation of the indicator.

Physical methods for cardiac output

Doppler echocardiography. This procedure measures blood flow in the ascending aorta. It entails separate estimations of flow velocity by ultrasound and aortic cross sectional area by echocardiography. Then:

$$\dot{Q} = f.\dot{v}.A \qquad (8.20)$$

where $\dot{Q}$ is cardiac output, f is the fraction of the cardiac cycle occupied by systole, $\dot{v}$ is mean aortic flow velocity during systole and A is aortic cross-sectional area. The instantaneous velocity is measured by the change in frequency when pulses of ultrasound waves of frequency 2 mHz from an emitter in the suprasternal notch are directed into the line of flow. The direction should be that associated with a smooth velocity : time curve which rises to a peak early in systole, a high frequency whistling sound when listening to the audible signal and the highest obtainable mean velocity when the signal is integrated over the duration of systole. The duration can be obtained separately by phono-cardiography. The cross-sectional area is usually 2 cm above the aortic orifice. At this site it is approximately 3 cm^2 in adults. The area should be estimated directly and not calculated from the diameter which by itself is insufficient since the cross section is not circular. The dimensions are those between the leading edges of the anterior and posterior echoes.

The method is based on the assumptions that the probe is in the line of flow and the flow is relatively uniform across a cylinder of blood extending outwards from the aortic orifice. In practice good agreement with other methods has been reported by a number of authors (e.g. Ihlen and colleagues). The method is appropriate for following changes in resting left ventricular output in an individual in whom only the mean flow velocity is relevant; it is less suitable for measuring absolute output and does not measure pulmonary blood flow if there are shunts. The method cannot be used when there is movement of the trunk, as, for example, during treadmill walking or stepping exercise.

Electrical bio-impedance cardiography. The method utilises the rate of change of thoracic impedance over the cardiac cycle to estimate stroke volume. Input electrodes are applied bilaterally to the side of the neck and to the lower thoracic cage and supplied by a constant current sinusoidal field generator. The impedance signal is recorded through pairs of electrodes placed respectively 5 cm below and above the input electrodes. The stroke volume is calculated using the relationship:

$$SV = \frac{dz/dt \text{ max.}}{z} \, t.PF \qquad (8.21)$$

where z is thoracic base impedance in ohms (Ω), dz/dt max. is maximal rate of change of impedance during systole (Ω/s), t is ventricular ejection time (s) and PF is an empirical personal factor which reflects the distance between the electrodes and other variables; it can be expressed in terms of age, sex, stature and body mass. This procedure measures both left and right ventricular outputs simultaneously. The method is not invalidated by exercise, is convenient and of good reproducibility; it is suitable for monitoring changes in cardiac output but the absolute accuracy is poor.

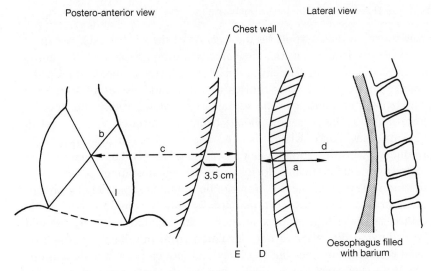

Fig. 8.18 Radiographic method for estimating heart volume. Only X-rays showing a clearly defined cardiac outline should be used. Dimensions are measured in cm. The length of the heart (*l*) is taken from the apex to the junction with the great vessels and the breadth (*b*) (which is nearly at right angles to the length) from the junction with the pulmonary conus to the junction with the diaphragm; the depth (*d*) is the maximal horizontal distance. The heart volume (HV) is given by:

$$HV = l \times b \times \left(\frac{A-a}{A}\right)^2 \times d \left(\frac{A-c}{A}\right) \times \frac{\pi}{6} \text{ cm}^3$$

where *A* is the anode to film distance, *a* and *c* are respectively the distances from the centre of the heart to the film as seen end-on in the lateral and posterio-anterior projections (D and E respectively). The chest wall to film distances are taken respectively as 0.5 and 3.5 cm.

Radiographic heart volume

The volume of the heart can be estimated from its dimensions on postero-anterior and lateral chest radiographs. The exposures are preferably triggered by the electrocardiogram. They are made after a full inspiration with the heart in diastole and, for the lateral view, the posterior border is delineated with barium sulphate gruel. The method is shown in Fig. 8.18. The volume includes the epicardial fat.

Inequality of ventilation–perfusion ratios

Classical three compartment model

Principle. Lung ventilation and perfusion are each subdivided into a part which in an ideal lung would be adequate for gas exchange, and a remainder; the latter reflects the extent to which the lung departs from the ideal model. Separation is effected using the alveolar air equation to calculate the oxygen tension of the idealised gas exchanging compartment. The excess ventilation per breath is the physiological deadspace; this comprises the anatomical and alveolar deadspaces. The physiological

Table 8.3 Three compartment model: summary

Compartment	Subdivision	Derivation
Physiological deadspace (V_{DS})	Anatomical deadspace (V_D,anat.) Alveolar deadspace (V_D,alv)	Fowler method (page 214) V_D, alv $= V_{DS} - V_D$,anat.
Ideal gas exchanging compartment		Alveolar air equation (page 252)
Physiological shunt ($\dot{Q}s$) also called venous admixture effect ($\dot{Q}Va$)	Anatomical shunt ($\dot{Q}s$,anat.) Alveolar shunt compartment ($\dot{Q}s$.alv)	Oxygen method (page 254) Inert gas methods $\dot{Q}s$.alv $= \dot{Q}s - \dot{Q}s$,anat.

blood shunt similarly comprises the anatomical shunt and the venous admixture effect. The compartments are described on page 190, and their derivations are summarised in Table 8.3.

Physiological deadspace

Derivation. The carbon dioxide content of mixed expired gas is represented as comprising carbon dioxide from deadspace gas which has the composition of inspired gas (so is effectively zero) and ideal alveolar gas in which the tension of carbon dioxide is that of the mixed arterial blood. Then by the mass balance equation:

$$Vt.F_{E}.co_2 = V_{A},t.F_{A},co_2 + (Vd + \alpha Vid).F_{I},co_2 \qquad (8.22)$$

where Vt is tidal volume, Vd is the physiological deadspace and V_{A},t is the alveolar component of the tidal volume. Vid is the deadspace of the mouthpiece, value box and instruments used in the collection of the expired gas and α is the fraction of Vid which enters the alveolar compartment, Fco_2 and Pco_2 are respectively the fractional concentrations and tensions of carbon dioxide and E, A and I refer to expired, ideal alveolar and inspired gas.

But:

$$V_{A},t = Vt - (Vd + \alpha Vid) \qquad (8.23)$$

and when breathing air, F_{I},co_2 is zero. On substitution and elimination the relationship then becomes:

$$Vt.F_{E},co_2 = (Vt - Vd - \alpha Vid)F_{A},co_2 \qquad (8.24)$$

or, multiplying both sides by the dry gas pressure in the lungs ($P_B - P_{H_2O}$)

$$Vt.P_{E},co_2 = (Vt - Vd - \alpha Vid)\, P_{A},co_2 \qquad (8.25)$$

then, on rearrangement:

$$Vd/Vt = (P_{A},co_2 - P_{E},co_2)/P_{A},co_2 - \alpha Vid/Vt \qquad (8.26)$$

251

The fraction α normally approaches unity but is reduced when, as in pulmonary embolism, there is a large alveolar deadspace. It may be derived using the relationship of Singleton and others:

$$\alpha = \left(\frac{P_{A,CO_2}}{P_{a,CO_2}}\right)^2 = \left(\frac{P_{E,CO_2}, Vt}{P_{a,CO_2}\,(Vt - Vd,\,\text{anat} - Vid)}\right)^2 \qquad (8.27)$$

where P_{a,CO_2} is the tension of carbon dioxide in the arterial blood and Vd, anat is the anatomical deadspace; the latter can be estimated by the Fowler method (page 214).

Practical aspects. The fractional concentration of carbon dioxide in mixed expired gas was formerly obtained by analysis of gas collected in a Douglas bag (page 22); it is now usually measured on-line using an infrared analyser or respiratory mass spectrometer sampling distal to a gas mixing chamber (Fig. 14.5, page 426). The fractional concentration of carbon dioxide in ideal alveolar air was formerly obtained by the Haldane−Priestley method which entailed analysis of gas collected at the end of a rapid forced exhalation down a long tube. Alternatively, a device for sampling the end tidal gas was used. These historical methods are illustrated in Fig. 3.1 (page 22). Alveolar carbon dioxide concentration is now obtained on-line by continuous sampling at the lips; the relevant concentration is that one-third of the way along the alveolar plateau − i.e. between the exhalation of at least 750 ml and the end of expiration. Where this condition is not met or the lung function is uneven the tension of carbon dioxide in arterial blood should be used instead. The methods are described on page 301. The instrument deadspace is estimated from its dimensions, or volumetrically by water displacement, and the tidal volume by one of the methods described in Chapter 3 (page 21).

Ideal alveolar gas

Derivation. The oxygen tension of ideal alveolar gas is that of a single chamber gas exchanger for which the respiratory exchange ratio is that of mixed expired gas and the tension of carbon dioxide is that for arterial blood. The oxygen tension is calculated using the alveolar air equation. This is based on the mass balance equation for the respired gases (equation 3.3, page 35). Allowance is made for movement of gas into or out of the lung on account of the volumetric transfers of oxygen and carbon dioxide seldom being equal (R effect).
From equation 3.2:

$$\dot{V}_I = \dot{V}_E \times F_{E,N_2}/F_{I,N_2} \qquad (8.28)$$

where F is fractional concentration of gas, in this case nitrogen, and $\dot{V}$ is ventilation minute volume, I and E refer to inspired and expired gas respectively.

But, neglecting the rare gases and inspired CO_2 the term F_{E,N_2} can be replaced by $(1 - F_{E,O_2} - F_{E,CO_2})$; and F_{I,N_2} by $(1 - F_{I,O_2})$. The relationship then becomes:

$$\dot{V}_I = \dot{V}_E \, (1 - F_{E,O_2} - F_{E,CO_2})/(1 - F_{I,O_2}) \qquad (8.29)$$

Similarly, the respiratory exchange ratio (R) can be written in the form:

$$R = (\dot{V}_E \times F_{E,CO_2})/(\dot{V}_I \times F_{I,O_2} - \dot{V}_E \times F_{E,O_2}) \qquad (8.30)$$

By combining equations 8.29 and 8.30 the ventilation terms can be eliminated; also since the respiratory exchange ratios for alveolar and expired gas are equal, fractional concentrations in alveolar gas (F_A) can be substituted for those in expired gas (F_E). Then on rearrangement:

$$F_{A,O_2} = F_{I,O_2} - \frac{F_{A,CO_2}}{R} + \frac{F_{A,CO_2}}{R} \times F_{I,O_2} \, (1 - R) \qquad (8.31)$$

or in terms of partial pressures:

$$P_{A,O_2} = F_{I,O_2} \times (P_B - P_{H_2O}) - \frac{P_{A,CO_2}}{R} + \frac{P_{A,CO_2}}{R} \times F_{I,O_2} \, (1 - R)$$
$$(8.32)$$

The respiratory exchange ratio is obtained by analysis of expired gas (page 36). The inspired fractional concentration of oxygen is 0.2093 when breathing air and is otherwise obtained by analysis. The alveolar tension of carbon dioxide is that used for calculating physiological deadspace (q.v.).

The uses and limitations of the alveolar air equation are considered on page 194. Its application to the measurement of the transfer factor for oxygen is described on page 320.

Practical aspects. The procedure is straightforward and reasonably accurate provided that attention is given to all the details (cf. page 50).

Anatomical shunt and venous admixture effect

Derivation of physiological shunt. Using the mass balance equation:

$$\dot{Q}_t \times C_{a,O_2} = \dot{Q}_{s,air} \times C_{\bar{v},O_2} + (\dot{Q}_t - \dot{Q}_{s,air}) \, C_{c',O_2} \qquad (8.33)$$

where $\dot{Q}_t$ is total cardiac output, $\dot{Q}_{s,air}$ is physiological shunt, i.e. breathing air, and C_{a,O_2}, $C_{\bar{v},O_2}$ and C_{c',O_2} are the contents of oxygen respectively in systemic arterial blood, mixed venous blood and blood leaving the pulmonary capillaries. The physiological shunt as a percentage of cardiac output is obtained by rearrangement:

$$\dot{Q}_{s,air}/\dot{Q}_t \, (\%) = [(C_{c',O_2} - C_{a,O_2})/(C_{c',O_2} - C_{\bar{v},O_2})] \times 100 \qquad (8.34)$$

It is expressed in terms of saturation of haemoglobin (S) by dividing numerator and denominator by the capacity of the blood for oxygen, then:

$$\dot{Q}s,air/\dot{Q}t \; (\%) = [(Sc',o_2 - Sa,o_2)/(Sc',o_2 - S\bar{v},o_2)] \times 100 \qquad (8.35)$$

Practical aspects. The saturation of oxygen in arterial blood (Sa,o_2) is measured directly. The saturation in the mixed venous blood ($S\bar{v},o_2$) is obtained in one of the following ways:

1 By analysis of mixed venous blood obtained at cardiac catheterisation.

2 From the dissociation curve following a rebreathing procedure for measurement of tension of oxygen in mixed venous blood (page 240).

3 By calculation via the Fick relationship (page 239) from measurements of consumption of oxygen, content of oxygen in systemic arterial blood and cardiac output.

4 From an assumed value for the difference in saturation between arterial and mixed venous bloods. The difference is assumed to be 22% at rest and rather more on exercise (see Fig. 13.7, page 398).

The saturation in pulmonary end-capillary blood (Sc,o_2) cannot be measured directly; however, the corresponding tension of oxygen when the subject is breathing air is almost the same as that in the alveolar gas (see Chapter 9). The tension in alveolar gas is obtained by use of the alveolar air equation; it is assumed to exceed by 0.1 kPa (1 mmHg) the tension in blood as it leaves the pulmonary capillaries so the latter is obtained by difference. The corresponding oxygen saturation is obtained from the blood dissociation curve for oxygen (Fig. 9.3; page 280). The validity of the assumed gradient for oxygen between alveolar gas and pulmonary end-capillary blood (in this case 0.1 kPa) is subsequently tested in the way described on page 321.

Derivation of anatomical shunt. The partitioning of the physiological shunt into components due to the anatomical shunt and to the venous admixture effect is achieved by the subject breathing 100% oxygen. This raises the tension in all ventilated alveoli to a level in excess of 13 kPa (100 mmHg); hence pulmonary exchange of oxygen takes place on the flat linear part of the dissociation curve. Under these circumstances the higher tension and content of oxygen in blood which has perfused well-ventilated alveoli compensate for the lower tension and content of blood from alveoli which are poorly ventilated (c.f. page 205). Most of the difference in tension of oxygen between mixed alveolar gas and systemic arterial blood is then due to admixture with venous blood which has either bypassed the lung or perfused alveoli that are not ventilated. The extent of this anatomic shunt is assessed while breathing oxygen. Under these circumstances, the high alveolar oxygen tension as well as fully saturating the pulmonary capillary blood, also raises the quantity of oxygen dissolved in the capillary plasma. Depending on the size of the shunt the amount of oxygen dissolved in the systemic arterial plasma can also be increased. The dissolved oxygen can be allowed for in equation 8.35 which then becomes:

$$\frac{\dot{Q}s,o_2\ (\%)}{\dot{Q}t} = \frac{h\ (Sc',o_2 - Sa,o_2) + s(Pc',o_2 - Pa,o_2)}{h\ (Sc',o_2 - S\bar{v},o_2) + s(Pc',o_2 - P\bar{v},o_2)} \times 100 \qquad (8.36)$$

where $\dot{Q}s,o_2/\dot{Q}t$ is the anatomical shunt, h is a factor which converts from saturation to quantity of oxygen combined with haemoglobin, s is the solubility of oxygen in plasma and the other terms are as defined above. When breathing oxygen Sc',o_2 is approximately 100% and Pc',o_2 is effectively alveolar oxygen tension. Hence in the absence of nitrogen:

$$Pc',o_2 \approx PB - PH_2O - Pa,co_2 \qquad (8.37)$$

where PB, PH_2O and Pa,co_2 are respectively barometric pressure the pressure of water vapour in the lung and the tension of carbon dioxide in arterial blood. This quantity, which is nearly equal to alveolar carbon dioxide tension, is obtained from analysis of systemic arterial blood. The arterial oxygen tension is measured concurrently.

If the anatomic shunt is relatively small then the tension of oxygen in the systemic arterial blood exceeds about 20 kPa (150 mmHg) and the term $(Sc',o_2 - Sa,o_2)$ is effectively zero. The relationship thus becomes:

$$\frac{\dot{Q}s,o_2}{\dot{Q}t}(\%) = \frac{s(PB - PH_2O - Pa,co_2 - Pa,o_2)}{h\ (100 - S\bar{v},o_2) + s(PB - PH_2O - Pa,co_2 - P\bar{v},o_2)} \times 100$$
$$(8.38)$$

Measurement of the anatomical shunt requires accurate measurement of the arterial oxygen tension during breathing oxygen. This is best done using an intra-arterial electrode which has been calibrated over the full range of oxygen tensions. Alternatively if drawn blood is used, it should be analysed immediately. The other component measurements, both for this determination and for the physiological shunt, present few difficulties especially if assumed values are used for the tension and saturation of the mixed venous blood. Reference values are given in Table 15.22 (page 511).

In addition to its determination by gasometric methods, the physiological shunt can be obtained from the proportion of the dose of a tracer gas which traverses the lung after injection in solution into the superior vena cava. Krypton-85 or xenon-133 can be used for this purpose; this and other methods are illustrated on page 233.

Practical aspects. The measurement of arterial oxygen tension during breathing oxygen requires careful calibration of the polarograph (page 41). In addition before the blood sample is taken for analysis the subject should have breathed oxygen for sufficient time to eliminate nitrogen from the lungs. The sample should be analysed immediately.

Multiple inert gas elimination technique (MIGET)

Derivation. The model used for this approach to uneven lung function is discussed on page 196. It assumes that lung ventilation and perfusion are continuous processes. The technique requires that gaseous equilibrium between alveolar gas and pulmonary capillary blood is achieved during a single passage of blood through the lung. The gas is dissolved and infused at a constant rate into a peripheral vein. Then for a lung compartment which is homogeneous with respect to its ventilation–perfusion ratio the quantity of gas which is exchanging between the alveoli and the pulmonary capillary blood is the same as that exchanging between the alveoli and the atmosphere. This quantity, expressed as a fraction of that in the mixed venous blood, is a function of the ventilation–perfusion ratio and the blood–gas partition coefficient for the gas in question. It is given by the following equation of Kety:

$$P_A/P_{\bar{v}} = P_{c'}/P_{\bar{v}} = \lambda/(\lambda + \dot{V}_A/\dot{Q}) \tag{8.39}$$

where the three partial pressure terms refer respectively to the alveolar gas, the mixed venous blood and the blood leaving the alveolar capillaries; λ is the blood–gas partition coefficient for the inert gas in question and $\dot{V}_A/\dot{Q}$ is the ventilation–perfusion ratio for the particular compartment. Then on rearrangement and after substituting arterial for end-capillary gas tension:

$$\dot{V}_A/\dot{Q} = \lambda\ (P_{\bar{v}}/P_a - 1) \tag{8.40}$$

where $P_a/P_{\bar{v}}$ is the ratio of the gas tensions in the arterial and mixed venous blood, hence, since the gas is inert, the ratio of the blood–gas concentrations; this is the fraction of the gas which is retained by the blood during its passage through the lungs. In practice six gases having different blood–gas partition coefficients are infused. Some gases which can be used are indicated in Fig. 8.19. During the infusion, when a steady state has been achieved, measurements are made of the gas concentrations in arterial blood and alveolar gas. The cardiac output and ventilation are measured concurrently. The analysis is performed for a 50 compartment model lung in which the ventilation–perfusion ratios range from zero (i.e. pure shunt) to nearly infinity. For the lung as a whole the mixed arterial concentration is a blood flow weighted mean of the values for the several compartments whilst the mean expired level is similarly a ventilation weighted mean of the compartmental values. The analysis identifies a numerical distribution of ventilation–perfusion ratios which is compatible with the arterial and alveolar concentrations of all gases concurrently.

Procedure. The six gases are dissolved in saline and infused into a vein in one arm or hand. The infusion rate in a resting subject is 3 ml of saline per min, or more during exercise, and the measurements of gas concentration in expired gas and arterial and mixed venous blood are normally made after 30 min. Expired gas and arterial blood are sampled directly. Systemic venous blood from the contralateral arm can be substituted for arterial blood but the infusion should then be given for 90 min to allow time for the venous gas tensions to rise to within 5% of the equilibrium values. Mixed venous blood is normally sampled from

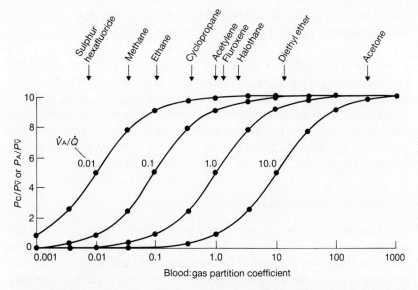

Fig. 8.19 Relationship between inert gas retention $Pc/P\bar{v}$ (or excretion $P_A/P\bar{v}$) and blood–gas partition coefficient, using a logarithmic scale for the abscissa. Four curves are drawn, each for homogeneous lung units with different $\dot{V}_A/\dot{Q}$ ratios. (Source: Wagner PD, Saltzman HA, West JB. *J Appl Physiol* 1974; **36**: 588–599.)

a catheter in the pulmonary artery. Alternatively cardiac output is measured with indocyanine green and the mixed venous gas concentrations are calculated by the Fick principle. The dye is injected via a catheter into the superior vena cava and the dye dilution curve is obtained for blood from the radial arterial catheter which is also used for blood gas analysis. This is performed using gas chromatography; if a number of determinations are envisaged the extraction of gases from blood should preferably be automated and the analyser connected in line to the computer.

A programme for the calculation including an algorithm for enforced smoothing of the $\log_e \dot{V}_A/\dot{Q}$ distribution curve and calculation of its mean and standard deviation or dispersion (respectively the first and second moments) has been developed by Evans and Wagner.

The reproducibility of the dispersion expressed as the coefficient of variation has been found to be approximately 8.5% when based on a single estimate and 6.1% for duplicates. The log dispersions of $\dot{V}_A/\dot{Q}$ with respect to both perfusion and ventilation (designated $\log$ SD$\dot{Q}$ and $\log$ SD$\dot{V}$) are reported together with the standard deviation of the difference between the measured gas retentions and excretions; this overall index of heterogeneity of lung function is given by:

$$\text{Disp R} - \text{E} = 100 \sqrt{\Sigma_1^n \frac{(\text{R} - \text{E})^2}{n}} \qquad (8.41)$$

where R and E are respectively the retentions and the excretions corrected for the physiological deadspace. The correction is made using a calculated deadspace which is compatible with the observed gas retentions and partition coefficients, cardiac output and ventilation minute volume; the derivation is given by Gale and colleagues.

Comment. The method is limited by the accuracy of present chromatographic techniques for gas analysis. In addition it does not provide a unique answer since the same arterial and alveolar concentrations could result from other distributions of ventilation and perfusion in the lung. However, these limitations are no greater than for other methods which attempt to describe in simple terms the complex gas exchanging function of the lung. This one is the most successful so far.

Regional $\dot{V}_A/\dot{Q}$ inequality

The isotope methods for assessing regional distribution of ventilation and perfusion are described on page 233. Regional $\dot{V}_A/\dot{Q}$ ratios can be calculated from these data but underestimate the extent of uneven lung function because intra-regional differences are not included. The procedures are nonetheless of great clinical value and are widely used.

Pulmonary blood shunt

The pulmonary blood shunt can be estimated as the difference between cardiac output and pulmonary blood flow. The method detects blood flow from the right side of the heart which bypasses ventilated alveoli. The shunt determined in this way, therefore, includes intracardiac right-to-left shunts, pulmonary arterio-venous fistulae and blood traversing collapsed or fluid-filled alveoli. The measurement does not include post-pulmonary shunts through bronchial veins, thebesian veins, anterior cardiac veins and portal-pulmonary venous anastomoses. These latter are included in the shunt estimated by the oxygen method (page 254).

Derivation. Pulmonary blood shunt is estimated from the proportion of an inert gas which remains in the blood during its passage through the lungs and is not lost into the alveoli. The blood is sampled in a peripheral artery and the proportion is obtained by comparing the dilution of the inert gas with that of a non-volatile indicator which does not enter the alveoli. The non-volatile indicator can be indocyanine green, cold saline, tritiated water or other substance; it measures total cardiac output. The volatile indicator is a gas dissolved in saline; ideally it should be one which disappears without trace when it enters the alveoli. Under these circumstances the proportion of indicator in arterial blood would be determined solely by the size of the shunt. In practice removal from the alveoli is incomplete; the remainder then exerts a back pressure which contributes to the gas present in the arterial blood drawn for analysis. The contribution of the back pressure can be determined by using two indicators having different partition coefficients, for example tritium (T_2) and krypton-85. However, the procedure is then too complicated for regular use except as part of the

258

multiple inert gas technique for ventilation perfusion inequality. As an alternative Murray and colleagues suggested using a single volatile indicator and making an empirical correction for the effect of back pressure. These workers employed xenon-133 which is widely used for study of regional lung function (page 233). Where that information is not required the indicator of choice is krypton-85 which has a low blood−gas partition coefficient and the energy of the emission is also low. Acetylene, nitrous oxide and freon-22 are other possibilities.

Procedure. The solution of indocyanine green is equilibrated with xenon-133 in a 30 ml syringe for long enough to raise its activity to 0.5 mCi/ml. The material is transferred to a smaller syringe through a millipore filter and 3 ml is injected rapidly into the superior vena cava from a catheter in a brachial vein. The dye dilution curve is obtained from the output of a densitometer attached to an arterial cannula and concurrently blood is collected in a 30 ml syringe over a period of 1 min. Two similar blood samples are collected sequentially, the first after 10 min for determining residual circulating radioactivity and the second after the subject has inhaled a 3 ml bolus of xenon-133 adminis- tered by injection into the mouthpiece whilst the subject is breathing air. The latter sample is used to estimate the relationship of the back pressure to the dose of xenon-133. The radioactivities of the delivery syringe before and after the injection and of the three collecting syringes are determined using a scintillation counter. The blood is then used to make serial dilutions of a further sample of dye, the densitometer is calibrated and cardiac output calculated (page 247). The pulmonary blood shunt is then given by:

$$\dot{Q}s/\dot{Q}t = \frac{SC \text{ measured} - SC \text{ back pressure}}{SC \text{ calculated}} \quad (8.42)$$

where SC is scintillation count in the relevant blood sample or in the case of the denominator the count which would have obtained if none of the gas had passed into the alveoli; the latter is given by SC injected/$\dot{Q}$t (dye). The limitations to the procedure are discussed by Murray and colleagues.

Intrabreath R index of $\dot{V}A/\dot{Q}$ inequality

This index was introduced by West and colleagues and preceded the multiple inert gas elimination technique (MIGET) which has recently been used to provide validation. The test was modified by Guy *et al.* who incorporated suggestions made by Meade and others. In its present form the index is the proportional change in ventilation−perfusion ratio per litre of expired gas over the middle half of a slow expiration from total lung capacity. The change is calculated from that in the respiratory exchange ratio; it reflects events taking place during the expiration including gas exchange and serial emptying of lung units having different ventilation−perfusion ratios. Theoretically the method

259

should not detect inequality between lung units emptying in parallel; however, in practice small differences in time constants can yield a result (e.g. Fig. 8.20).

Derivation. Respiratory exchange ratio is calculated from the alveolar air equation (equation 8.32, page 253); this can be rearranged in the form:

$$R = P_{A,CO_2}(1 - F_{I,O_2})/(P_{I,O_2} - P_{A,O_2} - F_{I,O_2} \times P_{A,CO_2}) \qquad (8.43)$$

The corresponding ventilation−perfusion ratios are then calculated using the mass balance equation for oxygen passing from alveolar gas to pulmonary capillary blood.

$$\dot{V}_A/\dot{Q} = bR(C_{a,O_2} - C_{\bar{v},O_2})/P_{A,CO_2} \qquad (8.44)$$

where $\dot{V}_A/\dot{Q}$ is the ventilation−perfusion ratio which corresponds to the measured respiratory exchange ratio (R). The term within the bracket is the difference in content of oxygen between arterial and mixed venous bloods; this is usually assumed to be $2\,mmol\,l^{-1}$ ($44\,ml\,l^{-1}$), equivalent to a difference in saturation of 22%. P_{A,CO_2} is the tension of carbon dioxide in alveolar gas; it is assumed to be equal to that in oxygenated venous blood. The constant term (b) is a factor which converts these quantities into the appropriate units; in SI units it is 2.58 and in traditional units 0.863.

The result can be displayed graphically as instantaneous respiratory exchange ratio against volume expired from total lung capacity

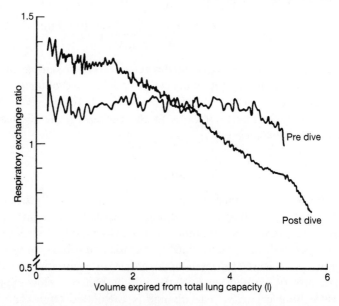

Fig. 8.20 Intrabreath R in a healthy man before and after onset of ventilation−perfusion inequality; this was caused by intravascular bubbles accumulating in the pulmonary circulation during decompression following a saturation dive. (Source: Thorsen I, Reed JW. Unpublished.)

(Fig. 8.20). The contribution of gas exchange to the relationship can be indicated by superimposing on the resulting curve that for $\dot{V}A/\dot{Q}$ ratio calculated for a single compartment lung having the same lung volume and average $\dot{V}A/\dot{Q}$ ratio as the subject being studied. Curves can also be calculated for $\dot{V}A/\dot{Q}$ ratios which differ by ±10% from that value.

Procedure. The subject breathes through a mouthpiece connected to a flow transducer as for the single breath nitrogen test of uneven lung function. The respired gas is sampled continuously from the mouthpiece and analysed for oxygen, carbon dioxide and nitrogen using a respiratory mass spectrometer. The output from the mass spectrometer should preferably be processed by computer. The subject breathes normally through the mouthpiece then slowly inhales air to total lung capacity and immediately exhales completely at a slow rate ($<0.5 \, \mathrm{l s}^{-1}$). Alternatively the procedure is compared with the single breath test of gas mixing using argon as the indicator gas (page 221). In this event the test expiration is preceded by the subject breathing out to residual volume and inhaling a bolus of argon with the air. The arterio-venous oxygen content difference is also needed in order to calculate instantaneous $\dot{V}A/\dot{Q}$ ratios (equation 8.44). It is best obtained by measurement of oxygen uptake and of cardiac output by the carbon dioxide re-breathing method. Alternatively it is estimated (see page 254).

Arterial–alveolar tension difference for nitrogen

The theoretical basis for this index of $\dot{V}A/\dot{Q}$ inequality is given on page 209. The index is obtained from measurements of the tensions of nitrogen in the alveolar gas and the arterial or peripheral venous blood. The latter is obtained by gas chromatography following extraction of nitrogen from the subject's blood. Calibration is performed by equilibration with known gas mixtures using tonometers in a water bath at 37°C and a modified Van Slyke apparatus. The method has the advantage that the nitrogen difference is not dependent on sequential emptying of different lung compartments but it is technically demanding and has been replaced by others described in this chapter.

Conclusions

Irregularities in the distribution of lung ventilation and perfusion can be assessed in a variety of ways. For ambulant patients, the distribution of ventilation can be checked using the lung volume index of uneven ventilation (page 222), the single breath nitrogen test, the nitrogen/argon test, or the closing volume (Figs 8.3 and 8.4). The modified procedures of Paiva and others should be considered for the diagnosis of bronchiolitis (page 219). For inequality of ventilation–perfusion ratios the intrabreath R index can be used. Alternatively, the expired-to-mixed venous tension difference for carbon dioxide can be partitioned into a deadspace component, the a-A $\mathrm{dCO_2}$ and the arterio-venous difference using the methods developed by Campbell, Jones and McHardy amongst others, which are described in this chapter.

For patients in hospital, or as part of a detailed assessment of ambulant patients the arterial blood can be sampled directly. The physiological deadspace and the physiological shunt can then be calculated when breathing air and also when breathing oxygen (page 253). The range of ventilation—perfusion ratios is best assessed by the multiple inert gas elimination technique; this should be considered for research purposes and when the venous admixture effect appears to be increased (page 254).

For patients in whom there may be localised areas of hypoventilation or pulmonary thrombo-embolism or in whom thoracic surgery is contemplated, the measurement of regional lung function should be undertaken. This is usually best done using a ventilation scan with ^{81m}Kr and a perfusion scan with ^{99m}Tc (page 238) or one of the other methods listed on page 230. In addition the lobar function can be assessed by analysis of bronchial air samples obtained during bronchoscopy (page 225).

Guide to references

The references (Chapter 18) are classified under subject headings of which the following are particularly relevant to the present chapter:

9: Exchange of Gas in the Lung

Introduction

External respiration between the lung and atmospheric air is a prelude to tissue respiration in mitochondria throughout the body. Passage of oxygen to the mitochondria is effected by the processes of ventilation and gas distribution, gas exchange, transport by blood and transfer within the tissues. At each stage the partial pressure of oxygen decreases compared with the previous stage so the flow of oxygen takes place as a series of cascades down a pressure gradient. The capacity of each stage can be expressed in terms of its conductance; this is the maximal rate (i.e. maximal quantity per unit of time) at which oxygen can be transferred per unit of pressure difference between the two ends of the stage under consideration. Some numerical values are given in Table 9.1. The first stage reflects alveolar ventilation. The conductance is low at rest mainly because much of the minute volume is wasted in ventilating the physiological deadspace. On exercise this convective conductance rises because the alveolar ventilation increases to a much greater extent than the deadspace ventilation. For the same reason the convective conductance increases with hypoxia. The alveolar ventilation and its distribution within the lung influence the alveolar oxygen tension that provides the head of pressure for the second stage, which is the transfer of oxygen across the alveolar capillary membrane. The transfer is determined mainly by the area and thickness of the alveolar capillary membrane, the volume of blood in alveolar capillaries and the kinetics of the reaction of oxygen with haemoglobin. These aspects are considered in the present chapter. The third and fourth stages are the transport of oxygen from the lungs to the tissue capillaries and the transfer from red blood cells into the tissues (page 396). Here the oxygen is used as a hydrogen acceptor (page 401) and for oxidation of substrate. The oxidative metabolism leads to the formation of carbon dioxide which returns along a similar series of cascades to the atmosphere.

Table 9.1 Representative mean oxygen tensions (Po_2) and conductances (G) for the several stages of oxygen transport in subjects assessed during rest and exercise at sea level and at an altitude of 5365 m (17 000 ft)

Circumstance Oxygen uptake	Rest 15 mmol min⁻¹			Exercise 100 mmol min⁻¹			Altitude 15 mmol min⁻¹		
	Po_2 (kPa)	(mmHg)	G (mmol min⁻¹ kPa⁻¹)	Po_2 (kPa)	(mmHg)	G (mmol min⁻¹ kPa⁻¹)	Po_2 (kPa)	(mmHg)	G (mmol min⁻¹ kPa⁻¹)
Inspired gas Convective G	20	(150)	2.2	20	(150)	15	9.4	(71)	3.9
Alveolar gas Alveolar capillary G	13.3	(100)	7.5	13.3	(100)	22	5.6	(42)	19
Pulmonary capillaries Tissue capillary G	11.3	(85)	3.8	8.7	(65)	25	4.8	(36)	30
Tissue capillaries Tissue G	7.3	(55)	7.5	4.7	(35)	71	4.3	(32)	15
Tissue cells	5.3	(40)		3.3	(25)		3.3	(25)	
Overall conductance			1.0			6.0			2.4

Overall conductance was obtained from the sum of the reciprocals of the individual conductances; the reciprocals are the resistances to the flow of oxygen across the stages. (Adapted from Otis AB. In Fishman AP, ed. *Handbook of Physiology*, Bethesda: American Physiological Society, Section 3, IV: 1–11, 1987.)

Alveolar ventilation

Gas exchange

Alveolar ventilation can be defined as that part of the minute volume which participates in gas exchange. It is best defined in terms of ventilation–perfusion ratios but in practice is usually determined on the assumption that the lung is homogeneous (page 194). The alveolar ventilation is the resultant of factors which control the minute volume (page 325) and the deadspace ventilation (page 192); they include the respiratory drive and the work of breathing. The latter is influenced by choice and allocation of breathing frequency and tidal volume. The efficacy of a given level of alveolar ventilation depends on how well its distribution within the lung matches the distribution of perfusion (page 204). In the greater part of the healthy lung the matching is satisfactory; in this circumstance the contribution of alveolar ventilation to gas exchange is relatively independent of the breathing pattern by which it is achieved.

Effect upon the composition of alveolar gas

The composition of the alveolar gas lies somewhere between that of inspired gas and gas in equilibrium with mixed venous blood. Within these limits the composition is determined by the rates at which oxygen and carbon dioxide in the alveoli exchange with the environment (i.e. alveolar ventilation) and, across the alveolar capillary membrane, with plasma in the alveolar capillaries (i.e. diffusion). When the level of alveolar ventilation is high, the tensions in the alveoli move closer to those of inspired air; when it is low, the tensions approach those of mixed venous blood. The product of alveolar ventilation and alveolar concentration of carbon dioxide is the rate at which carbon dioxide leaves the body in the expired gas. When the subject is in a steady state this is the same as the rate of evolution of carbon dioxide into the alveoli.

The relationship may be written in the following form:

$$F_{A,CO_2} = P_{A,CO_2}/(P_B - P_{H_2O}) = \dot{n}_{CO_2}(\text{or } \dot{V}_{CO_2})/\dot{V}_A \quad (9.1)$$

$$P_{A,CO_2} = a(\dot{n}_{CO_2} \text{ or } \dot{V}_{CO_2})/\dot{V}_A = a(\dot{n}_{O_2} \text{ or } \dot{V}_{O_2}) R/\dot{V}_A \quad (9.2)$$

where F_{A,CO_2} is the concentration of carbon dioxide in the alveolar gas and P_{A,CO_2} is the corresponding CO_2 tension (kPa or mmHg); $\dot{n}$ and $\dot{V}$ are the rates of exchange of the relevant gases in mmol min^{-1} and ml STPD min^{-1}, and R is the respiratory exchange ratio. $\dot{V}_A$ is the alveolar ventilation (l BTPS min^{-1}). The factor a is required by the arbitrary units of the other variables; in SI units it has the value 2.56 (or 2.58 for oxygen) and in traditional units 0.863.*

* $2.56 = 22.26 \times (101 - 6.3) \div \left(\dfrac{273}{310} \times \dfrac{713}{760}\right)$ $0.863 = (760 - 37) \div \left(\dfrac{273}{310} \times \dfrac{713}{760}\right)$

265

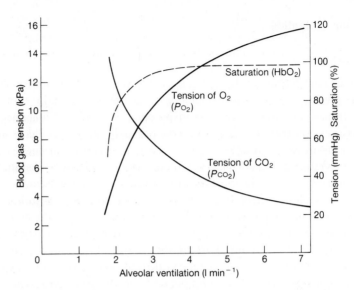

Fig. 9.1 Relationship of the composition of blood leaving the alveolar capillaries to the level of alveolar ventilation; for derivation see text. The tensions of oxygen and carbon dioxide are sensitive to small changes in alveolar ventilation. By contrast, on account of the shape of the dissociation curve, the oxygen saturation is relatively independent of the level of ventilation until this is greatly reduced.

The corresponding relationship for oxygen can be obtained by substitution in the alveolar air equation (page 252). These relationships are illustrated graphically in Fig. 9.1 which shows the tensions of oxygen and carbon dioxide to be expected in a healthy subject at rest under steady state conditions. They have been calculated for an oxygen consumption of 11 mmol min^{-1} (250 ml min^{-1}) and a respiratory exchange ratio at all levels of ventilation of 0.8; barometric pressure is 101 kPa (760 mmHg). The figure also shows the saturation with oxygen of blood leaving the alveolar capillaries. This has been derived from the dissociation curve (Fig. 9.3) on the assumption that the tension of oxygen in mixed end-capillary blood is equal to that in alveolar gas. This is nearly true in healthy subjects, but in patients with an increased range of ventilation–perfusion ratios the mean tension in the blood is less than that in the alveolar gas (see e.g. Fig. 7.13, page 208).

The figure shows that the *tensions* of oxygen and carbon dioxide in blood leaving the alveolar capillaries are sensitive to small changes in alveolar ventilation. By contrast, because the upper part of the dissociation curve is relatively flat, the *saturation* of haemoglobin with oxygen is nearly independent of the level of alveolar ventilation until this is greatly reduced. On account of these differences, a progressive reduction in alveolar ventilation causes hypercapnia before it gives rise to hypoxaemia.

Diffusion in the gas phase

Respirable gases are molecules having a diameter of approximately

266

3×10^{-10} m; at atmospheric pressure the average distance between the molecules is about 10 diameters and they move in random directions at high speed. The movement is due to the molecules having a limited kinetic energy which is a function of temperature. The kinetic energy is the product of mass and velocity squared ($1/2\,MV^2$) and at a given temperature is the same for all gases, hence the rate of diffusion of a gas is inversely proportional to the square root of mass or density; this relationship is now called Graham's Law. As well as varying with temperature the rate of diffusion is inversely proportional to barometric pressure. At constant temperature and pressure gas molecules of similar mass have similar average velocities; thus under normal ambient conditions the velocities of oxygen and carbon dioxide are both approximately $4\,\mathrm{m\,s^{-1}}$. The velocities of nitrogen and carbon monoxide are only slightly greater than that of oxygen. However, that of helium is about four times greater and of sulphur hexafluoride correspondingly less. The close proximity of the molecules leads to collisons occurring with a frequency of approximately 5×10^9 per s; the frequency is independent of the mass so the distance a particle travels between collisions, which is the mean free path, is a function of velocity. Compared with oxygen, helium has a long mean free path so diffuses relatively rapidly whilst sulphur hexafluoride has a short path and diffuses slowly. The collisions lead to the movement of individual molecules being in random directions so the movement in any one direction is slow relative to the average velocity.

For air the directional velocity is approximately $10\,\mathrm{mm\,s^{-1}}$. This is sufficient for movement of gas within the acinus where the distance between the respiratory bronchiole and the attendant alveoli is usually less than 1 mm.

Additional factors

Additional factors which influence the behaviour of gases include the extent to which they attract or repell each other and the composition of the gas mixture. The former is characterised by the potential energy of interaction which for symmetrical molecules can be described in terms of a model due to Lennard-Jones. It applies to a limited extent to dipolar molecules. The effect of gas composition is best seen in a mixture of two gases where gaseous diffusion can be described by a single diffusion coefficient; this is because any concentration gradient due to one gas diffusing faster than the other enhances the movement of the slower component and slows down that of the faster component. The equilibrium rate which is reached is nearly independent of the relative gas concentrations. The rate, however, is dependent on the molecular weights of the constituent gases. Thus at 37°C and 1 atmosphere pressure the binary diffusion coefficients for oxygen with nitrogen and oxygen with helium were calculated by Chang as respectively 0.22 and $0.79\,\mathrm{cm^2\,s^{-1}}$. Those for carbon dioxide with oxygen and with nitrogen were approximately $0.16\,\mathrm{cm^2\,s^{-1}}$. The derivation of the units

Exchange of gas in the lung

Table 9.2 Influence of carrier gas on effective mass diffusion coefficients for O_2 and CO_2 in tracheal (i.e. inspired) and alveolar gas, expressed for dry gas at body temperature

Carrier gas	D_{O_2} $(cm^2 s^{-1})$	D_{CO_2} $(cm^2 s^{-1})$	Ratio to D binary
N_2	0.240	0.177	1.1
He	0.530	0.438	0.68
SF_6	0.143	0.096	1.4

The coefficients were computed using a version of equation 9.3 in which gas concentration was expressed in terms of partial pressure. Then:

$$D = 1.935 \times 10^4 \, J(mmol\,cm^{-3}s^{-1}) \, \delta \, (cm)/\Delta P(mmHg)$$

where J is mass flux and δ is film thickness. The units simplify to cm^2/s. (Source: Chang H-K, Farhi LE _Respir Physiol_, 1980; **40**: 269–279.)

is indicated in the footnote to Table 9.2. Carbon monoxide behaved similarly to nitrogen. Where more than two gases were present in a mixture there was no similar tendency for the fluxes to equalise so no common coefficient was obtained; however, that for each substance was still influenced by the others. This could result in the flux being independent of the partial pressure gradient but in most circumstances a proportional relationship was obtained. The ratio was then the effective diffusion coefficient. Values of this quantity for oxygen and carbon dioxide in nitrogen, helium and sulphur hexafluoride are given in Table 9.2 together with the ratio of the coefficients to those for a simple binary system. The presence of carbon dioxide on average reduced the changes in the diffusivity of oxygen associated with the foreign gases compared with nitrogen.

The concept of diffusion coefficient was introduced by Fick who postulated that under steady state conditions the diffusional flux was proportional to the concentration gradient:

$$Jz = -D \, dC/dz \tag{9.3}$$

where J is mass flux, dC/dz is the concentration gradient in direction z and the constant term D is the diffusion coefficient. In practice gas concentration is often expressed in terms of partial pressure (P) or fractional concentration (F): then for gas species y:

$$Py = Cy/\beta g \tag{9.4}$$

$$Fy = Cy/(\beta g.Ptot) \tag{9.5}$$

where $Ptot$ is total pressure and βg is the capacitance coefficient which is the quantity of substance in undiluted gas in the units mmol/(volume × pressure). Values for βg are given in Table 9.3 (page 272).

Equation 9.3 is now known as Fick's first law. His second law related to non-steady state conditions when the concentration varies with time. Under these circumstances the principle enshrined in the law is that of conservation of mass.

268

Within the air spaces of the lung, movement of gas takes place by convective ventilation and diffusion. Convective ventilation arises from the respiratory muscles acting on the thoracic cage and hence indirectly on the tissue of the lung; the resulting bulk flow of gas penetrates deeply into the lung and replaces gas present in the larger airways. The penetration and distribution of the gas are determined by many factors; these are considered in Chapters 7 and 8.

Gas molecules move by diffusion between the ventilated parts of the lung and the alveolar capillary membrane. Diffusion also contributes to gas mixing within terminal lung units and dispersion of gas in lung airways; these processes account for approximately 10% of the overall resistance to movement of gases by diffusion within the lung.

The dispersion of gas can be across or along the line of flow (respectively radial and axial dispersion). Its extent depends on whether the flow is laminar or turbulent and on the flow velocity, the airway diameter and the diffusion coefficient of the gas.

Under conditions of laminar flow, the flow velocity is greatest at the centre of the airway and decreases progressively towards the periphery. The profile is parabolic and the flow penetrates the resident gas which is to some extent displaced radially (Fig. 7.3, page 185). Radial diffusion occurs into the displaced gas which is then carried back along the wall of the airway creating a zone of nearly still air. This process was first investigated by Taylor so was described as Taylor diffusion but Piiper and Scheid have proposed *Taylor laminar dispersion* which is more nearly correct. Radial dispersion occurs particularly in medium sized airways corresponding to Weibel's generations 8–12. Axial dispersion is mainly a feature of small airways and their attendant air spaces. The interrelations between radial and axial dispersion have been investigated using gas mixtures containing helium and sulphur hexafluoride. During inspiration the helium diffuses radially to a greater extent than the sulphur hexafluoride so the concentration of the latter gas in the small airways is relatively increased. Differences in axial diffusion also occur. Thus for a given penetration by bulk flow the subsequent alveolar penetration by diffusion is much less for aerosol particles and greater for helium than for air. The difference in alveolar penetration between air and helium is increased when the diffusion pathway is lengthened by emphysema and a similar change might be expected in diffuse interstitial fibrosis; the consequences for gas exchange in these conditions are considered in Chapter 16. Reduced alveolar penetration also occurs when the environmental pressure and hence the gas density are increased by a deep dive.

Under quiet resting conditions entry of tidal gas into the alveoli is almost entirely by diffusion. During exercise there is entry by bulk flow because the tidal volume increases. Some convective ventilation also occurs because the uptake of oxygen normally exceeds the output of carbon dioxide (i.e. respiratory exchange ratio <1.0). This process is maximal during apnoea following replacement of nitrogen in the lung with oxygen. In these circumstances the tension of carbon dioxide in the alveolar gas rises to the level of the mixed venous blood; thereafter the output of CO_2 almost ceases and is replaced by the storage of carbon dioxide in the tissues. But the uptake of oxygen continues; this process reduces the pressure in the alveoli relative to the mouth and causes gas to flow into the alveoli. So long as the gas is 100% oxygen the flow is adequate to maintain the uptake of oxygen without the need for respiratory movements. However, the presence of an inert gas interrupts the flow because its molecules accumulate in the lung; the tension of oxygen then falls progressively to the level of the mixed venous blood when uptake ceases. Uptake of oxygen in the absence of respiratory movement is called *diffusion respiration*; it is of use in the management of patients receiving assisted ventilation because, after the lungs have been flushed with oxygen, the respirator may be disconnected for short periods without the patient becoming hypoxaemic.

Within alveoli the mixing of gases is effectively instantaneous. Hence there is no significant concentration gradient or boundary layer at the gas-to-tissue interface; such a layer, if present, would hinder gas exchange. Instead conditions are optimal for exchange of gas across the alveolar capillary membrane.

Transfer of gas across the alveolar capillary membrane

Cells which form the alveolar epithelium fit closely together (page 85). They are lined by lipoprotein molecules arranged in the form of a net which has water repellent properties. The net is coated by a layer of surface active material containing lecithin; this is responsible for the low surface tension of the boundary layer (page 95). The epithelial cells mainly comprise proteins and electrolytes in an aqueous medium which exchanges freely with the lung interstitial fluid, the interior of the endothelial cells of the alveolar capillaries and the blood plasma. The volume of intra- and extra-cellular fluid in pulmonary tissue (lung water) is normally in the range 0.2–0.25 l. Gases enter the alveolar capillary membrane either by dissolving in the lipid layer or by passing through gaps in the lipid to dissolve directly in the aqueous component of the epithelial cells. The process of solution is practically instantaneous. The quantity of gas which dissolves depends on its solubility; this varies for different gases from a very low value for helium and other insoluble gases to a relatively high value for diethyl ether, with most other gases intermediate (e.g. page 272). For a given partial pressure a soluble gas builds up a bigger surface concentration within the alveolar cell than one which is insoluble; other factors being equal its rate of diffusion in solution is greater in consequence.

Once a gas has dissolved in the tissue of the alveolar wall it diffuses rapidly through the aqueous medium of the alveolar capillary membrane into the blood plasma. The exchange is confined to that part of the membrane which is bounded on the one side by alveoli which are ventilated and on the other by capillaries and small arterioles which contain blood. Approximately half the alveolar membrane normally meets this requirement; the other half either adjoins the interstices between the alveolar capillaries or constitutes those alveoli which are devoid of either ventilation or perfusion. However, Staub and others have demonstrated that some oxygen enters the blood in the pulmonary arterioles; similarly blood may exchange gas with respiratory bronchioles as well as with alveoli. Thus the site of gas exchange is difficult to define anatomically. Instead it is convenient to define alveolar vessels as those which exchange gas with the air-containing spaces of the lung. For the vessels to make a useful contribution the blood should be flowing, but the blood which is stationary may sometimes contribute to gas exchange, for example during measurement of transfer factor by the single breath method (page 292).

The rapid flow of gas through the alveolar capillary membrane reflects the short distances which are involved ($0.15-0.5\,\mu m$). The flow is assisted by factors which promote circulation of lung tissue fluid; these include thermal gradients due to variations in metabolic activity within the cells and movement imparted by respiration and the pulsatile flow of blood. The hypothesis that a chemical mediator contributes to the exchange of gas, which was suggested by Bohr (page 7) and revived by Gurtner, has little evidence to support it.

The factors which contribute to gas exchange through the alveolar capillary membrane include the molecular weight of the gas (see Graham's law page 267), the solubility (indicated above) and the area and thickness of the membrane. Then for the whole lung:

$$Dx = k \cdot \frac{A}{d} \cdot \frac{sx}{\sqrt{MWx}} \qquad (9.6)$$

where Dx is the overall rate of transfer of gas x in vols per unit of pressure gradient per unit time, k is the diffusion coefficient of the gas in the alveolar membrane (cm^2 per unit time) A and d are respectively the area and thickness of the membrane (cm), sx is the solubility of gas x in the lung tissue (vols/vol per unit gas partial pressure) and MWx is molecular weight. Values of s for different gases are given in Table 9.3.

The quantity Dx in appropriate units is the diffusive conductance of the alveolar capillary membrane for substance x. It is also called the diffusing capacity or transfer factor (page 277).

The rapidity with which gas traverses the alveolar capillary membrane contributes to the time to achieve nearly complete equilibrium after a stepwise change in alveolar gas concentration. Thus from equation 9.6, for an inert gas which moves by diffusion and does not react chemically in the blood, the time to 99% equilibrium varies with the square root of the molecular weight for the gas in question. Based on equation 9.9 which is given below, the 99% time for halothane (molecular weight 197.5) is of the order of 0.04 s and for hydrogen (molecular weight 2) approximately 0.004 s; these times are in the ratio $\sqrt{(197.5/2)}$:1 which is effectively 10:1. The times to equilibrium for most other inert gases lie within these limits. The times are very short compared with the transit time for blood through alveolar capillaries which at rest is about

Table 9.3 Molecular weight (MW), capacitance coefficient (mmol l^{-1}kPa^{-1}) and solubility (vol STPD, vol^{-1}atm^{-1}) in water at 37°C (β and s respectively), oil-to-water partition coefficient and the rate of diffusion (from equation 9.6) relative to that of oxygen for some respired gases (for sources see references)

Substance	MW	β	s	Partition coefficient	Rate of diffusion
O_2	32	0.0105	0.0239	5.0	1.00
C_2H_2	26	0.3301	0.749	–	34.8
A	40	0.0114	0.0259	5.3	0.97
CO_2	44	0.2514	0.567	1.6	20.3
CO	28	0.0081	0.0184	–	0.83
He	4	0.0037	0.0085	1.7	1.01
Kr	85*	0.0198	0.0449	9.6	1.15
N_2	28	0.0054	0.0123	5.2	0.55
NO	30	0.0180	0.041	–	1.76
N_2O	44	0.1710	0.388	3.2	13.9
Xe	133*	0.0375	0.085	20.0†	1.75

* Radioactive isotope.
† Fat-to-blood partition coefficient 8.0−9.8:1.

In the gas phase the value for β for an ideal gas at 37°C is 0.388 mmol l^{-1} kPa^{-1}. In blood, for gases which combined chemically, β is determined mainly by the slope of the dissociation curve.

0.75 s. The times to equilibrium for oxygen and carbon dioxide which react chemically with blood are somewhat longer and are considered below.

Role of gas solubility in blood

The instantaneous flow rate of gas across the alveolar membrane is described by the Fick equation (equation 9.3) which can be written in the form:

$$dQ/dt = Dx\,[P_{A,x_t} - Pc,x_t] \qquad (9.7)$$

where dQ/dt is the quantity of gas transferred instantaneously at time t. Dx is the diffusive conductance and the term within the bracket is the instantaneous partial pressure gradient. The quantity of gas can also be expressed in terms of solubility and partial pressure. Hence:

$$dQ/dt = sx,\text{blood}.dPx/dt.10^{-2}\,Vc \qquad (9.8)$$

where sx, blood is the solubility of gas x in red cells and plasma (ml per 100 ml per unit of gas partial pressure), dPx/dt is the rate of change of capillary partial pressure with time and Vc is capillary blood volume (ml). Equations 9.6, 9.7 and 9.8 can be combined and integrated with respect to time, then:

$$Pxt = P_{A,x} + (P\bar{v},x - P_{A,x}).\exp - \left(\frac{100\,kA}{60\,dVc} \cdot \frac{sx\ \text{tissue}}{sx\ \text{blood}\ \sqrt{MWx}}\right) t \qquad (9.9)$$

where $P\bar{v},x$ is the partial pressure of gas x in mixed venous blood as it enters the alveolar capillaries at time zero and the other terms are as defined above. This derivation is due to Forster and the intermediate steps are given by Wagner. The equation describes the change with time in the partial pressure of a gas entering or leaving the alveolar capillaries as an exponential function of the driving pressure (i.e. the alveolar−mixed venous partial pressure difference). The exponent term includes the ratio of the solubilities of the gas in lung tissue and blood. It is independent of both the individual solubilities and the alveolar partial pressure provided that these are independent of each other. This is the case for most inert gases: the ratio of the solubilities (expressed in the same units) is close to unity except for gases which are very soluble in fat. For carbon dioxide which combines chemically with constituents of blood, the ratio of the solubilities is also nearly independent of the partial pressure because the whole blood dissociation curve is effectively linear (page 207). When solubility is expressed in the units ml per 100 ml per mmHg, sCO_2 is approximately 0.07. Wagner has expressed βCO_2 as the ratio of the arterio-venous CO_2 content difference to the corresponding difference in partial pressure; these differences are respectively approximately 4 ml/100 ml and 5 mmHg giving a value for βCO_2 of 0.8. Hence the solubility ratio is of the order of 1/11. Based on this figure and after allowing for molecular weight the estimated time to 99% equilibrium of carbon dioxide across the alveolar capillary membrane comes out at 0.21 s. For oxygen sO_2 is approximately 0.003. The value of βO_2 at rest obtained using the same procedure as for βCO_2 comes out at 0.083; this results in a value for the ratio $sO_2/\beta O_2$ of 1/27 which is approximately 40% of that for carbon dioxide but only about 4% of those for inert gases which have a ratio of unity. Assuming this ratio and if the dissociation curve were linear the time to 99% equilibrium of oxygen across the alveolar capillary membrane in a resting subject would be 0.43 s. However, Forster and Wagner point out that the equilibrium time for oxygen is reduced by the curvilinearity of the dissociation curve and its dependence on other factors in blood. Carbon dioxide does not share these advantages: its dissociation curve is effectively linear and the chemical re-action with blood has several components some of which are relatively slow. Thus despite the high diffusivity of the carbon dioxide in solution the time to equilibrium across the alveolar capillary membrane exceeds that for oxygen. The process of transfer is described below.

Transfer of gas across the alveolar capillary membrane

Transfer involving chemical reaction with blood

Transfer of gases by diffusion alone severely limits the volume of tissue which can be supplied and the quantity of gas which can be transferred. The limitation was eased some 450 million years ago by the evolution of haemoglobin and the development of a system for its circulation round the body. In resting man the transfer of oxygen into the blood in the alveolar capillaries is confined to an aliquot of some 70 ml which is replaced with each contraction of the heart; the average residence time is 0.75 s. On exercise the volume of blood is greater but its residence time is less.

The transfer from plasma to erythrocytes occurs by diffusion. Gas tension gradients in the plasma are reduced by convective mixing due to respiratory movements and the pulsatile flow of blood.

Penetration of the red cell membrane is assisted by its large surface area and by migration of haemoglobin molecules between the surface and interior of the cells; the evidence for this facilitated diffusion is reviewed by Kreuzer. In addition, the corpuscles change their shape as they traverse the capillaries. This stirs the contents of the cells and causes changes in pressure which lead to movement of water and hence of gases in solution between the cells and plasma. By these means the penetration of the red cell membranes by gas molecules takes place rapidly and the cell contents are mixed effectively.

Gases combine chemically with haemoglobin at finite rates. The reactions are reversible so may be said to be opposed by back reactions which also have specific reaction rates. The stages of the reactions have been studied in particular by Roughton and his colleagues including Sirs. The rates of the forward reactions for oxygen, carbon monoxide and nitric oxide have been determined *in vitro* for both haemoglobin in solution (Table 10.5, page 318) and for intact red blood corpuscles; in the SI system the rates are expressed as conductances, in the units mmol min^{-1} per l of blood per kPa of plasma tension. The overall rate is then the product of the reaction rate, the driving pressure (i.e. the partial pressure difference) and the volume of blood in the alveolar capillaries. Variation in this quantity or in the concentration of haemoglobin will affect the rates of uptake of oxygen, carbon monoxide and possibly nitric oxide. The reaction rate varies with the temperature and acidity of the blood (page 281); for carbon monoxide it is also a function of the tension of oxygen in the plasma which therefore affects the rate at which carbon monoxide displaces oxygen and combines with haemoglobin (page 293). Use is made of the interaction between oxygen, carbon monoxide and haemoglobin in order to estimate the diffusing capacity of the alveolar capillary membrane and the volume of blood in the alveolar capillaries. The method is outlined on page 313.

Blood which has been refurbished in the alveolar capillaries is conveyed to the tissue capillaries by the circulation. It is replaced by mixed venous blood at a rate which is a function of the cardiac output; the latter influences the gaseous composition of the blood and hence the back tension exerted by gas in the alveolar capillaries. At the beginning of the capillary the back tension is that in mixed venous blood; for oxygen the mixed venous tension varies directly with cardiac output and inversely with metabolic rate. The cardiac output also influences the plasma back tension along the length of the capillary by determining the rate at which the plasma is replaced. Thus even in an ideal lung the rate of gas exchange is determined by a number of factors.

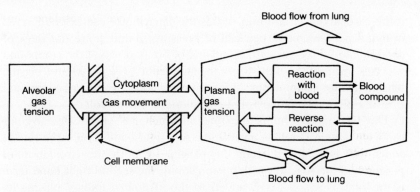

Fig. 9.2 Schematic representation of the processes which determine the tension of gases in the alveolar capillary plasma; for details see text.

Synthesis of factors affecting transfer of gas across the alveolar capillary membrane

When a unit of blood plasma enters a pulmonary capillary a very rapid movement of gas occurs across the alveolar membrane. In the case of an inert gas entering the plasma from the alveoli the plasma tension rises to the level of the alveoli within about 20 ms and thereafter remains virtually constant. The overall rate of uptake is then determined by the diffusion gradient, the solubility and the rate of blood flow. For a gas which combines with haemoglobin a similar initial rise in the plasma tension occurs; however, in the case of oxygen the gas tension does not immediately reach the level of the alveoli. Instead, within about 10 ms, a dynamic equilibrium is established in which the rate at which the gas traverses the alveolar membrane is balanced by the rate at which it combines with blood. The compound which is formed then tends to dissociate and this back reaction raises the plasma gas tension. The extent of the back reaction is proportional to the concentration of the compound, which increases during the transit of the blood along the capillary. Consequently the tension of oxygen in plasma rises progressively up to an equilibrium value which is usually attained within about 0.3 s. The factors which contribute to the transfer of gas are illustrated diagrammatically in Fig. 9.2. For a single chamber lung the overall rate may be described by an equation, developed by Meade, in which at any point in time:

$$Dm(P_A - P\bar{c}) = P\bar{c}(\beta\dot{Q} + \theta Vc) - (\phi CVc + P\bar{v}\beta\dot{Q}) \; \text{mmol min}^{-1}$$
$$(9.10)$$

where Dm is diffusing capacity of the alveolar capillary membrane in mmol min^{-1} per kPa of diffusion gradient;* P_A, $P\bar{c}$ and $P\bar{v}$ are respectively the tensions in kPa of gas in the alveoli, the alveolar capillary plasma and the mixed venous blood entering the alveolar capillaries; $\dot{Q}$

---

* The rate of transfer of gas substance may also be expressed in ml STPD min^{-1} mmHg^{-1} when the corresponding unit of volume is the ml and the capacitance coefficient is replaced by $s/760$ where s is the Bunsen solubility coefficient (Table 9.3).

is the cardiac output in l min^{-1}; β is the capacitance coefficient at 37°C in mmol per l of blood per kPa of pressure; θ and ϕ are the rates of combination of the gas with blood and of break-down of the compound which is formed; the units for θ are mmol min^{-1}l^{-1} per kPa of plasma tension and for ϕ mmol min^{-1}l^{-1} per unit of concentration of compound C in the blood; Vc is the volume of blood in the alveolar capillaries in l. The left hand term is the rate at which gas enters the alveolar capillary plasma from the alveoli; the first right hand term is the rate at which gas is removed from the plasma by both the circulation of plasma and the reaction with haemoglobin; the second right hand term is the rate at which gas is added to the alveolar capillary plasma by both the breakdown of the compound with haemoglobin and the entry of more gas in solution in the mixed venous plasma. The mean plasma tension cannot be measured directly; it can, however, be described in terms of the other variables.

It can be seen that the transfer of gas from the alveoli to the haemoglobin in the alveolar capillaries entails overcoming a series of hurdles or resistances. First, that imposed by the alveolar capillary membrane, next, the resistances imposed by diffusion within the blood and by the relatively slow combination of the gas with haemoglobin and lastly, the resistance set up by the back pressure of gas dissolved in the plasma. The latter comes both from gas which has passed through the membrane and from that evolved in the red cells by breakdown of the haemoglobin compound. These resistances act one after another and therefore summate, in series. By analogy with electric current, resistance is given by pressure (voltage) divided by flow rate (current) so resistance is equal to pressure per unit of flow rate. The diffusing capacity of the alveolar capillary membrane (Dm) is flow rate per unit of pressure, so that $1/Dm$ has the dimensions of resistance. Similarly when blood is flowing $\beta\dot{Q}$ is measured in terms of flow rate per unit of pressure, and so is θVc. The resistances set up by these two factors are $1/\beta\dot{Q}$ and $1/\theta Vc$ respectively. The resistance $1/Dm$ is interposed between the alveoli and the far side of the alveolar membrane. The other two resistances act between the membrane and the red cell, both maintaining a raised plasma tension of gas. They, therefore, act simultaneously and, as a first approximation, can be added together as $1/\theta\dot{Q} + \beta Vc$. The uptake of gas from the lung as a whole (i.e. flow rate per unit of pressure or Tl) is limited by the total resistance which is governed by the sum of the three individual resistances. Thus:

$$\frac{1}{Tl} = \frac{1}{Dm} + \frac{1}{\beta\dot{Q} + \theta Vc} \tag{9.11}$$

where Tl is the conductance or transfer factor of the lung for carbon monoxide.*

* Piiper and Scheid have shown that the corresponding exponential equation describing the total conductance across the alveolar capillary membrane is given by:

$$G = \dot{Q}\beta(1 - e^{-Tl/\dot{Q}\beta})$$

where G is conductance and the other terms are as defined in the text.

The overall rate of transfer of gas from alveoli to blood is the product of the transfer factor and the alveolar tension in excess of the back tension, hence from equation 9.11:

$$\text{Rate of transfer of gas from alveoli to blood} = \cfrac{1}{\cfrac{1}{Dm} + \cfrac{1}{\beta \dot{Q} + \theta Vc}} \times \left[\text{alveolar tension} - \text{back tension} \right] \quad (9.12)$$

The back tension is considered below. The second right hand term is the effective gas-pressure gradient (or transfer gradient) between the alveolar gas and the capillary blood; for oxygen it is also called the diffusion gradient but this usage is not strictly correct since the gradient is the resultant of several processes and is not solely due to diffusion. For carbon monoxide the transfer gradient is sometimes called the effective alveolar tension or the alveolar drive.

It should be noted that the term transfer factor is a general one, so to avoid ambiguity it may be necessary to indicate the substance and the beginning and ends of its transfer, e.g. $Tl,co(al \rightarrow c)$ where al and c refer respectively to the alveolar gas and the mean capillary blood. Alternative terms are diffusing capacity and diffusive conductance (see page 271). For gases which do not combine with haemoglobin θ is zero and Dm is large relative to $\beta \dot{Q}$; $1/Dm$ is then very small relative to $1/\beta \dot{Q}$ and may as a first approximation be neglected. The transfer factor then simplifies to $Tl = \beta \dot{Q}$. The appropriate back tension for the calculation of the effective alveolar tension in these circumstances is the tension of gas in the mixed venous blood entering the alveolar capillaries. These quantities may be substituted in equation 9.12 which then, after rearrangement, becomes the Fick equation for determining the cardiac output (page 239).

For carbon monoxide, nitric oxide and, to a lesser extent, for oxygen the rate at which the gas leaves the alveolar capillary plasma by combining with haemoglobin is fast relative to the rate at which it is removed by dissolving in circulating blood. Under these circumstances the term $\beta \dot{Q}$ is small compared with the term θVc and may as a first approximation be neglected. Roughton and Forster have pointed out that the relationship for the transfer factor therefore simplifies to:

$$\frac{1}{Tl} = \frac{1}{Dm} + \frac{1}{\theta Vc} \quad (9.13)$$

The appropriate back tension for calculating the rates of uptake of oxygen or carbon monoxide from alveolar gas by use of equation 9.12 is the tension exerted by the compound with haemoglobin. The value of the back tension at the point where the blood enters the alveolar capillary is the tension in mixed venous blood. The extent to which the back tension rises along the length of the capillary depends on the speed of the reaction with haemoglobin and the extent of dissociation of the compound which is formed. These features differ as between oxygen, carbon monoxide and nitric oxide. They are discussed below and are summarised in Table 9.4.

Table 9.4 Principal factors which limit the transfer of gases across the alveolar capillary membrane. Numerical values are given in Table 10.5 (page 318)

	Anatomical dimensions (Dm)	Diffusion within blood	Rate of reaction with haemoglobin (θVc)	Rate of back reaction (ϕCVc)
Oxygen	√	(√)	(√)	√
Carbon monoxide	√	(√)	√	—
Nitric oxide	√	(√)	—	—

The transfer factor of the lung for oxygen or carbon monoxide is also called the diffusing capacity. The latter term was introduced at a time when the rate of combination of gas with haemoglobin was believed to be practically instantaneous; in such circumstances the reaction rate θ would be very large, hence the term $1/(\beta \dot{Q} + \theta Vc)$ in equation 9.11 would be so small that it could be neglected; the diffusing capacity of the lung would then be equal to Dm which is the diffusing capacity of the alveolar capillary membrane. In practice the term is of material magnitude for oxygen on account of the back tension which develops, and for carbon monoxide on account of the slower reaction time for combination with haemoglobin. Thus for these gases the capacitance coefficient can be described correctly as a transfer factor but not as a diffusing capacity. In the case of nitric oxide the reaction with haemoglobin is rapid, approximately 280 times that for carbon monoxide, and the back reaction is extremely slow. However, Borland has found that the rate of transfer is influenced by haemoglobin concentration. Thus whilst the diffusing capacity for nitric oxide mainly reflects the diffusing characteristics of the lung membrane the diffusion of the gas from the plasma to the interior of the red cells also contributes significantly to the rate of gas exchange.

Gas exchange for oxygen

Reaction of oxygen with blood

Oxyhaemoglobin dissociation curve. The solubility or capacitance coefficient for oxygen in blood plasma is similar to that for water at 37°C; this is approximately $0.01 \, \mathrm{mmol \, l^{-1} \, kPa^{-1}}$ (Table 9.3), hence for a subject breathing air the quantity of oxygen dissolved in arterial blood is approximately $0.13 \, \mathrm{mmol \, l^{-1}}$ (0.3 ml per 100 ml). When breathing 100% oxygen the concentration increases to approximately $0.9 \, \mathrm{mmol \, l^{-1}}$ (2.0 ml per 100 ml). Human blood also carries up to 1.39 ml of oxygen in combination with each gram of haemoglobin. The normal concentration of haemoglobin monomer in blood and the normal capacity of blood for oxygen are both $9 \, \mathrm{mmol \, l^{-1}}$, equivalent to 14.6 g of haemoglobin and 20 ml of oxygen per 100 ml of blood.

Molecules of oxygen react with haemoglobin near the surface and in the interior of the red blood corpuscles. The reaction occurs in stages and is influenced by many components of the haemoglobin molecule. However, the details are not fully understood. The outcome is described by the oxygen haemoglobin equilibrium or dissociation curve (Fig. 9.3). The middle part of the curve can be represented by an empirical equation due to A.V. Hill:

$$\log y(1 - y) = \log k + n(\log Po_2) \tag{9.14}$$

where y is the fractional saturation of haemoglobin with oxygen, k is the dissociation constant and the exponent n is normally in the range 2.6–3.0. The equation can be used to obtain the $P_{50}o_2$ (page 281). Adair proposed that the reaction be treated mathematically as if it comprised four over-lapping stages each with its own rate of forward and back reaction and intermediate compounds:

$$Hb_4 + O_2 \rightleftharpoons Hb_4O_2 \tag{1}$$

$$Hb_4O_2 + O_2 \rightleftharpoons Hb_4O_4 \tag{2}$$

$$Hb_4O_4 + O_2 \rightleftharpoons Hb_4O_6 \tag{3}$$

$$Hb_4O_6 + O_2 \rightleftharpoons Hb_4O_8 \tag{4}$$

The equilibrium constants for the reactions are the ratios of the individual constants for the forward and backward reactions. Under physiological conditions the speed of the forward reactions has been shown to increase by a factor of 500 between the first and fourth stages. The values for the intermediate stages have been estimated but not measured directly. For whole blood the equilibrium positions of the reactions are described by the dissociation curve (Fig. 9.3 and Table 9.5); at its lower and upper ends the slope of the curve is due to reactions 1 and 4 respectively whilst in the middle it is due mainly to reactions 2 and 3. The flat top both tends to stabilise the quantity of oxygen in the arterial blood (cf. page 285) and contributes to the tension of oxygen in blood leaving the alveolar capillaries being nearly equal to that in the alveolar gas; how this is achieved is discussed below. The steep middle part of the curve ensures that a large proportion of the oxygen which is carried by the blood is delivered to the tissues at a relatively high tension. This attribute of haemoglobin is illustrated in the figure where the uptake of oxygen by haemoglobin is represented as taking place in the lung over a range of tensions of oxygen from 13.3 kPa (100 mmHg), as occurs when breathing air, to 6 kPa (45 mmHg) at an altitude of 3300 m equivalent to a subject breathing oxygen at a fractional concentration of 0.135 (13.5% O_2 in N_2); the corresponding saturations of haemoglobin with oxygen are 97% and 80%.

Unloading of oxygen occurs in the tissue capillaries at saturations which, near the venous ends of the capillaries, are less than those in the arterial blood by approximately 25% at rest and 50% during

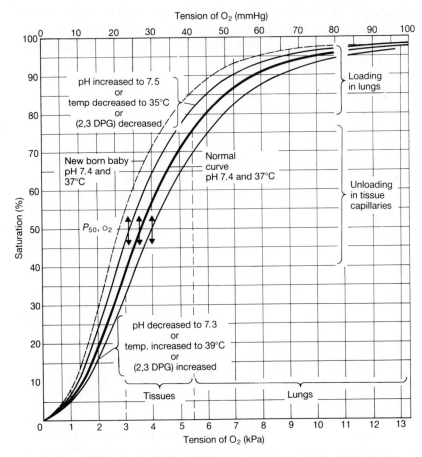

Fig. 9.3 Dissociation curves for oxyhaemoglobin compiled from data in the literature. The broad line is for pH 7.4 and 37°C (Table 9.5); the narrow lines show the effects of a change in pH or in body temperature.* The interrupted line is for a newborn baby. The brackets indicate the approximate saturations and tensions at which haemoglobin loads up with oxygen in the lung and unloads in the tissue capillaries. The tension at which haemoglobin takes up oxygen is reduced when the subject is breathing a hypoxic gas mixture or the lungs are underventilated. The tension in the tissue capillaries is reduced by a low cardiac output such as occurs in patients with restrictive cardiac disease; low values also obtain during strenuous exercise.

* The following relationships were used in the construction of the curves:

$$\log_{10}[Po_2, 37°C/Po_2, t°C] = 0.024\ (37 - t)$$

$$\log_{10}[Po_2, pH\ 7.4/Po_2, pHa] = -0.48\ (7.4 - a)$$

The curve for a newborn baby at pH 7.4 resembles that of an adult at pH 7.6. $P_{50}O_2$ is the tension of oxygen at which haemoglobin is 50% saturated with oxygen. (Source: Severinghaus JW. *J Appl Physiol* 1966; **21**: 1108–1116.)

moderate exercise. Due to the shape of the dissociation curve the corresponding tensions of oxygen are in the range 5.3–2.9 kPa (40–22 mmHg). Transport of oxygen is assisted by differences between the lungs and peripheral tissues with respect to the tension of carbon dioxide (*Bohr effect*), pH and temperature. In the tissues the pH is relatively low on account of production of carbon dioxide and, during exercise, of lactic acid; the temperature is relatively high as a result of metabolism. Both these changes shift the dissociation curve to the right; this has the effect of liberating oxygen from haemoglobin in the tissue capillaries. In the lung the temperature is lower and the pH is higher. These changes displace the dissociation curve to the left; they have the converse effect of increasing the uptake of oxygen by the blood at the tension which obtains in the alveoli.

Chemical reaction. The binding of oxygen to haemoglobin is influenced by the presence within the red cells of relatively large amounts of organic phosphate compounds including 2,3-diphosphoglycerate (2,3-DPG). This substance combines with haemoglobin, particularly in the reduced form, and by doing so weakens the attachment of haemoglobin for oxygen; mainly on this account the dissociation curve in its lower part is displaced to the right by an amount which is proportional to the concentration present. 2,3-DPG is absent from purified haemoglobin solution and is present in reduced amounts in combination with fetal haemoglobin; these features lead to the dissociation curve being displaced to the left. The displacement is conveniently described in terms of the oxygen tension at which the haemoglobin is 50% saturated with oxygen ($P_{50}O_2$). The $P_{50}O_2$ can be obtained using equation 9.14 and is normally approximately 3.6 kPa (27 mmHg) (Table 9.5); it is a function of the tension of carbon dioxide, the concentrations of hydrogen ions, chlorine ions, 2,3-diphosphoglycerate and the prevailing temperature.

Table 9.5 Relationship of oxygen tension to saturation for normal blood at pH 7.4 and temperature 37°C; the values were compiled by Severinghaus from data in the literature

Saturation HbO$_2$ (%)	Oxygen tension		Saturation HbO$_2$ (%)	Oxygen tension	
	kPa	mmHg		kPa	mmHg
1	0.25	1.9	85	6.6	49.8
2	0.45	3.4	90	7.7	57.8
4	0.76	5.7	91	8.0	60.0
6	1.0	7.5	92	8.4	62.7
10	1.4	10.3	93	8.8	65.7
15	1.7	13.1	94	9.3	69.4
20	2.1	15.4	95	9.9	74.2
25	2.3	17.3	95.5	10.3	77.3
30	2.6	19.2	96	10.8	81.0
35	2.8	21.0	96.5	11.5	86.0
40	3.0	22.8	97	12.2	91.6
45	3.3	24.6	97.5	13.3	99.6
50	3.55	26.6	98	14.8	111
55	3.8	28.7	98.5	17.2	129
60	4.2	31.2	99	21.2	159
65	4.5	34.0	99.5	30.0	225
70	4.9	36.9	99.8	46.7	350
75	5.4	40.4	99.9	66.7	500
80	5.9	44.5	99.95	93.3	700

The effects of the chemical variables are interrelated because they combine at a limited number of locations on the haemoglobin molecule.

The salt bridge between the imidazole group of β146 histidine and β94 aspartine is susceptible to pH changes in the physiological range and is believed to account for approximately half the normal Bohr effect. Half the remainder is due to oxygen-linked binding of chloride ions; amongst several effects this linkage alters the ionisation at the NH_2-terminal α amino group on the α chain of the haemoglobin molecule. The corresponding terminal on the β chain of the molecule appears to be the main site of incorporation of carbon dioxide to form carbamic acid; this site also binds 2,3-DPG which then diminishes the carbamino reaction. The relationships between these variables have been investigated by Rossie-Bernardi and by Kilmartin amongst others.

2,3-Diphosphoglycerate is formed from 1,3-diphosphoglycerate which is an intermediary in the metabolism of glucose. Thus the reaction of 2,3-DPG with haemoglobin provides a means whereby the rate of metabolism, the supply of substrate and the level of tissue oxygenation can influence the extent to which oxygen is released from haemoglobin in the tissue capillaries. The metabolic pathway is illustrated by the central column in Table 9.6. The equilibrium between 1,3- and 2,3-DPG is influenced by a number of factors all of which contribute to the red cell concentration of the latter substance. Circumstances in which

Table 9.6 Contribution of 2,3-diphosphoglycerate to shape of haemoglobin dissociation curve as described by $P_{50}O_2$

[2,3-DPG] reduced	Normal pathway	[2,3-DPG] increased
	Glucose	Increased metabolic rate
Hexokinase deficiency	↓	Pyruvatekinase deficiency
	1,3-Diphosphoglycerate	
DPG mutase deficiency	↑	
Increased pyruvatekinase activity		
Thyroxine deficiency		Thyroxine excess
Ageing and storage of red cells, acidosis	2,3-Diphosphoglycerate (DPG)	High altitude, alkalosis, right to left shunt, heart failure
Fetal Hb / Hb Milwaukee	$\begin{bmatrix} \text{Normal concentration} \\ \approx 4\,\text{mmol}\,l^{-1}\,\text{RBC} \end{bmatrix}$	Hb Chesapeake
Less Hb DPG complex	Combines with haemoglobin	More Hb DPG complex
$P_{50}O_2$ reduced	$P_{50}O_2 \simeq 3.6\,\text{kPa}\ (27\,\text{mmHg})$	$P_{50}O_2$ increased

the level is altered are indicated in the table. When the haemoglobin is normal the $P_{50}O_2$ varies proportionately. However, with some haemo-globin variants the binding of 2,3-DPG is abnormal and the $P_{50}O_2$ is altered in consequence. The $P_{50}O_2$ also declines with age but it is not known why. The decline influences the level of tissue oxygenation and hence performance during exercise. An example is given by Oski and his colleagues.

Reaction rate. The rate of combination of oxygen dissolved in plasma with intra-corpuscular haemoglobin is determined by a number of factors; the principal ones have been described in this chapter. They include (a) the permeability of the red cell membrane to oxygen and the rates of movement of molecules of oxygen and haemoglobin within the red cells, (b) the rates of chemical combination of oxygen with both reduced haemoglobin and the intermediary compounds of oxy-haemoglobin, (c) the rate of change of pH caused by the loss of carbon dioxide from the blood in the alveolar capillaries. The latter depends on the speed of dissociation of carbamino-haemoglobin and on the rate at which bicarbonate ions from the plasma pass into the red cells and dissociate under the influence of carbonic anhydrase. The overall rate at which oxygen reacts with haemoglobin is a function of these three groups of variables and their combined effect is not known precisely. Such measurements as have been made suggest that the rate of combi-nation of oxygen with haemoglobin is slow enough to limit the rate of transfer of oxygen when conditions for gas exchange are unfavourable. In addition the rate approaches zero when the haemoglobin is fully saturated with oxygen.

The transfer gradient for oxygen; role of the dissociation curve

The transfer gradient for oxygen at any point along an alveolar capillary is the difference in tension of oxygen between alveolar gas and plasma in equilibrium with red cells at that point, i.e.:

$$\text{transfer gradient for oxygen} = (P_{A,O_2} - P_{c,O_2}) \qquad (9.15)$$

where P_{A,O_2} and P_{c,O_2} are respectively the alveolar and instantaneous capillary plasma tensions of oxygen. Neither term is constant. The tension of oxygen in alveolar gas varies with ventilation minute volume (Fig. 9.1) and it is higher during inspiration than expiration, (Fig. 11.9, page 354). It is increased by breathing oxygen and is reduced by breathing gas in which the tension of oxygen is subnormal. The tension of oxygen in plasma in the alveolar capillaries also varies and is lowest at the point where gas exchange begins; the tension is then that in the mixed venous blood. It is particularly low during exercise (see Chapter 13) or when cardiac output is reduced by shock or cardiac disease. The mixed venous plasma tension is relatively high if the cardiac output is increased without a coincident increase in the metabolism, for example at high altitude, with an arteriovenous anastomosis or with cutaneous vasodilatation due to a warm environment. The plasma tension rises along the length of the alveolar capillary on account of the back reaction leading to the dissociation of oxyhaemoglobin (page 279). Normally the tension in blood as it leaves the capillary is equal to that in the alveolar gas. By contrast when the inspired oxygen tension is reduced an equilibrium across the membrane is probably not attained; instead the end-capillary tension is less than that in the alveoli. This end-capillary gradient is influenced by the shape of the dissociation curve and is discussed below. An increased end-capillary gradient can also occur during normoxia, but only when the transfer factor for oxygen is reduced (e.g. Fig. 9.4). In both circumstances the end-capillary gradient is larger during exercise. This is because the greater cardiac output leads to a more rapid flow of blood through the lungs; hence the time available for the exchange of gas (residence time) is reduced. In addition, there is a reduced O_2 tension in plasma entering the pulmonary capillaries during exercise, and this increases the quantity of oxygen which should be transferred.

The normal time course for exchange of oxygen along an alveolar capillary, when air is breathed at sea level, is illustrated in Fig. 9.4. Here the tension of oxygen in alveolar gas is assumed to be 13.3 kPa (100 mmHg) and the saturation of oxygen in mixed venous blood 70% for which the corresponding oxygen tension at pH 7.4 is 4.9 kPa

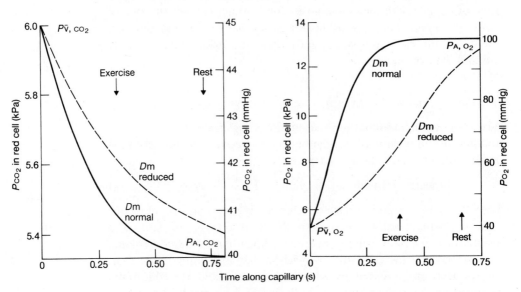

Fig. 9.4 Time course for the exchange of carbon dioxide and oxygen across the alveolar capillary membrane during breathing air. The curves were computed using the digital subroutines of Kelman for describing the O_2 and CO_2 dissociation curves. The values assumed for Dm,o_2 were 13.3 and 3.3 mmol min^{-1} kPa^{-1} (40 and 10 ml min^{-1} mmHg^{-1}); Dm,co_2 was 20 times Dm,o_2. The times when the blood was assumed to leave the capillary is indicated by the arrows. When both Dm is reduced and the transit time is shortened by exercise the blood is incompletely oxygenated; the associated tendency towards hypercapnia is usually corrected or reversed by an increase in ventilation. (Source: Wagner PD, West JB *J Appl Physiol* 1972; **33**: 62–71.)

(37 mmHg) (Fig. 9.3). The gradient for oxygen at the beginning of the alveolar capillary is then 8.4 kPa (i.e. 13.3−4.9) or 63 mmHg. This considerable gradient leads to a large flow of oxygen by diffusion from the alveolar gas into the plasma entering the alveolar capillaries. The tension of oxygen in the plasma and the saturation of haemoglobin with oxygen rise and the tension of oxygen in the alveolar gas diminishes in consequence. These changes reduce the transfer gradient and hence the rate of flow of oxygen. But exchange of gas is now taking place on the flat part of the dissociation curve where the addition of a small volume of oxygen is sufficient to cause a large rise in the tension of oxygen in the blood. The volume of gas which must be transferred to attain equilibrium is now within the capacity for diffusion of the membrane and the rate of reaction with haemoglobin; on this account, in healthy subjects breathing air at sea level, the transfer gradient at the point where the blood leaves the alveolar capillaries is of negligible proportions. The intermediate points can be calculated by the procedure of Bohr (page 7).

The normal situation can be contrasted with that when the alveolar oxygen tension is reduced for example by ascent to an altitude of 3500 m or, at sea level, by breathing oxygen at a fractional concentration of 0.135. Under these circumstances the alveolar oxygen tension is 6.9 kPa (52 mmHg). The saturation of oxygen in the mixed venous blood is now about 60% for which the corresponding tension, at a pH of 7.4, is 4.1 kPa (31 mmHg). The transfer gradient for oxygen at the beginning of the alveolar capillary is now 2.8 kPa (21 mmHg) or approximately one-third of that obtained during breathing air at sea level. Consequently, the rate at which oxygen passes by diffusion from the alveolar gas into the blood entering the alveolar capillaries is much less and the rate of reaction with haemoglobin is also slower. In addition, at the end of the capillary, the exchange of oxygen is still taking place on the steep linear part of the dissociation curve; the rate of transfer of oxygen which is necessary for the attainment of gaseous equilibrium then exceeds both the rate at which the oxygen can react with haemoglobin and the capacity for diffusion of the membrane. On this account, during hypoxia the tension of oxygen in the blood leaving the alveolar capillaries is lower than that in alveolar gas; the difference is small at rest but increases during exercise when it may exceed 1.3 kPa (10 mmHg) (page 284). A similarly increased transfer gradient can occur when the gas exchanging function of the lung is impaired by emphysema or diffuse interstitial fibrosis (Chapter 16).

Role of blood flow. The rate of pulmonary blood flow influences the transfer factor via its effect on the time for which blood is resident in the gas-exchanging vessels of the lung. The residence time is also called transit time but the latter term implies a continuous flow whereas in practice the flow is pulsatile in synchrony with cardiac systole. The volume of blood in the gas exchanging vessels approximates to the stroke volume. If the two volumes are equal the blood in the gas-exchanging vessels is replaced with each heart beat and is stationary during part of the time that gas exchange is taking place. This is more likely at rest than when the cardiac output is increased by exercise or other factors. The flow of blood contributes to gas transfer by promoting mixing within alveolar cell cytoplasm and alveolar capillary plasma and red cells. These beneficial consequences of an increase in blood flow partially offset the deleterious effect on gas exchange of the reduction in residence time which occurs concurrently. An increase in blood flow also increases the diameter and number of alveolar capillaries which are perfused; these changes improve the distribution of capillary blood flow ($\dot{Q}c$) with respect to the alveolar surface available for the exchange of gas, so the degree of $Tl/\dot{Q}c$ inequality is reduced. Such inequality is material at rest, when the transfer factor is less than half its maximal value. The transfer factor increases on exercise when the degree of $Tl/\dot{Q}c$ inequality diminishes. This aspect has been studied in particular by Hyde and others. As well as its effects on transfer factor a change in blood flow influences gas exchange via its effect on the mixed venous oxygen tension and hence on the transfer gradient and the bulk flow of oxygen into individual alveolar capillaries. A reduced cardiac output increases the gradient but it also calls for a higher alveolar ventilation in order to achieve gaseous equilibrium. An increased cardiac output relative to the metabolic rate has the converse beneficial effect. The two situations contribute to gas exchange respectively in shock (page 605) and at high altitude (page 395).

Summary. Gas exchange for oxygen is determined by the factors which influence both the transfer gradient and the transfer factor for oxygen. The former include the alveolar ventilation, the pulmonary bloodflow and the metabolic rate. The transfer factor is determined by the diffusion characteristics of the alveolar membrane (including the distributions of blood flow with respect to alveolar surface), the rates of association and dissociation of oxygen with intra-corpuscular haemoglobin (page 281), and the removal by the circulation of the oxygenated blood. The relationships between these factors is indicated in equation 9.12 and the present section. They have the effect that exchange of oxygen across the alveolar capillary membrane has normally ceased before the red cells reach the venous end of the pulmonary capillary. The transfer can be incomplete during strenuous exercise, at high altitude and as a result of diseases affecting the lung parenchyma; however, even in these adverse circumstances compensatory mechanisms, including an increase in ventilation, minimise the ill-effects. The process of transfer can be overwhelmed by pulmonary oedema and in this circumstance gas exchange will be seriously compromised. The measurement of transfer factor for oxygen is discussed on page 319.

Gas exchange for carbon dioxide

Carbon dioxide is normally present in arterial blood in a concentration of approximately $22\,\mathrm{mmol}\,\mathrm{l}^{-1}$ ($50\,\mathrm{ml}$ per $100\,\mathrm{ml}$); it exerts a tension of $5.3\,\mathrm{kPa}$ ($40\,\mathrm{mmHg}$). The content and tension in mixed venous blood are respectively approximately $24\,\mathrm{mmol}\,\mathrm{l}^{-1}$ ($54\,\mathrm{ml}$ per $100\,\mathrm{ml}$) and $6.1\,\mathrm{kPa}$ ($46\,\mathrm{mmHg}$). The carbon dioxide is transported by the blood in a number of forms; these include carbon dioxide in solution, carbamino-haemoglobin, and bicarbonate which is buffered by blood proteins including the haemoglobin and the plasma proteins. In resting subjects these forms account, respectively, for about 5%, 5% and 90% of the total quantity of carbon dioxide in the blood. There is also some carbon dioxide bound as carbamate to plasma proteins but this appears not to be of physiological significance. The underlying chemical reactions have been extensively investigated by Roughton and his many colleagues including Rossi-Bernardi, Perrella and Kilmartin, also Kloche and others. The reactions are summarised in Fig. 9.5 and in the following account. The relationships between the tension of carbon dioxide and the concentrations of bicarbonate and of hydrogen ions in blood are considered in Chapter 15.

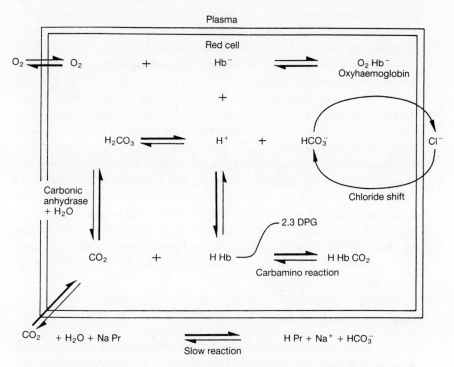

Fig. 9.5 Role of haemoglobin in the transport of carbon dioxide. The directions of the reactions are indicated for the tissue capillaries by broad arrows and for the alveolar capillaries by narrow arrows. In the tissue capillaries the oxygen is liberated from oxyhaemoglobin (O_2Hb^-) which reverts to the ionic form Hb^-; these ions are reduced to haemoglobin (HHb) by hydrogen ions (H^+) which are formed by dissociation of carbonic acid (H_2CO_3). The reduced haemoglobin accepts carbon dioxide to form carbamino-haemoglobin; it also combines with 2,3-DPG which reduces the extent of the carbamino reaction. In the tissues the bicarbonate in the plasma exchanges with the extra-cellular fluid.

Carbonic anhydrase and buffer systems

Carbon dioxide is formed in the tissues and thence passes rapidly by diffusion into the plasma in the tissue capillaries. Here some of the gas hydrates slowly to form carbonic acid; this dissociates into bicarbonate ions and hydrogen ions which displace sodium from combination with phosphate and protein in the plasma. The hydration reaction is mediated via a low energy form of the zinc-containing enzyme carbonic anhydrase (carbonic anhydrase I) which is present in the capillary endothelium. However, most of the dissolved carbon dioxide passes from the plasma into the red cells; here the greater part is hydrated through the mediation of the high energy form of carbonic anhydrase (carbonic anhydrase II).

In the red cells the hydration of carbon dioxide to form carbonic acid is the start of a series of reactions and migrations of ions of which some are shown in Fig. 9.5. The carbonic acid dissociates into bicarbonate ions and hydrogen ions; the hydrogen ions displace potassium ions from combination with haemoglobin in the interior of the red cell. This process is assisted by the dissociation of oxyhaemoglobin into oxygen, which passes into the tissues, and haemoglobin which takes up hydrogen ions more readily in its reduced than in its oxidised form. Subsequently the bicarbonate ions diffuse out of the red cells, where their concentration is high, into the plasma and the extra-cellular fluid where their concentration is lower; the participation of the extra-cellular fluid leads to the dissociation curve for carbon dioxide in the body, i.e. the *in vivo* dissociation curve, differing from that in the blood. This has been investigated by Michel amongst others. The bicarbonate ions which leave the red cells are replaced by chloride ions which are attracted into the red cells from the plasma by changes in electrical potential caused by the movement of bicarbonate. This exchange is called the chloride shift, or the Hamburger shift after its discoverer. It is an active process mediated by a carrier protein in the cell membrane and can be inhibited by drugs including salicylates and frusemide. The anion exchange leads to the uptake of carbon dioxide by blood in the tissue capillaries being shared between red cells and plasma, although the red cells contain the bulk of the protein upon which the process depends.

Carbamino-haemoglobin

As well as the reactions with water some carbon dioxide combines with reduced haemoglobin to form a compound of a carbamino type, i.e.:

$$HbNH_2 + CO_2 \rightleftharpoons HbNHCOOH \rightleftharpoons HbNHCOO^- + H^+ \quad (9.16)$$

In the tissue capillaries the forward reaction is facilitated by the quantity of reduced haemoglobin rising as the oxyhaemoglobin gives up its oxygen. The process is reversed in the lungs; hence the reaction contributes to the transport of carbon dioxide by taking it up from the tissues and releasing it in the lungs. It is believed to explain approximately 10% of the total transport in normal circumstances and up to 19% in the fetus, but these figures are subject to revision. The interaction between the transport mechanisms for oxygen and carbon dioxide was discovered by Christiansen, Douglas and Haldane and is known as the *CHD* or *Haldane effect*. The effect is related to the change in saturation of blood with oxygen; this aspect is shown in the O_2-CO_2 diagram (page 195) by the curvature of the isopleths for the carbon dioxide content of blood. The formation of carbamate occurs at terminal amino groups on the β chains of deoxygenated haemoglobin molecules and to a lesser extent on the α chains. However, the former reaction is diminished by 2,3-DPG which competes for the same sites (page 281); the organic phosphates do not compete for the sites on the α chains which in practice contribute equally with the β chains to the oxylabile carbamate transport of carbon dioxide.

Gas exchange in the lungs

In the lungs the chemical changes are the reverse of those which occur in the tissues. They are initiated by both the fall in the tension of carbon dioxide, which alters the position of equilibrium between dissolved carbon dioxide and carbonic acid, and the rise in the tension of oxygen which increases the concentration of oxyhaemoglobin; this reduces the quantity of carbamino-haemoglobin and also liberates hydrogen ions from reduced haemoglobin. The hydrogen ions in turn contribute to the release of carbon dioxide from bicarbonate. The temperature in the lungs is lower than that in the tissues by on average 0.5°C; this also contributes to the release of carbon dioxide. The CO_2 which is released diffuses rapidly in the aqueous phase of the lung tissue and thence into the alveoli. However, the lung water as well as being a conduit for carbon dioxide also smoothes the fluctuations of CO_2 tension which occur during the respiratory cycle; the stimulation of respiration from this source is reduced in consequence (page 344).

Rate of equilibration

The rate of diffusion of carbon dioxide across the alveolar capillary membrane has been estimated using radio-isotope labelled gases including $^{13}CO_2$, ^{16}O, ^{18}O and $C^{18}O_2$. The labelled oxygen exchanges rapidly with the oxygen in lung water so has a negligible plasma back tension. In two healthy male subjects the membrane diffusing capacity for $C^{18}O_2$ was found by Schuster to be on average $370\,\text{mmol}\,\text{min}^{-1}\,\text{kPa}^{-1}$ ($1102\,\text{ml}\,\text{min}^{-1}\,\text{mmHg}^{-1}$). From equation 9.6 the diffusivity of carbon dioxide should be greater than that for oxygen and carbon monoxide by factors of 20.3 and 24.6 respectively (Table 9.3). On this basis the values for Dmo_2 and $Dmco$ should be 18 and $15\,\text{mmol}\,\text{min}^{-1}\,\text{kPa}^{-1}$ which is consistent with other estimates. Hence the underlying hypotheses are likely to be correct.

The paradox of a relatively slow overall equilibration time for carbon dioxide despite its high diffusivity is due to the chemical processes. These are slower than those for oxygen, partly because the oxygenation of haemoglobin needs to be completed before carbon dioxide can achieve equilibrium between red cells and plasma. However, initially there is no similar equilibrium for hydrogen ions; instead the concentration in the red cells is less than in plasma due to the ions associating with bicarbonate ions prior to dehydration of carbonic acid (Fig. 9.5). The imbalance cannot be corrected directly because the red cell membrane is relatively impermeable to cations. Instead, the plasma carbonic acid is dehydrated slowly to yield additional carbon dioxide which diffuses into the red cells. Here the CO_2 is hydrated rapidly via the mediation of carbonic anhydrase II to reform hydrogen ions, and bicarbonate ions which return to the plasma. Chloride ions pass in the reverse direction. Crandall and others have evidence that the half time for this process is approximately 15 s. The delay may be responsible for the tension of carbon dioxide in the arterial blood sometimes being found to be less than that in the alveolar gas.

During its transit through the pulmonary capillaries the blood loses a large volume of carbon dioxide but the change in the tension of carbon dioxide is small (page 210). The relationship between these two variables is described by the CO_2 dissociation curve for the lung which is similar to that for drawn blood (Fig. 7.12, page 207). The curve over the physiological range is approximately linear; this is an advantage when there is a wide range of ventilation–perfusion ratios throughout the lung (Chapter 7). However, it renders more difficult the attainment of gaseous equilibrium across the alveolar capillary membrane, since there is no tailing off of the volume flow of gas as equilibrium approaches; in this the position differs from that for oxygen (page 285). The small tension difference and the linear dissociation curve contribute to the attainment of equilibrium across the alveolar capillary membrane being achieved relatively slowly, despite the high solubility and hence diffusivity of CO_2 in body fluids and the high activity of carbonic anhydrase present in the red cells. Under normal circumstances gaseous equilibrium is probably achieved at rest but not during heavy exercise; the likely time course is illustrated in Fig. 9.4. An end-capillary gradient can also occur if carbonic anhydrase is inhibited by acetazolamide, anion transport is depressed by salicylates or the lung parenchyma is damaged by disease. The deficiency in carbon dioxide excretion is normally made good by hyperventilation.

Gas exchange for carbon monoxide

Uptake of carbon monoxide by haemoglobin

Carbon monoxide resembles oxygen in its solubility and molecular weight (Table 9.3) and capacity to enter into reversible combination with haemoglobin. However, the affinity of haemoglobin for carbon monoxide is greater than for oxygen by a factor, the Haldane constant, which, in terms of the tensions of the two gases is approximately 230 (range 200–250). Then:

$$\frac{COHb}{O_2Hb} = M \frac{Pco}{Po_2} \qquad (9.17)$$

where the left hand term is the ratio of the concentrations of carboxy- and oxyhaemoglobin, and that on the right is the product of the ratio of the gas tensions and the Haldane constant M. When the gases are described in terms of their concentrations, the value for M is increased by the factor 1.3, which is the ratio of the solubilities (s) of the two gases (Table 9.3). Then:

$$\frac{[CO]}{[O_2]} = \frac{sco Pco}{so_2 Po_2} = \frac{1}{1.3} \frac{Pco}{Po_2} \qquad (9.18)$$

M is determined mainly by the ratio of the rates of association and dissociation of carbon monoxide with the intermediate compound of haemoglobin and oxygen Hb_4O_6 (cf. page 279). The rate of dissociation is relatively constant. The rate of association is labile and responsible for much of the observed variation in M. Factors which contribute include the prevailing temperature, pH and tension of carbon dioxide, which Sirs, in *in vitro* studies, has shown to form an intermediate complex with oxyhaemoglobin (CO_2,Hb_4O_6); compared with Hb_4O_6 this complex reacts at different rates with oxygen and with carbon monoxide. The reaction rate *in vivo* is difficult to calculate on account of the concentrations of the various substances not attaining equilibrium during the time of transit of the red blood corpuscles through the alveolar capillaries. Some aspects are discussed by Holland.

The high affinity of haemoglobin for carbon monoxide has the effect that when a low concentration of the gas is breathed for a long time the saturation of haemoglobin with carbon monoxide rises materially. For example, when breathing a gas mixture containing carbon monoxide in the fractional concentration of 0.001 made up in air (oxygen concentration 0.21) the saturation for both gases is 50%. The presence of carbon monoxide also alters the shape of the dissociation curve for oxygen (Fig. 17.2, page 626). On account of these features of the relationship of carbon monoxide with haemoglobin a relatively low concentration of carbon monoxide can endanger life.

Exposure to carbon monoxide

A small amount of carbon monoxide, approximately $18\,nmol^{-1}$ ($0.4\,ml\,h^{-1}$), is produced in the body during the breakdown of haem compounds. The process leads to a concentration of carboxyhaemoglobin in blood of approximately 0.7%. City dwellers exposed to environmental pollution by products of combustion including exhaust from petrol engines can have COHb levels of 2%, or more as a result of prolonged exposure at a busy city intersection or road tunnel. High concentrations of carbon monoxide are present in some industrial

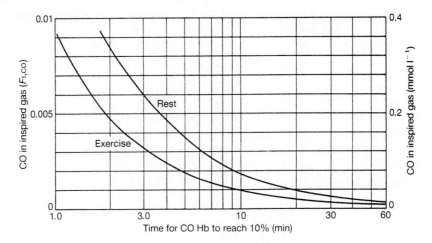

Fig. 9.6 Maximal concentrations of carbon monoxide in air which may be inhaled for different periods of time by healthy subjects without the saturation of Hb with carbon monoxide rising above 10%. The curves for rest and exercise have been constructed using ventilation minute volumes of 10 and $30 \, l \, min^{-1}$ respectively.

fumes and fuel gases. Alternatively the gas can be formed by metabolism following inhalation of methylene chloride used as a paintstripper. Smokers absorb carbon monoxide from cigarette smoke in which it is present in a fractional concentration of up to 0.06; this raises the blood level of carboxyhaemoglobin to an average of 5%, increasing to 14% in heavy smokers. The upper limit for safety is usually set at 15% carboxyhaemoglobin ($1.4 \, mmol \, l^{-1}$); however, 10% of carboxyhaemoglobin for which the corresponding alveolar concentration is about 50 parts per million ($2 \, \mu mol \, l^{-1}$) impairs the function of the nervous system; even lower concentrations can have a long-term effect (cf. page 626). For gas which is breathed continuously the concentration of 50 ppm should not be exceeded; for shorter exposures to higher concentrations the times should not exceed those indicated in Fig. 9.6. The speed of recovery from exposure to carbon monoxide is a function of the rate of dissociation of carboxyhaemoglobin which is mainly determined by the inspired oxygen tension (Table 17.5, page 627).

Transfer factor (diffusing capacity) for the lung for carbon monoxide

Carbon monoxide passes by diffusion from the alveolar gas into the plasma in the alveolar capillaries; from the plasma it passes into the erythrocytes where it combines with haemoglobin. At low tensions of carbon monoxide and normal tensions of oxygen the subsequent back reaction is relatively small so the plasma tension of carbon monoxide rises only very slightly during the residence time of the red cells in the alveolar capillaries. In these circumstances the transfer gradient is effectively the alveolar tension of carbon monoxide less the tension in mixed venous blood entering the alveolar capillaries. Thus the transfer gradient is effectively constant down the length of the capillaries and is not influenced by the rate of blood flow. In these circumstances, equation 9.11 simplifies to:

$$\frac{P_{A,CO} - P_{\bar{v},CO}}{\dot{n}_{CO}} = \frac{1}{Tl} = \frac{1}{D_m} + \frac{1}{\theta V_c} \qquad (9.19)$$

where $\dot{n}_{CO}$ is the rate of carbon monoxide uptake, $P_{A,CO}$ and $P_{\bar{v},CO}$ are the tensions of carbon monoxide in alveolar gas and mixed venous blood, Tl is the transfer factor (diffusing capacity) for the lung for carbon monoxide, D_m is the diffusing capacity of the alveolar capillary membrane, V_c is the volume of blood in the alveolar capillaries and θ is the reaction rate of carbon monoxide with oxyhaemoglobin. The term $1/Tl$ can be regarded as the resistance of the lung parenchyma to transfer of carbon monoxide; it is made up of the resistance of the membrane to diffusion $(1/D_m)$ and the resistance of the blood to combination with carbon monoxide $(1/\theta V_c)$. Roughton and others have demonstrated that the reaction rate is a function of the tension of oxygen and can be determined *in vitro*. On the assumption that this relationship also applies *in vivo*, the other terms can be obtained by the method which is described on page 313.

The transfer factor can, alternatively, be expressed per litre of alveolar volume when it is called the *transfer coefficient* or *diffusion constant*. This index is usually symbolised by K_{CO} or Tl/V_A where V_A is the alveolar volume in l BTPS. V_A is sometimes expressed in l STPD but this practice is not recommended. The index was introduced by Krogh as k_{CO} with the units l (BTPS) $\text{min}^{-1} \text{bar}^{-1}$ per l of alveolar volume. The two forms are linked by the relationship:

$$Tl/V_A(K_{CO}) = k_{CO} \frac{1000}{760} \times \frac{273}{310} \div 2.986 \, \text{mmol min}^{-1} \text{kPa}^{-1} \text{l}^{-1}$$

$$(9.20)$$

By analogy with electrical theory (page 183) the K_{CO} can be related to the time constant for the uptake of gas (τ,CO); this is the time in seconds for the alveolar concentration of carbon monoxide (expressed as $\log_e F_{A,CO},t$ as in equation 10.7, page 309) to fall exponentially to 37% of the initial value. The τ,CO is numerically equal to $60/K_{CO}$. The K_{CO} provides some indication of the density and volume of the alveolar capillaries (cf. Fig. 5.6, page 95); however, in any individual subject the K_{CO} varies inversely with the lung volume and, therefore, is less easy to interpret than the factor for the whole lung from which it is derived.

The technical advantage of carbon monoxide over oxygen for measuring the transfer factor has led to Tl_{CO} being used to estimate the transfer factor for oxygen. The method appears to have an acceptable accuracy (page 322). However, at least four different techniques can be used for measuring Tl_{CO} and each has its own assumptions and limitations; these are described in Chapter 10. The absolute values obtained by the different methods are concordant but not identical, so conclusions based on absolute values of Tl_{CO} should take account of the method. Factors which differ between the methods include the volume history prior to the measurement, the lung volume at which the measurement is made and the extent to which the result is influenced by uneven distribution of pulmonary ventilation and perfusion. The latter interaction is least when the measurement is made by the rebreathing method and somewhat greater using the breath holding method (paged 311). However, for other reasons the single breath method is the most widely used. It has provided the basis for the following account.

The transfer factor (diffusing capacity) for the lung during childhood increases with the growth of the lung (see page 460). In adult life it is related to body size and for a given size is usually higher in men than in women. The mean value in healthy adults is in the range 4.3−16 mmol^{-1}kPa^{-1} (13−48 ml min^{-1}mmHg^{-1}) (see footnote page 102). In a single subject *T*lco declines with age and varies with the depth of inspiration; the latter effect is approximately 10% per litre of lung volume or about 1.0 mmol min^{-1}kPa^{-1}l^{-1}. The transfer factor increases with activity by a factor of up to two compared with the value at rest. Due to a change in reaction rate (θ), the index is reduced in anaemia and increased in polycythaemia. It is diminished by smoking and varies with posture, being least in an upright and greatest in a head-down position. The transfer factor is reduced by diseases of the lung parenchyma and is abnormal in some patients with rheumatic and congenital heart disease (Chapter 16).

Alteration of the transfer factor is usually due to a change in either or both the volume of blood in the alveolar capillaries and the diffusing capacity of the alveolar capillary membrane. Their respective contributions are summarised in Tables 9.7 and 9.8 and are discussed in the next two sections. Other determinants of the transfer process, including

Table 9.7 Causes of variation in the transfer factor (*T*l) in subjects with normal lungs. *K*co varies in the same direction as *T*l except where indicated

Factors increasing *T*l	Factors decreasing *T*l	Principal variable
Exercise	Meals	
Lying down	Standing up and other causes of peripheral blood pooling	
Cold shower	Cutaneous vasodilatation	
Increased sympathetic tone from other causes		*V*c
(Müller manoeuvre)	Valsalva manoeuvre	
	Night (cf. day)	
	Smoking cigarettes	
Growth (children) [*K*co ↓]	Age (adults)	
Inspiration [*K*co ↓]	Expiration [*K*co ↑]	*D*m
Hypoxia	Breathing O$_2$ or CO	
Polycythaemia	Anaemia	
Goodpasture's syndrome (bleeding into the lung)		θ

Table 9.8 Effects of medical conditions on the transfer factor (Tl), the diffusing capacity of the alveolar capillary membrane (Dm) and the volume of blood in the alveolar capillaries (Vc). Factors affecting the reaction rate (θ) are included in Table 9.7. Kco varies in the same direction as Tl except where indicated. Features in parentheses are somewhat variable

Conditions	Dm	Vc	Tl	
Lung disorders				
Asthma	N or ↑	(N)	N or ↑	
Bronchits	(N)	(N)	N or ↓	
Emphysema	↓	(↓)	N or ↓	[Kco ↓]
Diffuse infiltrations	↓	(↓)	↓	
Restrictive pleural disease	↓	(N)	(↓)	[Kco ↑]
Loss of lung tissue	↓	N or ↓	↓	
Cardiovascular disorders				
Hyperkinetic states	N	↑	↑	
Low cardiac output	N	↓	↓	
Raised pulmonary venous pressure:				
Minimal	N	↑	↑	
Intermediate	↓	↑	N	
Material (also other causes of				
pulmonary oedema)	↓	↓	↓	

the residence times for blood in the alveolar capillaries, can contribute in some circumstances.

Volume of blood in the alveolar capillaries

The quantity that is measured is the volume of blood which exchanges gas with the alveoli. It includes blood in some small pulmonary arteries and veins as well as in capillaries. The volume exhibits fluctuations over the cardiac cycle. Changes in pulmonary blood volume are responsible for short-term variations in transfer factor (diffusing capacity) such as occur with posture, exercise and variation in body temperature. At rest the volume is least in an upright posture when it averages about 0.081 (80 ml); it increases progressively if the posture is altered from the vertical, through the horizontal to the head-down position. It increases linearly with the level of cardiac output during exercise and is decreased when blood is diverted to other parts of the body; this occurs in relation to meals, when the volume of blood in the splanchnic area is increased, and during exposure to heat, when there is dilatation of blood vessels in the skin. The volume of blood is reduced if the venous return to the heart is obstructed by a rise of the pressure in the thorax; this occurs during positive pressure breathing and when a subject performs the Valsalva manoeuvre by making an expiratory effort whilst the glottis is closed. The converse Müller manoeuvre of inspiration against a closed glottis can increase the pulmonary blood volume but not all subjects respond. The retention of blood in the veins of the legs by inflation of pressure cuffs around the thighs also decreases the volume of blood in the lung including that in the alveolar capillaries. Squeezing the legs and abdomen by immersion of the subject in water or inflation of an anti-gravity suit such as is used by flying personnel has the opposite effect.

The volume of blood in the alveolar capillaries is increased by a rise in the pulmonary venous pressure such as occurs in mitral stenosis; it is also increased by the considerable augmentation to pulmonary blood flow which occurs in some categories of congenital heart disease (page 602). The volume is usually normal in the early stages of chronic lung disease but declines in the later stages when there is destruction of lung tissue and pulmonary hypertension. The volume decreases slightly with age.

Diffusing capacity of the alveolar capillary membrane

The diffusing capacity of the alveolar capillary membrane for carbon monoxide is not relevant to exchange of gas in the normal lung because the uptake of gas is seldom limited by diffusion. However, the index provides a useful measure of the area of the membrane across which exchange of gas takes place and of the thickness of this membrane to which it is inversely related. The diffusing capacity of the membrane varies with lung volume since, at large volumes, the area of membrane is greater than at small volumes. Some of the evidence is reviewed by Stam and colleagues. The variability with lung volume is allowed for by making the measurement at total lung capacity. For a subject who is studied at one point in time, the diffusing capacity of the membrane is relatively independent of factors such as posture and the level of exercise which affect the volume of blood in the alveolar capillaries.

The diffusing capacity of the membrane is impaired when there is a reduction in the effective surface for gas exchange in the lung; it therefore decreases with age and in the presence of disease of the lung parenchyma in which either there is loss of lung tissue or parts of the lung are not ventilated. It is also reduced when there is thickening of the alveolar capillary membrane; this occurs as a result of proliferation of cells in sarcoidosis and other pulmonary granulomatoses. Thickening can also result from interstitial oedema due to pulmonary congestion.

The circumstances in which a low transfer factor is due to a reduced diffusing capacity of the alveolar capillary membrane can overlap with those in which it is due to a diminution in the volume of blood in the alveolar capillaries. However, except in some types of heart disease and in the late stages of chronic lung disease, a change in volume of blood is usually due to physiological processes which are reversible; by contrast a reduction in the diffusing capacity of the alveolar capillary membrane is evidence for lung pathology which is often irreversible. Tl reflects the sum of two resistances to gas uptake, imposed by (a) the alveolar membrane, (b) the rate of combination with blood, but it is not a reliable guide to the extent of abnormality in either one of these two factors on its own. Because of the relationship depicted in equation 9.13, Tl severely underestimates an isolated abnormality of Dm or Vc.

This is exemplified in mitral stenosis where a reduction in membrane diffusing capacity can be exactly matched by an increase in the capillary blood volume; the transfer factor is then within normal limits despite pathological variations in its components. However, such circumstances are uncommon. Usually the transfer factor provides the relevant information.

Gas exchange for nitric oxide

Nitric oxide is a sparsely soluble gas which combines with haemoglobin to form nitrosyl-haemoglobin and with oxyhaemoglobin to form methaemoglobin: the reactions are independent of oxygen tension. Nitric oxide can also oxidise to nitrogen dioxide but at low concentrations of nitric oxide (less than 40 ppm) this reaction is unimportant. The uptake of nitric oxide in the lungs is described by equation 9.11 (page 276). However, the rate of reaction with haemoglobin is rapid, approximately 280 times that of carbon monoxide so that for nitric oxide the chemical reaction component of the term $1/\theta Vc$ is effectively zero. Accordingly for this gas $1/\theta Vc$ is solely a measure of the diffusive resistance of the blood. In addition the rate of dissociation of nitrosyl-haemoglobin is extremely slow so the back tension in the capillary plasma is also negligible. In these circumstances the transfer factor for nitric oxide (Tl,NO) should be a better measure of the diffusing capacity of the alveolar capillary membrane than Tl,CO. This was first pointed out by Borland and Higenbottam. However, the dependence of Tl,NO on haemoglobin concentration (page 278) suggests that Dm,NO is also influenced by the diffusive resistance of the blood.

The solubility of nitric oxide is approximately twice that of carbon monoxide (Table 9.3) but the molecular weights are similar so from equation 9.6 the relative diffusivities ($Dm,NO/Dm,CO$) might be expected to be in the ratio 2:1. In practise the ratio has not been determined directly; however, the transfer factors for nitric oxide and carbon monoxide are in the ratio 4.3−5.3:1 which is consistent with the hypothesis. If this is confirmed the measurement of Tl,NO could make a valuable contribution to the assessment of lung function. Some aspects of the technique have been reviewed by Meyer and Piiper. The method of measurement including its use for obtaining Dm and Vc is described on page 317.

Guide to references

The references (Chapter 18) are classified under subject headings of which the following are particularly relevant to the present chapter:

10: Measurement of Transfer Factor (Diffusing Capacity) and its Subdivisions

Transfer factor for carbon monoxide (*T*lco), steady state, single breath and rebreathing methods.
Recommendations for standardisation.
Allowances for haemoglobin concentration and oxygen tension.
Measurement of diffusing capacity of the alveolar capillary membrane and the volume of blood in the alveolar capillaries.
Rate of reaction of carbon monoxide with blood.
Transfer factor for nitric oxide.
Transfer factor for oxygen (method of Riley and Lilienthal and derivations from *T*lco and from $\dot{V}_A/\dot{Q}$ distribution)

Introduction

The transfer factor (*T*l) links the rate at which gas can cross the alveolar capillary membrane to the pressure gradient from one side of the membrane to the other. It is therefore expressed as the quantity of gas (mmol or ml STPD) per min per unit of pressure difference (kPa or mmHg). *T*l is positively correlated with the area of that part of the membrane through which gas can pass into the blood and negatively correlated with the thickness. For a gas G, the relevant equation is:

$$T_{l,G} = \frac{\text{rate of uptake of G}}{P_{A,G} - P_{\bar{c},G}} \tag{10.1}$$

where $P_{A,G}$ and $P_{\bar{c},G}$ are the mean tensions of gas G in the alveoli and alveolar capillaries respectively. The transfer factor can be measured for oxygen, carbon monoxide or nitric oxide (page 274). That for oxygen is the most relevant but the measurement is not straightforward for the reasons which are described on page 321. The transfer factor for nitric oxide is of recent origin; it holds promise for the future (pages 297 and 317) but currently the method of choice is that using carbon monoxide. This gas has the advantages that the compound with haemoglobin (COHb) does not readily break down so unless there is a significant quantity of carbon monoxide in the mixed venous blood the tension of carbon monoxide in the plasma ($P_{\bar{c},G}$ in equation 10.1) can usually be taken to be zero. There are then only two variables to be determined — the rate of uptake and the alveolar gas tension. The rate of uptake is measured by analysing inspired and expired gas over a timed interval. The time can be about 10 s in the single breath (breath holding) method up to 20 s in the rebreathing method or several minutes in the steady state methods. A shorter interval is used for the single expiration method. The alveolar gas tension is obtained in one of several ways depending on which method is used. In many of the steady state methods, the $P_A,_{CO}$ is calculated from the concentration of carbon monoxide in the expired gas and a value for the physiological deadspace for carbon dioxide (Table 10.1).

The tension of carbon monoxide in pulmonary capillary blood is only slightly greater than that in the mixed venous blood. The latter is increased in heavy smokers and persons who have an environmental or occupational exposure. In such subjects the back tension may exceed 3 Pa (0.02 mmHg), equivalent to an alveolar concentration of $1.3 \, \mu mol \, l^{-1}$ (30 parts per million), and should be measured (page 313).

The various methods for measuring $Tl._{CO}$ do not give identical results, partly because of inherent inadequacies which will be described subsequently and partly because they estimate Tl at different lung volumes; the volumes affect the diffusion characteristics of the alveolar membrane. On average $Tl,_{CO}$ varies by approximately $1 \, mmol \, min^{-1} kPa^{-1}$ ($3 \, ml \, min^{-1} mmHg^{-1}$) per l change in alveolar volume and allowance for a volume difference can be made using this factor. Some features of the several carbon monoxide methods are summarised in Table 10.1. The single breath method is the procedure of choice.

Transfer factor (diffusing capacity) of the lung for carbon monoxide

STEADY STATE METHOD ($Tl,_{CO.SS}$)

This was the first method to be widely used. It is particularly suitable for young children. The measurement is made whilst the subject breathes a gas mixture containing a low concentration of carbon monoxide ($Fl._{CO} \approx 0.001$) made up in air. Breathing is continued for long enough

Table 10.1 Carbon monoxide methods for measurement of transfer factor ($Tl,_{CO}$)

Method	Version	Derivation of $P_A,_{CO}$*	Principal feature	Conditions (rest/exercise)	V_A*	Page
Steady state (tidal breathing of 0.1% CO)	Bates†	$P_A,_{CO_2}$	Uneven lung function causes error	Exercise		301
	Filley	$P_a,_{CO_2}$		Exercise	FRC	301
	Leathart	$P_{rebr}._{CO_2}$		Rest	$+0.5 \, Vt$	301
Single breath (breath holding)	Forster	$P_A,_{CO}$	Robust method	Either	0.95 TLC	302
Rebreathing	Lewis	$P_{rebr}._{CO}$	Corrects for uneven ventilation	Either	FRC $+0.5 \, Vt$	311
Single expiration‡	Nadel	$P_A,_{CO}$	Susceptible to volume history	Rest	Varies	
Multiple inert gas (MIGET)§	West	from $\dot{V}_A/\dot{Q}$	Corrects for $\dot{V}_A/\dot{Q}$ inequality	Either	FRC $+0.5 \, Vt$	322

* For terminology, see Chapter 2.
† Bates also used fractional CO uptake $(1 - F_E._{CO}/F_I._{CO})$; this was called conductance coefficient (ductance de CO) by Lacoste.
‡ The method is technically demanding and seldom used.
§ First used to obtain $Tl,_{O_2}$.

to achieve a steady state in which the quantity of carbon monoxide entering the alveoli from the inspired gas is equal to that taken up from the alveolar gas by the blood. One or 2 min is usually sufficient time. The expired gas is then collected for 1 min. The expired carbon monoxide concentration (obtained by analysis), and together with the ventilation minute volume are used to calculate the carbon monoxide uptake.

The alveolar carbon monoxide tension is usually calculated from the mixed expired concentration by making an allowance for the physiological deadspace. The deadspace is that measured for carbon dioxide; it is effectively equal to that for carbon monoxide. Then:

$$Vd/Vt = (P_{A,CO_2} - P_{E,CO_2})/(P_{A,CO_2} - P_{I,CO_2}) \qquad (10.2)$$

$$= (P_{E,CO} - P_{A,CO})/(P_{I,CO} - P_{A,CO}) \qquad (10.3)$$

hence:

$$P_{A,CO} = P_{I,CO} - \frac{P_{A,CO_2} \times (P_{I,CO} - P_{E,CO})}{P_{E,CO_2}} \qquad (10.4)$$

where Vd and Vt are physiological deadspace and tidal volume; P_I, P_A and P_E refer to the tensions of the designated gases (carbon dioxide and carbon monoxide) in inspired, alveolar and expired gas.

The tensions of carbon monoxide and carbon dioxide in the inspired and the expired gas are obtained by analysis; the tension of carbon dioxide in the alveolar gas is estimated in one of several ways. In the *Filley method* the tension of carbon dioxide is that in arterial blood. This is effectively the same as in the mixed alveolar gas, except when the range of ventilation−perfusion ratios is increased (see below). In the *Bates method* the alveolar gas concentrations are obtained by sampling the expired gas at the lips into a rapid analyser for carbon dioxide or carbon monoxide. The required gas concentration is that in the early part of the alveolar plateau (see for example normal capnigram, Fig. 8.7, page 226). This procedure can yield a representative value for the alveolar concentration during exercise, except when the distribution of lung function is uneven. It is unreliable at rest. In the *Leathart method* the alveolar carbon dioxide tension is obtained by rebreathing (page 47). The transfer factor is calculated using equation 10.1. An allowance for the back tension of carbon monoxide in the alveolar capillary plasma should be made in subjects who have smoked on the day of the test and when it is proposed to measure a subject's transfer factor several times at one session.

EFFECT OF UNEVEN LUNG FUNCTION

Uneven lung function is an important source of error in steady state methods. This is especially so at rest since the range of uncertainty in estimating the alveolar carbon monoxide tension is large relative to the transfer gradient. The error is less on exercise because this can improve the accuracy of estimation of $P_{A,CO}$ and increase the transfer gradient.

The result is still inaccurate if lung function is uneven. A low result by the method involving sampling the expired gas (Bates' method) is then evidence for either a transfer defect or uneven lung function. A low result by the method based on arterial blood (Filley method) is usually evidence for a transfer defect but this abnormality can be exaggerated if the lung function is uneven. The result can also be influenced by hyperventilation and by changes in bronchomotor tone induced by drugs. The subject has been investigated by Visser, Read, Haab and their respective collaborators amongst others.

Error due to uneven lung function is less of a problem using the single breath method because the transfer gradient is larger, but this method depends on analysis of an 'alveolar sample' which is probably not representative of the lung as a whole when there is uneven distribution of airways obstruction. This leads to a small underestimate of the true transfer factor. The error is somewhat reduced by the period of breath holding. The error is increased if the alveolar volume is underestimated. In patients with airflow limitation this occurs when the alveolar volume is obtained from the dilution in the lung of the single breath of test gas. In a study reported by Chinn and colleagues the degree of underestimation was 12%. The error can be largely overcome by estimating the alveolar volume as the inspired volume of test gas plus the residual volume measured independently by the multi-breath helium dilution method (page 150) or whole body plethysmography (page 157). However, this can lead to overestimation of the transfer factor in some patients with emphysema. Alternatively if the airflow limitation is partly reversible the error in using the single breath alveolar volume can be reduced by the patient inhaling a bronchodilator aerosol prior to the determination.

The error introduced by uneven distribution of lung ventilation, perfusion and permeability of the alveolar capillary membrane can be allowed for mathematically by using the multiple inert gas elimination technique (MIGET, page 322). The component due to uneven ventilation can be overcome mechanically by using the rebreathing method (page 311).

SINGLE BREATH (BREATH HOLDING) METHOD (Tl,co.sb)

The single breath method was proposed by Bohr and developed by Marie Krogh (1915) who obtained alveolar samples at the beginning and end of the period of breath holding. However, the samples came from parts of the lung having different expansion ratios so were not strictly comparable. The need for the first sample was avoided by Forster, Fowler and their colleagues with advice from Kety who suggested the inclusion of helium or other inert gas in the test gas mixture. The method is widely used on account of its good reproducibility, convenience for the subject and relative independence from uneven lung function. A version of the original method, which entailed using an independent estimate of residual volume to calculate alveolar volume (V_A), is recommended for routine laboratory investigations at rest and during exercise. Used with the single breath estimate of alveolar volume (V_A, eff), the method is recommended for respiratory surveys.

Outline

In this method a single breath of test gas is inhaled and held in the lung whilst the carbon monoxide disappears into the blood at a rate which is proportional to the alveolar carbon monoxide tension. Assuming that the lung is a single homogeneous gas exchanger the tension will decline exponentially during the time for which the breath is held. Consequently a semi-log plot of CO concentration against time will give a straight line with a slope proportional to Tl and inversely proportional to the volume (residual volume plus volume inspired) from which it is being absorbed. Only two points are required to define the straight line, the concentration at the start of breath holding and after a known time. The first of these is obtained by adding helium to the inspirate and the second by analysing an 'alveolar sample' at the end of breath holding. The optimal breath holding time is 10 s. Theoretically the inspiration and expiration of the gas sample should be instantaneous in which case the volume of the lung during the period of gas exchange would be constant. In practice the inspiration and expiration take a little time so allowance must be made for gas exchange taking place during these manoeuvres as well as during breath holding. The alveolar concentration of carbon monoxide at the start of the period of gas exchange is influenced by dilution of the test breath into the alveolar gas already present in the lung. The dilution is calculated from that of helium or other inert gas added to the test gas mixture. The helium is neither absorbed nor secreted into the lung so its dilution in an 'alveolar sample' reflects the initial dilution of the carbon monoxide, including the effect of any inequality due to the test inspirate not being distributed uniformly throughout the lung. The dilution of the helium can also be used to calculate the residual volume. However, in this event any uneven distribution of ventilation leads to underestimation of the volume and hence of the transfer factor compared with the single chamber model. The error can often be reduced by the prior inhalation of a bronchodilator aerosol (page 640). The alveolar oxygen tension during gas exchange is usually at its normal level but the test can usefully be extended by making an additional measurement with added oxygen. The two sets of results can be used to calculate the respective contributions to gas exchange of the diffusing capacity of the alveolar capillary membrane (Dm) and the volume of blood in alveolar capillaries (Vc). Dm and Vc can also be obtained from the concurrent measurement of Tl.co and Tl.no (page 318). Proposals for standardising the measurement of Tl.co have been made by the European Coal and Steel Community and the American Thoracic Society. These are incorporated in the present account.

Details of the single breath method

Apparatus. Measurement is commonly made using a spirometer with a capacity of 9 l, a kymograph with drum speed of $10\,\text{mm}\,\text{s}^{-1}$, a valve box with multiple connections, two bags of at least 6 l capacity and several bags of 1 or 2 l capacity made of material impervious to gases. The larger bags are mounted in a closed box (Donald, Christie box) and contain the gas to be inspired. The smaller bags receive the samples of alveolar gas for analysis. The equipment should meet the technical specifications given in Chapter 3. It can be combined with that for measurement of the total lung capacity (e.g. Fig. 10.1).

Gas analysis. The test gas mixture contains carbon monoxide (fractional concentration usually 0.003) and an inert gas. This is usually helium (fractional concentration in the range 0.02–0.14); alternatively neon is used when the gas is to be analysed by gas chromatography. For measurement of transfer factor the fractional concentration of oxygen is usually 0.17–0.18 in Europe and 0.21 in the USA with the remainder nitrogen.* For the additional measurement of Dm and Vc the remainder gas is oxygen. The 18% and 85% oxygen mixtures can be prepared by decanting into two tin-lined cylinders some gas from a master cylinder containing carbon monoxide at a fractional concentration of 0.018, with the remainder helium; the cylinders are then topped up respectively with air and oxygen. The procedure is described on page 49. These three gas mixtures are cheaper to produce than the four gas mixture which is needed when 21% oxygen is used.

Helium is analysed using a katharometer or one of the other methods described in Chapter 3. The katharometer should be fitted with a control unit to maintain a constant current through the detector. The instrument is slightly sensitive to carbon dioxide and water vapour and also responds to the ratio of the concentrations of oxygen and nitrogen in the gas samples. To enhance the specificity of the analysis the carbon dioxide and water vapour should be absorbed respectively by soda lime and anhydrous calcium chloride or copper sulphate. The gas sample should have the CO_2 removed first as the chemical reaction liberates water vapour which is then removed by the drying agent. This procedure reduces the volume of the sample so it increases the concentrations of the other gases; however, the helium and the carbon monoxide are concentrated to the same extent so the change does not interfere with their ratio which is needed for the measurement of transfer factor. When the dilution of helium is used for calculating the

* The transfer factor is influenced by the alveolar oxygen tension which is normally approximately $15\,\text{kPa}$. At sea level this tension can be approximated during breath holding by using an F_{I,O_2} of 0.17–0.18 as recommended in the European Coal and Steel Community's report *Standardized Lung Function Testing*. The alveolar oxygen tension during breath holding is then nearly independent of the volume inspired. The American Thoracic Society recommend an F_{I,O_2} of 0.21. At altitudes above sea level some oxygen enrichment is appropriate. Alternatively, the effect of P_{A,O_2} can be allowed for using equation 10.19 and the method outlined on page 313.

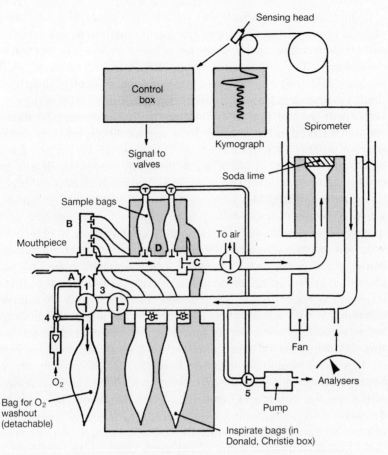

Fig. 10.1 Original resparameter (P.K. Morgan Ltd). Illustrating the combined
measurement of lung volumes by the closed circuit helium dilution method and transfer
factor by the single breath method. For the latter the subject breathes air or oxygen
through the port A of the valve box for up to 5 min, then after a complete expiration is
connected to the port B and inhales a predetermined volume of inspirate which is made
up in air or oxygen as appropriate. The port B then closes. After 8 s the port C opens
and a light flashes which is the signal for the subject to exhale. After the exhalation of
750 ml the port C closes; the port D then opens for the period of exhalation of a further
0.5 or 1 l; this gas passes into the sample bag which was previously evacuated. The
sample is subsequently transferred to the analysers by a pump. In the calculation an
allowance is made for the dilution of the sample during its collection. For the
measurement of lung volumes the taps are rotated via a common linkage into the
following positions:

$$1 \vdash, 2 \top, 3 \perp, 4 \dashv, 5 \top.$$

effective (single breath) alveolar volume, the expired concentration
should be reduced in proportion to the amount of carbon dioxide
which is absorbed (usually 5%). It is normally sufficient that the
katharometer should be calibrated for helium in dry air. For measurement of the diffusing capacity of the alveolar capillary membrane an
allowance should be made for the oxygen/nitrogen ratio of the mixture.
The correction factor varies between instruments so should be obtained
by calibration or from the manufacturers.

Carbon monoxide is analysed by infra-red absorption, a chemical
method or gas chromatography. The former method is well established
and yields accurate results when care is taken to calibrate and maintain
the detector. The detector has a useful life of on average 10 years. The
absolute calibration of analysers presents some difficulty because standard gas mixtures stored in high-pressure cylinders deteriorate on
account of the reaction of carbon monoxide with iron. The mixtures
should be stored in tin-lined cylinders and have their contents renewed
every 6 months. Alternatively fresh mixtures can be prepared in the
laboratory using a gas burette, a Wösthoff pump which has been
calibrated, or a closed circuit apparatus. The linearity of the analyser is
more important than the accuracy because the principal measurement
which is required is the ratio of the expired to the inspired carbon
monoxide concentration. The absolute concentration is only needed
when it is proposed to allow for the back pressure of carbon monoxide
in the blood (page 313). The procedure for checking the linearity is
illustrated in Fig. 10.2. The need for an accurate ratio requires that the
inspired gas should always be analysed concurrent with the sample of
expired gas; the concentration indicated on the inspirate cylinder will
be appropriate in some circumstances but this should not be relied on.
Infra-red analysers are sensitive to carbon dioxide and to water vapour
so these gases should be absorbed from the test gas prior to analysis.
Some analysers are also sensitive to oxygen which causes broadening
of the spectral absorption bands for carbon monoxide. This effect can
be allowed for by including an appropriate amount of oxygen in the
calibration gas. When the concentration of oxygen is also required it
should be determined by one of the methods described in Chapter 3.

Procedures. The transfer factor is influenced by the quantity of blood
in the lungs and the lung temperature both of which are affected by
metabolic and sympathetic nervous activity. The effects are minimised
by the subject being in a quiet relaxed state at the time of measurement.
This should preferably be at least 1 h after any meal or moderate
exercise and 4 h after consuming alcohol. The subject should preferably
not have smoked since the previous day. However, if the subject is a
very heavy smoker or has smoked within a few hours of the test the
mixed venous carbon monoxide tension should be measured; the procedure is given on page 313. In patients with airflow obstruction a
bronchodilator aerosol should preferably be administered if the lung
volume to be used in the calculation is that measured by the single
breath method (equation 10.11, page 310).

To make the measurement of transfer factor the subject is seated
upright in front of the apparatus and breathes air through the mouthpiece. A nose clip is worn. After a few normal breaths the subject
breathes out to residual volume, inhales rapidly to total lung capacity,
holds the breath for approximately 8 s then breathes out at a steady
rate. After exhalation of 0.75 l (range 0.7–1.0 l), a sample of 0.5–
1.0 l of alveolar gas is collected for analysis. The breath holding time is

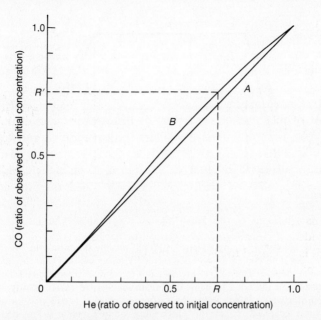

Fig. 10.2 Calibration of CO analyser. This diagram illustrates the procedure for calibrating a carbon monoxide analyser against a katharometer which has itself been calibrated for helium in air. An analogous procedure should be used for a meter calibrated for helium in oxygen. The inspirate gas mixture containing carbon monoxide and helium with 17% oxygen is passed through both gas meters before and after serial dilution with air. The readings so obtained are plotted as ratios of the initial concentrations. A linear relationship (line A) is evidence that the calibration is satisfactory and may be used without correction. A curvilinear relationship (line B) is evidence of the need for correction. For the ratio of the expired alveolar to the inspired concentration (R') the corresponding helium ratio (R) should be used. For the calculation of the diffusing capacity of the alveolar capillary membrane where a correction for back tension is required the true ratio of the initial to the final alveolar concentration of carbon monoxide is given by:

$$F_{A,CO_0}/F_{A,CO_t} = (F_{E,He}/F_{I,He} - R_B) \div (R - R_B)$$

(cf. equations 10.9 and 10.11), where R_B is the helium ratio corresponding to the measured back tension of carbon monoxide expressed as a fraction of the inspired tension.

Once a dilution curve has been constructed it can be used repeatedly provided the calibration is constant. This can be assessed by setting the meter on the inspirate mixture then performing one spot check at the dilution of maximal deviation from linearity.

usually obtained by the method of Jones and Meade which is given in Fig. 10.3.

Alternatively, the three phases of inspiration, breath holding and expiration can be treated separately as recommended by Graham and colleagues. Conventions for breath holding time which make no allowance for gas exchange continuing during the collection of the alveolar gas sample, including that of Ogilve and colleagues can lead to error in patients with airflow obstruction. Procedures which minimise the error have been recommended by the American Thoracic Society and European Coal and Steel Community (Table 10.2). The convention for breath holding time of the American Thoracic Society Epidemiology

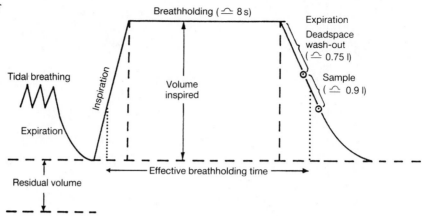

Fig. 10.3 Relationship of lung volume (l, BTPS) to time (s) during the breathholding manoeuvre for determining the transfer factor (diffusing capacity) for the lung by the single breath method. The subject breathes out to residual volume, inhales a vital capacity breath of the test gas, holds the breath for 8s then exhales slowly; after the exhalation of 750 ml a sample of 0.5 or 1.0 l of alveolar gas is collected for analysis. Criteria for a technically satisfactory curve are given in Table 10.2. Provided these are met the start of inspiration and of breath holding can be determined either by eye or by backward extrapolation from the linear part of the inspiratory limb of the curve (cf. Fig. 6.4, page 138). By the method of Jones and Meade the effective duration of breath holding is taken to include two-thirds of the time of inspiration and the time of expiration up to half-way through the period of sample collection.

Project gives systematically high results and is not recommended. Some of these methods have been assessed by Chinn and colleagues and by Crapo.

Calculation. The transfer factor for carbon monoxide is the uptake of this gas from the alveoli in mmol (or ml STPD) per min per unit of alveolar tension in excess of the equilibrium back tension. At normal tensions of oxygen the transfer gradient for carbon monoxide is effectively that between the alveolar gas and the mixed venous blood. Hence:

$$Tl,\text{co} = \dot{n}\text{co}/(P_{A,\text{co}} - P_{\bar{v},\text{co}}) \text{ mmol min}^{-1}\text{kPa}^{-1} \qquad (10.5)$$

where Tl,co is the transfer factor for carbon monoxide in SI units, $\dot{n}\text{co}$ is the uptake of carbon monoxide in mmol min^{-1} and $P_{A,\text{co}}$ and $P_{\bar{v},\text{co}}$ are the mean tensions of carbon monoxide (kPa) in alveolar gas and in equilibrium with the carboxyhaemoglobin of the mixed venous blood at the mean tension of oxygen in the alveolar capillary plasma.

At one point of time the relationship becomes:

$$Tl,\text{co} = \frac{dF}{dt} \times V_A/22.4 \ (F - F\bar{v})(P_B - P_{H_2O}) \text{ mmol min}^{-1}\text{kPa}^{-1}$$

$$(10.6)$$

where V_A is the alveolar volume in ml STPD, F is the instantaneous

308

Table 10.2 Summary of recommended procedures for measuring Tl,co,sb.

Condition of the subject	Rested, post-absorptive, seated for 10 min, preferably adequately bronchodilated and not having smoked or taken alcohol that day
$FI.co$	0.0025–0.003; if below this range the CO back tension should be allowed for.
$FI.o_2$	0.17–0.18 (or 0.21, page 304). (Time should be allowed after any previous test involving breathing O_2)
Inspired volume	>90% of largest measured vital capacity
Alveolar volume	Method should be stated. (VA,eff should always be calculated)
Washout volume	0.75–1.0 l (0.5 l if VC≤2 l)
Sample volume	0.5–1.0 l collected over <3 s into bag of volume ≤1 l
Time of inspiration	Normally <2.5 s; up to 4 s if there is airflow limitation
Breath holding	9–11 s (subject should relax against shutter)
Time of sample collection	<3 s
Effective breath holding time	Should preferably allow for time of sample collection (Jones Meade method)
Number of tests	At least two which meet above criteria (the average is used)
Interval between tests	4 min with subject seated throughout
Gas analysis	Before the analysis CO_2 should be absorbed then water vapour. Analyses should be linear and accurate to ±1%, both inspirate and 'alveolar' sample should be analysed.

(Sources: American Thoracic Society. *Am Rev Respir Dis* 1987; **136**: 1299–1307; Cotes JE, Chinn DJ, Quanjer PhH *et al. Eur Respir J* 1993; **6**, suppl 16: 41–53.)

fractional concentration of carbon monoxide in the alveolar gas, t is time in minutes, and $F\bar{v}$ is the fractional concentration of carbon monoxide which would obtain in gas equilibrated with the mixed venous blood at the mean tension of oxygen in the alveolar capillaries. ($PB - PH_2O$) is the pressure of dry gas in the lung (kPa) and 22.4 is the volume in l STPD occupied by one mole of gas.

On rearrangement and integration this relationship becomes:

$$Tl,co = VA/22.4(PB - PH_2O) . 60/t$$
$$\times \log_e[(Fo - F\bar{v})/(Ft - F\bar{v})] \text{ mmol min}^{-1}\text{kPa}^{-1} \quad (10.7)$$

where t is now the time of breath holding in seconds and Fo and Ft are the fractional concentrations of carbon monoxide in the alveolar gas at the beginning and end of this period.

In practice it is convenient to express the alveolar volume in l BTPS, to use logarithms to base 10 instead of to base e and to assume a constant barometric pressure. On substitution of the appropriate conversion factors the relationship becomes:

$$Tl,co = bVA/t \times \log_{10}[(Fo - F\bar{v})/(Ft - F\bar{v})] \text{ mmol min}^{-1}\text{kPa}^{-1}$$
$$(10.8)$$

where V_A is now in l BTPS. The value of b is 53.6 ($b = (2.30 \times 60 \times 826)/(22.4 \times 0.133 \times (760 - 47))$ where 2.30 converts from $\log_e$ to $\log_{10}$, 60 from s to min and 826 from l BTPS to ml STPD. Alternatively, when it is intended to report the result in the traditional units ml min^{-1} mmHg^{-1} the value of b is 160 (i.e. $53.6 \times 22.4 \times 0.133$, see Table 2.4).

The fractional concentration of carbon monoxide in the alveolar gas at the start of breath holding (Fo) is obtained from the dilution of the helium by the following relationship:

$$Fo = F_{I,CO} \times F_{A,He}/F_{I,He} \qquad (10.9)$$

where Fo is the initial alveolar concentration and $F_{I,CO}$ is the concentration of carbon monoxide in the inspired gas. $F_{A,He}$ and $F_{I,He}$ are the concentrations of helium respectively in the alveolar and the inspired gas.

When breathing air, the back tension of carbon monoxide in the blood is small enough to be ignored. Equation 10.8 then simplifies to:

$$Tl,co = bV_A/t \times \log_{10} \left(\frac{F_{I,CO} \times F_{A,He}}{F_{A,CO} \times F_{I,He}} \right) \text{ mmol min}^{-1}\text{kPa}^{-1} \quad (10.10)$$

where $F_{A,CO}$ is the fractional concentration of carbon monoxide in the alveolar gas at the end of breath holding (i.e. Ft in equation 10.8) and the other symbols are as defined above.

The alveolar volume during breath holding (V_A) is volume inspired (corrected to BTPS), plus residual volume obtained by an independent method (page 149). Effective alveolar volume is given by:

$$V_A,\text{eff} = (V_I - V_{ID}) \times F_{I,He}/F_{A,He} \text{ l BTPS} \qquad (10.11)$$

where V_A,eff is the effective alveolar volume, V_I is the volume of gas inspired in l BTPS, V_{ID} is the sum of the anatomical deadspace and the deadspace of the recording apparatus in l; other symbols are as defined above. The term within the bracket is the volume of inspired gas which enters the alveoli. The right hand term is the ratio of the concentrations of helium in the inspired and the alveolar gas; the latter should be corrected for any absorption of CO_2 prior to analysis (page 305) and for the deadspace of the sampling bag. A value is assumed for the anatomical deadspace; when expressed in ml it is approximately equal to the sum of the subject's age in years and body weight in pounds (kg $\times$ 2.2). Alternatively in adults a value of 0.15 l can be used instead. The instrument deadspace is obtained from its dimensions or by water displacement.

The time of breath holding is obtained from the kymograph record as described under procedure above and illustrated in Fig. 10.3.

Some procedural faults to be avoided when making the measurement are illustrated in Fig. 4.1 on page 80. Common errors in gas analysis are given in Table 10.3. With careful attention to these aspects and to those in Table 10.2 (page 309), the coefficient of variation of a single measurement of transfer factor or of Kco, including the within day and

Table 10.3 Common sources of error in gas analysis

Gas	Method	Common fault	Feature*
Oxygen	Paramagnetic	Cell mis-aligned	Zero error
Helium	Katharometer	Neglect of O_2 effect	Proportional error
Carbon monoxide	Infrared	Detector leaking	Alinearity

* Illustrated in Fig. 3.10, page 53. The errors can be avoided using a three point calibration when 1% accuracy is achievable.
(Source: Chinn DJ, Naruse Y, Cotes JE. *Thorax* 1986; **41**: 133–137.)

the between day variability (page 67) is approximately 5%; that of the single breath alveolar volume is approximately 3%. The corresponding reproducibilities for Dm and Vc, when analysed in the reciprocal form in which they are derived (page 313), are approximately 8%. These reproducibilities are reduced by the factor $1/\sqrt{2}$ when the determinations are made in duplicate.

REBREATHING METHOD (Tl,co.rb)

The procedure of rebreathing promotes mixing of gas in the lung and on this account, the method is increasingly being used for assessment of patients with uneven lung function. To achieve reasonable accuracy the rebreathing manoeuvre should be performed vigorously but this is beyond the ability of some patients. Feeble rebreathing can be used to obtain an approximate result in patients whose vital capacity is reduced below the level of 1.5 l required for the single breath method. The procedure resembles the single breath method in most respects except that rebreathing replaces breath holding. The inspired carbon monoxide concentration is usually 0.1%. The rebreathing bag initially contains a volume of gas equal to the subject's FEV_1. The subject is connected to it after a forced expiration and rebreathes for a period of 30–45 s at a frequency of $30\,min^{-1}$. The bag should empty with each inspiration. The contained gas is sampled continuously by a pump which circulates the gas through the analysers in the manner described. The change in concentration of the carbon monoxide in the bag is plotted on a semi-log scale against the time from the start of the rebreathing; the curve which is obtained resembles that for nitrogen in Fig. 8.5 (page 224); the linear part of the record is used for the calculation. This is performed using a version of equation 10.8:

$$Tl,co = b(VRV + Vbag)/(t_2 - t_1)$$
$$\times \log_{10}[(F_1,co - F\bar{v},co)/(F_2,co - F\bar{v},co)] \quad (10.12)$$

where VRV and $Vbag$ are the volumes of gas in l BTPS respectively in the residual volume of the lungs and in the bag at the start of the rebreathing procedure. The subscripts 1 and 2 refer to two points in time on the linear part of the exponential decay curve (cf. Fig. 8.5). The term in the left hand parentheses is the volume of gas from which carbon monoxide is absorbed during rebreathing; the assumption is made that it is also the effective alveolar volume. The volume is calculated from the dilution in the lung of helium present in the test gas mixture. This is done using a version of equation 10.11:

$$(V_{RV} + V_{bag}) = V_{bag} \times F_{I,He}/F_{A,He} \text{ l BTPS} \qquad (10.13)$$

where $F_{I,He}$ and $F_{A,He}$ are the fractional concentrations of helium in the bag before and at the end of the period of rebreathing; the latter is corrected for the absorption of carbon dioxide in the manner indicated on page 305. The method gives results which are significantly correlated with those by the single breath method but are systematically lower; this is mainly due to the measurement being made at a smaller lung volume, but other factors, including the recirculation of blood through the lungs during the rebreathing, also contribute to the difference.

ALLOWANCE FOR THE EFFECTS OF HAEMOGLOBIN
CONCENTRATION AND CAPILLARY OXYGEN TENSION

The transfer factor is determined by the diffusing capacity of the alveolar membrane (Dm), the volume of blood in the alveolar capillaries (Vc) and the reaction rate of carbon monoxide with oxyhaemoglobin (θ). The latter in turn is dependent on the haemoglobin concentration and on the tension of oxygen in the alveolar capillaries. These variables affect the transfer factor according to the following relationship which is based on equation 9.13 (page 277) and further amplified on page 316 below:

$$\frac{1}{Tl} = \frac{1}{Dm} + \frac{1}{\theta'[Hb]Vc} \text{ kPa mmol}^{-1} \text{min} \qquad (10.14)$$

where θ' is the reaction rate at the average normal concentration for haemoglobin monomer of 9 mmol l^{-1} (14.6 g dl^{-1}) and $[Hb]$ is the haemoglobin concentration as a fraction of normal. The units of the other variables are given on page 275. A material deviation of the haemoglobin concentration or of the oxygen tension from its normal level can lead to error in the interpretation of the transfer factor unless an appropriate allowance is made. This is best done by reporting the result adjusted to a concentration of haemoglobin of 9 mmol l^{-1} (14.6 g dl^{-1}) and an oxygen tension of 14.7 kPa (110 mmHg) for which the corresponding value for θ (θs) can be obtained using equation 10.19 and Table 10.4. When Dm and Vc are measured in the manner which is described below the transfer factor under standard conditions (Tl,s) can be obtained using equation 10.14 by substituting θs for $\theta'[Hb]$. Alternatively, when the transfer factor is measured at an oxygen tension of approximately 14.7 kPa but no data are available for Dm and Vc the correction is made using a version of the same equation:

$$Tl,s = Tl,obs(a + \theta s[Hb]) \div (a + \theta s).[Hb] \qquad (10.15)$$

where Tl,obs is the transfer factor at the subject's own haemoglobin concentration, θs and $[Hb]$ are defined above and a is the ratio

Dm/Vc. This ratio is determined in part by the numerical values chosen for the reaction rate of carbon monoxide with oxyhaemoglobin which is described below; a *Dm/Vc* ratio in SI units (mmol, kPa, min and l) of 230 and in traditional units (ml, min and mmHg) of 0.7 has been found empirically to provide a valid correction. Using the more recently determined value for θ given in Table 10.4, the ratio is larger and hence the predicted change in transfer factor with haemoglobin concentration is slightly increased.

MEASUREMENT OF THE DIFFUSING CAPACITY OF THE ALVEOLAR MEMBRANE AND THE VOLUME OF BLOOD IN THE ALVEOLAR CAPILLARIES

The procedure for the measurement of the diffusing capacity of the alveolar membrane (*Dm*) and the volume of blood in the alveolar capillaries (*Vc*) is based on their relationship to the transfer factor which is referred to above:

$$\frac{1}{Tl} = \frac{1}{Dm} + \frac{1}{\theta Vc} \text{ kPa mmol}^{-1} \text{ min} \tag{9.13}$$

Tl can be estimated by the method just described and values for θ can be determined independently, leaving two unknowns in this equation. If two equations can be drawn up (using different values for θ) then the two unknowns, *Dm* and *Vc* can be calculated.

The method of Roughton and Forster makes use of the fact that the reaction rate of carbon monoxide with oxyhaemoglobin (θ) varies inversely with the tension of oxygen. The transfer factor is measured at two levels of alveolar oxygen tension, the levels normally being near to those which obtain during breathing air and breathing oxygen. The corresponding values for the reaction rate (θco) are then obtained in the manner which is described on page 316 below. This procedure yields two values each for *Tl* and θco which when substituted in equation 9.13 provides two simultaneous equations; these are solved for *Dm* and *Vc*. A graphical solution is illustrated in Fig. 10.4.

The transfer factor when breathing air is calculated by use of equation 10.10 in which the back tension is neglected. When breathing oxygen, in order to make allowance for the high back tension due to dissociation of carboxyhaemoglobin (page 290), equation 10.8 is used instead. The following procedure is recommended:

1 The subject breathes oxygen for 5 min in order to raise the tension of oxygen in the alveolar gas. The back tension of carbon monoxide in the circulating blood is then determined. To this end the airway is switched to a bag containing 5 l of oxygen which is connected to the mouthpiece through a canister of soda lime for absorbing carbon dioxide. The subject rebreathes from the bag for a period of 4 min. By the end of this time almost complete gaseous equilibrium for carbon monoxide has been attained between the bag and the alveoli where the tension is that exerted by the carboxyhaemoglobin in the alveolar capillaries.

313

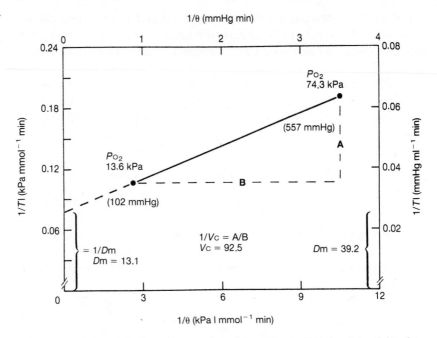

Fig. 10.4 Graphical solution to the equation $1/Tl = 1/Dm + 1/\theta Vc$ for determining the diffusing capacity of the alveolar capillary membrane and the volume of blood in the alveolar capillaries. The reciprocal of the transfer factor (diffusing capacity) for the lung $(1/Tl)$ is plotted against the reciprocal of the reaction rate $(1/\theta)$. The slope of the line is then the reciprocal of the volume of blood in the alveolar capillaries $(1/Vc)$ and the intercept is the reciprocal of the diffusing capacity of the alveolar capillary membrane $(1/Dm)$. Vc is here given in traditional units (ml). In SI units it is in l.

The gas in the bag is analysed for oxygen and carbon monoxide. From these data the tension of carbon monoxide exerted by the dissociation of carboxyhaemoglobin at any tension of oxygen can be calculated by use of the following relationship:

$$Pco = Po_2 \times Fco/Fo_2 \text{ kPa} \qquad (10.16)$$

where Pco is the tension of carbon monoxide exerted by carboxyhaemoglobin at an oxygen tension of Po_2 kPa; Fco and Fo_2 are the fractional concentrations respectively of carbon monoxide and oxygen in the gas sample. Alternatively the back tension can be obtained via the dissociation curve after direct measurement of the saturation of carboxyhaemoglobin using a CO-oximeter.

2 The transfer factor (diffusing capacity) for the lung is determined in the usual way except that the gas to be inhaled is made up in oxygen instead of air. The alveolar sample which is collected is analysed for oxygen as well as for helium and carbon monoxide. The back tension of carbon monoxide exerted by carboxyhaemoglobin at this tension of oxygen is then calculated by use of equation 10.16. From these and other data the transfer factor breathing oxygen is calculated by use of equations 10.8 and 10.9.

3 The subject breathes air for 10 min to flush the remains of the
previous inspiration from the lungs; the measurement of the transfer
factor is then repeated using the normal gas mixture in which the
helium and carbon monoxide are made up in oxygen at the fractional
concentration 0.17 with the remainder nitrogen. The alveolar sample
which is obtained is similarly analysed for oxygen as well as the other
gases and the corresponding transfer factor is calculated by use of
equation 10.10.

Measurement of
Dm and Vc

4 The values for the transfer factor at the two tensions of oxygen are
used to calculate the diffusing capacity of the alveolar capillary membrane and the volume of blood in the alveolar capillaries. This may be
done graphically as in Fig. 10.4, or by use of the following relationships:

$$Vc = \frac{\beta(P_1 - P_2)}{[Hb] \times (1/Tl_1 - 1/Tl_2)} \qquad (10.17)$$

$$Dm = \frac{1/\theta_1 - 1/\theta_2}{(1/\theta_1 \times 1/Tl_2) - (1/\theta_2 \times 1/Tl_1)} \qquad (10.18)$$

where, in SI or traditional units, Dm is the diffusing capacity of the
alveolar capillary membrane, Vc is the volume of blood in the alveolar
capillaries; [Hb] is the haemoglobin concentration as a fraction of
normal and β is defined overleaf; Tl_1 and Tl_2 are values for the transfer
factor for carbon monoxide measured using the gas mixtures made up
respectively with oxygen and with air; P_1 and P_2 are the corresponding
alveolar oxygen tensions in kPa or mmHg; θ_1 and θ_2 are the reaction
rates of carbon monoxide with oxyhaemoglobin which obtain in these
circumstances. An equation for the derivation of θ is given below,
together with an expanded version of equation 10.18 in which the
equation for θ is incorporated.

Comment

The procedure of Roughton and Forster for partitioning $1/Tl$ has been
used successfully to explore the effects of disease and other interventions
and has yielded intuitively sensible results (page 294). However, the
method is based on a number of assumptions of which some are, at
best, only approximately correct. The assumptions include that the
haematocrit is identical in pulmonary capillary and systemic venous
blood, the values for θco are identical in a rapid reaction apparatus
(see next section) and the pulmonary capillary blood and the derived
indices (Dm and Vc) are independent of the oxygen tension and
haemoglobin concentration. The effects of variations in one or more of
these relationships are currently being explored. That associated with
oxygen acting on the pulmonary circulation can be avoided by concurrent measurement of Tl,co and Tl,no. The latter measurement is
described on page 317.

The reaction of carbon monoxide with partially oxygenated blood is described by the following relationship:

$$Hb_4\,(O_2)_3 + CO \xrightarrow{l'4} Hb_4\,(O_2)_3\,CO$$

where the haemoglobin reactant has three of its four binding sites occupied by molecular oxygen, $l'4$ is the bimolecular reaction velocity constant for the binding of carbon monoxide to the fourth position on the haemoglobin molecule in the units $mmol\,l^{-1}s^{-1}$. The velocity constant is related to the reaction rate of carbon monoxide with blood (θco); this was first reported by Roughton and Forster in the units ml per min per mmHg per ml of blood containing haemoglobin at the average concentration of $14.6\,g\,dl^{-1}$. In SI units and making allowance for any haemoglobin which is already combined with carbon monoxide the reaction rate (θco) can be described by the following relationship:

$$\frac{1}{\theta co} = (\alpha + \beta P\bar{c},o_2) \div [Hb](1 - Sc,co/100)kPa\,mmol^{-1}\,min \quad (10.19)$$

where $P\bar{c},o_2$ is the mean tension of oxygen in plasma in the alveolar capillaries in kPa, [Hb] is the concentration of haemoglobin in blood as a fraction of normal and Sc,co is the mean percentage saturation of haemoglobin with carbon monoxide; the latter term, which is due to Meade, is only important after some carbon monoxide has been inhaled.

The parameters α and β, i.e. the coefficient terms, have been measured *in vitro* by the rapid mixing of suspensions of human red cells and carbon monoxide in solution. The procedure is technically difficult so only a few determinations have been made. The results for four subjects reported in 1957 and for five reported briefly in 1983, are given in Table 10.4. The latter determinations were made at physiological carbon monoxide tensions and appear to be the more reliable. They can be inserted into equation 10.19 for the derivation of θco at any level of $P\bar{c},o_2$. The latter term is obtained from a version of equation 10.25 (page 319) using measured or estimated values for the tension of oxygen in the alveoli, the consumption of oxygen and the diffusing

Table 10.4 Parameters of equation 10.19 relating θco to $P\bar{c},o_2$ for human blood at 37°C

	α		$\beta \times 10^{-3}$	
	SI	Traditional	SI	Traditional
Roughton and Forster (1957)*	$(1-3) \times 10^{-3}$	0.34–1.0	0.134	6.1
Forster (1987)	3.9×10^{-3}	1.30	0.09	4.1

* The range for α reflects different assumptions about the permeability of the red cell membrane. The lower values were used for estimating the effect of haemoglobin concentration upon *T*lco (page 312) and for deriving the reference values given in Chapter 15.

capacity of the alveolar capillary membrane for oxygen (Dm,o_2); the latter is linked to the Dm,co through their respective diffusivities (Table 9.3, page 272). Then on rearrangement:

$$P\bar{c},o_2 = PA,o_2 - 0.83 \, \dot{n}o_2/Dm,co \text{ kPa} \qquad (10.20)$$

where PA,o_2 is the mean tension of oxygen in the alveolar gas in kPa, Dm,co is the diffusing capacity of the alveolar capillary membrane for carbon monoxide in $\text{mmol min}^{-1}\text{kPa}^{-1}$, $\dot{n}o_2$ is the uptake of oxygen in mmol min^{-1} and 0.83 is the diffusivity of carbon monoxide relative to that for oxygen. When θ is obtained using pencil and paper it is convenient to substitute for Dm in equation 10.20 an estimate which is a multiple of the transfer factor breathing air. On the basis of the Roughton and Forster values for α and β the multiplier was thought to be approximately 1.5, but a value in the range 3−5 is more likely to be correct (see above). Alternatively, when the calculation is performed using a digital computer the equations 10.19 and 10.20 can be incorporated into that for the calculation of the diffusing capacity of the alveolar capillary membrane (equation 10.18). Then in SI units:

$$Dm = \frac{Tl_1 \times Tl_2 \times (P_1 - P_2) - 0.83\dot{n}o_2(Tl_2 - Tl_1)}{Tl_1 \times P_1 - Tl_2 \times P_2 - \alpha/\beta \times (Tl_2 - Tl_1)} \text{ mmol min}^{-1}\text{kPa}^{-1}$$

$$(10.21)$$

In traditional units the equation is the same except for the substitution of $\dot{n}o_2$ by $\dot{V}o_2$ (ml min^{-1}).

Comment

The 1987 values for α and β yield results for the volume of blood in the alveolar capillaries (Vc) that are 1−20% lower than those obtained using the 1957 values; the associated values for Dm are materially higher than those reported previously. If confirmed these observations indicate that the alveolar capillary membrane offers a minimal barrier to gas transfer compared to the diffusive resistance of the blood and the resistance of the chemical reaction of carbon monoxide with oxyhaemoglobin. The findings reduce the impact of measurements of Dm and Vc in disease since they suggest that Vc is the main determinant of Tl. If the new parameters are correct the reference values for Dm (Chapter 15) and the values for Dm used to calculate Table 9.1 and Fig. 9.4 would also alter. However, the reference values for Vc would not change to a material extent.

Transfer factor for nitric oxide

Background

Nitric oxide combines rapidly with haemoglobin and the compound so formed dissociates very slowly (Table 10.5). The reaction is not influenced by oxygen tension. These properties appear to be optimal for

Table 10.5 Some features of oxygen, carbon monoxide and nitric oxide which are relevant to gas exchange

	Molecular weight	Solubility at 37°C s	Rate of diffusion (a)	$P\bar{v}$ (kPa) (b)	$P50$ (kPa) (c)	Combination velocity (d)
O_2	32	0.024	1.0	5.3	3.5	47
CO	28	0.018	0.83	$(2-100) \times 10^{-4}$	1.5×10^{-3}	0.9
NO	30	0.041	1.76	8×10^{-7}	3.9×10^{-7}	255

(a) Rate relative to oxygen (from Table 9.3, page 272).
(b) Mixed venous tension at rest; range for CO includes smokers.
(c) Tension for 50% saturation reflects affinity for haemoglobin.
(d) With haemoglobin in solution (units $M^{-1}s^{-1} \times 10^{-5}$, cited by Meyer and colleagues).

measuring the diffusing capacity of the alveolar capillary membrane independent of blood flow and the reaction with haemoglobin. However, recent work suggests that diffusion within the blood could contribute to the result as could any reaction of nitric oxide with lung tissue if this were to take place. Nitric oxide also has other properties (page 203) but in low concentration can be used for measurement of transfer factor (Tl,NO) provided that only a short breath holding time is used (see below). The method was introduced by Borland and Higenbottam and developed by Piiper and his colleagues including Meyer amongst others.

Method

The methods which are available resemble those for carbon monoxide which have already been described. They are constrained by the possible biological and chemical reactivity of all but very low concentrations of nitric oxide; such concentrations can be analysed by a chemiluminescent method in which ozone is used to oxidise nitric oxide to nitrogen dioxide and photons of light; the latter are detected and quantified via a photomultiplier. The instrument can be used in conjunction with a single breath procedure similar to that used with carbon monoxide (page 304). The inspired concentration of NO is in the range 8–40 parts per million and the breath holding time in the range 3–8 s. At the present time measurements by the rebreathing method (page 311), can be made only in animal preparations. For this application relatively high concentrations of nitric oxide (e.g. 600 ppm) are analysed breath-by-breath using a respiratory mass spectrometer. The application of the rebreathing measurement to man must await the development of alternative detection systems sensitive to lower concentrations of test gas.

Values for Tl,NO and Tl,CO obtained during the same breath holding manoeuvre can be used to calculate Dm and Vc. To this end equation 9.13 is solved simultaneously for the two gases using appropriate values for Dm,NO $/Dm$,CO (approximately 2.0 from Table 10.5), θCO (from Table 10.4) and θ_{NO}; the latter has been given the value $1.5 \times 10^3\,\mathrm{mmol\,min^{-1}\,kPa^{-1}\,l^{-1}}$ by Borland. Then:

$$1/Tl,\mathrm{co} = 1/Dm,\mathrm{co} + 1/\theta\mathrm{co}.Vc \qquad (9.13)$$

$$1/Tl,\mathrm{NO} = 1/(2Dm,\mathrm{co}) + 1/\theta\mathrm{NO}.Vc \qquad (10.22)$$

from which it follows that:

$$Dm,\mathrm{co} = (\theta\mathrm{NO} - 2\theta\mathrm{co})/(\theta\mathrm{NO}/Tl,\mathrm{NO} - \theta\mathrm{co}/Tl,\mathrm{co}) \qquad (10.23)$$

$$Vc = 1/(\theta\mathrm{co}/Tl,\mathrm{co} - \theta\mathrm{co}/Dm,\mathrm{co}) \qquad (10.24)$$

Comment

The transfer factor for nitric oxide differs from that for carbon monoxide in a number of respects (Table 9.4, page 278). These lead to the proportion of the transfer factor which is represented by the membrane diffusing capacity being higher for nitric oxide than for carbon monoxide; the proportions have been estimated by Borland and Cox as respectively 40% and 18%. Thus even for nitric oxide the main constituent of the transfer factor is the diffusive resistance of the blood. Hence Tl,NO and Dm,NO are not interchangeable. The ratio $Tl,\mathrm{NO}/Tl,\mathrm{co}$ differs from $Tl,\mathrm{o_2}/Tl,\mathrm{co}$ (page 322) in apparently having a wide range (approximately 3–5) but whether the cause is technical or biological has still to be established. An early use for Tl,NO may be in the estimation of Dm and Vc since the method, which is summarised above, is not invalid in circumstances when oxygen exerts a pharmacological effect on the pulmonary circulation. Only one single breath manoeuvre is required so there is no error due to variation between two breaths as can occur with the original procedure.

Transfer factor for oxygen

METHOD OF RILEY AND LILIENTHAL

By this method the transfer factor or diffusing capacity for the lung for oxygen is obtained from the following relationship:

$$Tl,\mathrm{o_2} = \dot{n}\mathrm{o_2} \quad \text{or} \quad \dot{V}\mathrm{o_2}/(P_{A,\mathrm{o_2}} - P\bar{c},\mathrm{o_2}) \qquad (10.25)$$

where $Tl,\mathrm{o_2}$ is the transfer factor for the lung for oxygen, $\dot{n}\mathrm{o_2}$ or $\dot{V}\mathrm{o_2}$ is consumption of oxygen per min, $P_{A,\mathrm{o_2}}$ is the tension of oxygen in the alveolar gas and $P\bar{c},\mathrm{o_2}$ is the tension which under equilibrium conditions would be associated with the mean saturation of oxyhaemoglobin in the alveolar capillaries; the term within the parentheses is therefore the mean transfer gradient.

Procedure

The data required for the calculations are obtained during two periods of steady state exercise performed with the subject breathing respectively air and a hypoxic gas mixture (fractional concentration of oxygen usually 0.12). Mixed expired gas is collected during the 4th to 6th min, the volume and compositions are obtained by analysis and used to calculate the consumption of oxygen and respiratory exchange ratio (page 35). Arterial blood is sampled and the tensions of oxygen and carbon dioxide are obtained by analysis (page 43). The respiratory exchange ratio and the arterial carbon dioxide tension are inserted into the alveolar air equation for calculation of mean alveolar oxygen tension (page 252). Alternatively, at the cost of some loss of accuracy the P_{A,O_2} can be obtained by analysis of end tidal gas using a respiratory mass spectrometer or other rapid analyser for oxygen. When this is done the arterial oxygen tension is obtained via the oxygen dissociation curve from the arterial oxygen saturation measured using an ear oximeter (page 40).

Calculations

The consumption of oxygen and the tension of oxygen in alveolar gas are obtained in the manner described above. The mean tension of oxygen in the alveolar capillaries cannot be determined directly. Instead it is obtained by integration in the manner first described by Bohr. For this purpose, values are calculated for the tension of oxygen down the length of the capillary from estimates of tension at the two ends; a mean value is then obtained by integration. The integration is over a range of oxygen tensions which for convenience should lie in the linear part of the oxygen dissociation curve; this is usually achieved with an inspired oxygen concentration of 0.12. Use is then made of Piiper's equation:

$$Tl_{,O_2} = \frac{\dot{n}o_2 \text{ or } \dot{V}o_2}{Pc'_{,O_2} - P\bar{v}_{,O_2}} \log_e \frac{P_{A,O_2} - P\bar{v}_{,O_2}}{P_{A,O_2} - Pc'_{,O_2}} \qquad (10.26)$$

where $P\bar{v}_{,O_2}$, $Pc'_{,O_2}$ and P_{A,O_2} are respectively the tensions of oxygen in the blood entering and leaving the alveolar capillaries and in the alveolar gas. The tension of oxygen in the blood entering the alveolar capillaries is that of the mixed venous blood; the tension at the end of the capillary is obtained by a process of trial and error which was developed by Lilienthal and Riley. The method requires the measurement of the difference in the tension of oxygen between the alveolar gas and the arterial blood during normoxia and during hypoxia. The difference is partitioned into two compartments as follows:

$$(P_{a,O_2} - P_{a,O_2}) = (P_{A,O_2} - Pc'_{,O_2}) + (Pc'_{,O_2} - P_{a,O_2}) \qquad (10.27)$$

where $Pc'_{,O_2}$ and P_{a,O_2} are respectively the tensions of oxygen in the blood leaving the alveolar capillaries and the left ventricle. The left-hand term is then the A$-$a difference, the middle term is the diffusion gradient between the alveolar gas and the blood leaving the alveolar capillaries and the right hand term is the component due to the venous admixture effect.

The partitioning is done first for data obtained when the subject is breathing air, by assuming a value (usually 0.1 kPa or 1 mmHg) for the diffusion gradient; this permits calculation of Pc',o_2 by subtraction and hence of the venous admixture effect by use of equation 8.34. The same venous admixture is then applied to calculate the end-capillary oxygen tension (Pc',o_2) during hypoxaemia. The end-capillary tension so obtained is fed into the integration procedure for calculating the mean tension of oxygen in the pulmonary capillary blood; this, in turn, is substituted in equation 10.25 in order to calculate the diffusing capacity of the lung for oxygen. The value assumed for the diffusion gradient at the point where the blood leaves the alveolar capillaries when the subject is breathing air is next examined to find out if it is consistent with the diffusing capacity which is calculated from it. If this is not the case an alternative value is assumed and the process is repeated, until by trial and error, values are obtained which are mutually consistent.

Comment

The reproducibility of the method is surprisingly good considering the complexity of the procedure. This is a consequence of the shape of the dissociation curve by which when breathing air, the greater part of the tension difference for oxygen between the alveolar gas and the arterial blood can be attributed to uneven distribution of lung ventilation and perfusion; this component of the A−a difference is relatively independent of the value assumed for the diffusion gradient. By contrast, when breathing gas deficient in oxygen, most of the A−a difference is due to the diffusion gradient; the error which arises from incorrect estimation of the component due to venous admixture is then relatively small. However, despite their good reproducibility the results can be misleading on account of the underlying assumptions being in error. Thus:

1 When the spread of the ventilation−perfusion ratios is increased the alveolar air equation does not provide a correct estimate of the tension of oxygen in the alveolar gas (page 192).
2 The venous admixture effect which is needed for the calculation is that during breathing gas deficient in oxygen; this may differ from the value actually used which is measured during breathing air (page 200).
3 The Bohr integration as normally performed requires that blood shall flow at a uniform rate along the alveolar capillaries; however, there is now good evidence that the flow is pulsatile (page 247).
4 The reaction rate should be constant along the length of the alveolar capillaries; this is probably the case when the arterial oxygen saturation is lower than 90% but the numerical value for the transfer factor which is obtained under these conditions may then not relate to breathing air.

The errors which are introduced by the lung not behaving in an ideal way are now known to largely cancel out. On this account the values for Tlo_2 which are obtained during exercise are only slightly less than those obtained by other methods. This is not the case at rest when the values obtained using the single compartment model are materially lower. In this instance the difference is probably not technical but due to the distribution of the gas exchanging characteristic $Tl/\dot{Q}c$ being less uniform at rest than it is on exercise. These aspects have been investigated by Haab, Piiper, Wagner and West and their respective colleagues whose studies demonstrate the fundamental importance of the measurement. Unfortunately, it remains unsuitable for routine use.

DERIVATION FROM Tl,CO

The transfer factor for oxygen would be expected to exceed that for carbon monoxide on account of the gases differing in their diffusivity and rates of reaction with haemoglobin (Table 10.5, page 318). These differences can be allowed for by substitution into equation 9.13 (page 277) of the appropriate conversion factors:

$$\frac{1}{Tl,o_2} = \frac{1}{1.23\ Dm,\text{CO}} + \frac{1}{\theta o_2 Vc} \tag{10.28}$$

where 1.23 is the rate of diffusion of oxygen relative to that for carbon monoxide and θo_2 is the reaction rate for oxygen with reduced haemoglobin; the latter varies with oxygen tension but can be allocated the value obtained by Staub and his colleagues of $0.9\ \text{mmol min}^{-1}\,\text{kPa}^{-1}$ ($2.73\ \text{vol/vol min}^{-1}\,\text{mmHg}^{-1}$). A slightly higher rate has been found by Yamaguchi and colleagues. However, a lower rate may be more appropriate. Part of the discrepancy appears to be due to the measurement being greatly influenced by the conditions under which it is obtained.

The derived value for Tl,o_2 is that for the conditions of measurement of Tl,CO and they need to be appropriate for the particular application. If steady state conditions are of interest the Tl,CO should be measured by the steady state method. The accuracy of the method has been validated empirically by concurrent measurements using carbon monoxide and an isotope of oxygen; these studies have shown that the theoretical conversion factor of 1.23 does apply in practice. However, the model used for the derivation assumes that the lung function is homogeneous which is not necessarily the case.

ESTIMATION FROM $\dot{V}A/\dot{Q}$ DISTRIBUTIONS

Background

The multiple inert gas elimination technique describes the distribution of pulmonary ventilation and perfusion in terms of 50 compartments having ventilation−perfusion ratios which range from zero to infinity. The distribution is independent of diffusion because the test gases all achieve gaseous equilibrium in which the tensions in the alveoli and in blood leaving the alveolar capillaries are equal. During exercise under hypoxic conditions this is not the case for oxygen (page 285). Instead

the end capillary tension is less than the alveolar tension both for the
lung as a whole and for the individual compartments. The tension
difference for the whole lung is used in the method of Riley and
Lilienthal. A more accurate estimate of Tl,o_2 can be obtained by
weighting the diffusing characteristics of the compartments according
to their blood flow; this is done by assuming that the ratio $D/\dot{Q}\beta$
is constant for all compartments, where D is diffusing capacity, $\dot{Q}$ is
blood flow and β is the whole blood capacitance coefficient for oxygen
(page 272). In hypoxia β is assumed to be constant.*

For any compartment the end capillary oxygen tension gradient is
calculated making the assumption that the process of equilibration is
exponential, then for compartment j:

$$(P_{Aj} - P_{c'j}) = (P_{Aj} - P\bar{v})e^{-D/\dot{Q}\beta} \qquad (10.29)$$

where the terms within the parentheses are, on the left the end capillary
oxygen tension gradient and, on the right the transfer gradient. The
exponent is defined above. This approach is due to Piiper.

Method

The subject is prepared by the insertion of systemic arterial and peripheral venous catheters and the application of sternal electrodes for
electrocardiography. A thermistor for measurement of temperature in
the lung parenchyma is placed in the lower oesophagus or a Swan-
Ganz catheter sited in the pulmonary artery. The procedure is then
carried out during the 6th to 8th minutes of exercise with the subject
breathing a hypoxic gas mixture (e.g. $F,o_2 = 0.11$). Measurements are
made of ventilation, gas exchange, the arterial blood gas tensions,
blood pH, haemoglobin concentration, haematocrit and deep body
temperature. Inert gases are infused and sampled using the multiple
inert gas elimination technique (page 255). Cardiac output is also
obtained from the inert gas measurements and used with the oxygen
uptake and the arterial oxygen content to calculate the mixed venous
oxygen tension by the mass balance equation (equation 8.11, page 239).
Alternatively, the latter tension is obtained by analysis of mixed venous
blood sampled via the Swan-Ganz catheter.

Calculation

The distributions of ventilation and perfusion are obtained by the
procedure of West (page 255). These are used to calculate the oxygen
and carbon dioxide tensions in blood leaving each compartment and
hence the oxygen tension in mixed pulmonary venous blood. If the
model is correct the calculated tension should be equal to the measured
arterial oxygen tension.

* β for oxygen is given by $(Ca,o_2 - C\bar{v},o_2)/(Pa,o_2 - P\bar{v},o_2)$ which is the slope of the
oxygen dissociation curve (Fig. 9.3, page 280). The quantity is different from that for
plasma which is given in Table 9.3 (page 272).

Initially the computation is performed assuming equilibrium across the alveolar capillary membrane. The compartmental end capillary oxygen tensions are then those calculated for the gas compartments. Subsequently the calculations are repeated using equation 10.29 with different values of $D(Tl,o_2)$ in order to simulate the effect of different degrees of diffusion limitation. The *in vivo* Tl,o_2 is assumed to be that at which the calculated and measured arterial oxygen tensions are equal.

Comment

The procedures and calculations are formidable but in a dedicated laboratory they can now be carried out semi-automatically using analysers which are connected on line to a suitably programmed computer. The method has been developed by West, Wagner, Gale and others. The resulting values for Tl,o_2 provide a standard with which the results by other methods can be compared (e.g. page 321). The maximal values come close to those predicted by Weibel and colleagues based on morphometric measurements.

Guide to references

The references (Chapter 18) are classified under subject headings of which the following are particularly relevant to the present chapter:

11: Control of Respiration

Introduction

Breathing is regulated to maintain nearly constant the tensions of oxygen and carbon dioxide and the concentration of hydrogen ions in arterial blood and cerebral extracellular fluid. The regulatory mechanisms operate over a wide range of levels of metabolism and altered acid−base balance, and during phonation, eating and drinking. Controlled changes in breathing form part of the homeostatic responses to many circumstances including hypoxaemia, hypercapnia, hyperthermia, pregnancy and diseases of the lungs and the cardiovascular system.

Breathing is controlled by the activity of networks of neurones in the medulla and pons. These respiratory centres initiate rhythmic contractions of the respiratory muscles, co-ordinate the responses to speech and swallowing and respond to sensory information from receptors in the lungs, carotid bodies and other parts of the brain. The motor pathway is via the spinal cord, the phrenic nerves, which innervate the diaphragm, and the nerves which supply the intercostal, abdominal and other respiratory muscles. Their action is influenced by the elastic recoil, resistance to movement and inertance of the lung and chest wall, all of which are monitored by receptors in the thorax. The activity of the respiratory centres can be overridden by spinal cord reflexes in response to local sensory inputs and by voluntary action emanating from higher centres in the brain.

Pattern of breathing

The respiratory control system determines the pattern of breathing and the lung volume from which it starts (i.e. functional residual capacity). The pattern embraces the volume−time profile of the entire breath of which the principal dimensions are the tidal volume and the separate durations of inspiration and expiration. These attributes exhibit slight

325

variation from breath to breath; the principal variable is the duration of inspiration, whilst at any level of ventilation the mean inspiratory flow rate is relatively constant. This is illustrated in Fig. 11.1 where flow rate is described by the slopes of the lines relating tidal volume to time of inspiration or expiration. The range of normal variation is represented by the thickened portions of the lines. An increase in minute volume is achieved by an increase in inspiratory and expiratory flow rates and by shortening of the time of expiration. The time of inspiration (t_I) is much less affected. Thus during moderate exercise or hypoxia t_I is at the resting level. However, t_I diminishes when tidal volume exceeds about half the vital capacity. The reduction is due to the Hering−Breuer inflation reflex which is described below. The duration of inspiration is also reduced during hyperthermia (page 338). With this exception the pattern of breathing during increased ventilation under steady state conditions is independent of the stimulus. The pattern can be summarised for the whole breath by the relationship of ventilation to tidal volume which is illustrated in Fig. 11.2. The constancy of the pattern is evidence for the different respiratory drives converging before they influence the central pattern generator. However, the constant pattern is not achieved immediately; instead the initial response varies depending on the stimulus. When this acts via the carotid chemo-

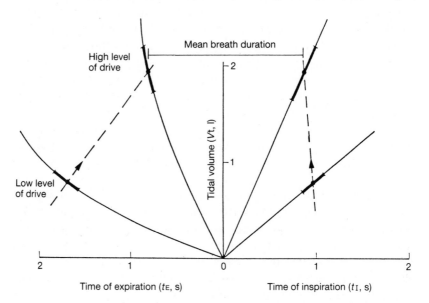

Fig. 11.1 Idealised relationship of the durations of inspiration and expiration to the tidal volume of healthy subjects during exercise and breathing mixtures of carbon dioxide in air. The two pairs of continuous lines are for low and high levels of drive with the thickened portions showing the mean values and the variation between breaths under steady state conditions. The arrows show the direction of change as the level of drive is increased: there is an increase in tidal volume and a reduction in the mean duration of each breath which is due mainly to shortening of expiration. In the circumstances indicated the time of inspiration is relatively constant but it is reduced by hyperthermia. (Source: Kay JDS, Petersen ES, Vejby-Christensen H. *J Physiol (Lond)* 1975; **521**: 657−669.)

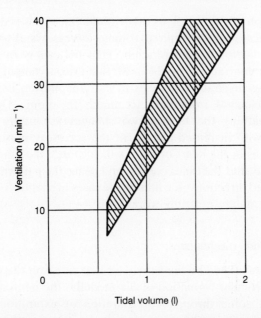

Fig. 11.2 Relationship of exercise ventilation to tidal volume in healthy adults of
European descent. For steady state conditions Hey and colleagues found the average
values of m and c to be respectively 28.3 (SD 5.7) and 0.32 (SD 0.13). The tidal volume
is also related to vital capacity (Fig. 15.30, page 509) and to ethnic group (Table 15.9,
page 473).

receptors the first response is usually a shortening of the time of
expiration (t_E) hence an increase in respiratory frequency. When the
stimulus acts via central chemoreceptors, for example while breathing
carbon dioxide in oxygen, the initial response is an increase in tidal
volume without much change in respiratory frequency. In this event
the apparent constancy of breath duration is due to converse changes
in its components: t_E decreases as might be expected but t_I increases.
The latter change is responsible for the initial increase in tidal volume.
The subject has been investigated by Gardner amongst others.

Inspiration is effected by contraction of inspiratory muscles and any
increase in flow rate is due to more rapid contractions. Expiration is
normally passive and results from the elastic recoil of the lung overcoming the thoracic resistance. The volume–time relationship during
passive expiration has been described by Brody as:

$$Vt_x = Vo \cdot e^{-t_x \cdot (RC)^{-1}} \qquad (11.1)$$

where Vt_x is volume at time t_x, Vo is volume at the start of expiration
and RC is the product of compliance and resistance which is the time
constant of the lung (page 183). In a normal adult at rest the time
constant is approximately 0.4 s (compliance $2.0 \, l \, kPa^{-1}$, thoracic resistance $0.2 \, kPa \, l^{-1} s$). A complete expiration will occupy approximately
four time constants or 1.6 s; this is somewhat less than is normally
observed at rest. The difference is due to expiration being slowed
down by contraction of the inspiratory muscles. Progressive shortening

327

of the duration of expiration as tidal volume increases is due to airway resistance decreasing as inspired volume increases and to progressive removal of constraints on expiration. Thus the calibre of the larynx is increased by contraction of the posterior cricoarytenoid muscle, the activity of the inspiratory muscles in early expiration is reduced and the subject changes from nose to mouth breathing. During nearly maximal breathing the former two changes are partly reversed in conjunction with increased activity of the accessory muscles of expiration. Diseases of the heart or lungs which change the lung compliance and resistance alter the time constant and hence the pattern of breathing in the expected directions (see illustrative cases in chapter 16). However, the mechanisms are not fully worked out.

Central nervous mechanisms

Breathing is regulated by the activity of nerve cells in the pons and the respiratory reticular formation of the medulla; the neurones discharge rhythmically, some throughout inspiration or expiration and others either early or late in the respiratory cycle including the change-over from inspiration to expiration and vice versa. They constitute a central pattern generator (CPG) which controls respiration through its action upon upper respiratory motor neurones in the medulla. However, the mechanism of rhythm generation remains unknown. The most comprehensive model is that of von Euler and colleagues which is presented in the following account. The starting point is the occurrence of sustained inspiratory activity or apneusis; this was first observed by Lumsden (1923). It occurs on blocking the vagi in decerebrate cats which have bilateral lesions of their 'pneumotaxic' centres (now called the nuclei parabrachialis medialis). The observation led to the concept that rhythm generation is due to modulation of central inspiratory activity by information from stretch receptors, chemoreceptors and other afferents. The model neglects the possibility that information from chemoreceptors could also contribute a direct tonic inspiratory drive to upper respiratory motor neurones; this has been suggested by Sears.

Functional anatomy

The nucleus of the tractus solitarius in the dorsomedial part of the medulla receives afferent fibres from the lungs and extrathoracic airways via the vagus nerves; the fibres make extensive connections within the nucleus particularly to its dorso- and ventrolateral parts. The dorsolateral subnuclei also receive afferent information from the chest wall and diaphragm via the contralateral dorsal columns of the spinal cord and the lateral funiculus. The ventrolateral subnuclei have a substantial innervation from neurones with an inspiratory rhythm located in the contralateral ventral medulla. Additional information from higher centres in the brain stem is received via corticofugal fibres and from carotid chemoreceptors via the glossopharyngeal nerves (Fig. 11.3).

328

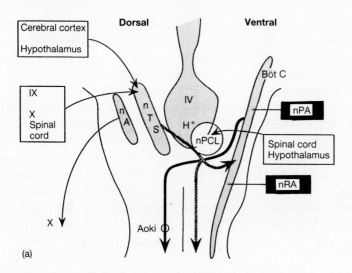

(a)

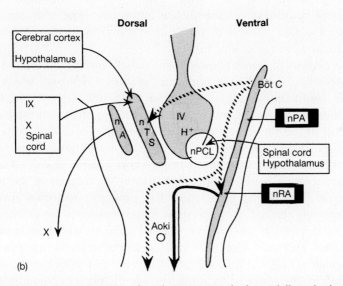

(b)

Fig. 11.3 Some inputs and outputs of respiratory centres in the medulla and spinal cord. In (a) the broad arrows indicate pathways which are active mainly during inspiration and in (b) those active during expiration. nA = nucleus ambiguus; nPCL = nucleus paragiganto cellularis lateralis; nPA = nucleus paraambigualis; nTS = nucleus of tractus solitarius; Böt C = Bötzinger complex; nRA = nucleus retroambigualis.

The nucleus of the tractus solitarius is rich in inspiration-related neurones. The Rα neurones of Baumgarten and Kanzow have a discharge pattern which resembles that of phrenic motor neurones; like them their activity is inhibited by activation of the inspiratory off-switch mechanism which is described below. Conversely the Rβ neurones are activated by lung inflation via stimuli from pulmonary stretch receptors. The neurones are connected with those which supply the external intercostal muscles which have an inspiratory function; in

329

addition they connect with other medullary neurones and with phrenic motor neurones in the spinal cord. The dorso-medial group of neurones also includes neurones which discharge early in expiration. The nucleus ambiguus contributes motor neurones which supply the laryngeal muscles via the vagi.

The majority of respiration-related neurones lie in a ventral column which in order from above downwards forms the Bötzinger complex, the nucleus paraambigualis, the nucleus retroambigualis, the nucleus retrofacialis and the Aoki group of inspiration-related relay neurones in the 1st and 2nd segments of the spinal cord. The nucleus retroambigualis contains mainly premotor neurones which make synaptic contacts with motor neurones in the spinal cord; the latter supply expiratory internal intercostal muscles. The bulbar expiration-related (E-R) neurones are active mainly towards the end of expiration especially when it is prolonged. They appear to be activated by E-R neurones in the Bötzinger complex. Other neurones from this region of the brain stem inhibit, during expiration, the inspiration-related activity of neurones from the nucleus ambigualis. The early expiratory neurones of the nucleus of the tractus solitarius in the dorsomedial group could have a similar function.

The nucleus paraambiguus contains mainly inspiration-related (I-R) premotor neurones. The majority are premotor neurones which cross to the contralateral side of the brain stem and activate the motor neurones of the phrenic nerve and inspiratory intercostal muscles. In the case of the intercostal motor neurones the activation is direct via bulbo-spinal pathways but in the case of the phrenics some of the premotor neurones are relayed in the Aoki centres described above. This innervation is in addition to that from the nucleus of the tractus solitarius. The discharge of most I-R premotor neurones increases progressively throughout inspiration. Other neurones are active at the start of inspiration; they make synaptic contact with and appear to inhibit the expiratory premotor neurones present in the nucleus retroambigualis. The early-burst I-R neurones may also modulate the activity of adjacent late-onset I-R neurones within the nucleus paraambigualis.

Central inspiratory activity

According to the von Euler hypothesis the drive to respiration is a continuous phenomenon which is inhibited periodically to allow expiration to take place in a mainly passive manner. There is no equivalent expiratory drive so the system is asymmetrical. The inspiratory activity originates in local neuronal circuits which do not give rise to peaks of electrical activity so are not readily identifiable. Their location is not known but it probably includes the nucleus paragiganto cellularis lateralis (nPCL) which is near to the nucleus retrofacialis in the ventral respiratory group of neurones. The nPCL adjoins the CO_2-sensitive region of the floor of the 4th ventricle and is connected to the nucleus of the tractus solaritarius which in turn receives brain stem inputs from peripheral chemoreceptors. It also has rich connections with other brain stem nuclei and with the spinal cord. Some of the neurones contain serotonin, catecholamines, and other pharmacologically active substances. Inactivation of the nucleus by local cooling has been shown to cause apnoea.

The central inspiratory activity increases in intensity with time during each inspiration then stops at the onset of expiration. The increase is believed to be due to progressive synaptic excitation and not to declining inhibition. The time profile as reflected by activity in the phrenic nerve resembles that of the volume change described in the preceding section. Both have a relatively linear profile but variable duration. The inspiratory activity is influenced by the level of central excitation; this is reduced by sleep, anaesthesia, sedative drugs and appropriate hypnotic suggestion. It is also reduced by hypoxia acting on the central nervous system in the manner described below. The central excitation is increased by exercise and by stimulant drugs. These differ in their specificity, from convulsant drugs which are nonspecific, to progesterone which appears to affect only the drive to inspiration (page 469). The intensity of inspiratory activity is also influenced by stimuli from chemoreceptors and sensory nerve endings. The strength of the stimulus influences the total phrenic discharge per unit time; the half time for the resulting inspiration is similar following stimulation from hypoxia (via the peripheral chemoreceptors), hypercapnia and exercise. The half time is reduced when the stimulus is hyperthermia which also changes the pattern of breathing (page 338).

Duration of inspiration

Inspiration is terminated by inhibition of the discharges from inspiratory premotor neurones. The inhibition arises within the brain stem but is modulated by afferent information of which the most important is that from the lungs and carotid body. In most laboratory animals the principal inspiratory off-switch mechanism is the *Hering–Breuer inflation reflex*. The stimulus is lung inflation which is detected by slowly adapting stretch receptors in the airways (page 88); the afferent signals are transmitted up the vagi and lead to inhibition of inspiration and prolongation of the subsequent expiration. The stimuli also lead to an increase and then, if they are continued, a decrease in the calibre of the larynx and trachea. A similar response follows an increase in intercostal muscle tension, which activates their tendon organs, but the relevance of the response to control of breathing in normal circumstances is not known. These response are modified by the action of J receptors (also called C fibre receptors) whose function is described on page 334.

The Hering–Breuer reflex is well developed in many mammals and in newborn babies. In adults the inhibition has a high threshold and is normally only demonstrable at tidal volumes in excess of 1 l despite the receptors responding to all levels of volume change. Denervation of

331

the lungs, which occurs during heart–lung transplantation, is not as-sociated with any apparent deviation from the normal pattern of resting ventilation either when the subject is awake or during the several stages of sleep. The effects of denervation have been studied by Shea and colleagues amongst others. Their observations weaken the von Euler hypothesis for respiratory regulation as applied to man; however, the major role which the hypothesis attributes to the pulmonary stretch receptors might be shared with tendon organs and other non-pulmonary afferents. If so, this has still to be demonstrated. The threshold for activation of the Hering–Breuer reflex may not hold for the calibre of the larynx and trachea which Cohen and others have shown to be regulated by the Hering–Breuer mechanism at all levels of tidal volume.

The Hering–Breuer inflation reflex is inactivated by inhalation of local anaesthetic aerosol or carbon dioxide in high concentration. It is partially inactivated by hypoxia, hypercapnia in the physiological range, and exercise which raise the threshold volume at which the inflation reflex operates. The reflex is facilitated by an increase in the rate of rise in central inspiratory activity such as occurs with hyperthermia. It is also facilitated by vibration applied to the chest wall; this can activate intercostal muscle spindles. Both types of stimuli increase the frequency of breathing by reducing the duration of inspiration.

The duration of inspiration is not only reduced by activity of stretch receptors but also by activation of other pulmonary receptors. Stimu-lation of rapidly adapting *lung irritant receptors* produces shallow rapid breathing by reducing the duration of the respiratory cycle and hence the tidal volume. However, the ventilation may increase because of both an increase in peak activity in the phrenic nerves and additional deadspace ventilation resulting from the tachypnoea. The stimulus to the irritant receptors can be an inhaled irritant substance such as ammonia gas or histamine. Deflation of the lungs by suction applied to the trachea, external compression or controlled pneumothorax can exert a similar effect. Pulmonary J receptors can also cause tachypnoea; they are considered below.

The excitability of the inspiratory off-switch is correlated with the rate and the volume of inspiration; these features appear to influence the activity of the $R\beta$ neurones of the dorsomedial group referred to above. The cut off itself could be effected by late-onset inspiration-related neurones such as are present in the dorsomedial and ventral groups of respiratory neurones. However, the evidence for this is mainly circumstantial.

Expiration

Inspiratory muscle activity continues into the early part of expiration thus opposing the expiratory effect of lung elasticity and slowing the rate of expiration. The contraction is a positive feature of breathing and not a mere tailing off of the previous inspiration because it is associated with a switch in activity of premotor neurones; there is inhibition of neurones which fire during inspiration and activation of others which fire during early expiration. Expiratory muscles do not contract during this period but will do so subsequently if the drive to ventilation is increased. Then contraction is accompanied by firing of expiratory premotor neurones in the nucleus retroambigualis but the linkage is less strong than is the case for inspiration. The E-R neuronal activity is increased in response to hypercapnia. The associated change in the pattern of breathing is described on page 89.

The duration of expiration (t_E) is a function of the end inspiratory volume which is partly determined by the Hering–Breuer mechanism. It is also influenced by the tailing off of inspiratory muscle activity and by laryngeal calibre. The calibre in turn is under reflex control from pulmonary stretch receptors.

Central chemoreceptors

The central inspiratory activity is augmented by tonic stimulation from chemosensitive areas present on the ventrolateral surface of the medulla. The area has been called the ventrolateral medullary shell. The chemosensitive cells have not been identified and the mechanism by which the signal is developed remains in doubt. The effective stimulus appears to be hydrogen ion concentration, which varies with the tension of carbon dioxide, and the response is transmitted via cholinergic nerves which are stimulated by acetylcholine; the response to hydrogen ions is blocked by atropine. It is also blocked by cooling or applying local anaesthetic to the overlying surface of the medulla; this projects to the nucleus paragiganto cellularis, the retrofacial nucleus and the nucleus of the tractus solitarius; here the signal summates with afferent information from other sources including the skeletal muscles. The action of the central chemoreceptors has the effect of protecting the central nervous system from changes in hydrogen ion concentration including those which result from strenuous exercise (page 404). The subject has been explored by Loeschcke and others including Schlafke.

Central effects of hypoxia including the role of endorphins

Hypoxia affects central inspiratory activity both directly and indirectly, but the direct action is apparent only after inactivation of the carotid chemoreceptors. Hypoxia then depresses central inspiratory activity, reduces tidal volume and can cause tachypnoea: the tachypnoea resembles that associated with hyperthermia (page 338). The site of hypoxic depression overlies the central chemoreceptors. The depression is probably due to hyperpolarisation of respiratory neurones caused by changes in concentration of neurotransmitter substances, for hypoxia reduces the concentrations of excitatory neurotransmitters including monoamines and acetylcholine, whilst the concentrations of the inhibitory substances γ-aminobutyric acid (GABA), adenosine and

Table 11.1 Some mediators of hypoxic respiratory depression

Mediator	Antagonist
γ-Aminobutyric acid (GABA)*	Bicuculline
Adenosine	Theophylline
Endogenous opioids	Naloxone

* Synthesis is enhanced and degradation impeded by lactacidosis.

endogenous opioids are increased. The actions of the inhibitory neurotransmitters can be reduced by antagonists which block the relevent receptors (Table 11.1).

Each of the individual blocking agents has been shown to reverse the hypoxic depression only partially, so it must therefore be due to more than one inhibitor. However, whilst hypoxia depresses the level of inspiratory activity, the sensitivity of the central receptors to hypercapnia is not affected, and a normal increase in activity in response to a rise of Pco_2 or cH is retained.

In adults central hypoxic depression of respiration occurs only with severe hypoxia and is normally more than compensated by peripheral drive from chemoreceptors. By contrast in the newborn depression occurs with lesser degrees of hypoxaemia but can be alleviated by naloxone. This suggests that it is due in part to endogenous opioids (page 352).

The production of these opioids is stimulated by some anaesthetic agents and by high tensions of carbon dioxide. Consequently naloxone can alleviate carbon dioxide respiratory depression. Endorphins also contribute to the respiratory depression observed in patients with a very high airway resistance (page 685) but they do not contribute to the control of breathing in normal circumstances. This subject has been investigated by Edelman and colleagues. They have pointed out the many barriers to clear understanding; these include the multiple actions and the dose-dependent interactions of the many substances which are involved. Thus in the case of cerebral hypoxia the respiratory depression is preceded by hypoxic vasodilatation which causes transient reductions in central Pco_2 and cH and hence in central chemoreceptor drive. Subsequently the production of lactic acid is increased; this both stimulates central chemoreceptor drive and leads to accumulation of the inhibitory substance GABA.

Pulmonary C fibre receptors

Paintal described juxta-capillary receptors (J receptors) in the lung parenchyma which are served by small non-myelinated nerve fibres in the vagi. Receptors with the same innervation occur in the airways and the two together have been designated *pulmonary and bronchial C fibre receptors* by the Coleridges. The effect on the central pattern generator of afferent impulses from these receptors is to shorten expiration and increase respiratory frequency, but this effect is concealed by impulses from the slowly adapting pulmonary stretch receptors (PSR), which shorten inspiration, and can only be revealed by cooling the vagi to 4–8°C. When cooled, the vagi no longer conduct impulses from the PSR, an observation made by Head in 1889, when he described a paradoxical inspiratory response to inflation of the lung under these circumstances. Pissari and others have shown that C fibre and stretch receptors must both be inactivated before the slow deep breathing of vagotomy develops fully. It is now known that some of the effects formerly attributed to stimulation of PSR are really due to C fibre receptors.

J receptors are stimulated by pulmonary congestion, embolism and infection and by a number of chemical substances (Table 11.2). The response comprises apnoea at full inspiration followed by rapid shallow breathing; in addition there is usually bradycardia and hypotension. Bronchoconstriction, somatic motor inhibition and increased airway secretion can also occur.

The initial apnoea is due to generalised inhibition of respiratory activity involving the inspiratory and expiratory premotor neurones in the nucleus of the tractus solitarius and α and δ motor neurones supplying the intercostal muscles. The mechanism of the subsequent shortening of the time of expiration appears not to have been established. Experimental stimulation of C fibre receptors causes rapid shallow breathing resembling that observed in many abnormal conditions of the pulmonary parenchyma (Table 11.2). However, a causal association appears not to have been established. By contrast there is evidence for the C fibre activity being increased during exercise by the increase in pulmonary blood flow.

Table 11.2 Conditions which can activate bronchial and/or pulmonary C fibre receptors (see Coleridge and Coleridge for further details)

*Intrapulmonary condition**	*Lung autocoids†*
Diffuse pulmonary infiltration	Bradykinin
Increased pulmonary blood flow	Histamine‡
Lung inflation	Prostaglandins‡ ($F_2\alpha$, E_1, E_2, I_2 etc.)
Pulmonary anaphylaxis	Serotonin
Pulmonary embolism‡	
Pulmonary inflammation	*Other substances*
Pulmonary oedema	Ammonia‡
Raised pulmonary venous pressure‡	Capsicum‡
	Carbon dioxide
*Anaesthetic agents**	Chlorine
Chloroform	Ozone*
Ether	Phenyl diguanide‡§
Halothane	Sodium dithionite
Trichlorethylene	Sulphur dioxide†‡
	Tobacco smoke†‡

* Mainly pulmonary receptors (J receptors).
† Mainly bronchial receptors.
‡ Irritant receptors also active.
§ Effect not demonstrable in man.

During the breathing of carbon dioxide C fibre receptors contribute to the increase in frequency of breathing. Thus the frequency is increased by cooling the vagi to block afferent fibres from pulmonary stretch receptors and decreased only when all vagal afferents are interrupted. The mechanism whereby carbon dioxide activates the C fibre receptors is not known.

Spinal mechanisms

The efferent nerve impulses from the respiratory reticular formation converge upon the respiratory motor neurones in the spinal cord; here they summate with impulses from other sources including *Golgi tendon organs* and muscle spindles in the intercostal muscles and diaphragm. The tendon organs are tension receptors. They provide a safety mechanism whereby an undue increase in tension in an intercostal muscle can inhibit the α motor neurone which is causing the muscle to contract. The tendon organs also supply information to higher centres in the brain stem, and may contribute to the inspiratory off-switch mechanism by this route (page 331).

The *muscle spindles* are length receptors; they consist of sensory nerve endings joined to small muscle fibres enclosed in a fusiform sheath (Fig. 11.4). The endings respond to stretching of the central portion of the spindle. The intrafusal muscle fibres are innervated from the spinal cord by unmyelinated fibres from γ motor neurones. The sensory endings communicate through afferent nerves with the α motor neurones in the spinal cord that supply the respiratory muscles.

Sears suggests that the spindles act in the following way. At the start of inspiration nerve impulses from the respiratory reticular formation activate both the γ and the α motor neurones. The discharge of the γ motor neurones leads to contraction of the intrafusal muscle fibres; this causes traction on the sensory endings in the spindles. Concurrently the discharge of the α motor neurones contracts the extrafusal fibres

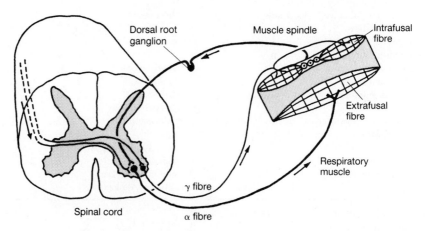

Fig. 11.4 Diagram illustrating the role of the muscle spindles in regulating the contraction of the respiratory muscles. For details see text.

of the respiratory muscles. When the contraction is accompanied by shortening of the muscle the length of the spindle and hence the traction which is exerted on the sensory ending is reduced. The discharge from the ending reflects the balance between the two forces. When the shortening of the extrafusal fibres lags behind that of the spindles the discharge from the sensory endings stimulates the α motor neurones to increase the strength of contraction of the respiratory muscles. When the respiratory muscles shorten at a greater rate than the spindles the stimulation of the α motor neurones is reduced. Hence the strength of the contraction of the respiratory muscles is modified by the extent to which it causes movement of the chest wall. In support of this Newsom Davis and Sears have found that the reflex arc from extrafusal fibre to respiratory muscle has a latency of 33−85 ms which is shorter than the minimal voluntary reaction time. The muscle spindles can also be stimulated by vibration applied to the chest wall and by this means they may contribute to the inspiratory off-switch mechanism (page 331). However, Matthew's has suggested that their main role is as sensory receptors with access to consciousness.

Respiratory sensation

The tendon organs and muscle spindles probably contribute both to motor activity and to respiratory sensation produced, including that by resistive and elastic loads. These can be induced respectively either by inserting an orifice in the breathing circuit or by breathing from a closed container. Receptors in costo-vertebral and costo-sternal joints play only a minor role and intrapulmonary receptors do not normally contribute. The sensations arise from changes with respect to time, volume, pressure and muscle tension; they have been summarised by Campbell and Howell as length−tension inappropriateness. The principal site of detection is normally the diaphragm but, depending on circumstances, the intercostal muscles, the muscles of the upper airways and the accessory muscles of respiration can also contribute to sensation. The afferent pathways from the relevant dorsal horn cells of the spinal cord extend to the cerebral cortex but the details of the innervation appear not to have been worked out. The normal limits of sensation are indicated in Table 11.3. They relate to changes in lung volume and pressure, and in resistive and elastic loading of respiration. In common with other types of sensation the threshold for *detecting* a resistive load is proportional to the background or initial resistance; this is codified in Weber's law which can be expressed as:

$$\Delta\phi/\phi = k \qquad (11.2)$$

where ϕ is the background resistance and $\Delta\phi$ the smallest detectable change. The value of the Weber fraction for an added resistive load is approximately 0.2−0.3. This holds for both normal subjects and those in whom the background resistance is increased by histamine or asthma. However, the detection of resistance loads is impaired by additional

Table 11.3 Approximate detection limits for respiratory sensations; compiled from a number of sources by Zechman and Wiley (1986)

Aspect*	Detection threshold†	Conditions for detection
ΔPmouth	0.05 kPa	Suboptimal when ΔP confined to upper airways
ΔRaw,insp	0.07 kPa l^{-1} s^{-1}	Optimal at mid-inspiration
ΔE,insp	0.1 kPa l^{-1}	Optimal at end inspiration

* For explanation of symbols see Table 2.3, page 15.
† For pressure in traditional units (cmH$_2$O) multiply by 10.2.

elastic loads. The relevance of Weber's law to the assessment of bronchodilatation is considered on page 148.

Estimation of *magnitude* of an added load is additionally influenced by a personal factor which Guz and colleagues amongst others have shown to be consistent over a wide range of stimuli involving different receptor sites. Subjects who give a high rating to one type of stimulus also tend to do so for others. The sensitivity can be described in terms of Stevens' psychophysical power law which has the form:

$$\Psi = k\phi^n \tag{11.3}$$

where Ψ is the perceived magnitude of the load, ϕ is the physical magnitude, k is the constant of proportionality and n is an exponent that provides an index of the sensitivity with which a sensation is perceived. The exponents for judging the relative sizes of a pressure, volume or minute volume usually exceed unity implying that the perceived magnitude increases as the stimulus gets larger. By contrast the exponents for resistive and elastic loads are typically less than unity implying that the perceived magnitudes are relatively less for large than for small loads.

Assessment of the perceived magnitude of resistive loads is influenced by the effort required to overcome them. On this account the assessment is influenced by curarisation of the muscles or by muscle fatigue.

The respiratory sensations which have been discussed arise from physiological information that is needed for the regulation of breathing. They contribute with other information to the sensation of breathlessness which in turn is an important determinant of exercise limitation. This aspect is discussed on pages 387 and 405.

Body temperature

A rise in deep body temperature increases ventilation relative to metabolism. There is an increase in inspiratory and expiratory flow rates and a rise in respiratory frequency. The latter is due to shortening of the times of both inspiration and expiration. Thus the breathing pattern differs from that associated with increased chemoreceptor drive to breathing (page 326). The effect of temperature is additive with other stimuli. It is mediated mainly via thermal receptor cells in the hypothalamus. Indirect evidence suggests that the cells project to the nucleus of the tractus solitarius and the nucleus paragiganto cellularis lateralis (Fig. 11.3). A rise in body temperature occurs during prolonged exercise when it causes an increase in ventilation relative to metabolism and a shift towards an increase in respiratory frequency. The same stimulus is responsible for thermal panting in dogs and some other animals.

Thermal panting is probably mediated by the local production in the hypothalamus of 5-hydroxytryptamine. This substance also initiates cutaneous vasodilatation and reduces the metabolism of muscle tissue. The responses are inhibited by noradrenaline, its precursor dopamine and the dopamine agonist apomorphine. The panting is associated with a reduction in the concentration of dopamine in the hypothalamus and panting is enhanced by the dopamine antagonist haloperidol.

Following denervation of the carotid bodies in experimental animals panting occurs in response to hypoxia. This form of tachypnoea bears the same relationship to dopamine metabolism as was described above for hyperthermia. The similarity has led Bonora and Gautier to conclude that they share a common hypothalamic mechanism. The mechanism is readily overridden by respiratory drive from the carotid chemoreceptors.

Hyperthermia increases the activity of all metabolising cells and hence the metabolic rate. Amongst its effects is an increase in the rate of firing of slowly adapting pulmonary stretch receptors, but the suggestion that this contributes to thermal polypnoea has not been confirmed. An increased heat load also stimulates cutaneous receptors particularly in the skin area supplied by the trigeminal nerve. Both the central and the cutaneous receptors contribute to the homeostatic responses to hyperthermia; these include increased sweating and an increase in skin blood flow. These changes can affect the capacity for exercise (page 397). A raised temperature can also cause a respiratory alkalosis and reduce the capacity of haemoglobin to transport oxygen.

Increases in body temperature in response to infection or experimental administration of pyrogen also influence respiration. During the time when the body temperature is rising the respiratory frequency often falls unless ventilation is increased by shivering. The effect is modulated by prostaglandins released into the hypothalamus and blocked by anti-inflammatory drugs including salicylates and indomethacin. When given early in the fever these drugs can increase the respiratory frequency. Salicylates can also increase the respiratory frequency by a direct action on the brain stem. Cooling the skin or immersing the limb or trunk in cold water induces an immediate strong inspiration. In the newborn this can initiate breathing. During immersion it can contribute to drowning. Under a cold shower the gasp response can be followed by hyperventilation with washout of carbon dioxide and an increase in the functional residual capacity. However, prolonged cooling depresses the ventilation and can cause severe hypercapnia. The effects of temperature on breathing have been reviewed by Cooper and Veale.

Diving response

Cooling of the face or submersion of the face in cold water has a number of effects which are loosely described as the diving response. The stimuli appear to be local cooling and pressure applied to the territory of the trigeminal nerve including the skin of the face and the mucous membrane of the nose; the extent of the exposure influences the response. This is integrated in the medulla and persists after decerebration. The central site is closely related to that which mediates the chemoreceptor drive to respiration (Fig. 11.3, page 329). The response is well developed in aquatic mammals and is of modest proportions in man. The respiratory component includes apnoea if the water enters the nose; alternatively if the immersion is premeditated there is a reduction in respiratory drive. This manifests itself as transient reductions in ventilation and in the ventilatory responses to carbon dioxide and cyanide which normally stimulate the carotid bodies. There is an increase in maximal breath holding time. The response is not elicited by immersing the face in warm water.

In addition to reducing the drive to respiration the cold stimulus causes a reflex increase in bronchomotor tone. This increases the airways resistance which in turn impairs the distribution of ventilation with respect to lung perfusion (page 198). The bronchoconstriction is not associated with collapse of the lungs which can occur in diving mammals with very mobile chest walls.

The respiratory response to cold facial immersion contributes to the cardiovascular response which is fully developed only when apnoea is present. There is then increased sympathetic vasoconstrictor activity to the blood vessels supplying skeletal muscles; this reduces muscle blood flow. There is a reduction in sympathetic outflow to the skin; this opens subcutaneous arteriovenous anastomoses and thereby diverts blood flow away from the skin. The effects of these changes is to raise systemic blood pressure, which, by stimulating aortic baroceptors, results in bradycardia. In diving mammals but not apparently in man there is reduced metabolic activity in the liver and other tissues not immediately necessary for hunting during submersion. In summary the principal effect of the diving response is to prolong the breath holding time; this can contribute to survival. In man the response is not well developed. Thus its presence does little to support the hypothesis that during his evolution man passed through an aquatic phase.

Peripheral chemoreceptors

The carotid bodies monitor the tension of oxygen, the tension of carbon dioxide and/or the hydrogen ion concentration in arterial blood. The information is transmitted via the carotid sinus nerves to the nucleus of the tractus solitarius and other centres in the brain (Fig. 11.3). By this means the carotid bodies contribute a chemoreceptor drive to respiration; this has been investigated in depth and is described in the next section. The aortic bodies appear not to have a respiratory function.

The carotid bodies are small nodes which are closely related to the carotid bulb from which they obtain a rich blood supply. The node diameter is normally 1–2 mm but it is increased by chronic hypoxia such as occurs as a result of residence at high altitude or chronic lung disease. The nodes have a glomerular structure with a connective tissue stroma containing clusters of cells surrounded and invaded by large glomerular capillaries. The capillaries can be bypassed by arterio-venous anastomoses. The glomerular cells are of two types. The type I cells are relatively large (diameter 8–12 μm), have vesicles containing catecholamines in their cytoplasm, make contact with other type I cells and have a rich covering of nerve endings. Most of the nerve endings arise from sensory neurones with cell bodies located in the petrosal ganglion of the glossopharyngeal nerve (9th cranial nerve). The type II cells have long thin cytoplasmic processes that envelop and insinuate between type I cells; they resemble the Schwann cells which protect and nourish nerve axons. The blood vessels are innervated from the superior cervical ganglion of the sympathetic nervous system and local parasympathetic ganglion cells which are supplied by the carotid sinus branch of the glossopharyngeal nerve.

The type I cells or the adjacent nerve endings respond to hypoxia which increases the rate of firing of afferent nerve fibres in the carotid sinus nerves. Most of the fibres are myelinated but non-myelinated fibres also respond. The association between the nerve discharge and oxygen tension is weak at tensions in excess of approximately 13 kPa (100 mmHg). Below this level the rate of firing varies inversely with oxygen tension. The rate is also influenced by the coexisting arterial tension of carbon dioxide and/or concentration of hydrogen ions. When these are increased the response to hypoxia is augmented in a multipli-cative fashion; when they are reduced the response to hypoxia is diminished or absent. However, for the response to hypoxia to be suppressed the carbon dioxide tension must be very low. The response latency is of the order of 0.3 s and the time to peak nerve discharge in the range 1–3 s. The pattern of firing is mainly random but exhibits a periodicity at the frequency of breathing up to maximum of 20 min^{-1} for oxygen and 70 min^{-1} for carbon dioxide and/or hydrogen ion con-centration. The oscillations contribute to the regulation of breathing. As well as hypoxic hypoxia the chemoreceptors respond to stagnant hypoxia associated with a reduction in systemic blood pressure and histotoxic hypoxia such as follows the administration of cyanide (page 625). There is little response to a reduction in delivery of oxygen caused by anaemia or inhalation of carbon monoxide (page 625).

The glomus cells have a high metabolic rate and require a high ambient oxygen tension for the full oxygenation of their contained cytochrome; they therefore become short of oxygen when the tension in the arterial blood is reduced or the flow of blood to the capillary network is decreased. Either event leads to anaerobic metabolism in the node and local production of metabolites which stimulate the adjacent nerve endings.

A number of transmitter substances appear to contribute to the response. Dopamine is released from the glomus cells in response to hypoxia but has a mainly inhibitory effect on chemoreceptor activity. By contrast the effects of released noradrenaline and adenosine are mainly excitatory. The noradrenaline probably acts by redistributing blood flow within the glomeruli. This raises the sensitivity to hypoxia and hypercapnia and contributes to the increase in ventilation which occurs during exercise. The glomus cells also contain encephalins, vasoactive intestinal peptides and substance P which are released by hypoxia; the encephalins reduce and the latter two substances enhance the ventilatory response to hypoxia. The substance P antagonist [D-Pro^2, D-Trp$^{7.9}$] SP has been shown by Prabhakar and colleagues to reduce the response of the carotid body to hypoxia but not to hyperoxic hypercapnia: these authors suggest that substance P is closely related to the transmitter substance for the response to hypoxaemia.

The response to hypercapnia probably has different intermediaries which Lahiri and colleagues have suggested are independent of mitochondrial oxygen metabolism. The hypercapnic response may also have a different central distribution to expiratory as well as to inspiratory premotor neurones.

Chemoreceptor drive to respiration

Lack of oxygen in the arterial blood depresses the central nervous system; at the same time it increases the flow of sensory stimuli from the peripheral chemoreceptors to the respiratory reticular formation. Hyperoxia has the opposite effect. Abrupt changes in the concentration of oxygen in the inspired gas are followed within a few seconds by changes in ventilation; the latter initially mirror the changes in peripheral and/or central chemoreceptor activity (Fig. 11.5) but are subsequently diminished or may be reversed by alterations in the tensions of carbon dioxide which are consequent on the initial change in ventilation.

The secondary adjustments are most marked at rest when they lead to the steady state ventilation during moderate hypoxaemia not being materially changed compared with breathing air, whilst during oxygen breathing the ventilation is usually increased. The changes which underlie this paradoxical behaviour are illustrated in Fig. 11.6. Inhalation of gas deficient in oxygen causes an immediate increase in ventilation; this increases the excretion of carbon dioxide from the lung and reduces the tension of carbon dioxide in arterial blood. Hence the stimulus to inspiration from carbon dioxide decreases and the ventilation declines towards that which obtained when breathing air. Converse changes occur during the inhalation of 100% oxygen. There is then an immediate decrease in ventilation minute volume, so less carbon dioxide is excreted and the tension of carbon dioxide in the arterial blood rises; this change stimulates breathing. The rise in the tension of carbon dioxide

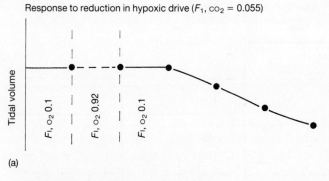

Response to reduction in hypoxic drive ($F_I, {CO_2} = 0.055$)

(a)

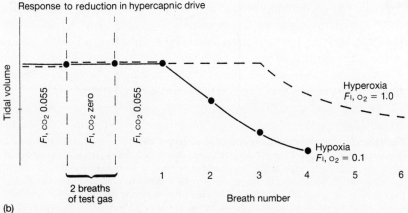

Response to reduction in hypercapnic drive

(b)

Fig. 11.5 Response of ventilation to a brief change in the concentration of oxygen or carbon dioxide in inspired gas. In (a) the carbon dioxide is held constant whilst the oxygen is increased sufficiently to greatly reduce the peripheral chemoreceptor drive. The reduction in ventilation is detectable two breaths later. In (b) the oxygen is held constant whilst the carbon dioxide is reduced. During hypoxia, when the chemoreceptor drive is intact, the reduction in ventilation is again detectable two breaths later; when the peripheral chemoreceptor drive is eliminated by breathing oxygen, the reduction is only detectable after four breaths. The delay represents the additional time needed for the blood to reach the central chemoreceptors. (Source: Cunningham DJC, Lloyd BB, Miller JP, Young JM. *J Physiol (Lond)* 1965; **179**: 68P–70P.)

also dilates cerebral arterioles and increases the flow of blood to the brain. This change causes a rise in cerebral oxygen tension which is in addition to that due to the initial enrichment of the inspired gas with oxygen. The two processes combine to increase the concentration of oxyhaemoglobin in the blood in the cerebral capillaries; less reduced haemoglobin is then available to take up and transport dioxide from the brain in the form of carbamino-haemoglobin. The tension of carbon dioxide in the medulla rises in consequence and this change further increases the hypercapnoeic drive to respiration. At rest, the increase more than compensates for the reduction in peripheral chemoreceptor drive caused by the hyperoxia; on this account, the steady state ventilation at rest when breathing oxygen exceeds that when breathing air by about $2 \, l \, min^{-1}$.

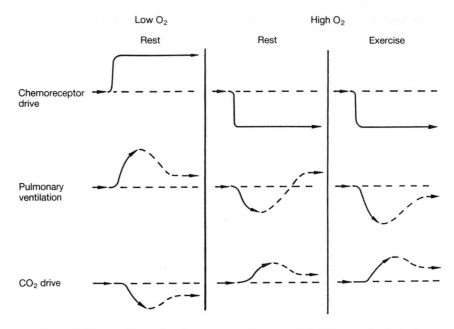

Fig. 11.6 Diagram illustrating the sequence of events which follows a change in the chemoreceptor drive to respiration. Inspiration of gas deficient in oxygen increases the drive; this stimulates respiration. The resulting increase in ventilation washes out carbon dioxide from the blood; this decreases the overall stimulus to breathing. The ventilation then declines to a new equilibrium value where the increased chemoreceptor drive is nearly offset by the reduced drive from carbon dioxide. When breathing oxygen converse changes take place. However, they are partly offset by a concurrent increase in the carbon dioxide drive due to a reduction in the buffering capacity of blood perfusing the brain. At rest this change causes an increase in the ventilation above that when breathing air. On exercise the effect is concealed by the relatively greater importance of the chemoreceptor drive.

During exercise the factors which contribute to transport of carbon dioxide are similar to those at rest. But the peripheral chemoreceptor drive is increased by a rise in blood noradrenaline and other factors (page 356). On this account, when oxygen is administered during exercise, the reduction in chemoreceptor drive exceeds the gain in hypercapnoeic drive so ventilation decreases and the tension of carbon dioxide rises. The rise can be material, of the order of 1.3 kPa (10 mmHg) and occurs in healthy subjects as well as in patients with lung disease. The hypercapnia is evidence for the major role of chemoreceptor drive in regulating the respiration during exercise.

The signal from the chemoreceptors is in the form of afferent discharges in the carotid sinus nerves. These reflect the mean oxygen and carbon dioxide tensions in the arterial blood and the fluctuations in tension of carbon dioxide which occur throughout the respiratory cycle. Changes in the mean level of discharge are responsible for much of the chemoreceptor drive to respiration. The possibility that the oscillations also contribute was suggested by Yamomoto and explored amongst others by Torrance, Semple, Guz and their respective collaborators. They have shown that the timing of the peak discharge in relation to the breathing cycle can influence respiration. Peaks in late expiration or early inspiration prolong the relevant inspiration whilst peaks at other times prolong the next post-expiratory pause. These reactions may contribute to control of breathing during sleep and when the rhythm of breathing is disturbed by speech or coughing. In addition the rate of increase of discharge which accompanies the upstroke of the Pa_{CO_2} oscillation could contribute to the increase in ventilation which occurs during exercise. This aspect is discussed on page 354. Chemoreceptor drive is also important when central drive to respiration is reduced or the ability of the respiratory apparatus to increase ventilation is impaired. In such circumstances the continuance of respiration may depend solely upon the chemoreceptor drive. If this is removed by administration of oxygen the breathing becomes reduced and may cease altogether (page 579). The assessment of chemoreceptor drive is described in Chapter 12.

Hypercapnic drive

Hypercapnic drive to respiration is mediated via the carotid and central chemoreceptors (Fig. 11.5). There may also be receptors which monitor the tension of carbon dioxide in pulmonary venous blood, for such receptors exist in birds and their presence in mammals has been deduced from the discharge pattern of selected single fibres in the vagus nerve. However, no receptors have been found in humans and study of patients following heart–lung transplantation does not suggest a role for pulmonary venous receptors in the control of breathing. The stretch receptors in the walls of bronchi can be inhibited by carbon dioxide in the respired gas (page 332) but this observation has yet no physiological significance. The effective stimulus to the known receptors is either tension of carbon dioxide or hydrogen ion concentration at the receptor site and the response is critically influenced by the coexisting tension of oxygen. For peripheral chemoreceptors either CO_2 tension or hydrogen ion concentration is an effective stimulus; the response is dependent on and interacts with that to oxygen. This is discussed below. For central chemoreceptors the usual mediator is carbon dioxide which diffuses readily to the receptor site; the response is independent of oxygen tension except to the extent that hypoxaemia depresses central nervous activity. However, the response is modulated by concurrent changes in blood flow to the central medulla which appears to increase more in the presence of hypoxia and hypercapnia than blood flow to other parts of the brain.

Study of the ventilatory responses to carbon dioxide is complicated because they are influenced by the way in which the gas is administered. Rebreathing from a bag containing oxygen produces progressively increasing hypercapnia with hyperoxia. In these circumstances the peripheral chemoreceptors are inactive, the arterial carbon dioxide tension does not vary over the respiratory cycle and the ventilatory response is that to a raised carbon dioxide tension at the central chemoreceptors

345

(page 333). It relates to conditions of hyperoxia when the buffering of carbon dioxide by haemoglobin is reduced (page 288). Breathing mixtures of carbon dioxide in air stimulates both central and peripheral chemoreceptors; however, the resulting increase in ventilation raises the alveolar oxygen tension and hence reduces the hypoxic drive unless the inspired oxygen tension is adjusted concurrently. In addition the increase in ventilation increases proportionally the quantity of carbon dioxide delivered to the lungs; this delays the attainment of a steady state for up to 20 min during which time the renal excretion of bicarbonate is increased. If several gas mixtures are used consecutively the resulting acid–base changes can modify the ventilatory response.

The effects of carbon dioxide in man have mostly been investigated using one or other of these techniques and considerable ingenuity has been applied to achieve our present understanding. Recently Cummin and Saunders have re-introduced an alternative technique using a constant CO_2 mass load and this could lead to further advances.

Hypercapnic drive extends over a wide range of tensions of carbon dioxide from an upper limit when carbon dioxide depresses central nervous activity to a lower limit when the ventilation is apparently independent of the carbon dioxide tension. Respiratory depression occurs as a result of inhaling high concentrations of carbon dioxide ($F_1CO_2 > 0.08$). Dissociation of ventilation from carbon dioxide tension occurs following voluntary overbreathing which increases the elimination of CO_2 and lowers the alveolar carbon dioxide tension. In between these limits the ventilatory response to hypercapnia can be described by a linear equation:

$$\dot{V}A = S(P\text{A.}CO_2 - B) \tag{11.4}$$

where $\dot{V}A$ is alveolar ventilation ($l\,min^{-1}$), $P\text{A.}CO_2$, is alveolar carbon dioxide tension (kPa or mmHg) and S and B are constants. Breathing air the sensitivity to carbon dioxide (S) is normally in the range 7.5–52 $l\,min^{-1}\,kPa^{-1}$ (1.0–7.0 $l\,min^{-1}\,mmHg^{-1}$). The constant term B is approximately 4.7 kPa (35 mmHg). The respiratory sensitivity to carbon dioxide varies inversely with the tension of oxygen (Fig. 11.7). It is also affected by other circumstances (Fig. 11.8(a)). Thus increased sensitivity occurs in response to noradrenaline, progesterone, almitrine, persistent hyperventilation, reduction in carotid blood flow and following administration of neurotransmitter substances of which some are considered on page 342. Reductions in sensitivity occur during sleep and anaesthesia and with propranolol, dopamine, encephalins and other substances. It is also reduced when the work of ventilating the lung is increased as a result of disease of the lung or the chest wall. However, if the disease process affects only the mechanical functions of the lung and not the control system the response will be within normal limits when expressed in terms of the work which is performed on the lung (page 375).

The intercept B is related to the concentration of bicarbonate in blood plasma (Fig. 11.8(b)); it is reduced when the concentration is

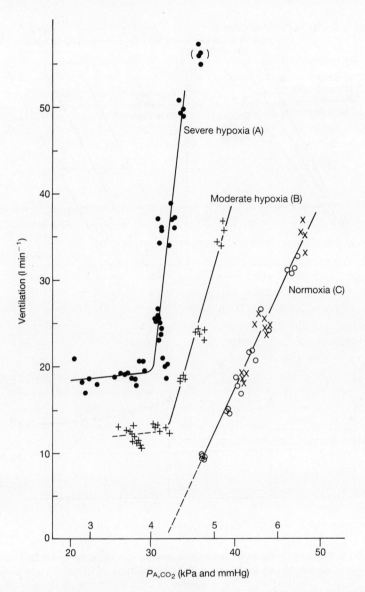

Fig. 11.7 Relationship of ventilation to alveolar tension of carbon dioxide (P_{A,CO_2})
under steady state conditions of: (A) severe hypoxia (P_{A,O_2}, 4.9 kPa, 37 mmHg);
(B) moderate hypoxia P_{A,O_2} (6.3 kPa, 47 mmHg); (C) normoxia. During hypocapnic
hypoxia the ventilation is nearly independent of P_{A,CO_2}. (Source: Nielsen M, Smith M.
Acta Physiol Scand 1951; **24**: 293–313.)

decreased by metabolic acidosis or by persistent overbreathing such as
occurs at high altitude, in pregnancy and with some diseases of the
lung parenchyma. It is also reduced by exercise. The threshold is
increased if the blood bicarbonate is raised, either by the ingestion of
bicarbonate or by a depression of respiration sufficient to cause the
retention of carbon dioxide in the arterial blood. This occurs, for
example, in some patients with an obstructive type of ventilatory
defect. The threshold is increased during sleep and as a result of the

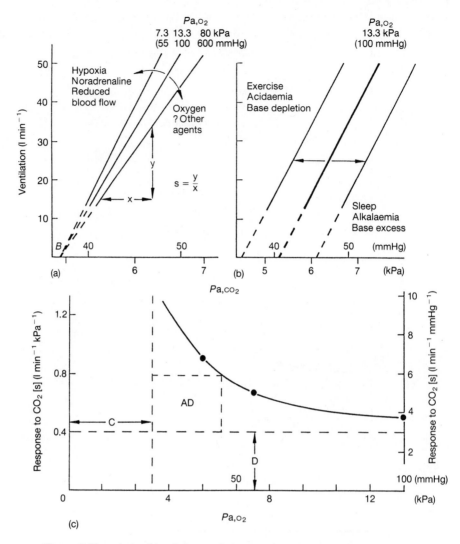

Fig. 11.8 The relationship of the ventilation minute volume to the end-tidal or arterial
tension of carbon dioxide for a subject breathing mixtures of CO_2 and O_2 in nitrogen.
(a) The regression lines for different tensions of oxygen converge on the point *B*. The
response to carbon dioxide (*S*) at any tension of oxygen is calculated in the manner
indicated. (b) Some of the factors which, under steady state conditions, determine the
value for *B*. Somewhat higher values obtain during rebreathing. (c) The relationship of
the response to carbon dioxide (*S*) to the tension of oxygen. *D* is the response of
ventilation to carbon dioxide when the subject is breathing gas containing oxygen in a
fractional concentration of approximately 0.95. *C* is the oxygen tension at which the
response to carbon dioxide is infinite and *A* is another factor which describes the
response of ventilation to hypoxaemia. (Source: Lloyd BB, Cunningham DJC. In
Cunningham DJC, Lloyd BB, eds. *The Regulation of Human Respiration*. Oxford:
Blackwell Scientific Publications, 331−349, 1963.)

administration of sedative drugs including morphine and codeine. It is
also affected by changes in the concentration of hydrogen ions in
arterial blood. The intercept is independent of oxygen tension and
many of the other factors which influence respiratory sensitivity.

The multiplicative interaction between the effects of hypoxia and hypercapnia upon ventilation have been described in many ways, some of which have been listed by Severinghaus. For steady state conditions Lloyd and Cunningham have used the following empirical hyperbolic equation:

$$\dot{V}\text{E} = D[A/(Pa,\text{o}_2 - C) + f](Pa,\text{co}_2 - B) \ \text{l min}^{-1} \quad (11.5)$$

where $\dot{V}\text{E}$ is the ventilation minute volume in l BTPS min^{-1}, Pa,o_2 and Pa,co_2, in kPa (or mmHg) are the tensions of oxygen and carbon dioxide in arterial blood and B is the intercept for carbon dioxide (see above). D is the ventilatory response to carbon dioxide in oxygen and has the units l BTPS min^{-1} kPa^{-1} (or mmHg^{-1}), A is the tension of oxygen at which the response to carbon dioxide is twice that which obtains when breathing 100% oxygen and C is the tension of oxygen at which the stimulant effect of hypoxaemia reaches its maximal value. f is 7.5 in SI units and 1 when traditional units are used. The tension C is believed to be that at which there is a zero tension of oxygen in the chemoreceptor cells. The term within the right hand brackets is the effective stimulus to respiration by carbon dioxide. The remaining terms, which are illustrated in Fig. 11.8(c) describe the response of the subject to this stimulus under the conditions of measurement.

The factor D, which is the ventilatory response to hyperoxic hypercapnia, is usually in the range 5−22.5 l min^{-1} kPa^{-1} (0.7−3.0 l min^{-1} mmHg^{-1}). The response is related to the vital capacity of the subject and for men and women of European descent may, on average, be described by the following relationship of Patrick and Cotes:

$$D = 7.5 \, [0.89 + 0.35\text{VC, SD } 0.58] \ \text{l min}^{-1} \text{kPa}^{-1} \quad (11.6)$$

where VC is the vital capacity in litres and 7.5 converts between SI and traditional units. For people of some other ethnic groups the value for D is reduced (page 477).

Hypoxic drive to respiration

The response of ventilation to hypoxaemia is mediated solely by peripheral chemoreceptors. It can be described in terms of the factors A and C which are defined above. These factors have values which are usually of the order of 2.7−6.7 kPa (20−50 mmHg). The procedure for measurement is described on page 380. The response is reduced in people who are born and grow up at high altitude, subjects with mountain sickness and patients with cyanotic congenital heart disease (page 360); an intermediate response is observed in some athletes. The response to hypoxia is less labile than that to hypercapnia. For example it is not affected by an alteration in the acid−base balance of the blood and is relatively less affected by partial obstruction to the lung airways. At the onset of isocapnic hypoxia there is a brisk ventilatory response which declines after a few minutes to an intermediate level. The decline appears to be due to adenosine exerting a central inhibitory action; the inhibition can be reversed by aminophylline acting as an

349

adenosine antagonist. The residual response does not adapt with time. Thus the chemoreceptor drive continues to operate when the activity of the respiratory centre is depressed by narcotic agents or cerebral hypoxia to such an extent that carbon dioxide no longer exerts its central stimulant effect. In these unfavourable circumstances the maintenance of spontaneous respiration and, indeed of life itself, depends entirely upon the chemoreceptor drive.

Sleep

During sleep ventilation is often reduced and the pattern of breathing modified. The changes are due to a reduction in central inspiratory activity, a diminished response to chemoreceptor drive and a loss of tonic activity in the muscles of respiration. Mild hypoxaemia and hypercapnia develop and are aggravated if periods of apnoea occur. These effects can be cumulative. Susceptibility to them is influenced by genetic and environmental factors; their joint occurrence can increase the risk of infants succumbing to sudden infant death syndrome, and of adults developing chronic hypoventilation. These considerations have led to intensive study of the physiology and pathophysiology of sleep and to the development of methods for its assessment (page 364). Disturbed sleep may occur in some people (p. 577) and also occurs at high altitude (p. 359).

Stages of sleep

The important observation that sleep can take two radically different forms was made by Aserinsky and Kleitman in 1953. They observed that typical quiet sleep is interspersed by periods of altered activity including rapid eye movements, hypotonicity and alterations in the pattern of breathing. The rapid eye movement sleep (REM sleep) is preceded by quiet or non-rapid eye movement sleep (NREM sleep); this can be subdivided into four stages of progressively increasing depth. The cycle duration is usually 90–120 min. Light NREM sleep (stage 1) is characterised by unconsciousness from which the subject is readily roused; the electroencephalogram (EEG) exhibits a low voltage and high frequency resembling that when the subject is awake. In stage 2 sleep the EEG frequency is more variable and the subject is less easily roused. Approximately half of adult sleep is of this pattern. In stages 3 and 4 the EEG voltage is high and the frequency slow, hence the designation slow wave sleep. Arousal is further diminished. In rapid eye movement sleep the EEG reverts to a low voltage and high frequency pattern. There are alternate periods of hypotonicity when postural muscle tone is greatly diminished and of rapid eye movements. The latter are associated with twitching movements of the face and limbs, dreaming and autonomic and respiratory disturbances. The subject is easily roused from sleep but the arousal is often of brief duration.

Non-REM sleep is believed to be due to withdrawal of tonic discharges

from the ascending reticular formation which normally maintain the
waking state. This is supplemented by inhibition from higher centres.
The decreased neural activity affects the respiratory premotor neurones
in the pons and medulla; their firing is reduced or suppressed altogether
and their responsiveness to sensory inputs is diminished. REM sleep
is associated with rhythmic synchronous discharges of the pontine
neurones; these cause synchronous rapid eye movements, twitching
movements of the limbs and face and variable respiratory activity.
Other neuronal discharges activate the EEG and inhibit postural muscle
tone. The inhibition involves both α and γ motor neurones. The
intercostal muscles and the muscles of the upper airways can be virtually
paralysed in consequence. In the diaphragm tonic activity is greatly
reduced but rhythmic contractions persist. This relative sparing of the
diaphragm has been attributed to it having a relatively low density of
muscle spindles.

Ventilation and gas exchange

During all stages of sleep the ventilation and tidal volume are reduced
compared with the waking state. The reductions exceed that in the
rate of metabolism which is approximately 10%. During NREM sleep
the arterial carbon dioxide tension increases by 0.3−0.9 kPa
(2−7 mmHg) and the oxygen tension falls by a similar amount. During
much of REM sleep the ventilation is similarly reduced, but there are
periods of apnoea during which the arterial oxygen tension falls further.

The respiratory frequency is usually normal whilst the rhythm varies
depending on the stage of sleep. In stages 3 and 4 of NREM sleep the
rhythm is regular. In stages 1 and 2 the frequency often fluctuates in a
regular manner so the rhythm is periodic. In REM sleep both the
frequency and the rhythm vary with the highest frequency and greatest
variability occurring in proximity to periods of marked hypoventilation
on apnoea. The extent of the changes varies with the frequency of eye
movements.

The changes in ventilation during sleep are consistent with alterations
of sensitivity to hypercapnia and hypoxaemia. The responses are depressed in all stages of sleep, the depression being greatest during
REM sleep with frequent eye movements (Table 11.4). The depression
is practically reversed during hypoxia (page 584).

The respective contributions of rib cage or diaphragm to ventilation
vary with the type of sleep. During NREM sleep the rib cage contributes
rather more than when awake but during REM sleep the rib cage
component is reduced or even absent. There is then paradoxical retraction of the intercostal spaces during inspiration: this is particularly
conspicuous in infants. At the same time the tone of the diaphragm is
reduced; this reduces the functional residual capacity. The reduction
can result in closure of small airways which persists during inspiration
and thus contributes to hypoxaemia (page 193). Closure is particularly
likely to occur in older subjects (page 488) and patients with diseases
which affect small airways (e.g. chronic bronchitis page 529).

Table 11.4 Some features of different sleep states compared with being awake

	NREM		REM
	2	3–4	
EEG voltage	—	↑	—
EEG frequency	—	↓	—
Arousal	↓↓	↓↓↓	↓
Muscle tone	↓	↓↓	Nil
Tidal volume	↓	↓	↓↓
Rib cage contribution	↑	↑	↓↓
Respiratory frequency	—	—	↑
Hypercapnia/hypoxaemia	↑	↑	↑↑
Respiratory responsiveness	↓↓	↓↓	↓↓↓↓

An additional cause of hypoxaemia is obstruction of the oropharynx or larynx; this can occur during REM sleep on account of loss of tone and reduced inspiratory activity in the respective abductor muscles. The muscles include the genioglossus, tensor palati and medial pterygoid muscles which contribute to the patency of the oropharynx, and the posterior cricoarytenoid and cricothyroid muscles which abduct the larynx. During REM sleep with frequent eye movements the virtual paralysis of these muscles can contribute to *sleep apnoea/hypopnoea syndrome* in which the airway is occluded, though phasic diaphragmatic contractions persist. The role of drugs is considered subsequently (page 620). Other predisposing factors are listed in Table 11.5.

Respiratory control at birth

During intra-uterine life the fetus performs breathing movements which are irregular and occur at a high frequency. These are associated with periods of rapid eye movement and are unrelated to maternal or fetal blood–gas tensions. Near to term periods of slower more regular breathing also occur interspersed with apnoea. The movements are often confined to the diaphragm but can be associated with closure of the glottis when they present as hiccups. At birth the level of respiratory activity increases abruptly and there is also increased respiratory movement in the larynx; this contributes to an increase in end-expiratory pressure in the lung which assists lung expansion.

Table 11.5 Factors which can predispose to sleep apnoea/hypopnoea syndrome*

Small cross-sectional area of glottis, pharynx or larynx

Obstruction from supine posture, thick neck, myxoedema, tonsils, adenoids, nasal polyp, local tumour, macroglossia, posteriorly displaced mandible

Impaired muscle function associated with hypotonia and increased pharyngeal compliance; can occur with poliomyelitis, encephalitis, neoplastic or vascular lesion of central nervous system

* Can also predispose to snoring or to inspiratory flow limitation (page 126).

The onset of respiration is due to a number of factors of which one is increased central stimulation from afferent nerves supplying the skin and respiratory tract. There may also be a reduction of the central inhibition of respiration caused by endorphins which are produced in the placenta during intra-uterine life (page 695). This source of inhibition is removed at birth. In addition a rise in the plasma concentration of noradrenaline at birth increases the activity of peripheral chemoreceptors. This occurs just prior to delivery and enables the infant to respond to hypoxic drive. The response initially takes the form of an increase in ventilation. This persists during quiet sleep but during rapid eye movement sleep (REM sleep) or when awake the hyperventilation dies away. However, hypoxia still drives ventilation for brief inhalation of 100% oxygen reduces it. The respiratory responses to carbon dioxide and to cold are initially depressed by hypoxia. The transition to normal adult responses to hypoxia and hypercapnia takes 2−3 weeks. During this time the respiratory control system is relatively labile and vulnerable to both hypoxia and to mechanical difficulties. The latter can arise from accumulation of fluid in the lung or from the chest wall being so compliant that it is subject to paradoxical inward movement during inspiration. This reduces the effectiveness of diaphragmatic contraction. The capacity of the diaphragm to perform work is also reduced by its immaturity. These difficulties are aggravated by hypoxia; they can be partly compensated by the metabolic rate of the newborn infant diminishing in response to cold or hypoxia, which is not the case in adults. In addition the chest wall is protected against paradoxical movement by the intercostal tendon inhibitory reflex being well developed at birth (cf. page 331). The inhibitory response to stimulation of pulmonary stretch receptors (Hering−Breuer reflex) may also be increased.

The particular features of respiratory distress syndrome of the newborn and sudden infant death syndrome are discussed elsewhere (pages 524 and 350).

Ventilation during exercise

Moderate exercise

During exercise the ventilation increases to deliver additional oxygen and eliminate excess carbon dioxide. Under steady state conditions the control mechanism is tuned to maintain the tension of carbon dioxide in arterial blood at its resting level. This carries the implication that during moderate exercise the alveolar ventilation is proportional to the carbon dioxide output. On account of the deadspace increasing with tidal volume the ventilation is also linearly related to the latter variable. The carbon dioxide output reflects the rate of energy expenditure and the relative proportions in which fat and carbohydrate are metabolised. The proportions can be influenced by diet.

The close association between ventilation and carbon dioxide output

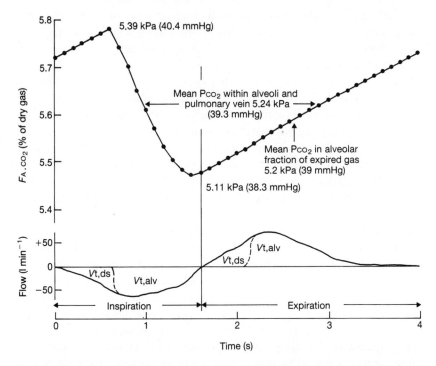

Fig. 11.9 Alveolar carbon dioxide tension (P_{A,CO_2}) over one respiratory cycle showing a linear rise during the expiratory phase. The lower tracing shows that to obtain the mean P_{A,CO_2} the optimal time for sampling the alveolar gas is shortly after mid-expiration. $V_{t,ds}$ and $V_{t,alv}$ are respectively the deadspace and alveolar fractions of the tidal volume. (Source: DuBois AB, Britt AG, Fenn WO. *J Appl Physiol* 1952; **4**: 535–548.)

suggests that hypercapnic drive should be the principal cause of the increase in ventilation. The signal appears to be the rate of increase of arterial carbon dioxide tension with time during the upstroke of respiratory oscillation in Pa_{CO_2}. During expiration the slope is independent of ventilation and varies directly with the rate at which carbon dioxide is delivered to the lungs (Fig. 11.9). The delivery increases from the second or third breath following the start of exercise. Cross and colleagues in studies on dogs have found that the associated rise in the slope of the upstroke is correlated with the respiratory changes including a shortening of t_E and an increase in tidal volume. Thus the slope of the upstroke can explain much of the increase in ventilation during moderate exercise. However, nearly the same relationship between ventilation and CO_2 output can be achieved after separate elimination of most of the components in the respiratory control system. There appears to be a superfluity of control mechanisms of which some are described below; their respective contributions under normal circumstances remain in doubt.

The change in ventilation with respect to time during exercise of a few minutes duration can be described in terms of five components. There is an initial abrupt increase at the onset: this is followed by a rising phase and an exercise phase which is normally a plateau. On

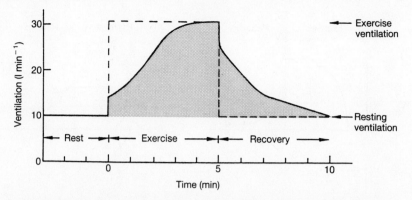

Fig. 11.10 Diagram illustrating the changes in ventilation during a 5-min period of test exercise in a healthy subject. The changes are described in the text. In addition using the terminology of Hugh Jones and Lambert the area which is shaded represents the excess exercise ventilation (EEV). During moderate exercise the part of the EEV which is incurred during recovery is approximately equal to the ventilation deficit at the start of exercise; the two areas bounded by the curve and the interrupted lines are therefore of equal size. Further details are given on page 367.

cessation of exercise there is an initial abrupt decrease followed by a decline (Fig. 11.10). The initial increase occurs within a few seconds and is accompanied by an increase in cardiac output. This led Wasserman and others to suggest that the initial increase in ventilation might be a consequence of the cardiovascular changes. However, study of the recipients of heart−lung transplants excludes this as the only mechanism. The traditional explanation due to Krogh and Lindhard is that the central nervous activity which initiates the exercise also stimulates the respiratory reticular formation. In support of this hypothesis coupling between the spinal pathways to the legs and to the respiratory muscles has been demonstrated by Eldridge and colleagues. But other evidence again suggests that this cannot be the only mechanism; thus Adams and colleagues found an immediate increase in tidal volume in response to electrically induced leg exercise in patients with transection of the spinal cord at the level of the 6th thoracic vertebra. The pattern of the response was slightly different from that of normal subjects in whom the initial increase was in respiratory frequency not tidal volume but the effect on minute volume was similar. The rising phase of ventilation was also similar in the two conditions which suggested that impulses from the active muscles (or the joints on which they acted) did not contribute to that part of the response either.

The rising phase is undoubtedly influenced by concurrent changes in arterial blood gas tensions including a transient rise in the tension of carbon dioxide and fall in the tension of oxygen. These features were first observed by Matell (Fig. 11.11). The response is mediated in part via the carotid chemoreceptors and the speed of the response, expressed as the half time for the increase in ventilation, has been shown by Whipp and colleagues to vary with the background oxygen tension. During hypoxia the response is speeded up and during hyper-oxia slowed down. It is also slowed down following depression of

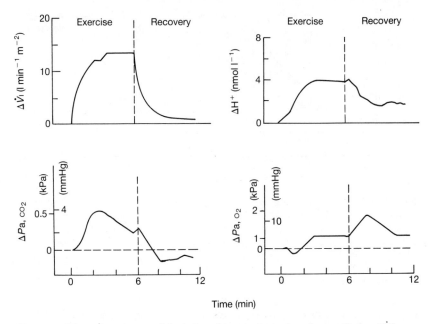

Fig. 11.11 Mean time course of deviations from resting values for ventilation ($\dot{V}$I), hydrogen ion concentration [H⁺] and arterial tensions of carbon dioxide and oxygen (Pa,co₂ and Pa,o₂) during and after moderate exercise in five healthy subjects. (Source: Matell G. *Acta Physiol Scand* 1963; **58**: suppl. 206, 1–53.)

chemoreceptor activity by intravenous infusion of dopamine (page 342) or denervation of both carotid bodies.

Acute inhibition of peripheral chemoreceptor activity by breathing oxygen also reduces the plateau phase of the ventilatory response to exercise. The resulting hypercapnoea limits the reduction by stimulating the central chemoreceptors. Possibly on this account chronic denervation of the carotid bodies can be associated with a normal ventilation in the steady state.

Additional factors that contribute to the ventilatory response include increases in the plasma concentrations of noradrenaline and potassium (page 344). These increases occur during the first 2 min of exercise. Later in the exercise the deep body temperature rises and this also stimulates ventilation. The rise in temperature is preceded by an increase in cardiac frequency. Cortical drive also contributes in some circumstance, for example when disproportionate respiratory effort is required on account of partial curarisation of the respiratory muscles. This observation was first made on himself by Moran Campbell.

Strenuous exercise

During moderate exercise the subject attains relatively stable levels of ventilation and gas exchange though not necessarily of cardiac frequency. The blood concentration of lactic acid remains at near to its baseline level. During strenuous exercise, as a result of rapid glycolysis, more lactic acid is produced by the active muscles than can be metabolised concurrently. The resulting lactacidaemia, which can be transient or persistent, can raise the blood hydrogen ion concentration. The extra ventilation flushes additional carbon dioxide from the lungs. The changes do not disturb the relationship of ventilation to carbon dioxide output, which remains linear, but relative to oxygen uptake the ventilation increases (Fig. 11.12).

The oxygen uptake at which the increase occurs (Fig. 11.12) reflects the rise in blood lactate; this was first pointed out by Owles. The inflection has been called the anaerobic threshold but this is inappropriate (page 401). The disproportionate increase in ventilation is due to the additional hydrogen ions stimulating the carotid chemoreceptors. The increase is reversed instantly by breathing oxygen and this suggests that central chemoreceptors do not normally contribute to the response. Heavy exercise makes additional demands on the respiratory muscles including the diaphragm which, during electrical stimulation, can be made to incur an oxygen debt. However, during spontaneous breathing the energy of contraction is provided by oxidative glycolysis (page 401). In some circumstances the pulmonary venous pressure rises during heavy exercise and this stimulates pulmonary J receptors (C fibre receptors) which reflexly increase the respiratory frequency. For example, cardiogenic tachypanoea is a feature of patients with mitral stenosis (Fig. 16.20, page 605) and cardiac insufficiency secondary to ischaemic heart disease (page 605). Whether or not these receptors also contribute to the normal ventilatory response to exercise is

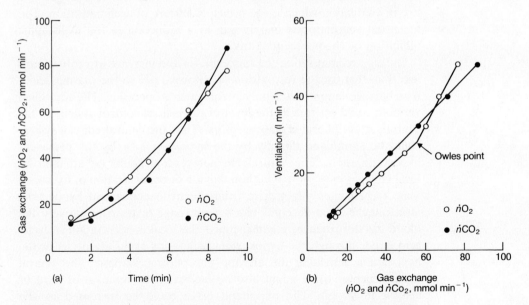

Fig. 11.12 Ventilation and gas exchange during progressive exercise in a healthy subject breathing air. (a) In relation to time (and hence to work rate) the carbon dioxide output increases more than the uptake of oxygen (hence the respiratory exchange ratio rises). (b) The increased CO_2 output is linearly related to and due to the increase in ventilation. On this account beyond Owles point (oxygen uptake $56 \, \text{mmol} \, \text{min}^{-1}$) the ventilation is increased relative to the oxygen uptake.

357

considered on page 334. The pattern of breathing during normal
exercise is described on pages 325 and 372.

High altitude

Acclimatisation

Ascent to high altitude is accompanied by a reduction in barometric
pressure and hence in the tension of oxygen in inspired gas (Fig. 17.1,
page 611). The resulting hypoxaemia stimulates the carotid chemoreceptors and increases the chemoreceptor drive to respiration (page
342). Ventilation increases in consequence. The hyperventilation is
somewhat greater than with an equivalent chemoreceptor drive at sea
level because the reduced air density decreases the airflow resistance
and hence the work of breathing (page 111). The hyperventilation
causes hypocapnia; this partly inhibits the chemoreceptor drive and
reduces the hyperventilation compared with what it would have been
in the absence of hypocapnia (page 345). The hypocapnia also reduces
the plasma concentrations of carbonic acid and hydrogen ions (cH),
which constitutes respiratory alkalosis (page 520). This is partly compensated by increased renal excretion of sodium bicarbonate. Consequently the plasma cH rises and the plasma pH falls towards the
normal sea level values; these are restored within about a month. The
change in plasma bicarbonate influences the ventilatory response to
carbon dioxide (Fig. 11.8, page 348). It also contributes to a progressive
rise in ventilation which is the principal feature of acclimatisation. The
increased ventilation is mainly due to a reduction in the hypocapnic
inhibition of chemoreceptor drive.

During acclimatisation the half time for the increase in ventilation is
less than that for the restoration of a normal pH so the plasma acid–
base balance cannot be the only factor which is operating. The additional
variable could operate at the level of the central control system or the
central or peripheral chemoreceptors. Thus the central control system
could be stimulated directly by the hypoxaemia or by the persistent
hyperventilation. The central chemoreceptors could be affected by
local changes in tension of carbon dioxide or concentration of hydrogen
ions; the changes might arise from the hypoxaemia and hypocapnia
affecting the local cerebral blood flow (page 334). Alternatively the
blood gas disturbances might increase the local concentration of lactic
acid either through the hypoxaemia facilitating rapid glycolysis or the
hypocapnia activating the enzyme phosphofructokinase. The central
chemoreceptor drive might also be facilitated by removal of local or
central inhibition. The peripheral drive could be increased by the
hypoxaemia depleting the chemoreceptor stores of dopamine which
would otherwise exert an inhibitory effect (page 342). The central
response to the chemoreceptor drive could also be modified by the
other changes. One or more of these mechanisms probably contribute
to acclimatisation but the actual details remain in doubt.

Oxygen transport

Acclimatisation has the effect of raising the alveolar oxygen tension compared with the unacclimatised state. The residual hypoxaemia also contributes directly or indirectly to other compensatory changes. The most direct effect is on the kidneys where the production of erythropoietin is increased. The hormone stimulates the production of red blood cells; this in turn raises the blood haemoglobin concentration and increases the capacity of the circulation to deliver oxygen to the tissues. The transport of oxygen by haemoglobin is also affected by the hypoxaemia increasing the red cell concentration of 2,3-diphosphoglycerate. This facilitates the unloading of oxygen in tissue capillaries (Fig. 9.3, page 280). However, in the short term the effect is to some extent nullified by the initial respiratory alkalosis which has the converse effect. The haematological changes also influence the capacity of the blood to transport carbon dioxide (Fig. 9.5, page 287). Additional changes occur in the tissues which increase their ability to utilise oxygen. The density of capillaries which serve active muscles is increased as is the number and density of mitochondria. There is a rise in the concentration of enzymes which contribute to oxidative metabolism (page 401). These features contribute directly to the capacity for exercise. There are also indirect benefits from the hyperventilation exerting a training effect on the respiratory muscles. This increases the vital capacity and the maximal breathing capacity compared with the unacclimatised state. Most of the changes persist for a few weeks after descent from altitude so residence at altitude can be used to secure a temporary increase in exercise performance at sea level (page 396).

During exercise at altitude the ventilation is increased by hypoxaemia and acclimatisation. However, the hypoxia also reduces the oxygen transfer gradient across the alveolar capillary membrane and this impairs the normal uptake of oxygen by haemoglobin (page 285). During strenuous exercise the resulting transfer defect aggravates the hypoxaemia which further increases the ventilation. When this is increased to its maximal extent it limits the capacity for exercise (page 393). Under these conditions the bulk flow of gas to and from the lungs, expressed in $mmol\,min^{-1}$ or $l\,STPD\,min^{-1}$, approaches its sea level value.

Sleep

At altitude the hypoxaemia and resulting hypocapnia modify the normal changes which occur during sleep. The latter are described beginning on page 350. On the first night following the ascent there is an increase in very light sleep (stage 1), a reduction in slow wave sleep (stages 3 and 4) and an increased number of arousals. These are due to hyperpnoea associated with the termination of periods of apnoea. The alternating hyperpnoea and apnoea was first described by Cheyne and Stokes. The initial stimulus is hypoxia which causes more profound hypoxaemia and hence greater peripheral chemoreceptor drive during sleep than when the subject is awake. The hyperventilation causes pronounced hypocapnia which leads to cessation of breathing. During the apnoea the arterial tension of oxygen falls and that of carbon dioxide rises; the chemoreceptor drive then increases and initiates the next period of hyperventilation. Cheyne Stokes breathing is very common on ascent to altitudes in excess of 1800 m (6000 ft); the symptom improves with acclimatisation. Elderly subjects are particularly susceptible. The disturbed sleep is associated with lassitude and often with morning headache. The condition is alleviated by oxygen in low dosage (page 616). It can also be improved by slightly increasing the arterial carbon dioxide tension, for example by breathing through a mask which acts as an external deadspace. The condition can be avoided by prior treatment with acetazolamide; this prevents the development of a respiratory alkalosis by promoting the renal excretion of bicarbonate.

Blunting of the hypoxic response

The normal adaptation to high altitude is centred round the process of acclimatisation and the additional changes which are described above; they have the effect of materially increasing the capacity for exercise and in the case of acute exposure, of permitting survival in conditions which might otherwise be lethal (page 610). The secondary changes can also reduce the level of acclimatisation which is required. Thus long-term residence at high altitude is associated with a decline in the ventilatory response to hypoxia. This blunting of the hypoxic response is acquired in early adolescence by children living at high altitude. It can also develop after about 20 years in persons who move to high altitude as adults. The blunting can be reversed by return to sea level. In persons with cyanotic congenital heart disease similar changes occur though the blunting is then often irreversible and not responsive to correction of the cardiac defect. Weill has found that the blunting affected particularly oxygen tensions in the range 5−9 kPa (40−70 mmHg). Extreme hypoxia still elicits marked hyperventilation. Thus blunting represents a displacement of the ventilatory response to hypoxia not an inhibition. Blunting is associated with a somewhat increased ventilation during normoxia and a paradoxical response to breathing oxygen which then increases ventilation instead of depressing it. The blunting can be accompanied by a reduced ventilatory response to carbon dioxide. Both features are usually acquired but genetic constitution also contributes. Thus when tested at sea level, the ventilatory response to carbon dioxide has been found to be reduced in New Guinea highlanders and men from Nepal, and the acute response to moderate hypoxia is reduced in the Himalayan bar-headed goose and the South American llama both of which are very tolerant of high altitudes. Blunting of the hypoxic response was produced experimentally in cats by Tenney and Ou. The blunting appeared to be initiated by stimuli from higher suprapontine centres in the brain. The peripheral chemoreceptors could also contribute since chronic hypoxia leads to hypertrophy of the glomus tissue and to accumulation of dopamine which inhibits chemoreceptor activity. However, the ventilatory response to stimulation of the chemoreceptors by doxapram was found by Forster and colleagues not to be reduced in life-time residents at high altitude. Thus the mechanism remains in doubt.

Blunting of the hypoxic response is accompanied with relative hypercapnia, and by increased hypoxaemia which in some subjects leads to gross polycythaemia and other features of chronic mountain sickness (page 617). This syndrome has aspects in common with other conditions of chronic hypoventilation including Pickwickian syndrome (page 579) and sleep apnoea/hypopnoea syndrome (page 581).

Guide to references

The references (Chapter 18) are classified under subject headings of which the following are particularly relevant to the present chapter:

12: Assessment of Respiratory Control

Introduction

The respiratory control system is described in the previous chapter. In a wide range of circumstances, it operates to maintain normal tensions of oxygen and carbon dioxide. Faulty respiratory control leads to inappropriate levels of ventilation or an abnormal pattern of breathing; the changes alter the levels of the arterial blood gases which in turn can have consequences for all bodily organs and systems, particularly the central nervous system (page 621). The changes can present in a number of ways of which the most immediate are hypoxaemia, hyper- or hypocapnia, breathlessness or somnolence. Subsequently adaptations occur in response to the changes in carbon dioxide tension (page 520) or to hypoxaemia and the latter can be complicated by right heart failure (page 541) and by polycythaemia which in turn, predisposes to intra-vascular thromboses. In otherwise healthy persons the risk of a fault arising in the respiratory control system is influenced by environmental factors including those which predispose to obesity, and by the genetic constitution. The fault can also arise in the course of many pathological conditions, particularly those which affect the respiratory reticular formation in the brain. The conditions are described in Chapter 16 (pages 579–586).

Is the control faulty?

The first stage in the assessment of respiratory control is to measure, in the clinic, the arterial oxygen and carbon dioxide tensions. Normal values exclude gross abnormalities but are compatible with minor changes during sleep or exertion. Abnormal values are not diagnostic of disturbed respiratory control but can also occur in many other circumstances. The principal causes of hypoxaemia are listed in Table 17.1 (pages 612 and 613) and of an abnormal arterial carbon dioxide tension in the pages cited above. Having measured the arterial blood gases during the day, the next step could be to monitor the arterial oxygen saturation during sleep or to undertake polysomnography. Alternatively, or subsequently, measurements might be made during exercise with a veiw to exposing faults not apparent at rest. Having detected a fault a subsequent step might be to test the components of the control system and then to act on the information which has been obtained.

Arterial blood gases

The arterial blood should be sampled via an indwelling arterial cannula (page 38) after the elapse of approximately 30 min for the subject to have recovered from the cannulation procedure. The subject should be at rest, relaxed and in a post-absorbtive state (page 77). The analyses should be performed using one of the methods described previously (pages 39–47).

Interpretation of the arterial blood gas tensions and cH depends on a knowledge of the normal levels, or reference values; for adults under quiet resting conditions these are summarised in Table 15.22, page 508. Usually only minor changes occur during moderate steady state exercise (Fig. 13.7, page 398).

The tension of oxygen in arterial blood is low in newborn babies (page 453). It rises to a steady level at about the third week of extrauterine life and thereafter remains fairly constant into adulthood. Subsequently the tension declines with age due to the lung function becoming progressively more uneven (page 489). The decline can be described by a linear regression equation such as that of Rayne and Bishop:

$$Pa,o_2 = 0.133 \ [104 - 0.24 \ \text{Age (yr), SD 7.9}] \ \text{kPa} \qquad (12.1)$$

where 0.133 converts from traditional to SI units. This relationship applies only to those who live at sea level; lower figures are normal at lower barometric pressures. The linear model is almost certainly an oversimplification of the change with age but the information from which to construct a better model appears not to exist at the present time. The situation could change now that measurement can be made non-invasively. The normal tension of oxygen varies inversely with body mass and is reduced by uneven lung ventilation/perfusion ratios such as are caused by smoking, chronic bronchitis or emphysema (page 529). The tension exhibits circadian variation and is less during sleep than in the waking state (page 350). There is also a small monthly oscillation in women, with relatively high values in the luteal phase of the menstrual cycle when progesterone stimulates respiration (page 469).

The tension of carbon dioxide in arterial blood resembles that of oxygen in being relatively low in newborn babies. Subsequently the resting level stabilises at around 5.3 kPa (40 mmHg) when the subject is awake; it increases somewhat during sleep (page 350). The level falls in response to increased respiratory drive such as that associated with a reduced inspired oxygen tension or an increased blood concentration of progesterone. During moderate steady state exercise the arterial carbon dioxide tension can deviate upwards or downwards from the resting level; the deviations reflect alterations in the respiratory control and in the tension of carbon dioxide in mixed venous blood, which depends on the blood flow through the exercising muscles. Thus the circumstances need to be taken into account when deciding whether or not the arterial blood gases are abnormal.

Respiratory control during sleep

Respiratory control during sleep is described on page 350. Disturbed sleep associated with periods of apnoea or hypopnoea is relatively common amongst patients with some respiratory, cardiovascular and other disorders (page 579). If left untreated the hypoventilation can contribute to clinical deterioration. This has led to the establishment of clinical sleep laboratories and to many physicians conducting simplified sleep studies. The subject has been reviewed by the American Thoracic Society amongst others.

Terminology

Polysomnography refers to studies which aim to relate the ventilation and arterial blood gases to the stages of sleep. Simplified studies aim to identify disturbances to ventilation and/or arterial oxygen saturation during sleep but do not relate these to the stage of sleep. Physiological studies of respiratory drive and responsiveness as outlined later in this chapter can also be performed during sleep: when these are undertaken the study should include measurements of the stage of sleep.

Indications

The indications of the American Thoracic Society are given in Table 16.19 (page 583).

Circumstances of the study

Overnight attendance at a sleep laboratory can be an ordeal for the subject who will usually sleep fitfully in consequence. A preliminary visit to the laboratory and an explanation of what is involved will make the study more acceptable to the subject. Alternatively the measurements can be made in a normal hospital bed; this should be connected by an electric cable to the recording instruments which should be in a separate room. Subjects who fall asleep by day can also be studied during a daytime nap. The nap should be of more than 2 h duration and include rapid eye movement sleep (REM sleep) as well as non-REM sleep; the subject should be supine for at least part of the study.

Optimal reproducibility is achieved by making definitive measurements on a second night following a practice session but for clinical purposes the information obtained on a single night is usually adequate. In some centres the night is divided into two parts, the first for making the diagnosis of sleep apnoea and the second for assessing the response to treatment (page 715).

Respiratory control during sleep

Methods

The stage of sleep is assessed from the electrical activity of the brain, the presence or absence of rapid eye movements, the level of muscle tone during REM sleep and the occurrence of movements associated with arousal (page 350). Electrical activity is recorded by electrodes in the position C_3, C_4, A_1 and A_2 of the 10−20 International System described by Jasper; the electroencephalogram leads C_3/A_2 or C_4/A_1 are interpreted (cf. Table 11.4, page 352).

Rapid eye movements are identified using electrodes situated close to the outer canthus of each eye; the electrodes are placed obliquely with the right hand one a centimetre above and the left hand one a centimetre below the horizontal. General muscle tone and movement can be monitored for any skeletal muscle other than the respiratory muscles. Arm or leg electrodes can be used for this purpose. However, the submental muscle of the chin is often preferable on account of its accessibility. Electrodes are placed one on the chin and one on each side below the lower border of the mandible. Only one of the latter is used at any one time for recording the electromyogram. The second is in reserve in case the first is dislodged.

The arterial oxygen saturation can be recorded using an ear oximeter; this has adequate accuracy and response time but is liable to become dislodged. Alternatively a finger pulse oximeter can be used. Gas tensions in arterial blood are seldom monitored because this can only be done by arterial catheterisation. Indirect recording of tissue oxygen tension via a cutaneous electrode is not satisfactory because the tissue tension only responds slowly to a change in ventilation. The mean tissue carbon dioxide tension can be recorded satisfactorily in this way.

Ventilation is monitored in one of several ways, depending on the extent and accuracy which is required. At its simplest the respiratory frequency is monitored at the nose or mouth using a thermistor or rapid analyser for carbon dioxide. Alternatively the breath sounds are recorded using a laryngeal microphone, or the thoracic excursions are registered using a potentiometer or mercury strain gauge. However, the signals are qualitative and insensitive to small changes in the pattern of breathing. The alternative of collecting the respired gas using an oronasal mask is unsatisfactory during sleep. Instead the ventilation should be measured semi-quantitatively using magnetometers or a jerkin inductance plethysmograph. The system which is used should monitor movement of the abdomen as well as the thorax and should be calibrated before and at the end of the session (page 26). If the two calibrations agree then the results can be interpreted with some confidence and, if not, at least the best will have been done in the circumstances.

The ventilatory monitor should permit the identification of periods of apnoea. When these are of central origin the respiratory muscles are relaxed, but when they are due to obstruction the respiratory muscles continue to contract. When the subject is awake a propensity to obstructed breathing can sometimes be identified from the presence of a saw tooth pattern on the maximal flow volume curve. However, the association is not a close one. The two types of apnoea can be differentiated by recording the activity of the diaphragm or the intrapleural pressure. These two pieces of information can be obtained concurrently using an oesophageal catheter connected to a pressure transducer and incorporating an electrode for recording the diaphragmatic electromyogram. Alternatively Sackner has suggested the use of a neck inductive plethysmograph. This consists of one or two inductive transducer bands 2.5 cm wide; they are positioned around the neck to produce a display of *P*pl waveform with respiration. The cardiovascular changes during sleep are secondary to the respiratory ones. They should be recorded using the chest lead CM5 of the electrocardiogram.

Reporting results

Polysomnography produces a superabundance of information and one needs to be selective in its use. The usual clinical requirement is to identify sleep apnoea or hypopnoea. Apnoea is commonly defined as the absence of air movement for 10 s or longer. Such periods can be identified from the ventilation record, and the number and total duration obtained by addition. Periods of hypopnoea can sometimes be identified and quantified in a similar manner, but the onset of hypoventilation cannot be recognised without a knowledge of the level of arterial blood gases, which is seldom available during sleep; this limits the value of hypopnoea as an indicator of abnormality. The effect of the disturbed sleep upon arterial oxygen saturation can be obtained from the output from the oximeter. It can be expressed as the total time for which the saturation is less than a specified level, for example 80%, or for which saturation has fallen by a specified amount, for example 4%. An analysis along these lines can often be carried out automatically. A more detailed analysis is likely to start with identification of the different stages of sleep; these are then related to the periods of apnoea and the extent of desaturation. However, the need for this information should first be established. Often only the occurrence of apnoeas and their diagnosis as central or obstructive are of practical importance. When there is obstruction the site and the mechanism should be established so that appropriate treatment can be given. The relevant factors are summarised in Table 11.5 (page 352).

The interpretation of sleep studies is likely to be improved by further standardisation of the methods, including definitions of the relevant indices. This will simplify the documentation of normal sleep and the compilation of reference values for people of different ages. Such studies are likely to identify other reference variables or characteristics predisposing to sleep apnoea. These in turn will affect how the tests are used.

Some indications for submitting a patient to polysomnography are given on page 581, whilst the underlying physiology is discussed on page 350. The prevention of post anaesthetic obstruction is considered on page 618.

Respiratory control during exercise

For study of respiratory control an exercise test can often reveal an increase in respiratory frequency which cannot be detected in other ways. Such an increase may be demonstrated in mitral stenosis, early left ventricular failure and some diseases of the lung parenchyma. This and other aspects of ventilation during submaximal exercise are considered in this section. The broader physiological response to exercise is considered in subsequent chapters.

Submaximal exercise ventilation

During strenuous exercise the ventilation is greatly influenced by the rate of rapid glycolysis and hence lactacidaemia. This reflects the adequacy of the muscle blood flow and the activity of the mitochondrial enzymes in the muscles (see Chapter 13). Disturbance of the bellows function of the lung sets an upper limit for the exercise ventilation and tidal volume. On the other hand during submaximal exercise the ventilation is determined mainly by interaction between the respiratory control system, the mechanical function of the lungs and chest wall and the function of the lung as an organ of gas exchange. When the mechanical and gas exchanging functions are normal, the exercise ventilation reflects the activity of the control system. When the lung function is abnormal the level of ventilation is also influenced by the extent of uneven distribution of pulmonary ventilation and perfusion, by hypoxaemia and by shallow breathing secondary to pulmonary fibrosis. The level of ventilation during submaximal exercise is usually expressed relative to the uptake of oxygen, but the rate of external work and the output of carbon dioxide can also be compared with ventilation.

Step test of Hugh-Jones and Lambert. During exercise of a few minutes duration the ventilation exhibits an abrupt followed by a slow increase, a steady level and an abrupt followed by a slow decline (page 354). The steady level and the extent to which the recovery phase is prolonged can be assessed very simply by measuring the ventilation each 30 s during stepping exercise of standard intensity performed for 5 min. The exercise is preceded and followed by measurement of resting ventilation; after exercise the measurements are continued until the initial level is restored. The rate of work is 57 W ($350 \, \mathrm{kp\,m\,min^{-1}}$) or occasionally 33 W ($200 \, \mathrm{kp\,m\,min^{-1}}$).

The stepping is performed on and off a box of height 0.2 m, the height is varied by adding an appropriate number of wood tiles which should be suitably secured. The frequency of stepping is adjusted using a metronome. The work rate is calculated by adjusting the height and frequency according to the following relationship:

$$\text{work level} = h \times f \times w \times 0.163 \text{ watts} \qquad (12.2)$$

where h is the height of the step in metres, f is the frequency of stepping per min and w is the body weight of the subject in kg. The interrelationship between the alternative units of work is given on page 16. For subjects of different weights, settings for the step height and the frequency of stepping which will provide the desired work level can be read off a nomogram (Fig. 12.1). The rate of stepping is paced by a metronome which is set at four times the desired number of steps per min to allow for the movement of both feet on and off the box. During the exercise in order to achieve the desired work level the subject should move the weight of the body through the height of the step. To this end the trunk should be held erect and the subject should preferably not grip any support with the hand as this has the effect of reducing the amount of work which is performed during the test. The ventilation in the 4th and 5th min of exercise usually provides an adequate description

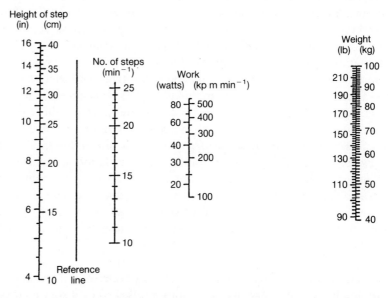

Fig. 12.1 Nomogram for obtaining a predetermined rate of vertical work during stepping exercise. A ruler is laid across the two right hand scales at the body weight of the subject and the desired rate of vertical work. The point where the ruler crosses the reference line is marked with a soft pencil. Any straight line through this point linking the left hand scale, which is the height of the step, with the next scale, which is the rate of stepping, will yield the desired work level. In practice the ruler is swivelled about the reference point until a convenient combination of step height and rate of stepping is obtained.

of the ventilatory response but it does not reflect the initial phase or the recovery period. These components are included in the excess ventilation which is illustrated in Fig. 11.10 (page 355). The latter index is obtained by subtracting from the total volume of gas breathed throughout the exercise and recovery that which would have been breathed had the subject remained at rest. The excess ventilation may be used to calculate a standardised ventilation which is given by:

$$SV = \dot{V}\text{rest} + EEV/t \text{ l min}^{-1} \qquad (12.3)$$

where SV is standardized ventilation, $\dot{V}$rest is resting ventilation, EEV is excess exercise ventilation (page 355) and t is the duration of exercise in minutes. The exercise ventilation and standardised ventilation are equal except when the recovery is delayed by a need to repay an oxygen debt incurred during the exercise. This occurs in mitral stenosis or other conditions where the cardiac output is inadequate for the needs of the exercise. In other circumstances if the subject is unable to exercise for long enough to reach a steady state the standardised ventilation may be substituted for the exercise ventilation. Representative values are given in Fig. 12.2. The test has the advantage over the use of a fixed height and frequency of stepping that the result is nearly independent of the body weight of the subject.

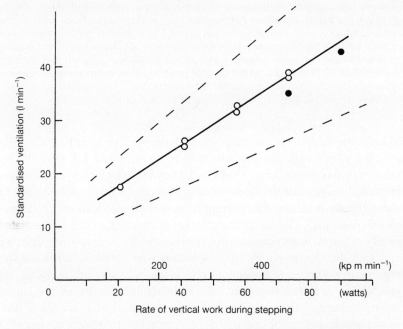

Fig. 12.2 The ventilatory response to exercise of healthy subjects during the performance of the Hugh-Jones step test. The subjects include male and female laboratory personnel and industrial workers (open circles) and athletes (closed circles). Ninety-five per cent of the observations lie within the interrupted lines which are drawn at a distance of twice the standard deviation about the mean regression. For men and women respectively the test is usually performed at rates of work of 57 and 49 watts (350 and 300 kpm min^{-1}); for the former the consumption of oxygen is on average 60 mmol min^{-1} (1.4 l min^{-1}). The consumption at other rates of work is indicated in Fig. 14.3, page 421. (Source: Gandevia B. *Am Rev Respir Dis* 1962; **85**: 378.)

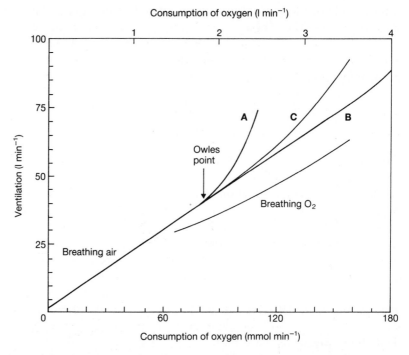

Fig. 12.3 Relationship of ventilation to consumption of oxygen during progressive treadmill exercise up to the maximum which the subjects could achieve. At the time subject A was untrained and had a low capacity for exercise, subject B was a world class middle distance runner, subject C who was assessed by Asmussen and Nielsen was well trained; his response to breathing oxygen was also recorded. During moderate exercise breathing air the ventilatory responses were similar for all three subjects; they diverged during strenuous exercise due to the onset of rapid glycolysis at different rates of work which reflected the exercise capacities of the subjects. The ventilation was reduced by breathing oxygen (cf. Figs 11.5 and 11.6, pages 343 and 344).

Ventilation relative to consumption of oxygen. The ventilation during exercise varies with the consumption of oxygen (see Fig. 12.3). The relationship is linear up to *Owles point* beyond which the ventilation is increased relative to the consumption of oxygen; this is mainly due to rapid glycolysis raising the concentration of hydrogen ions in the arterial blood (page 402). The rectilinear portion of the relationship is illustrated in Fig. 12.4; it is similar for progressive and for steady-state exercise and may be described by the coefficient and constant terms of the regression equation (equation 12.4 below), but this, whilst useful for prediction, is not convenient for reporting the results of individual subjects. Instead the ventilation can be reported at a specified consumption of oxygen, for example 45 or 67 mmol min^{-1} (1.0 or 1.5 l min^{-1}) for men as has been recommended by a committee of the International Labour Organization, and 45 mmol min^{-1} (1.0 l min^{-1}) for women. The values are obtained by interpolation in the manner illustrated in Fig. 12.4. The ventilatory response to exercise was formerly reported as the ventilation per 100 ml of uptake of oxygen, i.e. the *ventilation equivalent*. The index is calculated on the assumption that the ventilation

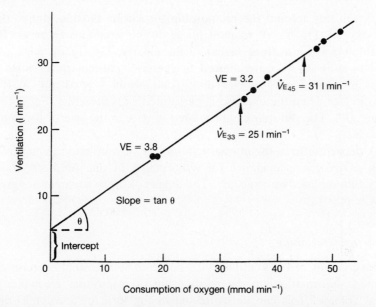

Fig. 12.4 Ways of reporting ventilation during exercise. Graph shows ventilation and consumption of oxygen for a patient with chronic lung disease during progressive exercise. The result is described accurately by the slope (θ) and intercept of the regression line or by the ventilation at specified uptakes of oxygen (e.g. $\dot{V}E$ 33 or $\dot{V}E$ 45): it is described incorrectly by the ventilation equivalent (VE, see text) which varies depending on the oxygen uptake at which the calculation is made.

is proportional to the consumption of oxygen, which is not the case, and yields a variable result depending on where on the regression line the calculation is made (Fig. 12.4). It is best abandoned in favour of the procedure which is described above.

The ventilation during exercise is influenced by both physiological and psychological factors. They have the effect that when the subject performs the exercise for the first time, or in warm surroundings, or is apprehensive, unduly high values are often recorded. On this account the use of duplicate determinations is desirable but not essential. Rather greater errors are introduced when the consumption of oxygen is estimated from the rate of performance of external work in the manner described below.

At sea level for healthy adult males during moderate exercise with the legs the ventilation may be described empirically in terms of the consumption of oxygen:

$$\dot{V}E = 0.5\dot{n}o_2 + 2, \text{ SD } 5.4\, l\,min^{-1} \qquad (12.4)$$

where $\dot{V}E$ is ventilation minute volume in $l\,BTPS\,min^{-1}$ and $\dot{n}o_2$ is consumption of oxygen in $mmol\,min^{-1}$. When the consumption of oxygen is expressed in $l\ min^{-1}$ the coefficient term is 22 (i.e. $0.5 \times 10^3 \div 22.4$). A similar relationship obtains for carbon dioxide but the coefficient term is greater. However, with exercise of increasing severity the output of carbon dioxide increases relative to the consumption of oxygen so that the respiratory exchange ratio rises (Fig. 11.12, page

371

357). On this account the relationship for carbon dioxide, unlike that for oxygen (Fig. 12.3), remains linear during strenuous exercise. The ventilation is on average higher in the elderly (Fig. 15.19, page 491) and in subjects who are unused to exercise, particularly at rates of consumption of oxygen exceeding 45 mmol min^{-1} (1.0 l min^{-1}). It is also higher when the exercise is performed with the arms (Fig. 15.19, page 491). The differences are related in part to the size of the active muscles.

A departure from the normal relationship of ventilation to consumption of oxygen is evidence for abnormality in one or more of the variables outlined on page 367. The details of the assessment are given in Chapter 14.

Pattern of breathing

Measurement of the ventilatory response to submaximal exercise can provide information on the relationship of respiratory frequency to tidal volume. This can be expressed in the form of a volume−time diagram (Fig. 11.2, page 327). However, due to variation between breaths the construction of this diagram requires more information than can conveniently be processed during a routine exercise test. Alternatively, the average tidal volume and frequency for each half minute can be used to describe the relationship of exercise minute volume to tidal volume (Hey plot Fig. 11.1, page 326) or that of exercise respiratory frequency to ventilation (Fig. 12.5). The relation-

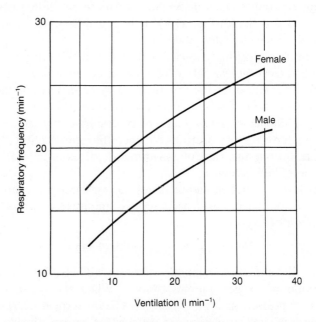

Fig. 12.5 Average relationship of respiratory frequency to minute volume during exercise for healthy adult male and female subjects of European descent. The difference between the sexes is due to men on average having larger vital capacities. This anatomical factor can be allowed for by using the index Vt 30 which is described in the text.

ships should preferably be constructed using average tidal volumes and frequencies calculated for whole numbers of breaths rather than for fixed time intervals but this is not essential. The Hey plot yields the tidal volume at a minute volume of $30\,l\,min^{-1}$. This index varies directly with forced vital capacity:

$$Vt\ 30 = 0.13\ FVC + 0.87,\ SD\ 0.22\ l \qquad (12.5)$$

where $Vt\ 30$ is tidal volume at a minute volume of $30\,l\,min^{-1}$ and FVC is forced vital capacity. The relationship is independent of age, gender and ethnic group. It is unaffected by many chronic lung diseases including chronic bronchitis and diffuse interstitial fibrosis. It also holds for most cases of emphysema. A reduction in $Vt\ 30$ relative to the volume expected for the patient's forced FVC is evidence of tachypnoea which can be caused by stimulation of pulmonary J receptors (C fibre receptors). Tachypnoea associated with mitral stenosis and with subacute beryllium disease is illustrated in Figs 16.13 and 16.20 (pages 566 and 605) respectively.

The role of the $Vt\ 30$ in the assessment of patients with lung disease is considered on page 432.

Tests of control function

The principle of testing is to alter a component of the drive to respiration and measure the response. The alteration can take the form of reducing or augmenting an existing stimulus to breathing or introducing a new one. The response can be the change in ventilation or in respiratory work. The relationship of the response to the change in respiratory drive should be available in the form of a dose–response curve which should be linear or capable of linearisation by an appropriate transformation (page 60). The respiratory sensitivity is then described by one of the parameters of the regression equation (e.g. m in the equation $y = mx + c$, where y and x are respectively the response and the change in the stimulus, cf. page 381).

In practice the response can be influenced by the conditions of testing, which can introduce either bias or variability, whilst the change in the stimulus is seldom clear cut. These sources of error can be overcome but the measures needed are often technically demanding or lengthen the procedure or have other disadvantages. Thus the tests which are chosen usually represent a compromise between what is ideal and what is practical and are likely to vary with circumstances.

The stimulus

Central or peripheral? The stimulus can be directed to either or both the peripheral chemoreceptors and the central control system. The central control system can be stimulated directly by the subject breathing a gas mixture containing carbon dioxide in oxygen. Direct stimulation can also be effected by hyperthermia. Uncomplicated peripheral stimulation is provided by mild hypoxia and by substances such as progesterone for which the respiratory effect is mediated solely via the chemoreceptors. In other circumstances, of which the commonest is hypoxia with hypercapnia, there is both central and peripheral stimulation, with the latter having the shorter latency (Fig. 11.5, page 343).

Direction of change. The stimulus used to study the control function can take the form of a reduction or an increase in the respiratory drive. A reduction in respiratory drive has the advantage that very little or no additional load is imposed on the respiratory system. Thus the load is only slightly increased on switching to breathing a hyperoxic gas mixture from breathing air at rest (Fig. 11.6, page 344). When the initial state is one of hypoxia and/or exercise the load is reduced by breathing oxygen (Fig. 12.3). The respiratory drive can also be reduced by hypnosis or by inducing a state of hypocapnia and/or alkalaemia through voluntary over-breathing or ingestion of sodium bicarbonate. However, the first and third of these are more suited to studying mechanisms of respiratory control than for quantitative assessment. The control function can be assessed in terms of the onset of breathing and the associated rise in alveolar carbon dioxide tension following a period of breath holding or involuntary apnoea.

An increase in respiratory drive can be induced by exercise; it can also be achieved by breathing a hypoxic or hypercapnic gas mixture, by raising the body temperature or by reducing the blood pH usually through the ingestion of ammonium chloride. However, the last of these is of limited usefulness for assessing the control function.

External stimuli are another possibility, for example an intravenous injection of cyanide can stimulate the carotid body but this substance is unsuitable for routine use. Other specific respiratory stimulant or depressant drugs might be used but their potential for testing the control function appears not to have been explored.

Complicating factors. Any change in respiratory drive of sufficient magnitude to alter the alveolar ventilation inevitably has secondary effects. An increase in ventilation which is not due to hypercapnia leads to the excretion of additional carbon dioxide and reduces the hypercapnoeic drive to breathing. Depending on circumstances it may also reduce the hypoxic drive. A change in respiratory drive which causes hypoventilation can have the opposite effects. These feedback mechanisms can be interrupted by measures to maintain the constancy of one variable whilst monitoring the effect of another. The simplest procedure entails rebreathing a mixture of carbon dioxide in oxygen. The oxygen tension is then maintained at above the threshold for stimulating the carotid body so the effect which is observed is that of central hypercapnia with hyperoxia. Alternatively the respiratory effects of varying degrees of hypoxia or hypercapnia can be assessed at a constant tension of the other variable. This isocapnic technique was introduced by Cunningham, Lloyd and colleagues at Oxford; it is effected by monitoring the end tidal or alveolar gas concentrations and, in the light of the findings, making appropriate adjustments to the composition of the inspired gas.

The response

Ventilation. The response to a change in respiratory drive is usually assessed in terms of its effect on ventilation. This is acceptable in normal circumstances, though because the properties of the lungs and the chest wall differ between individuals, some of the variability in the ventilatory responses is due to factors in the thorax. The effect of this thoracic component is increased in patients with obesity, with skeleto-muscular disorders and in those with airway obstruction in whom the control function may be normal but the ventilatory response reduced (see e.g. Fig. 12.6). Procedures for assessing the ventilatory responses to carbon dioxide and to hypoxia are given on page 379.

The procedures depend on having a measurable stimulus, and in the case of carbon dioxide this is usually obtained by imposing relatively high tensions which do not occur normally. The effects of carbon dioxide tensions within the normal range can be studied by the constant input technique. This entails delivering a constant quantity of carbon dioxide to the lung each minute and not a constant concentration of CO_2 as is used in the steady state method.

The ventilatory responsiveness is indicated by the relationship between ventilation and P_{A,CO_2}. Thus the method ignores any breath-by-breath or within breath fluctuations in respiratory drive; these can be assessed by one of the methods described below. In addition a

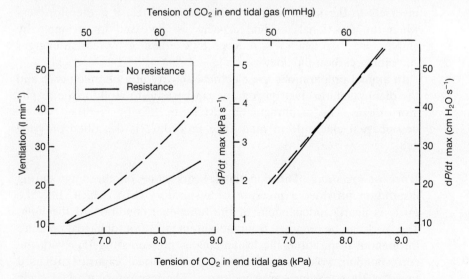

Fig. 12.6 Effect of respiratory resistance upon the ventilation minute volume and the (dP/dt)max during rebreathing carbon dioxide in oxygen. (Source: Matthews AW, Howell JBL. *Clin Sci* 1976; **50**: 199–205.)

single measurement session can extend for more than an hour and during this time the acid−base balance can change as a result of renal compensation for the respiratory acidosis which is imposed. However, despite these disadvantages the method has contributed greatly to present knowledge of chemoreceptor drive, particularly the major role of hypoxaemia and how the resulting hypoxic drive is modulated by carbon dioxide and other stimuli.

Respiratory drive. In persons with normal lungs Milic Emili has shown that the drive can be represented by the average flow rate during inspiration. This is the tidal volume divided by the time of inspiration (Vt/tl); the relationship between these variables is illustrated in Fig. 11.1 (page 326). However, the index is of limited usefulness in patients with lung disease for whom the $Po.1$ or dP/dtmax should be used instead. These indices are due respectively to Milic Emili and to Howell and their collaborators. The $Po.1$ is the suction developed at the mouth 0.1 s after the start of inspiration when this is made against a closed shutter. The dP/dtmax is the maximal rate of rise of pressure at the start of inspiration made against a breathing valve selected to have a finite opening pressure. The $Po.1$ has the advantage of being definable in absolute units and requiring only very simple equipment; it has the disadvantage of interrupting the breathing and hence only being applicable to a small proportion of breaths. The dP/dtmax cannot easily be calibrated in absolute units but it is derivable from every breath and on this account is the more reproducible index. An example is given in Fig. 12.6. The thorax is stationary during the measurement so the suction is independent of factors which influence the rate of movement of the lungs, including the resistance and compliance of the lungs and chest wall. However, at a constant level of drive the suction is related inversely to the initial length of the muscle fibres; it is therefore less when the functional residual capacity is increased for example by emphysema than when it is reduced by exercise or by rebreathing gas containing carbon dioxide.

In animal preparations the electrical activity in a phrenic nerve and the diaphragmatic electromyogram can be used to monitor the respiratory drive. The diaphragmatic EMG can also be recorded via an oesophageal electrode in man. The procedure is described on page 578.

Work of breathing. The non-elastic work done on the lungs during inspiration provides a measure of respiratory drive which, like the $Po.1$, is nearly independent of the functional condition of the lung. The work can be obtained from measurements of oesophageal pressure throughout inspiration; the instantaneous pressures together with the corresponding volumes above functional residual capacity are used to delineate a volume−pressure curve. The inspiratory work is given by the area of the inspiratory part of the curve; this is illustrated in Fig. 5.18 (page 127). The method provides a means for validating of entailing intubation of the oesophagus.

Oxygen cost of breathing. The consumption of oxygen by the respiratory muscles reflects the respiratory drive. The consumption can be estimated from measurements of the uptake of oxygen made at two or more levels of ventilation minute volume. In the procedure devised by Campbell, Westlake and Cherniack the subject rebreathes from a closed circuit spirometer which is fitted with an absorber for carbon dioxide and is equipped to record on a kymograph. The spirometer is filled with oxygen then, after allowing time for equilibration the ventilation and uptake of oxygen are recorded. The carbon dioxide is administered by arranging that the subject rebreathes from a length of wide-bore tubing introduced between the mouthpiece and the spirometer circuit. In terms of ventilation the oxygen cost is given by:

$$\text{oxygen cost} = [\dot{n}o_{2(2)} - \dot{n}o_{2(1)}]/[\dot{V}_{E(2)} - \dot{V}_{E(1)}] \text{ mmol} \, l^{-1} \qquad (12.6)$$

where $\dot{n}o_2$ is the uptake of oxygen in $\text{mmol} \, \text{min}^{-1}$, $\dot{V}_E$ is the ventilation minute volume in $l \, \text{min}^{-1}$ and (1) and (2) refer respectively to measurements made when breathing 100% oxygen and mixtures of carbon dioxide in oxygen. In practice the oxygen cost is not a linear function of the ventilation but increases disproportionately as the level of ventilation rises. Therefore, the ventilation should be reported separately, as is done on page 129; alternatively, the results can be presented graphically (Fig. 5.19, page 128). The work and the oxygen cost of breathing are increased with disease of the lung or the chest wall. The increase can cause hypoventilation (page 574). By contrast the oxygen cost is within normal limits if the hypoventilation is due to reduced activity of the respiratory centre but the lung is normal. For such cases the result should be expressed in terms of the hypercapnoeic drive to respiration:

$$\text{oxygen cost} = \frac{[\dot{n}o_{2(2)} - \dot{n}o_{2(1)}]}{[Pa,co_{2(2)} - Pa,co_{2(1)}]} \text{ mmol} \, \text{min}^{-1} \text{kPa}^{-1} \qquad (12.7)$$

where Pa,co_2 is the tension of carbon dioxide in arterial blood in kPa and the other terms are as defined above. This index provides a measure of the activity of the respiratory centre which is independent of the structural integrity of the lungs and thoracic cage.

Apparatus. Ventilation is usually measured with a pneumotachograph or vane anemometer which should be calibrated. However, these techniques entail the use of a mouthpiece which could itself affect the ventilation; where this is relevant to the outcome a jerkin plethysmograph should be used instead. The measurement of ventilation is considered in Chapter 3 (page 21). Test gas mixtures are made up, mixed and stored in high pressure cylinders (page 48). The accuracy of the mixtures should be checked by analysis. Alternatively for the isopnoeic technique the gases are mixed on-line using a bank of rotameters

(Fig. 3.8, page 49). The apparatus used for measuring the physiological response to exercise is described on page 426.

The test gas mixture is usually contained in a bag-in-box (Donald,
Christie box, Fig. 8.1, page 215). The subject breathes or rebreathes
from the bag while his ventilation is being recorded from the displacement of air into or out of the box. The rebreathing technique requires
a bag of 6 to 8 l capacity and the steady state measurements a bag of
approximately 100 l capacity. But the latter is not critical as the bag can
be refilled during the procedure. If the box contains two bags the
subject can be switched between gas mixtures. Switching between bags
should be timed so that the subject inhales the new gas mixture from
the start of the breath. Thus a hand-operated tap on an inspiratory
airline should be turned during expiration. An automated tap can be
triggered by a signal reflecting instantaneous volume or flow during the
respiratory cycle. If the trigger is linked to the changeover from expiration to inspiration an allowance may need to be made for the time of
closure of the shutter. The measurement by differentiation of the
maximal rate of rise of pressure at the start of inspiration (dP/dtmax)
entails the use of a breathing valve with a finite opening pressure. This
can be constructed by adding a weight to a value flap or by making use
of the surface tension which develops between the flap and the valve
seating. The rate of rise of pressure reaches its maximal value early in
the inspiration so the airway closure need only be transient. However,
error can arise due to the presence of abrupt transients in the pressure
signal. These can often be eliminated from the differentiated signal by
reducing the frequency response of the differentiator to approximately
10 Hz. Alternatively if the differentiation is performed on a computer
or microprocessor the transients can be removed by appropriate
programming.

Conditions of measurement. In everyday life the respiratory drive varies
from breath to breath in response to the many factors which influence
it; this is reflected in cyclical variations in the pattern of breathing
which have been recorded by Priban and by Newsom Davis amongst
others (see e.g. Fig. 11.1, page 326). The drive diminishes on closing
the eyes and increases momentarily with every external stimulus. It is
very susceptible to suggestion both intrinsic and external. Thus to
obtain a representative result both the findings for a number of breaths
should be averaged and the conditions of measurement should be
standardised. This is particularly important at rest when steady state
measurements tend to be unreliable because some subjects hyperventilate if they become aware that interest is being taken in their breathing.
Subjects are less likely to hyperventilate while reading a bland book or
during exercise, which itself provides an alternative focus of interest.
In addition, since the drive to respiration is normally increased during
exercise, an assessment which is made under these conditions may
reveal an abnormality which is not detectable at rest. The precautions
to be taken when making a steady state assessment have been summar-

378

ised by Severinghaus; for example, the subject should be in a post-absorbtive state, unstimulated by caffeine, alcohol, or extraneous sights or sounds. Before the test the subject should empty the bladder, adopt a comfortable posture, take trouble over the adjustment of the mouthpiece, nose clip and other respiratory apparatus then relax for 30 min. During the test the subjects should preferably not think about their breathing or if they do should wait for each breath to come naturally and not consciously try to influence it. When the test entails switching between gas mixtures, this should be done in such a way that the subject is not aware of its occurrence; the gases should be of the same temperature and humidity, and there is a distinguished precedent for their all being scented with the same perfume!

Ventilatory response to carbon dioxide

The response is the increase in ventilation per unit increase in tension of carbon dioxide (Fig. 11.8, page 348). The derivation requires measurements of ventilation at a minimum of two levels of carbon dioxide tension. Under these circumstances:

$$S = \frac{\dot{V}_{E(1)} - \dot{V}_{E(2)}}{Pa,co_{2(2)} - Pa,co_{2(1)}} = \frac{\Delta \dot{V}_E}{\Delta Pa,co_2} \, \mathrm{l\,min^{-1}\,kPa^{-1}} \text{ (or mmHg}^{-1})$$

$$(12.8)$$

where S is the response of ventilation to carbon dioxide, $\dot{V}_E$ is the ventilation minute volume in $\mathrm{l\,min^{-1}}$ and Pa,co_2 is the tension of carbon dioxide in the arterial blood in kPa or mmHg. The subscripts (1) and (2) refer respectively to measurements made at high and low tensions of carbon dioxide. When the range of ventilation–perfusion ratios is within normal limits, the tension of carbon dioxide may be obtained by the sampling and analysis of the end-tidal gas (Fig. 3.1, page 22); in other circumstances the tension in the arterial or arterialised venous blood should be obtained by one of the methods described in Chapter 3.

The measurement is usually made by the *rebreathing method of Read*. The subject rebreathes from a bag which initially contains between 3 and 5 l of gas comprising carbon dioxide in a fractional concentration of 0.05 with the remainder oxygen. The duration of rebreathing is 4 min or until the concentration of carbon dioxide has risen to 0.09. The bag is contained in a Donald, Christie box which is connected to a dry gas meter, spirometer or pneumotachograph for measurement of ventilation. The tension of carbon dioxide in the end-tidal gas is assumed to be the same as that in the bag; the latter is measured with an analyser having a response time of less than 0.2 s. The ventilatory response to carbon dioxide is the slope of the relationship of ventilation to tension of carbon dioxide over the range where this is linear; alinearity is often apparent at low tensions of carbon dioxide and either these points or the first 45 s of rebreathing should be excluded from the analysis. The reproducibility is influenced by the number and accuracy

379

of the measurements of ventilation minute volume. Determinations made using finite numbers of whole breaths are to be preferred to those made over periods of 30 or 15 s. Repeating the test after an interval of 10 min will improve the accuracy. However, some subjects develop a headache so the use of duplicates may be inadvisable, especially where there is a need for serial measurements. Values for the index in healthy subjects are influenced by the size of the lung and by ethnic group; reference values are given on page 349. The procedure also yields the response time for the increase in ventilation and the tension of carbon dioxide in the mixed venous blood (page 47). The relationship of ventilation minute volume to tidal volume during breathing carbon dioxide can be recorded concurrently (see pattern of breathing, page 325). The tidal volumes are, on average, higher than those obtained by other methods.

When the *steady state method* is used the subject breathes one of two appropriate concentrations of carbon dioxide in oxygen for 20 min. Fractional CO_2 concentrations of 0.03 and 0.06 can be used. On each occasion the ventilation is measured over the last 5 min and if arterial blood is to be collected, it is sampled over 2 min. The circumstances of the test should meet the conditions of measurement described above.

For the *constant flow method* a constant flow of carbon dioxide in the range $0-0.8 \, l \, min^{-1}$ is delivered into wide bore tubing 3 cm proximal to the inspiratory valve adjacent to the mouthpiece. The concentrations of oxygen and carbon dioxide at the mouth and in the mixed expired gas are monitored using a respiratory mass spectrometer. The CO_2 concentrations at the mouth during expiration are used to estimate the arterial carbon dioxide tension (see e.g. Fig. 11.9, page 354). By this method the ventilatory response to carbon dioxide is found to increase during exercise. The method has been developed by Saunders and others including Cummin.

Peripheral chemoreceptor drive

The drive from carotid chemoreceptors varies inversely with oxygen tension starting from a tension of approximately 25 kPa (200 mmHg). Below this upper limit the chemoreceptors also respond to carbon dioxide; the response interacts with that to oxygen. The interaction can be described using the relationship of Lloyd and Cunningham (equation 11.5, page 349). The equation is illustrated in Fig. 11.8 (page 348). Its solution entails determining the four constants, A, B, C and D which together describe the ventilatory responses to hypoxia and hypercapnia. In subjects with a normal range of ventilation−perfusion ratios this may be done by an isocapnic technique. The subject breathes oxygen to which controlled quantities of carbon dioxide are added through rotameters. The flow rate is adjusted to maintain the ventilation minute volume at a predetermined level in the range $20-60 \, l \, min^{-1}$. The constancy of the ventilation is checked breath by breath using a pneumotachograph and integrator with automatic re-zeroing between breaths. The test is continued until a steady level has been established. The hypercapnic drive to respiration is then reduced by the operator decreasing the rate of flow of carbon dioxide. At the same time the chemoreceptor drive is increased by the addition of nitrogen at a rate which is determined by trial and error to keep the level of ventilation constant. During this procedure five determinations are made of the tensions of oxygen and carbon dioxide in the end-tidal gas or the arterial blood; one determination is also made at a lower level of ventilation. These data are used to calculate the indices A, B, C and D. Their magnitude in healthy subjects and the direction of change in patients with lung disease are discussed in Chapter 11.

The response to hypoxic drive can also be obtained by the isocapnic technique of Weil in which the ventilation is related to the alveolar oxygen tension during hypoxia of increasing intensity. The tension of carbon dioxide in the alveolar gas is kept constant. This shortens the test but has the effect that the level of P_{A,CO_2} which is adopted inevitably affects the hypoxic response. The latter is obtained from:

$$\dot{V}_E = \dot{V}_0 + 7.5\ A(w)/(P_{A,O_2} - 32)\ \mathrm{l\,min^{-1}} \qquad (12.9)$$

where P_{A,O_2} is the tension of oxygen in the alveolar gas in mmHg and 7.5 converts to kilopascals. The response term $A(w)$ is similar to the product term AD of Lloyd and Cunningham.

The ventilatory response to hypoxia can also be expressed in logarithmic form or in terms of the extent of desaturation of the arterial blood measured by oximetry. An isocapnic rebreathing test using the latter approach has been developed by Rebuck and Campbell.

How the tests are applied

Central inspiratory activity

This is assessed after the peripheral chemoreceptors have been inactivated by the subject breathing air enriched with oxygen at a fractional concentration in excess of 0.3. The oxygen can be delivered via a mouthpiece, mask or nasal prongs, when the flow rate should be at least $4\,\mathrm{l\,min^{-1}}$ (page 634). The tension of carbon dioxide should not be artificially increased through the use of an oxygen mask with a large deadspace. The response can be in terms of any of the variables which have been discussed. In patients with an acute chest illness superimposed on chronic lung disease the assessment is normally performed at the bedside by measurement of the arterial carbon dioxide tension during the course of oxygen therapy (page 629). However, the tension is also influenced by the mechanical derangement (page 375).

Central chemoreceptor drive

This is assessed by measuring the ventilatory response to carbon dioxide in the absence of peripheral chemoreceptor drive. The latter is eliminated by the subject breathing a test gas containing oxygen in a fractional concentration of not less than 0.3. The stimulus is a rise in the tension of carbon dioxide in the cerebrospinal fluid or arterial blood. The response is the increase in ventilation or the increase in respiratory drive. For convenience and in order to economise in the use of oxygen the measurement of choice is the ventilatory response obtained by the rebreathing method which is described on page 379. This can be combined with measurement of respiratory drive (q.v.).

Peripheral chemoreceptor drive

The *level* of peripheral chemoreceptor drive is assessed by measuring the immediate response to eliminating the peripheral drive by substituting 100% oxygen for the respired air. The response is usually measured in terms of ventilation (e.g. Fig. 11.5, page 343). The results of the test are influenced by the level of chemoreceptor drive and the rate at which the test gas mixes with and replaces the alveolar gas. For healthy subjects during exercise the response is usually analysed over three to five breaths starting two breaths after the changeover. For studies at rest or for subjects in whom the distribution of the inspired gas is uneven, periods of 15 s for gas replacement and of 30 s for measurement are more appropriate. The findings in healthy subjects are illustrated schematically in Fig. 11.6 (page 344) and by examples in Figs 11.5 and 12.3 (pages 343 and 370). The procedure can identify subjects in whom the chemoreceptor drive is diminished or absent. In healthy subjects the procedure can also be used to assess the respiratory sensitivity to hypoxia. For this purpose instead of using 100% oxygen the drive is increased by the administration of three breaths of nitrogen.

The *responsiveness* to peripheral chemoreceptor drive is usually assessed in terms of the ventilatory response to hypoxia. This is assessed by one of the methods described on page 380.

Comment. The causes and presenting features of abnormal respiratory control are summarised in Chapter 16 (page 579). The conditions are important clinically and are usually assessed semi-qualitatively through measurement of the tensions of oxygen and carbon dioxide in arterial blood at rest or of the arterial oxygen saturation by oximetry during sleep or during exercise. The sleep studies may need to be extended to polysomnography which relates the ventilatory and blood gas changes to the stage of sleep (page 364).

In healthy persons the levels of ventilatory sensitivity to hypoxia and hypercapnia vary over a wide range. An individual's sensitivity is important in the event of his developing chronic lung disease when it is a factor determining if progression of COPD takes place in the direction of the type A or the type B (page 542). However, the chances of a healthy individual being affected in one of these ways is small and there have been few attempts at longitudinal (prospective) studies. The responsiveness is of more immediate importance in relation to athletic training, to residence at high altitude (page 358) and to exposure to hyperbaric conditions through deep sea diving or work in a compression chamber (page 411). However, even for these applications few prospective studies have been undertaken. The techniques are available and they should probably be used more often than is the case at present.

Guide to references

The references (Chapter 18) are classified under subject headings of which the following are particularly relevant to the present chapter:

13: Factors which Limit Exercise

Introduction

Exercise depends on the contraction and relaxation of voluntary muscles. Such contraction can be short-lived (a kick), sustained (carrying an infant in the crook of one's arm), or repeated (walking), and can be isometric (tug-of-war) or isotonic (standing erect from squatting, or lifting a weight) but in most normal activities it is a combination of all of these. It is intermittent contraction repeated over many minutes which constitutes normal dynamic exercise and is the concern of this chapter. Ability to sustain the exercise for periods of hours requires additional features. Dynamic exercise usually involves many muscle groups, albeit simultaneously or serially, and the intensity of exercise can be assessed by measuring the work done in unit time. But the external work is not the only outcome of exercise; muscle contraction also produces heat, and extra work is done by raising limbs against gravity, by overcoming internal friction in muscles and joints, and by the circulation and the respiratory muscles. In fact external work accounts for only about a quarter of the total energy dissipated during exercise. The source of this energy depends on the duration of exertion, but in exercise lasting for more than a few seconds the energy comes mainly from aerobic catabolism of muscle glycogen, and of glucose and fatty acids carried to the active muscles in the bloodstream. The muscles are able to exceed the quota set by aerobic catabolism, for a limited period, by obtaining energy from rapid glycolysis which is non-oxidative metabolism of glucose and glycogen. The process was formerly incorrectly called anaerobic metabolism. The penalty incurred from rapid glycolysis is the production of lactic acid for which the body has a poor tolerance, and its accumulation prevents any further increase in exertion. During the recovery period extra oxygen is absorbed (the so-called oxygen debt) to dispose of the lactic acid and also to rebuild the stores of ATP and phosphocreatine in the muscles and of oxygen in myoglobin. Thus neither the external work done nor the uptake of oxygen *during* exertion can give a true account of the intensity of the exertion. However, during exercise which can be sustained for long periods (steady state exercise), the uptake of oxygen rises with the intensity of external work up to a limit beyond which increasing the work-load causes no further increase in oxygen uptake. This is the *maximal oxygen uptake* and it is widely used as a measure of exercise capacity.

Anatomical, physiological and psychological determinants of exercise capacity

The principal anatomical determinant of exercise capacity is body size. This influences the dimensions of the oxygen transport system, the mass of muscle which can be brought into use, and the mechanical conditions under which the muscle operates. Body size is influenced by genetic factors and environmental factors including diet, anabolic steroid drugs and the level of habitual activity. The genetic factor is very important and after allowing for age, is the largest single determinant of the capacity for exercise of healthy subjects. The amount of habitual activity determines the subject's place on the continuum between work hypertrophy and disuse atrophy. It also influences the production of growth hormone. This is particularly relevant during the adolescent growth spurt (page 465).

For aerobic exercise the physiological determinant is the oxygen transport chain which conveys oxygen from the atmosphere to the mitochondria in the active muscles. The stages comprise ventilation of the lungs (also called external respiration), diffusion from lungs to blood, circulation of oxyhaemoglobin, diffusion of oxygen across the capillary−muscle membrane and within the muscle, and incorporation of oxygen into the mitochondria. A similar transport chain conveys carbon dioxide in the reverse direction. The capacities of the different components of the chain are approximately matched. Thus, in one study, differences in aerobic power between groups of subjects were associated with similar differences in lung function, total body haemoglobin, cardiac interval (hence stroke volume) during exercise, total body potassium (hence body cell mass) and muscle size (Fig. 13.1). The matching can be disturbed by a number of factors such as, for the lungs, having asthma in childhood or, for the muscles, the techniques of body building. The matching is never perfect so the stages do not contribute equally to exercise limitation. Instead the principal limiting factor in normal circumstances is now believed to be the rate of diffusion of oxygen across the capillary−muscle membrane. This is greatly influenced by the mean capillary oxygen tension which is determined by the ability of the circulation to deliver blood to the muscle capillaries. This means that the limit is set by the circulation. By contrast the lungs normally have spare capacity; this is called upon at high altitude and is used up in the early stages of many lung diseases. All these aspects are considered subsequently. They are summarised in Table 13.1.

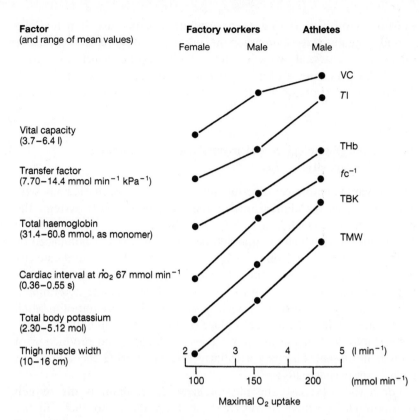

Factors which limit exercise

Factor (and range of mean values)	Factory workers		Athletes
	Female	Male	Male

Vital capacity (3.7–6.4 l)

Transfer factor (7.70–14.4 mmol min^{-1} kPa^{-1})

Total haemoglobin (31.4–60.8 mmol, as monomer)

Cardiac interval at $\dot{n}o_2$ 67 mmol min^{-1} (0.36–0.55 s)

Total body potassium (2.30–5.12 mol)

Thigh muscle width (10–16 cm)

Maximal O$_2$ uptake

Fig. 13.1 Concordance between variables which relate to the maximal oxygen uptake. For details see text. (Source: Cotes JE, Davies CTM. *Proc Roy Soc Med* 1969; **62**: 620–624.)

Table 13.1 Determinants of exercise limitation

Determinant	Conditions which render it critical
Ventilation capacity	Altitude, hyperbaria, resistance breathing Lung diseases, pulmonary congestion
Ventilation/perfusion	Lung diseases
Gas transfer in lungs	Altitude Lung diseases, pulmonary oedema
Oxygen content of blood	Anaemia Haemoglobin inactivated chemically
Cardiac output	A normal limiting factor Sedentary life style, cardiac disorders, reduced blood volume
Muscle blood flow	Lack of use Distribution of cardiac output altered by extraneous factors
Oxygen transfer from muscle capillaries	A normal limiting factor
Intramuscular oxygen	The amount depends on all of the above The tension is rarely a limiting factor
Intramuscular metabolism	Increased rapid glycolysis from any cause

When there is lung disease or other cause of incapacitating breathlessness on exertion, both exercise and oxygen uptake are limited by symptoms and the exercise capacity depends on the tolerance of discomfort; this varies from subject to subject. In normal subjects oxygen uptake is not so limited, and maximal oxygen uptake is in reality a submaximal measurement (see above). Psychological factors are still important since verification of $\dot{n}o_2$max requires that the subject should perform work beyond the aerobic maximum for a limited time. Many persons of a sedentary disposition are reluctant to exert themselves to the required extent.

For exercise which is symptom-limited any of a number of symptoms may be responsible (page 405). However, the predominant sensation usually relates to some component of the cardio-respiratory or skeleto-muscular systems. In most circumstances that sensation is dyspnoea.

Breathlessness

The sensation of dyspnoea

Dyspnoea is an uncomfortable awareness that breathing is difficult and entails increased effort, coupled with an anxious forboding that the effort could become unbearable. The quality of the sensation can vary depending on the cause, which might be cardiac failure, status asthmaticus or an artificial resistive or elastic hindrance to breathing. During exercise the sensation occurs when the ventilation is increased and usually leads to the subject making a response; this can be voluntary or involuntary. It can involve altering the pattern of breathing as was pointed out by Marshall and colleagues amongst others. Dyspnoea is a feature of most chronic disorders of the lung and its recognition can contribute to diagnosis. The onset of dyspnoea is the principal reason why such a patient restricts his activity.

A diagnosis of respiratory disability should not be made unless exercise is limited by dyspnoea, but exertional dyspnoea has other causes, such as anaemia and heart disease, and can present as angina. In addition the dyspnoea can lead to the subject adopting an unduly sedentary life style which can further reduce the capacity for exercise.

Minor degrees of dyspnoea are described as breathlessness and the two sensations are regarded as one for purposes of rating; this is done using a questionnaire, visual analogue scale, modified Borg scale or psychological tests.

Scores for breathlessness

In patients with lung disease the *grade of breathlessness* can be assessed clinically from answers to standard questions on what activities give rise to the sensation. However, breathlessness is not the only mode of limitation and the scores more nearly describe the exercise tolerance. The questions are usually based on those of Fletcher; an extended

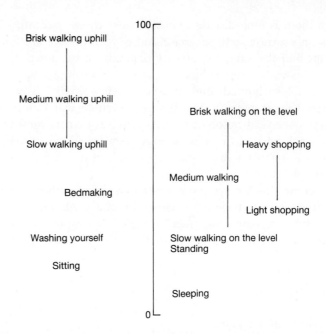

Fig. 13.2 Diagram for rating the ability to take exercise. The subject marks the central vertical line at what he considers to be the appropriate point; the ability score is the distance in cm from the origin (o). (Source: McGavin CR *et al. Br Med J* 1978; **ii**: 241–243.)

version of his clinical grades of breathlessness is given in Table 16.4 (page 517). The grading can also be performed using the *oxygen cost diagram* of McGavin and colleagues in which the score is related to the average energy cost of the activity in question (Fig. 13.2). A more extensive summary of the energy costs of activities is given in Fig. 13.3. The degree of breathlessness can be recorded using a *visual analogue scale* (Fig. 13.4). The scale is valuable for recording within subject changes in breathlessness, for example during the course of a progressive exercise test. It is a less reliable guide to the absolute level of breathlessness since subjects differ in the way in which they apportion their scores. The difficulty is overcome in the *Borg scale for breathlessness* which provides more information to the subject (Table 13.2).

The quality of the respiratory sensation can also be rated using an appropriate questionnaire and questionnaires can be used to elicit psychological information. For example a *semantic differential score* was used by Morgan and others to assess attitudes to general health breathlessness, and related factors (Table 13.3). The *hospital anxiety and depression scale* used by Tyrer, Zigmund, King and others can also contribute relevant information.

Mechanisms of breathlessness

A typical breathlessness score for a healthy subject performing progressive exercise tests is given in Fig. 13.5. However, subjects differ in

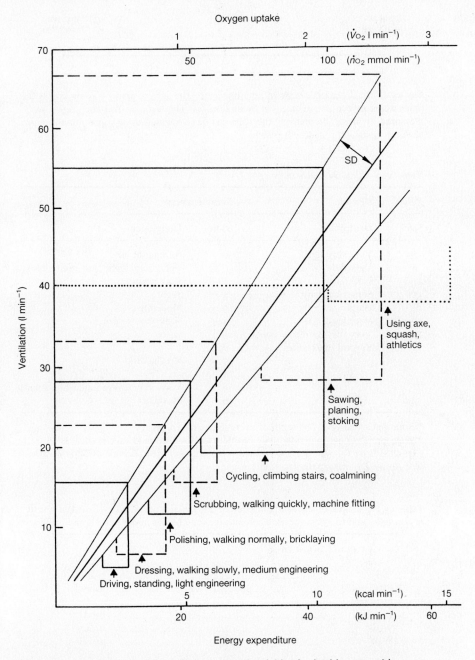

Oxygen uptake

Fig. 13.3 Average energy and ventilatory costs of activities for healthy men with an indication of the between-subject variation (given by the vertical and horizontal lines). In women the ventilatory costs are similar but the energy costs are approximately 10% lower. Ventilation is increased by age, smoking, respiratory symptoms and other factors; it is below average in persons who are physically fit. (Source: Cotes JE. *Br J Ind Med* 1975; **32**: 220–223.)

their responsiveness. Adams, Guz and colleagues have found that when healthy subjects perform a standard exercise task some of them assess their degree of breathlessness at a higher grade than the majority,

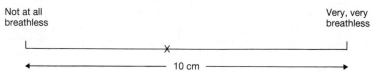

Fig. 13.4 Visual analogue scale of breathlessness. The subject marks a 10 cm line at the point which reflects the intensity of breathlessness. The distance from the origin can be measured by hand; alternatively the scale can be automated using a potentiometer or chain of lights controlled by a switch.

Table 13.2 Category scales of Borg

Perceived exertion		Breathlessness	
Score*	Description	Score†	Description
7	Very very light	0	Nothing at all
9	Very light	0.5	Very, very slight (just noticeable)
11	Fairly light	1	Very slight
13	Somewhat hard	2	Slight
15	Hard	3	Moderate
17	Very hard	4	Somewhat severe
19	Very very hard (the limit)	5	Severe
20	Beyond endurance	6	
		7	Very severe
		8	
		9	Very, very severe (almost maximal)
		10	Maximal

* Scale linear: score is one-tenth of average cardiac frequency.
† Scale proportional (a similar scale can be used for perceived exertion).
(Sources: Borg G. *Med Sci Sports Exerc* 1982; **14**: 377−381; Burdon JGW *et al. Am Rev Respir Dis* 1982; **126**: 825−828.)

Table 13.3 Example of semantic differential: 'my general health'. This is one of a series of concepts used to assess the patient's attitudes and beliefs about himself and his illness

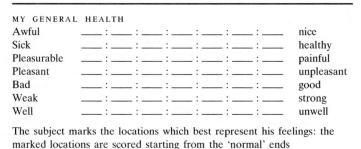

MY GENERAL HEALTH

Awful	___ : ___ : ___ : ___ : ___ : ___ : ___	nice
Sick	___ : ___ : ___ : ___ : ___ : ___ : ___	healthy
Pleasurable	___ : ___ : ___ : ___ : ___ : ___ : ___	painful
Pleasant	___ : ___ : ___ : ___ : ___ : ___ : ___	unpleasant
Bad	___ : ___ : ___ : ___ : ___ : ___ : ___	good
Weak	___ : ___ : ___ : ___ : ___ : ___ : ___	strong
Well	___ : ___ : ___ : ___ : ___ : ___ : ___	unwell

The subject marks the locations which best represent his feelings: the marked locations are scored starting from the 'normal' ends

(Source: King B, Cotes JE. *Thorax* 1989; **44**: 402−409.)

and that these subjects also have increased perception of other sensations. Such persons would appear to be at greater risk of developing respiratory disability than those who are less sensitive. The increased perception needs to be distinguished from other causes of disproportionate breathlessness, for example psychiatric illness or psychologi-

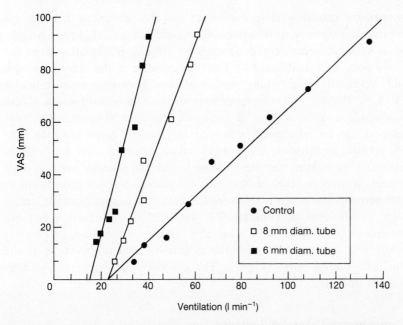

Fig. 13.5 Breathlessness during a progressive exercise test rated using a visual analogue scale (VAS). Scoring was each min using an illuminated scale controlled by one finger. The figure shows the effect of breathing through a resistance. A moderate resistance tube (diameter 8 mm, length 25 mm) increased the slope of the relationship whilst a high resistance also reduced the threshold level of ventilation at which breathlessness was first experienced. (Source: Crack MC. PhD Thesis, University of Newcastle upon Tyne, 1988.)

cal difficulties in relation to a claim for industrial compensation. Increased breathlessness is also a feature of pulmonary congestion such as can occur with mitral stenosis and left heart failure; these conditions are described on pages 603 and 605.

Pulmonary congestion is associated with shallow breathing due to increased activity of intrapulmonary receptors (cf. page 340). The elimination of stimuli from this source is achieved by interrupting the vagi. By doing this Guz and his colleagues were able to reduce the breathlessness of a patient with sarcoidosis. Nadel and his colleagues in elegant studies on unsedated dogs have observed a similar reduction in the tachypnoea (and hence probably the breathlessness) caused by inhalation of histamine.

Breathlessness during exercise or in response to chemoreceptor stimulation depends on the precise circumstances. It is usually greater during cycle ergometry than at the same level of ventilation on a treadmill. It is greater when ventilation is driven by hypercapnia or hypoxia than by exercise. However, there is normally a direct association between the drive and the response. But hypercapnia or hypoxia are not themselves the cause of dyspnoea for Adams and colleagues were able to show by varying the inspired gas mixture that there was an association between ventilation and breathlessness but not between peripheral carbon dioxide drive and breathlessness. In the case of oxygen the results were less clear cut and the possibility that hypoxia contributed directly to breathlessness could not be ruled out. Breathlessness is not necessarily dependent on afferent information from the lungs since it is unaffected by local anaesthesia of the airways, and it still occurs after heart−lung transplantation. Following neuromuscular blockade Banzett and colleagues have shown that breathlessness is also independent of the activity of respiratory muscles. By contrast breathlessness can be influenced by involuntary central respiratory drive to the respiratory muscles. It is not related to voluntary drive to the same extent. Thus Adams and others have found that breathlessness is *most* intense if a given level of isocapnic ventilation follows stimulation of chemoreceptors, is *less* if this ventilation occurs during exercise, and is *least* if this level of ventilation is achieved by voluntary effort. In summary, breathlessness is a manifestation of involuntary respiratory effort and appears to reflect the degree of reflex activation of the medullary respiratory complex. The evidence has been reviewed by Adams and Guz.

Components of exercise limitation (see also Table 13.1)

Ventilatory capacity

Exercise is not primarily limited by ventilation unless either the ventilatory capacity is reduced or the ventilatory cost of exercise is increased. But the ventilatory capacity contributes to the breaking point when the exercise gives rise to lactacidaemia; this is the case in normal circumstances and when the cardiac output is for any reason reduced (page 406).

Limitation by ventilation becomes inevitable when the exercise ventilation approaches the subject's ventilatory capacity. This is defined for each breath by the maximal flow−volume curve and for a number of breaths by the maximal breathing capacity (MBC). The maximal flow−volume curve puts upper limits on the respiratory flow rates at different lung volumes: it leads to the pattern of breathing being modified with respect to frequency, tidal volume and functional residual capacity to achieve maximal ventilation in the prevailing circumstances. An example is given in Fig. 13.6.

The maximal breathing capacity normally provides an upper limit to the maximal exercise ventilation. This led George Wright to use the ratio of these variables as an index of breathlessness:

$$\text{dyspnoeic index} = \frac{\text{exercise ventilation}}{\text{maximal breathing capacity}} \times 100\% \qquad (13.1)$$

The appropriate denominator is the maximal voluntary ventilation (MVV) measured when the subject is breathless; however, because this is difficult to obtain, it can be replaced by the MVV at rest or by the indirect MBC. The latter was defined by Kennedy as 40 times forced expiratory volume (FEV 0.75, page 135). Alternatively MVV

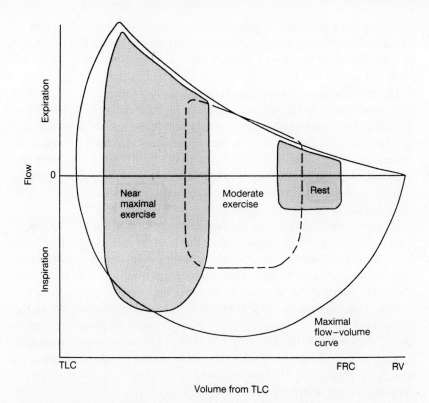

Fig. 13.6 Representative flow–volume curves for patients with chronic obstructive lung disease. The outer line represents the maximal curve (MEFV). This can be compared with the normal curve given on page 116. The inner curves are for rest, moderate exercise and near maximal exercise. In the latter circumstance the tidal volume (represented by the width of the curve) is less than for moderate exercise but the flow rates are greater; flow is limited by dynamic compression of lung airways. (Adapted from: Potter WA, Olafsson S, Hyatt RE. *J Clin Invest* 1971; **50**: 910–919.)

can be estimated from the forced expiratory volume (FEV_1). This is often done using the empirical relationship of Gandevia and Hugh-Jones:

$$\text{maximal breathing capacity } (l\,min^{-1}) = 35\ FEV_1\ (l) \quad (13.2)$$

Alternative relationships are given in Table 6.3 (page 136).

In healthy subjects the dyspnoeic index at the breaking point of exercise is usually in the range 70–90% but is often higher in athletes. It rises to, or may exceed, 100% when the density of the respired gas is reduced by ascent to altitude or by replacing the nitrogen in the inspired gas with helium. There is then an increase in the maximal breathing capacity compared with breathing air at sea level, but for reasons which are not yet understood, the ventilation at the breaking point of exercise rises even further, giving a higher dyspnoea index. Thus, at altitude both the maximal breathing capacity is increased and a larger proportion of it is available for use during exercise; the maximal exercise ventilation is much increased and may attain a value twice that observed at sea level. This change goes some way to accommodating the increase in hypoxic chemoreceptor drive which occurs at altitude. However, it is not sufficient to prevent exercise being limited by breathlessness at a lower level of energy expenditure than would be achieved at sea level.

The maximal breathing capacity is reduced by disease of the lung or the thoracic cage. It is also reduced by binding the chest or by immersion in water. In deep-sea divers and workers in caissons MBC is reduced by breathing gas at raised pressures (page 124). Under all these conditions the dyspnoeic index tends to be high. At the same time the maximal exercise ventilation is invariably less than in normal circumstances and capacity for exercise of the subjects can be reduced in consequence.

Unless there is nervous or deliberate hyperventilation the finding of a high dyspnoea index suggests that the exercise task has really been limited by ventilatory ability. This is the case for most patients with chronic lung disease (e.g. Table 13.8, page 407). A low dyspnoeic index can occur if the ventilatory capacity on exercise is less than it is at rest. This happens in some patients with mitral stenosis in whom the compliance of the lung falls during exercise, and in those asthmatics who experience bronchoconstriction during exercise. In other circumstances a low dyspnoeic index at the breaking point of exercise is usually evidence for the intervention of a non-respiratory factor; a common factor is apprehension.

Pulmonary gas exchange

This stage in the oxygen transport chain does not contribute to limitation of exercise in normal subjects but can do so in exceptional circumstances. In healthy subjects exercising at sea level the oxygen saturation of arterial blood is usually considered to be effectively constant and independent of the intensity of exercise. This view is an oversimplification since a minor degree of desaturation occurs in some subjects; the extent of the change varies with the rate of work and with the ventilatory response to exercise. Thus it is greatest in athletes, particularly those with a blunted ventilatory response to exercise, and in subjects in whom the ventilation is impeded by an external resistance or by strapping applied to the chest. The hypoxaemia is due to ventilation–perfusion inequality. The consequent reduction in oxygen transport is normally very small. This is because the upper part of the haemoglobin dissociation curve is relatively flat (Fig. 9.3, page 280), so that over a wide range of oxygen tensions, the blood leaving the lung is almost saturated with oxygen. For example, halving the tension of oxygen in the blood leaving the alveolar capillaries from 14 to 7 kPa (105–53 mmHg) only causes a change in the saturation from 98% to 87%; this is equivalent to a reduction in oxygen combined with haemoglobin of $1.0 \, \text{mmol} \, \text{l}^{-1}$ or $22 \, \text{ml} \, \text{l}^{-1}$. This degree of exercise hypoxaemia may occur in patients with impaired lung function. However, the associated reduction in exercise capacity is secondary to ventilatory impairment (page 406). The hypoxaemia is another consequence of that impairment but is of variable extent, being inversely related to the ventilation. For this reason the hypoxaemia seldom limits exercise directly while air is being breathed.

If oxygen is breathed the exercise capacity is increased (page 407), but again the mechanism appears to be a reduction in the ventilatory cost of exercise (page 406), not the relief of hypoxaemia, though this could be a factor in reducing breathlessness (page 391). However, impaired gas exchange can contribute to limitation of exercise when the inspired oxygen tension is reduced. This is due to the exchange of oxygen taking place on the linear part of the oxygen dissociation curve (page 285). The hypoxaemia due to a low oxygen tension is then aggravated by failure of the blood passing through the alveolar capillaries to reach equilibrium with alveolar gas. This diffusion limitation occurs during strenuous exercise at very high altitudes. Its occurrence has been demonstrated by West, Wagner and colleagues.

An important component of the gas transfer defect is the time for which red cells are in contact with alveolar gas. The time is probably reduced during hypoxia because this condition increases the cardiac output. When the hypoxia is due to high altitude there is an initial increase in cardiac output which is reversed by acclimatisation. The acclimatisation also reduces the alveolar to end-capillary oxygen tension difference and these two events are probably related: the improvement in gas exchange is then due to the acclimatisation prolonging the transit time of blood perfusing the alveolar capillaries.

Oxygen content of blood

This component of the oxygen transport chain directly affects the capacity for exercise. The haemoglobin content of blood in males expressed as haemoglobin monomer, is on average $9 \, \text{mmol} \, l^{-1}$, equivalent to $14.6 \, \text{g} \, \text{dl}^{-1}$. The concentration is rather less in females. The corresponding maximal oxygen content of the blood (the oxygen capacity) is $9 \, \text{mmol} \, l^{-1}$ or $20 \, \text{ml} \, \text{dl}^{-1}$. Under normal circumstances the arterial blood carries nearly this amount of oxygen. The oxygen content is less when either the inspired oxygen tension or the haemoglobin concentration is reduced. It is also diminished when some haemoglobin is inactivated, for example by conversion to met- or carboxy-haemoglobin. The availability of the remaining oxygen can be reduced by a change in the shape of the haemoglobin dissociation curve as occurs following breathing carbon monoxide (Fig. 9.6, page 292). Any of these circumstances can impair the ability of the blood to transport oxygen and hence the capacity for exercise. The extent of the limitation is influenced by other factors. For example, hypoxaemia due to ascent to high altitude is associated with a reduction in air density which itself can affect performance in various ways (page 410). Similarly in anaemia the reduced haematocrit lowers blood viscosity and this can increase the maximal cardiac output. As a result some subjects can achieve a normal maximal oxygen uptake despite a low haemoglobin concentration but on average the maximal uptake is reduced when the haemoglobin concentration falls below approximately 80% of its normal level; in men this is equivalent to a haemoglobin concentration of $12\,g\,dl^{-1}$.

An increase in the oxygen content of blood can have the converse effect of raising the capacity for exercise. This occurs following contraction of the spleen which releases erythrocytes into the circulation. It also occurs when oxygen is inhaled because the quantity of dissolved oxygen carried in the blood plasma is then increased from 0.3 to $2.0\,ml\,dl^{-1}$. A modest rise in red cell count has a similar effect. A marked rise has the haemodynamic disadvantage of increasing the blood viscosity and hence reducing the cardiac output. Ascent to altitude increases haemopoiesis; this exerts a beneficial effect on exercise capacity which persists for a short time following return to sea level conditions. Some athletes have made use of this reaction to increase their performance.

The stimulus to erythropoiesis is increased production by the kidneys of the bone marrow stimulating hormone erythropoietin. The hormone has recently become available commercially as recombinant erythropoietin (r-HuEPO).

Circulation of blood

The maximal oxygen uptake in the lungs has been found by Saltin and others to be linearly related to the delivery of oxygen to the muscles. The amount delivered is the product of muscle blood flow, arterial oxygen saturation and haemoglobin concentration. The last two are relatively constant so the muscle blood flow is the principal variable. This observation appeared to confirm the traditional view that exercise is normally limited by the capacity of the circulation and not by the ability of the muscle to use the delivered oxygen.

Recent work by Wagner and colleagues has shown this to be an oversimplification. Thus for a given oxygen delivery the maximal oxygen uptake in the muscles has been found to be related to the mean oxygen tension in the muscle capillaries and hence to be governed by the rate of transfer of oxygen across the capillary walls. The two sets of observations are compatible because the muscle blood flow influences many of the determinants of oxygen transfer across the capillary–muscle membrane (see extraction of oxygen below). During exercise the muscle blood flow is the resultant of cardiac output and its distribution within the body.

Cardiac output

The cardiac output is determined by the left ventricle ejecting into the systemic circulation the blood which it receives via the lungs from the periphery. Thus the venous return to the heart is very important. It is increased during exercise as a result of venoconstriction and the pumping actions of both the active muscles and the intrathoracic pressure swings. The resulting cardiac output is linearly related to the uptake of oxygen; for healthy subjects walking on a treadmill it is described approximately by the following relationship which is derived from the data of Reeves and others:

$$\dot{Q}_T = a\dot{n}o_2 + 3.4, \text{ SD } 0.9 \, \text{l min}^{-1} \qquad (13.3)$$

where $\dot{Q}_T$ and $\dot{n}o_2$ are respectively the output of the heart and the rate of consumption of oxygen. The coefficient a is the increase in cardiac output per unit increase in oxygen uptake. Its numerical value in SI units is 0.37 l per mmol or in traditional units 6.1 l per l. Taking into account the oxygen content of blood (9 mmol l^{-1}, or 20 ml dl^{-1}) the value of a is evidence that during exercise effectively all the additional cardiac output goes to the active muscles (which include the heart itself). Depending on a person's age and size the maximal cardiac output ranges from 10 to 35 l min^{-1}; it is increased by physical training and reduced by inactivity. It is also reduced by valvular disease of the heart, heart failure and conditions in which the total blood volume is reduced.

Cardiac output is the product of stroke volume and cardiac frequency. In a supine posture stroke volume is at its maximal value which is normally in the range 50–100 ml, or 150 ml in athletes. It decreases when the subject is upright. In this posture during progressive exercise starting from rest the stroke volume increases and attains its maximal value at an oxygen uptake of approximately 40% of the maximal oxygen uptake (Fig. 13.7). The stroke volume is increased by physical training which increases the quantity of muscle in the right as well as the left ventricle. The cardiac frequency is nearly linearly related to the oxygen uptake; its maximal value is effectively independent of physical training but declines with age. It has been described by Åstrand:

$$fc_{max} = 210 - 0.65 \text{ age (years)}, \quad \text{SD } 19 \, \text{min}^{-1} \qquad (13.4)$$

where fc_{max} is maximal cardiac frequency during exercise. Thus the increase in cardiac output associated with physical training is entirely due to an increased stroke volume.

Muscle blood flow

At rest the cardiac output is distributed between the brain, splanchnic area, heart and other organs with relatively little going to the skeletal muscles. Blood flow to the skin depends on the ambient temperature. During exercise sympathetic tone increases, the blood levels of adrenaline and noradrenaline rise and vagal tone diminishes. Metabolites produced in the active muscles stimulate the local autonomic nervous system. Thus cardiac output increases, muscle arterioles dilate and capillaries open up. These changes increase the blood flow to active muscles by up to 20 times compared with the blood flow at rest. At the same time the blood flow to the splanchnic area and other non-essential

397

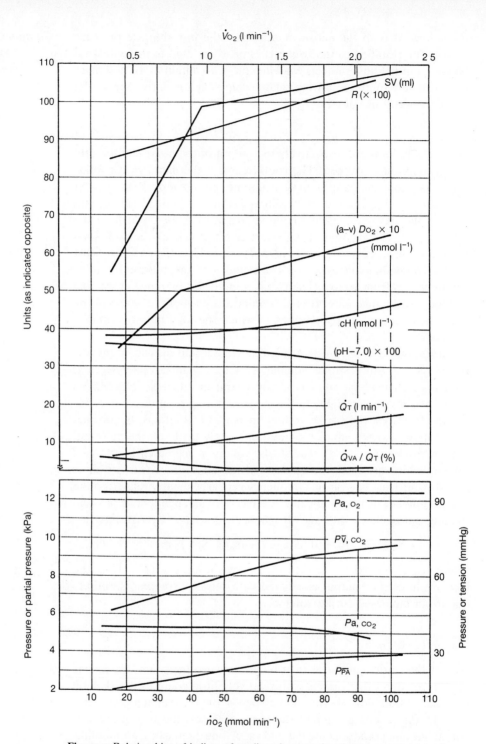

Fig. 13.7 Relationships of indices of cardio-pulmonary function to consumption of oxygen during exercise in an upright posture. The data are for untrained male subjects and are based mainly on the observations of Damato and Higgs and their respective collaborators. The pulmonary arterial pressures are measured from the xyphoid process; lower pressures are recorded when the reference point is the 4th rib at the sternum.

regions is reduced. The extent of the redistribution in blood flow is greatly influenced by physical training. It is also influenced by the prevailing ambient temperature and humidity. A cool dry environment maximises the blood flow to the muscles. By contrast a warm humid environment causes an increase in skin blood flow which is probably achieved at the expense of that to the muscles (page 412). The muscle blood flow does not reach such high levels when the cardiac output is for any reason impaired (see cardiac output above) or when the distribution of blood is affected by pharmacologically active substances, arterio-venous shunt or in other ways. Ingestion of alcohol and pregnancy are common examples.

Extraction of oxygen from blood

Oxygen which is delivered to the muscle capillaries passes into the muscle fibres as a result of dissociation of oxyhaemoglobin and diffusion of oxygen across the capillary−muscle membrane. The membrane is made up of the capillary endothelium, extracellular fluid and sarcolemma. The process of transfer was first considered in detail by Krogh and by Stainsby and Otis. It is the obverse of that in the lung which is summarised by equation 9.10, (page 275). In the muscle capillaries the dissociation of oxyhaemoglobin is assisted by the local conditions including the temperature, hydrogen ion concentration and tension of carbon dioxide; these variables are all higher in muscle capillaries than in the alveoli (see e.g. Fig. 9.5, page 287). The diffusing capacity of the capillary−muscle membrane is influenced by the membrane area and thickness, which depend on the number and degree of distension of perfused muscle capillaries. The perfusion rate determines the time for which the blood is in contact with the capillary−muscle membrane (i.e. the transit time). The transfer gradient is the difference in oxygen tension between the muscle fibres and the capillary blood.

On the basis of the Krogh model the local muscle oxygen tension was formerly assumed to vary inversely with distance from the nearest capillary; the model also assumed that the capillary oxygen tension declined progressively along the length of the capillary starting from the arterial end. However, recent work has shown that the model is incorrect. Ellsworth and Pittman have shown that the capillary oxygen tension varies on account of gas exchange with adjacent arterioles, venules and other capillaries. In addition, Honig and colleagues have demonstrated that the oxygen tension within muscle fibres is relatively uniform and independent of proximity to capillaries or distance from the centre. This aspect is discussed under the heading 'intramuscular oxygen tension' below. It has the effect that the mean intramuscular oxygen tension during exercise is approximately 0.5 kPa (3 mmHg) which is much less than that in venous blood leaving the muscle. Due to the low intramuscular tension the mean oxygen tension of muscle capillary blood is effectively equal to the transfer gradient. Almost all of it is available to promote diffusion of oxygen across the capillary−

Table 13.4 Muscle capillary oxygen tension at rest and during cycle ergometry at three inspired oxygen concentrations. The results are means for six non-smoking males (mean age 23.8 years)

	No exercise	Submax. exercise	Maximal exercise		
Inspired O_2 concentr.	0.21	0.21	0.21	0.15	0.12
O_2 uptake (mmol min^{-1})	NR	123	199	157	124
(l min^{-1})		2.75	4.46	3.53	2.79
Pao_2 (kPa)	11.9	12.4	12.7	7.4	5.0
(mmHg)	89.0	93.4	95.4	55.5	39.8
$P\bar{c}.mu,o_2$ (kPa)	NR	NR	5.1	4.0	3.3
(mmHg)			38.5	30.3	24.5
$Pf\bar{v},o_2$ (kPa)	3.8	2.6	2.2	1.9	1.6
(mmHg)	28.5	19.5	16.8	14.4	12.0
$\dot{V}E$ (l min^{-1})	NR	70	151	136	126
fc (min^{-1})	87	149	184	180	176

$Pc.mu,o_2$ and $Pf\bar{v},o_2$ are respectively muscle capillary and femoral venous oxygen tension. Other abbreviations are given in Table 2.2 (page 13)
NR = not recorded.
(Source: Roca J, Hogan MC, Story D *et al. J Appl Physiol* 1989; **67**: 291–299.)

muscle membrane. Thus the gradient is defended by both the oxygen delivery, which in trained subjects is high, and by the low oxygen tension at which the muscles operate.

A large transfer gradient is needed because the surface area for exchange of gases across the capillary–muscle membrane is relatively low. The diffusing capacity of the membrane is low in consequence. The large gradient partially compensates for this but the compensation is not complete, hence the capillary–muscle interface is an important determinant of exercise capacity. This has been demonstrated by Wagner and colleagues who studied healthy male subjects performing exercise at different ambient oxygen concentrations. The numerical results are summarised in Table 13.4. The maximal oxygen uptake at different inspired oxygen concentrations was *proportional* to the muscle mean capillary oxygen tension ($Pc.mu,o_2$) calculated using a Bohr integration; it was linearly related to tensions of oxygen in both the blood leaving the exercising muscles ($P\bar{v}.mu,o_2$) and the mixed venous blood.

Intramuscular oxygen tension

Oxygen molecules enter the muscles by diffusion across the capillary endothelium and sarcolemma; they then either enter into combination with cytochrome C in the mitochondria or combine with myoglobin. Diffusion into mitochondria occurs freely because there are many mitochondria and their total surface area is approximately 200 times greater than that of the muscle capillary membrane. However, most of the oxygen which traverses the sarcolemma combines immediately with myoglobin in the adjacent sarcoplasm. The myoglobin resembles haemoglobin in having a high capacity for oxygen. However, the molecular weight is small (approx. 17000) and the molecule has a hydrophilic surface so it is highly mobile within the sarcoplasm. The diffusivity is as much as one-tenth of that of molecular oxygen and this together with its high oxygen content makes myoglobin an efficient distributor of oxygen within the muscle fibres. The resulting oxygen tension in the fibres varies with the rate of metabolism. In one study of dog gracilis muscle Gayeshi and Honig found average tensions of approximately 2 kPa (13 mmHg) at 25% of maximal oxygen uptake falling to 0.2 kPa (1.7 mmHg) at 95% of the maximum. The range of tensions throughout the muscle also diminished with the intensity of exercise and at maximal exercise the tension was effectively identical throughout. These muscle oxygen tensions are higher than that required for oxidative metabolism in the mitochondria; the latter is less than 0.07 kPa (0.5 mmHg) and probably of the order of 0.01 kPa (0.1 mmHg). Thus even during maximal exercise at sea level the metabolism is not limited by the oxygen tension falling below the critical level for electron transport and oxidative phosphorylation. This finding has led to a revision of the traditional view that exercise is normally limited by the onset of *anaerobic* metabolism in the active muscles.

Intramuscular metabolism

Muscular contraction is effected by the combination of two contractile proteins actin and myosin. The reaction is triggered by calcium ions migrating from the sarcoplasmic reticulum into the sarcoplasm where they activate myofibular ATPase. The migration is due to nerve stimulation. The reaction consumes energy. This is supplied by hydrolyses of adenosine triphosphate (ATP) or other phosphate compound having a high energy of hydrolysis. The reaction with ATP can be represented as:

$$\text{ATP} + \text{actin} + \text{myosin} + \text{H}_2\text{O} \xrightleftharpoons{\text{Ca}^{2+}} \text{actinomysin} + \text{Pi} + \text{ADP} + \text{energy} \quad (13.5)$$

where Pi is inorganic phosphate and ADP is adenosine diphosphate. ADP can be used to generate more ATP but at the cost of reducing the available energy in the fibre:

$$2\text{ADP} \xrightleftharpoons[\text{kinase}]{\text{adenyl}} \text{ATP} + \text{AMP} \quad (13.6)$$

where AMP is adenosine monophosphate.

The quantity of ATP in skeletal muscle is approximately 7 mmol kg^{-1} which is sufficient for only a very brief contraction. The ATP can be replaced instantly by transfer of high energy phosphate contained in creatine phosphate:

$$\text{CP} + \text{ADP} \xrightleftharpoons[\text{kinase}]{\text{creatine}} \text{ATP} + \text{C} \quad (13.7)$$

401

where C is creatine and P is phosphate. However, the molar concentration of phosphocreatine in muscle is only about four times that of ATP so replenishment of ATP from this source is inevitably short term. In the long term the energy for replenishment is effected by oxidation of foodstuffs but ATP can be utilised at a faster rate than it can be renewed by oxidative phosphorylation alone. Thus an additional source of energy is needed: this is provided by the rapid breakdown of glucose by a process which does not involve oxygen. The process was formerly called anaerobic glycolysis but 'nonrobic' or rapid glycolysis are more appropriate terms. Each molecule of glucose is split in two by the mediation of enzymes and energy which comes from the degradation of two molecules of ATP. The reaction yields six molecules of ATP so the net gain is four molecules after allowing for priming. The other end product is two molecules of either lactate or pyruvate depending on the level of mitochondrial activity. The process is summarised in Table 13.5.

Glycolysis takes place in the sarcoplasm and sarcoplasmic reticulum and it is triggered by activation of the enzyme phosphofructokinase. Activation is effected by the synergistic actions of a number of substances including most of those which participate in the reactions. Positive effectors include relatively high concentrations of ADP, AMP, glucose 6-phosphate, fructose 1,6-diphosphate, ammonium radicals and inorganic phosphate; negative effectors include relatively low concentrations of ATP, creatinephosphate and hydrogen ions. Calcium ions which are concentrated in the sarcoplasm as a result of the contraction may contribute through inhibiting fructose 1,6-diphosphatase; the

Table 13.5 Stages in glycolysis

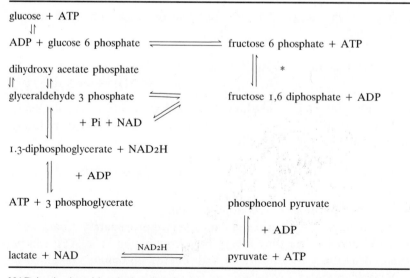

NAD is nicotinamide adenine dinucleotide, also called coenzyme; in its reduced form this substance is designated NADH or more correctly NAD2H. The rate limiting step (indicated by *) is controlled by the activation of phosphofructokinase (PFK). This process and also the other abbreviations are described in the text.

inhibition in turn leads to a rise in concentration of the enzyme's substrates. Calcium ions also promote glycogenolysis by converting the inactive enzyme glycogen phosphorylase b to its active form phosphorylase a. Thus the various metabolic pathways are interdependent.

The end product of glycolysis is either pyruvate or lactate depending on the mitochondrial activity. When the mitochondria can accept and oxidise the available NADH the end product is pyruvate which in turn is oxidised in the mitochondria. When the quantity of NADH more than saturates the mitochondrial enzymes the oxidation is effected in the sarcoplasm by the concurrent reduction of pyruvate to lactate. This process of rapid glycolysis occurs during the first 30s of moderate exercise when it is an important source of energy for regenerating ATP. Energy is also supplied by glycogenolysis and subsequent to 30s by oxidative glycolysis. Most of the lactate produced during the initial rapid glycolysis remains in the muscle; a variable quantity can pass into the blood and is taken up by the liver. Hence the lactate is either oxidised or resynthesised into glucose.

The process of glycolysis can be summarised as follows:

$$\text{glucose} + 2Pi + 2ADP \underset{\text{glycolysis}}{\overset{\text{rapid}}{\rightleftharpoons}} 2 \text{ lactate} + 2ATP + 2H_2O \tag{13.8}$$

$$\text{glucose} + 2Pi + 2ADP + 2NAD \underset{\text{glycolysis}}{\overset{\text{oxidative}}{\rightleftharpoons}} 2 \text{ pyruvate} + 2ATP + 2NAD2H + 2H_2O \tag{13.9}$$

The oxidation of pyruvate takes place in the mitochondria via a series of transformations which are described collectively as the Kreb's cycle or as the tricarboxylic or citric acid cycle. The outcome can be summarised as follows:

$$CH_3CO\ COOH + 5NAD \rightarrow 3CO_2 + 5NAD2H + \text{energy} + 3H_2O \tag{13.10}$$

The hydrogen ions in turn transfer from association with NAD to association with oxygen via an electron transport chain within the mitochondrial membrane. The chain involves flavoprotein and a series of cytochromes. It can be represented as:

$$NAD2H + \tfrac{1}{2}O_2 \xrightarrow[\text{flavoprotein}]{\text{cytochrome}} NAD + H_2O + \text{energy} \tag{13.11}$$

The principal substrates for muscle metabolism are glucose, free fatty acids and glycogen. The glycogen is phosphorylated to glucose which is then oxidised in the manner described above.

Muscle glycogen normally supplies most of the energy for strenuous exercise. The glycogen stores are depleted by prolonged exercise and in these circumstances free fatty acids make up some of the deficit but the exercise capacity is reduced.

The processes of glycolysis are severely impaired in patients with difficiency of muscle phosphorylase (McArdle's disease). These patients are unable to oxidise muscle glycogen. Consequently the maximal oxygen uptake is reduced. The reduction is associated with low levels of muscle NADH, an inability to produce lactate and reduced availability of pyruvate during exercise. There is also an accumulation of ADP and its breakdown products; they include inorganic phosphorus, AMP, inosine $5'$-monophosphate, ammonia and adenosine. These substances contribute to fatigue and muscle cramps; they also cause reflex vasodilatation in the active muscles and hence increase the cardiac output. The exercise capacity can be improved and the exercise cardiac output restored towards normal by provision of alternative substrates including glucose or fructose by intravenous infusion and free fatty acids by mobilisation from fat depots. This can be done by administration of noradrenaline or in other ways.

McArdle's syndrome is also associated with an increase in the ventilation during exercise; this causes hypocapnia so is in excess of the metabolic requirements. The hyperventilation occurs in the absence of lactacidaemia or a rise in muscle hydrogen ion concentration. It appears to be due to increased central drive to respiration.

Blood lactate and exercise limitation

In healthy subjects at rest the concentrations of lactic acid and pyruvic acid in the blood are approximately 0.9 and $0.04 \, \text{mmol} \, \text{l}^{-1}$ (8 and $0.4 \, \text{mg} \, \text{dl}^{-1}$). During mild exercise the lactate concentration is either unchanged or may fall slightly if the subject has been fasting. During moderate exercise the lactate concentration can rise transiently due to rapid glycolysis occurring in the active muscles at the start of exercise. During strenuous exercise the concentration rises progressively to reach a level of $6-14 \, \text{mmol} \, \text{l}^{-1}$ ($50-130 \, \text{mg} \, \text{dl}^{-1}$) at the breaking point of exercise. Much of the increase reflects the insufficient capacity of the mitochondrial enzymes to recycle NADH; the latter is closely related to but not identical with the ability of the oxygen transport chain to deliver oxygen to the mitochondria. In addition some of the increased concentration of lactate is due to its being in equilibrium with pyruvate, which also becomes more plentiful. The amount can be calculated on the assumption that the ratio of the concentrations of oxidised to reduced coenzyme is the same during exercise as it is at rest. The increment of lactate concentration which cannot be accounted for in this way has been called by Huckabee and Sendroy the 'excess lactate'.

The rise of lactate concentration during progressive exercise usually coincides with Owles' point; this is when ventilation starts to increase more rapidly than oxygen uptake and continues to outstrip it progressively more and more until the breaking point of exercise is reached (Fig. 12.3, page 370). High maximal lactate concentrations, with accompanying metabolic acidosis, are observed when the exercise level exceeds that which can be sustained by oxidative glycolysis (Figs 13.9 and 13.7). Lower maximal concentrations are observed when the exercise is limited mainly by the ability of the respiratory apparatus to ventilate the lungs. These two types of exercise limitation are compared below.

The breaking point of exercise

Exercise of progressively increasing intensity is nearly always limited by the sensations to which it gives rise. The commonest of these is breathlessness; others are fatigue, giddiness, ischaemic pain (angina or intermittent claudication) and pains in joints. The breathlessness is usually associated with a high dyspnoeic index (equation 13.1, page 392) which is due to the subject either having insufficient ventilatory reserve or attaining his aerobic capacity. These two modes of exercise limitation are described in Table 13.6.

The best guides to differentiation are the cardiac frequency, the concentration of lactic acid in blood at the breaking point of exercise and the rate at which the ventilation and the consumption of oxygen revert to their resting levels after exercise. The latter normally reflects the concentration of lactic acid in the blood which, when it is increased, declines exponentially at such a rate that, at any concentration above resting, the excess falls by 50% in about 10 min. However, the rate of recovery is also influenced by hyperventilation of psychological origin and by other factors. On this account, whilst a rapid recovery of ventilation after strenuous exercise is evidence for limitation by the respiratory system, a slow recovery should be interpreted in the light of other evidence. One such guide is the uptake of oxygen which, for exercise that is limited by respiration, usually reverts to its initial resting level within 3 min. For exercise which is limited by the capacity of the oxidative pathways, consumption of oxygen during the first 10 min of recovery is elevated by the need to reoxidise the lactic acid that was formed by rapid glycolysis during the course of the exercise. The consumption in excess of resting is the *oxygen debt*. It is influenced

Table 13.6 Physiological changes at the breaking point of exercise

Feature	Mode of limitation	
	Aerobic metabolism	Ventilatory capacity
Symptoms	Dyspnoea and fatigue; recovery is slow	Dyspnoea; recovery is rapid
Dyspnoeic index	40–100%	60–130%
Cardiac output	Maximal	Not maximal
Cardiac frequency	150–200 min^{-1}	<150 min^{-1}
Blood lactic acid concentration	6–14 mmol l^{-1}	<6 mmol l^{-1}
Arterial blood gases	Pa_{O_2} normal (or reduced) Pa_{CO_2} reduced (cH increased)	Normal or reduced Raised, normal or reduced
Diaphragmatic EMG	Usually normal	Evidence of fatigue
Ventilation and oxygen intake during recovery	Decline slowly	Revert rapidly to resting level

relatively little by hyperventilation of psychological origin so may be used to differentiate between this condition and the slow recovery of ventilation that is associated with marked lactacidaemia.

The principal factor limiting exercise in different conditions

The circumstances in which exercise is limited primarily by the internal oxygen transport system and primarily by the respiratory apparatus are tabulated in Table 13.7. In the first case the limitation in healthy subjects is mainly within those muscles which are active; hence the maximal oxygen uptake may be increased by a change in the mode of exercise which recruits additional muscle groups. The cardiac output is then also higher but the maximal output of the heart sets the limit in patients with mitral stenosis and other conditions in which the maximal cardiac output is reduced.

The limit is set by the respiratory system when either the ventilatory capacity is reduced or hypoxaemia on exertion increases ventilatory drive. A reduction in ventilatory capacity occurs in normal subjects under conditions of raised barometric pressure and in patients with disease of the lung or chest wall. Hypoxaemia leading to an increase in ventilation occurs in normal subjects at high altitude and at simulated altitude in a decompression chamber, while in diseased subjects hyperventilation occurs in cyanotic congenital heart disease and as a result of emphysematous or proliferative disease of the lung parenchyma. Both a ventilatory defect and an increase in the ventilatory cost of exercise can occur in patients with chronic obstructive pulmonary disease (COPD). The physiological features of the breaking point of exercise in the latter condition are illustrated in Table 13.8.

A material reduction in the quantity of haemoglobin which is available

Table 13.7 The principal factor limiting exercise in different conditions

Limiting factor	Conditions
Internal O_2 transport system	Healthy subjects at sea level Patients in whom the cardiac output is reduced Subjects with severe anaemia
Respiratory system (a) Increased ventilation on exercise	Healthy subjects at altitude or when breathing mixtures of air and N_2 Patients with disease of the lung parenchyma or cyanotic congenital heart disease
(b) Reduced ventilatory capacity	Healthy subjects under conditions of raised barometric pressure Patients with restriction of lung expansion
(c) Combination of (a) and (b)	Patients with airflow limitation or interstitial fibrosis

Table 13.8 Physiological features of the breaking point of exercise in COPD patients: mean data for 12 men (57 years, $FEV_{1.0}$ 0.94 l, FVC 1.50 l) during cycling and hand cranking breathing air and oxygen

	Cycling		Cranking
	Air	O_2	Air
Work rate (W)	50*	68*	40*
$\dot{V}_E$,max.ex (l min^{-1})	30.8	29.6	30.5
Dyspnoeic index (%)	97	95	97
V_t,max.ex × 100 ÷ VC (%)	43	45	44
f_R,max.ex (min^{-1})	30	28	29
f_C,max.ex† (min^{-1})	105	111	109

* Significant difference between work rates.
† Mean for three of the subjects.

for the transport of oxygen inevitably reduces the capacity for exercise. This is the case in patients with severe anaemia. However, with moderate anaemia the reduced oxygen capacity of the blood may be offset by an increase in stroke volume leading to an increase in cardiac output. At normal ambient temperatures there may then be no change in the relationship of the exercise cardiac frequency to the uptake of oxygen or in the capacity for exercise. However, at high ambient temperatures the submaximal cardiac frequency is increased and the capacity for exercise is reduced. A diminished capacity for exercise is also observed when carbon monoxide reduces the oxygen capacity of the blood (page 290); the reduction is often a result of smoking (page 483).

Effect of breathing oxygen

The inhalation of oxygen in place of air during exercise reduces the chemoreceptor drive to respiration, even though when breathing air the tension of oxygen in the arterial blood may be within normal limits; the mechanism is discussed on page 342. Inhalation of oxygen also decreases the need for rapid glycolysis, and hence the extent of any lactacidaemia, by increasing the quantity of oxygen which is carried to the tissues in solution in the blood plasma. The reduction in chemoreceptor drive acts at all levels of oxygen uptake (but see Fig. 11.6, page 344); the effect of lactacidaemia only occurs at beyond Owles' point (page 357). The two effects together reduce the level of ventilation during strenuous exercise in all the conditions which have been discussed. The effect of oxygen in a healthy subject is illustrated in Fig. 12.3 (page 370) and in patients with lung disease in Table 13.8 and Fig. 17.5 (page 640). By reducing the ventilation the inhalation of oxygen increases the intensity of exercise which can be undertaken without incapacitating breathlessness; thus, in appropriate circumstances, its administration from a portable apparatus provides a means for increasing the capacity for exercise of healthy subjects and also of patients whose breathlessness on exertion is due to disease of the heart or lung. The indications for the inhalation of oxygen during exercise, the possible complications and the equipment which may be used are discussed in Chapter 17 (see e.g. pages 623 and 639).

Physical training

A subject who increases his or her level of habitual activity initiates structural and functional changes which improve the capacity for exercise. The response depends on the intensity and duration of the stimulus but any increase in activity is beneficial. The required duration varies inversely with the intensity. For exercise of high intensity 10−20 min per day 3 days per week is very effective but for low intensity exercise, for example walking, or where the training is for endurance, longer times are needed. Maximal training in a normal sedentary subject can increase the capacity for exercise by approximately 20%. The associated structural and functional changes are summarised in Table 13.9. They have the effect that during submaximal exercise the cardiac frequency is reduced (Fig. 13.8), the rise in the lactate concentration occurs at a higher rate of work (Fig. 13.9) and thus Owles' point occurs at a higher

Table 13.9 Summary of the effects of physical training on ability to perform dynamic exercise

	Structural changes	Functional changes
Lungs*	Lung size ↑† Transfer factor ↑†	Respiratory muscle strength ↑ Vital capacity ↑ Maximal breathing capacity ↑
Blood	Total body haemoglobin ↑	Blood volume ↑
Heart	Muscle hypertrophies	Contractility ↑ Stroke volume ↑
Muscle capillaries	Number ↑	Blood flow ↑‡ Mean oxygen tension ↑‡
Muscle fibres	Diameter ↑ Number ↑ Proportion of type 1 ↑§	Power ↑
Mitochondria	Number ↑ Oxidative enzymes ↑	Oxidative capacity ↑
Skeleton	Bone diameter ↑† Mineral content ↑ Cartilage thickness ↑	Strength ↑
Respiratory control	—	Sensitivity to hypoxia ↓
Exercise ventilation	—	Submaximal ↓‡ Maximal ↑

* See page 472.
† During period of growth.
‡ At constant O_2 uptake.
§ These slow twitch (red) fibres (rich in myosin adenosine triphosphatase) are developed by endurance training.

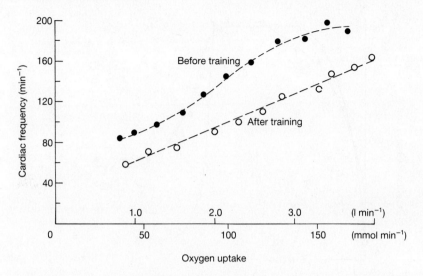

Fig. 13.8 Exercise cardiac frequency before and after a period of physical training. (Source: Brown A, Cotes JE, Mortimore IL, Reed JW. *Ergonomics* 1982; **25**: 793–800.)

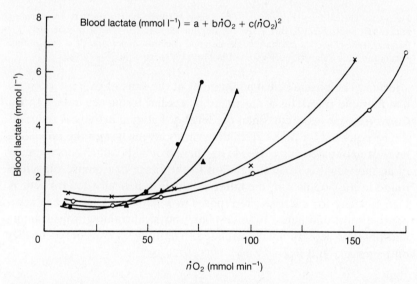

Blood lactate (mmol l^{-1}) = $a + b\dot{n}O_2 + c(\dot{n}O_2)^2$

Fig. 13.9 Blood lactate concentrations during steady state exercise in normal subjects. The oxygen uptake at a specified lactate concentration (e.g. 4 mmol l^{-1}) is correlated with and can be used to estimate the maximal oxygen uptake. (Source: Mortimore IL. PhD Thesis, University of Newcastle upon Tyne, 1982.)

oxygen uptake. The ventilation below Owles' point is insensitive to training in adult life (Fig. 12.3, page 370). However, differences in $\dot{V}E45$ between groups of subjects are correlated with the levels of *habitual* activity (e.g. Table 15.9, page 473), and there is some evidence that submaximal exercise ventilation may be reduced by activity in childhood. During maximal exercise the cardiac output, ventilation and consumption of oxygen are all increased by training but the maximal cardiac frequency and maximal blood lactate concentration are less

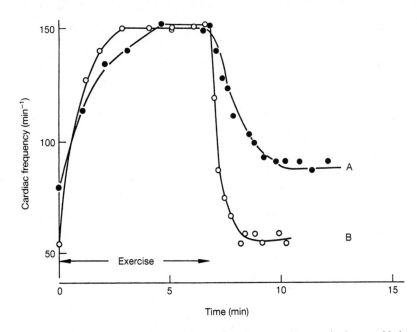

Fig. 13.10 The cardiac frequency during exercise of comparable severity in a world-class athlete (B) and subject having a low capacity for exercise (A). In the athlete the frequency rises faster at the start of exercise and declines sooner once it is over. Other results for these subjects are illustrated in Fig. 12.3 (page 370).

affected. The physiological adaptations at the start of exercise occur at a more rapid rate. This is illustrated by cardiac frequency in Fig. 13.10. Converse changes occur when the level of habitual activity is reduced.

The potential for physical training varies inversely with the prevailing level of habitual activity. However, the maximal possible improvement in an individual is small in relation to the range of exercise capacities found in the population; the latter is largely genetically determined. A high capacity for exercise predisposes to a person taking part in competitive sport and hence to undertaking physical training; thus training and physical activity are interrelated. The topic is considered further on pages 472 and 644.

High altitude

The hypoxia associated with ascent to high altitude reduces the capacity for exercise. However, the reduction is offset by acclimatisation, and by physical training which is a consequence of the increased activity associated with mountaineering. The reduced air density further increases the ventilatory capacity; this is illustrated in Fig. 5.16, page 124. On the other hand performance can be impaired by mountain sickness, disturbed sleep and exposure to extreme cold. Some of these features are summarised in Table 13.10. The effects on the lungs are described on pages 471 and 617.

The process of acclimatisation is mainly due to the hypoxia and consequent hypoxaemia stimulating the carotid bodies to increase the

Table 13.10 Some effects of alteration in barometric pressure

	Reduced pressure	Increased pressure
Lungs*		
Total lung capacity	↑ †	↑
Ventilatory capacity	↑	↓ ‡
Transfer factor	↑ †	↓ §
Respiratory control		
Sensitivity for CO_2	↑	↓
Sensitivity to hypoxia	↓ †	—
Exercise ventilation	↑	↓
Cardiac function	↓ (↑ †)	—
Blood		
Volume	↓	—
[Haemoglobin]	↑	—
[2,3-Diphosphoglycerate]	↑	—
Arterial O_2 tension	↓ ‡	(↑)
Muscle oxidative capacity	↑	—
Function of nervous system	↓	↓

* See pages 471 and 617.
† Effect long term.
‡ Principal effect (for details see text).
§ After deep saturation dives to >300 m.

chemoreceptor drive to respiration. The process is described on page 358. The hypoxaemia also impairs the transfer of oxygen across the alveolar capillary membrane. The impairment is most marked during acute hypoxia and is ameliorated by acclimatisation; the mechanism is discussed on pages 285 and 358.

Raised barometric pressure

Hyperbaria is normally associated with an increase in density of the respired gas. This increases the work of breathing, reduces the ventilatory capacity and can reduce the capacity for exercise. The subsequent decompression can lead to the formation of intravascular bubbles which can cause uneven perfusion of the lungs (Fig. 8.20, page 260). However, as with hypobaria there are some compensatory features; they include training of the respiratory muscles and general physical training when work is done in water. In addition there is often hyperoxia; this occurs when the respired gas is compressed air and with some gas mixtures used for saturation dives. During air dives these different effects of hyperbaria largely cancel out and the exercise capacity is at its sea level value. An example is given in Table 13.11. The underlying physiological changes are compared with those of high altitude in Table 13.10. The changes in ventilatory capacity are illustrated in Figs 5.16 and 5.17 (pages 124 and 125); some related changes which may be secondary to the accompanying physical activity are given on page 473.

Table 13.11 Effects of three atmospheres pressure upon lung function and exercise performance. Mean results for eight subjects breathing air

	1 ATA	3 ATA	*P*
Forced expiratory volume (FEV$_1$, l)	4.40	3.79	<0.01
Maximal voluntary ventilation (l min^{-1})	187.5	92.2	<0.01
Exercise capacity (W)	245	269*	<0.05
Maximal exercise ventilation (l min^{-1})	96.4	76.8*	<0.01
Maximal cardiac frequency (min^{-1})	190	191	NS

* Change from 1 ATA due to pressurisation raising the ambient O_2 partial pressure.
(Source: Craik MC. PhD Thesis, University of Newcastle upon Tyne, 1988.)

Following a deep saturation dive (depth > 300 m) both the capacity for exercise and the transfer factor can be reduced. Thorsen and colleagues have shown that the former change is related to the profusion of intravascular bubbles in the pulmonary circulation. The occurrence of oxygen toxicity could be a contributing factor. The mechanisms of these and other complications of hyperbaria are considered on page 630.

Hyperthermia

The body responds to a rise in hypothalamic temperature by increasing cutaneous blood flow and thus promoting the loss of heat from the skin. Heat is lost mainly by evaporation of sweat; during exercise this is supplemented by increased evaporative loss from the lungs.

In the skin the blood flow and the volume of blood in superficial vessels are both increased: this is effected by redistribution of blood volume and flow from other tissues. At the same time the blood pressure falls and the stroke volume diminishes; the cardiac frequency at rest and during submaximal exercise increases in consequence. These changes can reduce the quantity of blood available for the muscles; there is then less oxidative glycolysis than at normal temperatures and the capacity for exercise falls (page 412). The reduction was observed by Wyndham and colleagues to be associated with increased rapid glycolysis and lactacidaemia. However, this is not a constant feature in studies of hyperthermic exercise. Other factors contribute to the exercise limitation of which one may be the effect of a raised body temperature upon the function of the motor cortex.

The additional heat-load that accompanies prolonged exercise progressively raises body temperature and this limits endurance. At the same time the hyperthermia enhances respiratory drive (see page 338) and increases ventilation, changing the pattern of breathing towards rapid shallow breaths so that deadspace ventilation is also amplified. Hyperventilation is further stimulated by an increase in respiratory sensitivity to CO_2, which is a consequence of the metabolic adaptation to hyperventilation (page 346).

The effects of a high ambient temperature are offset by heat acclimatisation. The changes include a reduction in basal metabolism, an increase in blood volume, hypertrophy of sweat glands and a reduction in the salt content of the sweat which is produced.

Hypothermia

A cold environment causes reflex constriction of superficial blood vessels in the skin and dilatation of arterio-venous anastomoses in the deeper subcutaneous tissues. These changes maximise the insulating properties of the subcutaneous fat. They also divert blood to the lungs where both the transfer factor is increased and the distribution of pulmonary blood flow is disturbed. The latter change causes hypoxaemia which increases the chemoreceptor drive to respiration. The ventilation is then increased relative to the consumption of oxygen. At the same time the oxygen consumption is increased by shivering.

Breathing very cold air causes bronchoconstriction and this response is well developed in subjects with hyper-reactive airways (page 174). It can occur in most subjects if the air is cold enough (e.g. $-50°C$). The bronchoconstriction increases the work of breathing and so reduces any cold-induced hyperventilation. In addition if the deep body temperature falls, the central respiration activity is depressed. In these circumstances the ventilatory cost of exercise can be reduced. Peripheral hypothermia further impairs the ability to perform exercise by reducing the mobility of joints, impairing sensation and reducing the oxidative capacity of enzyme systems in the muscles. These adverse consequences of a cold environment can often be prevented: they are only very slightly amenable to cold acclimatisation.

Guide to references

The references (Chapter 18) are classified under subject headings of which the following are particularly relevant to the present chapter:

14: Assessment of the Physiological Response to Exercise

Introduction

Assessment of the physiological response to exercise is undertaken for two principal reasons: (a) to define what changes occur in healthy subjects and (b) to investigate the deviation from normal in patients with limited exercise tolerance. The comparison of normal with possibly abnormal results should take into account the age, gender and body size of the subjects; it should also take into account some measure of intensity of exertion either absolute or relative. The obvious choice might appear to be the rate of accomplishing external work on, for example, a cycle ergometer, and in trained subjects this correlates with the physiological changes. But in untrained or overweight subjects the correlation is relatively weak. The usual approach is to monitor the physiological changes in ventilation, cardiac frequency and related variables as they develop during progressive exercise and to relate them to one another and to the oxygen uptake which is a physiological index of the rate of energy expenditure. The carbon dioxide output also reflects the metabolic rate, but it is used less often because it is influenced by the alveolar ventilation.

The measurement of oxygen uptake entails analysis of the respired gas, and except for field studies, is now undertaken in an exercise laboratory. The exercise is then performed on an ergometer which is usually a treadmill, cycle or step. Simple tests of exercise performance which do not entail measurement of oxygen uptake can be performed outside the laboratory. Such tests can be used to assess a person's physical condition and to monitor the progress of a patient in relation to treatment. The 12 min dash and the 12 min walk are the distances a healthy person can run or a patient can walk in 12 min. These tests are best performed respectively on a running track and a hospital corridor; they can also be performed on a treadmill adapted so that the speed can be controlled by the subject. Tests of performance can also be undertaken using a cycle ergometer or stepping exercise on a box or flights of stairs.

Table 14.1 Respiratory indications for an exercise test

Investigate disproportionate breathlessness
Identify the mechanism of exercise limitation
Complement or increase the sensitivity of tests for lung disease
Assess suitability for rehabilitation, oxygen therapy etc.
Assess response to bronchodilator therapy or other treatment
Measure residual ability with view to employment or leisure pursuits
Measure disability with view to pension/compensation

Performance tests share with other forms of test exercise a risk that the subject may sustain an injury or develop myocardial ischaemia or other abnormality during the procedure. The risk can be reduced by preliminary assessment and appropriate monitoring and any ill effects can be minimised by effective early treatment. These aspects are best provided for in an exercise laboratory where it is usually simpler to perform a standard exercise test that includes electrocardiography (and also gas analysis) than to have the patient undertake a 12 min walk. Thus in respiratory medicine an exercise test is usually directed to assessing the cardiorespiratory response to progressive exercise. The 12 min (or 6 min) walk is also used. The emphasis is different in cardiology where ergocardiography is used extensively without measurement of oxygen uptake. In addition the measurement of aerobic capacity may be required for the proper surveillance of persons whose jobs entail intermittent very heavy work.

In relation to lung function the principal reasons for carrying out an exercise test are given in Table 14.1. The test provides information on the performance of the lungs under the stress of exercise, including respiratory control, pattern of breathing, ventilation, distribution of $\dot{V}_A/\dot{Q}$ and gas exchange; it enables the physician to see the patient when he is breathless and to note how quickly he recovers, while detailed results can indicate the extent to which exercise is limited by bellows function, gas mixing, or other abnormalities. Exercise can increase the sensitivity of individual lung function tests. Thus in early asbestosis the transfer factor may fail to increase to a normal extent during exercise at a time when the test result is still within normal limits at rest (page 712). The effects of incipient pulmonary congestion can often be detected only during exercise (page 599). In addition an exercise test is needed to demonstrate the presence of exercise-induced airflow limitation (page 176), and to distinguish hysterical hyperventilation from hyperpnoea due to cardiac insufficiency.

Ergometric methods and their limitations

Cycle ergometry

The essential feature of a cycle ergometer is a flywheel which is restrained by a friction belt or electromagnet. The rate of energy expenditure is the work done in unit time which is the product of the load on the flywheel and the distance through which it is moved per min; this is the circumference of the flywheel multiplied by the number of revolutions per min. When the load is applied by a friction brake the chosen work levels are achieved by the subject rotating the crank in time with a metronome, but this requires practice. The effect of fluctuations in cycling rate is less using electromagnetic braking because this is adjusted continuously throughout the exercise to keep the rate of work constant. The subject then unconsciously adopts the frequency of cycling which requires least effort. The calibrations of the breaking mechanism should be checked by driving the ergometer with an electric motor and relating the gauge readings to the work done.

The rate of work is expressed in watts which are linked to the basic units through the following relationships (see also Table 2.5, page 17):

Force = mass × acceleration: e.g. 1 newton (N) = $1 \, \text{kg} \, \text{m} \, \text{s}^{-2}$

work or energy = force × distance: e.g. 1 joule (J) = $1 \, \text{N} \, \text{m}$

rate of work or power = work ÷ time: e.g. 1 watt (W) = $1 \, \text{J} \, \text{s}^{-1}$

For a flywheel which is restrained by a loaded belt the rate of work was formerly expressed in kilopond metres per min where the kilopond (kp) is the force acting on the mass of 1 kg at the normal acceleration of gravity. Then:

$$\text{rate of work} = \pi d \times f \times l \, \text{kp} \, \text{m} \, \text{min}^{-1} \qquad (14.1)$$

where d is the diameter of the flywheel in metres, f is the frequency of rotation per min and l is the load in kg. Then since:

$$1 \, \text{kp} \, \text{m} = 9.81 \, \text{J} \qquad (14.2)$$

$$1 \text{ watt} = 1 \, \text{J} \, \text{s}^{-1} = \frac{60 \, \text{kp} \, \text{m} \, \text{min}^{-1}}{9.81} \qquad (14.3)$$

$$1 \, \text{kp} \, \text{m} \, \text{min}^{-1} = 9.81/60 = 0.1635 \, \text{watt} \qquad (14.4)$$

where 981 is the gravitational acceleration in cgs units.

The consumption of oxygen during cycling is linearly related to the work done against the flywheel, but also varies with body mass since the work of moving the legs is greater in heavy than in light subjects. For healthy subjects in an upright posture performing steady state exercise,* the consumption of oxygen per min is described approximately by the following relationship:

$$\dot{n}_{O_2} = [11.8 \, W + 6.84 \, M - 94 \, (\text{RSD } 90)] \div 22.4 \, \text{mmol} \, \text{min}^{-1} \qquad (14.5)$$

where $\dot{n}_{O_2}$ is the consumption of oxygen in $\text{mmol} \, \text{min}^{-1}$, W is the rate of work in watts, M is the body mass of the subject in kg and RSD is the standard deviation about the regression line. If the consumption of

---

* In the steady state the exchanges of oxygen and carbon dioxide over the intermediate stages of their transportation between the tissues and the environment are effectively constant. Attaining a steady state usually takes 3–4 min from the start of exercise.

417

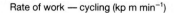

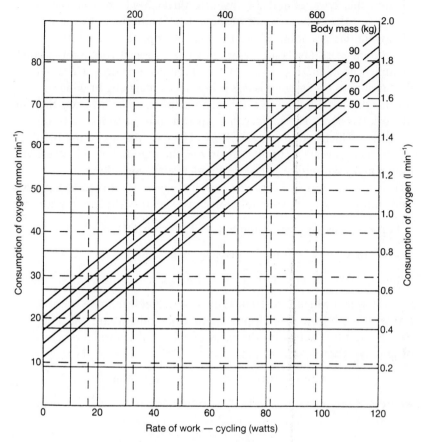

Fig. 14.1 Graphical solution to equation 14.5 relating the O_2 consumption to the rate of work during cycling. (Source: Cotes JE. *Ergonomics* 1969; **12**: 415–427.)

oxygen is expressed is $ml\,min^{-1}$ the factor 22.4 should be omitted. This relationship is illustrated in Fig. 14.1. However, for an accurate assessment the consumption of oxygen should be determined directly.

Treadmill exercise

The modern treadmill is a continuous belt which is moved across a smooth platform by an electric motor. The platform is provided with handrails and the mouthpiece is supported on a gantry whose position is linked to the incline of the platform. The speed of the belt and the angle of incline are adjustable, the former usually over the range 0–14.5 kph (0–9 mph), the latter from horizontal to an incline of 1 in 6 (17%). The belt moves towards the exercising subject who, at the start, should stand on the platform facing in the appropriate direction with the belt stationary. As a safety measure a chain is hooked across the platform behind the subject at the height of the buttocks or a safety harness is worn. The operator starts the motor with the gear in neutral, then slowly and progressively rotates the belt until the desired speed is attained. The subject is instructed to stand erect with head up take long steps and lift the feet only to the extent which is required for normal walking. The alternative practise of starting up the treadmill and having the subject step onto it off the side platform should be reserved for those who are agile and experienced. The handrail can be held at the start of exercise but if the measurements are to relate to a particular treadmill setting, the rail should be released before measurement is begun. As an additional precaution there should be a safety button within reach of the subject which can be used to decelerate the belt. An abrupt stop to the forward motion is undesirable as this can lead to the subject being propelled forward by his kinetic energy.

The rate of doing external work is a function of the body mass of the subject and the speed and incline of the belt. The work rate determines the rate of consumption of oxygen and the relationship between the relevant variables can be described empirically (e.g. Fig. 14.2). The coefficient of variation is approximately 20%. The oxygen uptake is reduced in subjects who are familiar with the procedure or who do much walking (e.g. Table 14.2). Outside the laboratory it is increased when the terrain is rough or the surface soft as is the case with bog, soft sand or snow. Thus the consumption of oxygen should be measured directly except when only an approximate estimate is needed.

Stepping exercise

Stepping exercise can take the form of box stepping, walking up stairs or climbing a ladder. In the exercise laboratory these forms are represented respectively by the standardised step test of Hugh-Jones and Lambert (page 367) and the Harvard pack test (page 438), a motorised escalator and a ladder mill in which work is also done with the arms. The exercise resembles treadmill walking in that (1) over a range of step frequencies the energy expenditure is linearly related to body mass, and (2) at a constant rate of external work heavier subjects expend more energy than lighter ones because of the internal work done in moving the legs and trunk. For a given rate of external work the energy expenditure is greater than that for cycle ergometry. Examples of energy expenditure during different forms of ergometry are given in Fig. 14.3.

Choice of ergometer

For assessing the cardiorespiratory response to exercise the choice is between a cycle ergometer and a treadmill. Box stepping is not satisfactory on account of the movement of the subject. Some features of the two forms of exercise are listed in Table 14.3. Usually the treadmill will be the instrument of choice because the exercise is more familiar to the subject. The principal exception is when it is proposed to sample the arterial blood gases during the exercise, or to monitor the pulmonary arterial pressure. In this circumstance the cycle ergometer has the

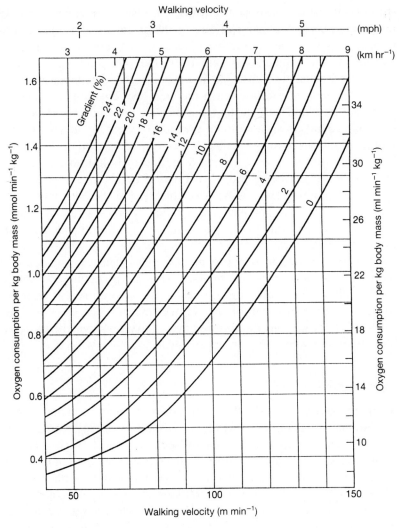

Fig. 14.2 Graphical solution to the relationship of Givoni and Goldman describing the oxygen cost of treadmill walking per kg body mass:

$$\dot{n}O_2 = \frac{44.6}{294} \eta M \, [2.3 + 0.32 \, (V - 2.5)]^{1.65} + G[0.2 + 0.07(V - 2.5)]$$
$$\times \text{RSD } 4.86 \, \text{mmol min}^{-1}$$

where $\dot{n}O_2$ is oxygen uptake in mmol min^{-1}; η is the terrain factor which for treadmill walking is 1.0, M is body mass (kg), G is gradient as percentage (100 × sine of angle of incline), V is velocity (km h^{-1}). To convert to O_2 uptake in l min^{-1} divide by 44.6 and to kcal h^{-1} multiply by 294. (Source: Givoni B, Goldman RF. *J Appl Physiol* 1971; **30**: 429–433.)

overriding advantages that the subject is seated and the arms are virtually immobile. Cycle ergometry with hand grips instead of pedals is used to study the responses to exercise with the arms. Box stepping can be used to study physical fitness including fitness for work (e.g. Harvard pack test, page 438). The aerobic capacity is usually best assessed on a treadmill since for subjects who do not cycle regularly the capacity by this method is greater than on a cycle ergometer.

Table 14.2 Mean values for the ventilation and the consumption of oxygen of men of weight 70 kg (154 lb) walking on a treadmill (A) for first time and (B) after practice, or when walking in a relaxed manner

Treadmill settings			Ventilation l BTPS min⁻¹		O_2 consumption mmol min⁻¹ (l min⁻¹)			
Speed		Incline						
m min⁻¹	(mph)	%	A	B	A		B	
60	(2.25)	—	22	17	42	(0.94)	31	(0.70)
107	(4)	—	33	29	66	(1.47)	58	(1.30)
60	(2.25)	10	37	31.5	75	(1.67)	63	(1.40)

(Source: Cotes JE, Meade F. *Ergonomics* 1959; **2**: 195−206.)

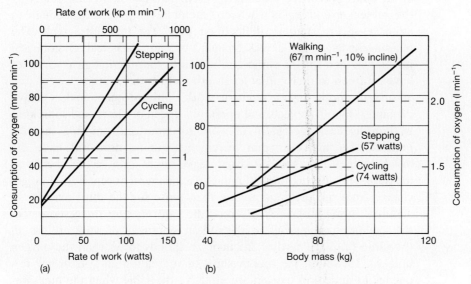

Fig. 14.3 (a) Average relationships for healthy males of the consumption of oxygen during cycling and stepping exercise to the rate of work (calculated from equations 14.1 and 12.2, page 368). For walking if the work is calculated from the rise and fall of the centre of gravity of the body per step, the relationship to energy expenditure is similar to that for cycling. (b) Average relationships of the consumption of oxygen to body mass for subjects performing standardised exercise: walking at 67 m min⁻¹ (2.5 mph) up an incline of 1 in 10, stepping at 57 watts (350 kp m min⁻¹) and cycling at 73.5 watts (450 kp m min⁻¹). (Sources: Cotes JE, Meade F. *Ergonomics* 1960; **3**: 97−119; Cotes JE, Davies CTM, John C. *J Physiol (Lond)* 1967; **190**: 29−30P.)

However, the latter is suitable for experienced cyclists. A ladder mill should be considered for investigation of levels of power output in excess of those which can be attained using other types of ergometry.

Exercise protocols

Cardiorespiratory response to submaximal exercise. A submaximal exercise test should identify the responses of the subject independent

Table 14.3 Physiological features of treadmill and cycle ergometry in respiratory patients. In instances marked with an asterisk the differences are also apparent in healthy persons

Aspects	Treadmill compared with cycle
Maximal oxygen uptake and ventilation	Greater*
Exercise desaturation†	More marked
Breathlessness score†	Lower
Submaximal $\dot{V}_E, V_t, f_c$	No material difference*

† Relative to oxygen uptake.
(Source: King B, Craik MC, Stevenson IC *et al. Clin Sci* 1987; **73**(suppl. 17): 3P.)

of the exact procedure which is adopted. This condition can be met by the subject exercising at each ergometer setting for long enough to attain a steady state as defined on page 417 (usually 4 min). The measurements are made over the next 1 or 2 min. Classical physiological practice is then for the subject to rest until the physiological variables have returned to their initial levels after which the exercise is repeated at one or more higher rates of work. This protocol makes heavy demands on both subjects and operators. It can be shortened somewhat by limiting each increment of work to 4 min and omitting the rest periods. Alternatively 3 min increments can be used but have the disadvantages that the steady state is never fully established and measurements during the first min of each increment represent a bigger change from the previous minute than those for the third minute. In addition during progressive exercise the half times for the responses of the several physiological variables to an increment of work are not all the same (e.g. the cardiac frequency responds faster than the oxygen uptake). However, the relationships of ventilation and of cardiac frequency to uptake of oxygen are effective the same when the measurements are made during progressive submaximal exercise with 1 min increments and during steady state exercise. This observation has led to the widespread use of progressive exercise with 1 min increments for assessing the cardiorespiratory response to submaximal exercise. But it has to be recognised that the result is not completely independent of the protocol. For example, in respiratory patients the extent of arterial desaturation at one rate of work is less during steady state than during progressive exercise. This can be important if the study is directed to exploring the mechanism. However, for routine assessment of patients a laboratory should adhere to a single protocol unless there is good reason for changing it. The aim will normally be to complete the submaximal test within 10 min. This gives time for the physiological adaptation to occur and is sufficiently short that the subject is not fatigued unduly. Some subjects can then perform a second test for measurement of the aerobic capacity in the same exercise session (page 433). As an alternative to using 1 min increments the rate of work can be increased continuously. In addition the physiological responses can be monitored each breath instead of each minute or half minute but the results tend to be variable unless smoothed by averaging.

To achieve an exercise duration of between 5 and 10 min the initial work level and the increment each minute should each be adjusted to the exercise capacity of the subject. Average protocols which have been found appropriate for a wide range of subjects are summarised in Table 14.4. They are in two parts, a submaximal protocol and a maximal protocol which can follow on or be taken separately. The distinction applies more to persons with a normal exercise capacity than to patients with lung disease. For the former group maximal exercise can be a disagreeable experience whilst for the latter it is often a tolerable everyday event. Maximal exercise is considered on page 433.

Ergocardiography. This procedure is widely used by cardiologists in the diagnosis and management of vascular disease of the heart. It also has other uses. The procedure entails exercise of progressively increasing intensity starting from rest and the end point is either the onset of clinical abnormalities (Table 14.6, page 425), the attainment of a predetermined cardiac frequency, usually 85% of the maximum predicted from equation 13.4 (page 397), or the attainment of a work rate equivalent to 80% of the expected maximal oxygen uptake. When based on a treadmill, the settings are often those set out in the Bruce protocol. This and some other protocols are given in Table 14.5.

The associated energy expenditures (oxygen uptakes) are indicated in Fig. 14.4. If a cycle ergometer is used the rate of work can be increased by equal increments each minute (for example 10 or 20 W per min) or logarithmic increments can be used.

Aerobic capacity. See page 433.

Table 14.4 Work protocols for assessing the cardiorespiratory response to exercise and maximal oxygen uptake

Test	Cycle ergometer			Treadmill		
	Healthy person		Patient (Combined)	Healthy person		Patient (Combined)
	Submax.	Max.		Submax.	Max.	
Starting point	Rest	W at R = 1.0 −20 W	Rest	3 kph	Incline ≥4°	2.0 kph Incline 4°
Increment per min	15 W	20 W	10 W	1 kph 1°*	1°	0.5 kph 1°
End point	R = 1.0	$\dot{n}O_2$max	$\dot{n}O_2$max (SL)†	R = 1.0‡	$\dot{n}O_2$max	4 kph‡ $\dot{n}O_2$max (SL)†

W = watts; kph = kilometres per hour; SL = symptom-limited.
* From 4 kph onwards increments of velocity and incline can alternate.
† Alternatively exercise can be terminated at $\dot{n}O_2 = 45$ mmol min^{-1}.
‡ Treadmill can be inclined to 4° at this point and exercise continued.

Ergometric methods and their limitations

Table 14.5 Treadmill protocols for cardiovascular stress testing (ergocardiography); the stages are of 3 min duration except where indicated

Time (min)	Bruce		Wolthuis		Balke	
	Speed (mph)	Incline (%)	Speed (mph)	Incline (%)	Speed (mph)	Incline (%)
0	1.7*	10	3.3†	0	3.3†	1‡
3	2.5	12		5		4
6	3.4	14		10		7
9	4.2	16		15		10
12	5.0	18		20		13
15	5.5	20		25		16

* 3.3 mph is 5.3 kph (the conversion factor is 1.61, Table 2.5, page 17).
† One or more stages at lower speeds are recommended for subjects who are not robust.
‡ Incline is increased at 1% per min.
For sources, see caption to Fig. 14.4.

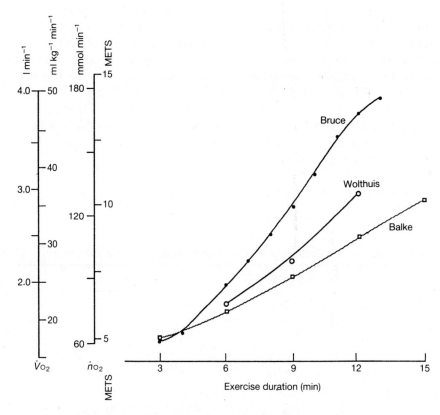

Fig. 14.4 Approximate relationships of oxygen uptake to exercise duration using different protocols. The relationships were obtained for men of mean body mass 80 kg. For these subjects, the resting metabolic rate, referred to as one metabolic equivalent (MET) was 12.5 mmol min^{-1} (0.28 l min^{-1} equivalent to 3.5 ml kg^{-1} min^{-1}).
(Sources: Pollock ML, Bohannon RL, Cooper KH *et al. Am Ht J* 1976; **92**: 39–46; Wolthuis RA, Froelicher VF Jr, Fischer J *et al. Am J Cardiol* 1977; **39**: 697–700.)

Table 14.6 Some cardiovascular indications for discontinuing an exercise test. Any association with cardiovascular disease should be verified

Features	Pallor with sweating
	Ischaemic pain (e.g. angina)
Electrocardiogram	ST depression > 0.2 mV
	Ventricular ectopic beats
	Coupled 2 or more
	Consecutive > 2
	Single > 7 per min
Blood pressure	Failure to increase with load
	Excessive increase (>210/150 mmHg)
	Decline > 10 mmHg, systolic

Safety precautions

An exercise test which is conducted by trained staff in a properly equipped laboratory is unlikely to cause harm to the patient. But safety precautions are essential. The ergometer, particularly the treadmill, should contain appropriate safety features (page 418) and be electrically earthed. The laboratory should be free from clutter and there should be good access to the subject. Provision should be made for a couch, an alarm button for summoning medical help, a resuscitation trolley (which should be checked and the drugs renewed every 6 months), and a cardiac defibrillator. Before embarking on exercise studies it is recommended that all subjects over the age of 40 should be questioned about previous heart attacks, angina, paroxysmal nocturnal dyspnoea and episodes of peripheral oedema. If any of these are reported then current heart failure and material hypertension (i.e. over 200/110) should be excluded.

A 12 lead electrocardiogram (ECG) should be obtained at rest on subjects with positive features and those who are at increased risk. The latter category is likely to include the obese, heavy smokers and all whose age exceeds 55 years. The existence of myocardial ischaemia should lead to a review of the need for the test. Contraindications are likely to include advanced disease and a grossly abnormal ECG chest lead V5: the latter is relevant because it or the related lead CM5 should be monitored continuously during the exercise. The cardiovascular indications for discontinuing the exercise test are given in Table 14.6. The indications are based on those used for ergocardiography (page 423) and should be strictly adhered to. However, their occurrence on one occasion does not preclude further testing since both the subject's condition may change and some features, particularly ventricular ectopic hearts, can be caused by apprehension.

Cardiorespiratory response to exercise

The cardiorespiratory response to exercise describes the adaptations of ventilation, cardiac frequency and related variables to several levels of

The physiological response to exercise

submaximal exercise. The exercise is usually progressive for the reasons given above (see exercise protocols, page 421). This section describes how the test should be conducted, the indices which are obtained and how they can be interpreted.

Equipment and calculations

The *equipment* used for assessing the cardiorespiratory response to exercise is illustrated in Fig. 14.5. It has evolved from a mouthpiece and Douglas bag (Fig. 3.1, page 22) to a computerised console, but whilst the change has improved the convenience and safety of the procedure, it has had less effect on the accuracy. This may account for the continued use of traditional equipment in some laboratories. The principal features of the measurements are the ergometer, breathing circuit, analysers, electrocardiograph, calculations and display. Automation has affected all of these and allows the display of the cardiorespiratory responses each half minute, or each breath during the test and the presentation of printed conclusions as soon as the test is completed. Results for single breaths are subject to error unless the equipment is of high quality, and are variable between breaths unless smoothed by averaging. This can be done over a number of breaths, when the scatter is less than when averaging is with respect to time; alternatively a running average can be used. The averaging procedure should be disconnected when it is proposed to assess the immediate response to a change in the rate of work or to a change from one inspirate to another. The reliability of the results depends on features listed in Table 14.7 and on the accuracy and frequency of calibration. The latter aspects are discussed in Chapter 3 and aspects of safety on page 425.

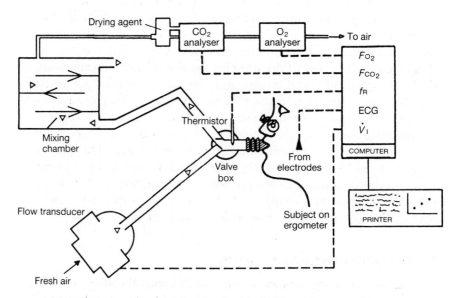

Fig. 14.5 Equipment for assessing the physiological response to exercise.

Table 14.7 Operational features of equipment for assessing the cardiorespiratory response to exercise

Ergometer		
Cycle	Adjustable cranks and saddle programmable up to 600 W	Calibration linear tolerance $< 2\%$
Treadmill	Speed 0–25 kph, incline 0–25°, emergency deceleration	Belt velocity uniform
Breathing circuit		
Mouthpiece	Area $> 5\,cm^2$, volume $< 15\,ml$	Clean between subjects
Valve box	Volume $< 50\,ml$	
Douglas bag	Wide bore connections, suspend vertically	Gas tight, flush before use
Gas meter	Free from cyclical error, should not pass unregistered gas	Volume tolerance $< 2\%$
Flow meter		Calibration should be linear
Mixing chamber	Volume $> 4\,l$, should mix (!)	
Overall resistance	$<0.01\,kPa\,l^{-1}\,s$ at $100\,l\,min^{-1}$	
Gas analysis		
Oxygen	Paramagnetic, zirconium oxide, mass spectrometer	
Carbon dioxide	Infra-red, mass spectrometer	Tolerance $< 1\%$
Electrocardiograph		
Should display and store ECG, count fc, other features optional		Counted fc should be checked
Data processing		
Allow for time delays in analysers; have appropriate time averaging (e.g. of fc); adjust for gas temperature and humidities; average gas volumes over whole breaths; use appropriate equations; store raw data		Use model lung (twin cylinder pump with predetermined ventilation and gas concentrations) as overall check

The *displays* should include the relationships of ventilation and cardiac frequency to uptake of oxygen. They should preferably also include the relationships of ventilation to tidal volume, ventilation to output of carbon dioxide, carbon dioxide output to oxygen uptake and respiratory exchange ratio to uptake of oxygen (Fig. 14.6). The *analyses* should include calculations of linear equations to describe the relationships over their linear portions. Linearity can be assessed by the computer programme comparing the slopes and residual variation about regression lines obtained using data points from different parts of the range. The upper limit of linearity on the $\dot{V}\text{E}/\dot{n}o_2$ plot defines Owles' point and that on the $\dot{n}co_2/\dot{n}o_2$ plot the anaerobic threshold of Wasserman and colleagues. The linear equations are used to identify, by interpolation, the ventilation, cardiac frequency and respiratory exchange ratio at specified levels of uptake of oxygen, for example 45 and

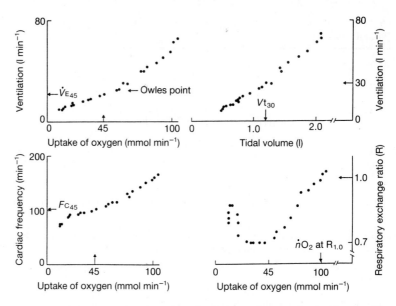

Fig. 14.6 Intermediate results of a submaximal progressive exercise test in a healthy subject showing the derivation of the indices fc_{45}, $\dot{V}_{E45}$, Vt_{30} and $\dot{n}_{O_2}$ at $R = 1.0$. For details see text.

67 mmol min^{-1} (1.0 and 1.5 l min^{-1}). In SI units the indices at the former level are designated respectively $\dot{V}_{E45}$, fc_{45} and RER$_{45}$; in traditional units they are $\dot{V}_{E1.0}$, $fc_{1.0}$, RER$_{1.0}$. Similarly the tidal volume at a minute volume of 30 l min^{-1} is designated Vt_{30} and the oxygen uptake at a respiratory exchange ratio of unity is designated $\dot{n}_{O_2}$ at RER$_{1.0}$. The computer programme can also identify maximal values for the indices; these should normally relate to the last or penultimate half minute of exercise. The indices and the relationships from which they are derived are listed in Table 14.8.

The operator should check any computer-based indices against the graphical displays. These will normally show a narrow scatter about the individual relationships (e.g. Fig. 14.6). However, the inspection may reveal initial hyperventilation, abberant points, wide variability or curviliniarity which could influence the result. An example is given in Fig. 4.1 (page 80). The observer should also note if Owles' point and Wasserman's point have been correctly identified. For the latter the reproducibility of the oxygen uptake was reported by Beaver and others as 3.8%. The oxygen uptakes at the two points are not identical and their physiological basis remains unclear (page 401).

The basic cardiorespiratory information can be supplemented by *additional measurements*. The most used procedure is oximetry, for the non-invasive detection of hypoxaemia developing during exercise. The measurement is best made using an oximeter applied to a finger tip or ear lobe; the part should be fully vasodilated (page 36). The cardiac output can be measured by the rebreathing method (page 241) or by an indicator dilution method (page 247). Pulmonary arterial pressure can be measured using a strain gauge pressure transducer and Swan-

Table 14.8 Indices of the cardiorespiratory response to exercise*

Relationship	Indices
Ventilation on oxygen uptake ($\dot{V}E/\dot{n}O_2$ or $\dot{V}E/\dot{V}O_2$)	$\dot{V}E_{45}$†, $\dot{V}E_{67}$, $\dot{n}O_2$ at Owles' point, $\dot{V}E$max, $\dot{n}O_2$max
Cardiac frequency on oxygen uptake ($fc/\dot{n}O_2$ or $fc/\dot{V}O_2$)	fc_{45}, fc_{67}, fcmax
Ventilation on tidal volume ($\dot{V}E/Vt$)	Vt_{30}, Vtmax‡
Respiratory exchange ratio on oxygen uptake (RER/$\dot{n}O_2$ or RER/$\dot{V}O_2$)	RER$_{45}$, $\dot{n}O_2$ at RER$_{1.0}$, RERmax
Ventilation on CO_2 output ($\dot{V}E/\dot{n}CO_2$ or $\dot{V}E/\dot{V}CO_2$)	Slope ($\Delta\dot{V}E/\Delta\dot{n}CO_2$)
CO_2 output on oxygen uptake ($\dot{n}CO_2/\dot{n}O_2$)	$\dot{n}O_2$ at anaerobic threshold of Wasserman and colleagues

* Ventilation volumes are in l BTPS, gas exchange is in mmol min^{-1} (or l STPD min^{-1}) and cardiac frequency is per min.
† In traditional units $\dot{V}E$ 1.0: these and the other indices are described in the text.
‡ Vtmax reaches a peak before the attainment of maximal exercise; in respiratory patients it may then decline.

Ganz catheter with its tip placed in a pulmonary artery. Alternatively a rigid catheter can be used with a view to also obtaining the wedge or pulmonary venous pressure. The pulmonary vascular pressures are best interpreted as resistances for which the cardiac output is also needed, so the two measurements should be made concurrently. Measurements of arterial blood gas tensions are then also likely to be required (page 39).

The *extent of breathlessness* during exercise can be reported or it can be recorded using a Borg or visual analogue scale (page 387); for the latter the method of scoring should be automated (page 33).

Conduct of the submaximal exercise test

Outpatients attending for an exercise test should be advised to come suitably clad and to have with them flat shoes with soft soles and heels. They should not have had a recent heavy meal and preferably not have smoked on the day of the test. The procedure should always be preceded by a clinical appraisal and, if appropriate, by electrocardio-graphy (page 425). For respiratory patients the forced expiratory volume and vital capacity should be available at the time of the test; the FEV_1 provides an indication of the likely maximal exercise ventilation and the FVC the maximal tidal volume. The subject should have been weighed recently. In the laboratory the operator starts the session by calibrating the ventilation meter and gas analysers and checking that the safety equipment is in order. A check is made that the subject's condition has not changed materially since the clinical appraisal. The blood pressure is recorded using a sphygmomanometer. The time of the most recent bronchodilator therapy should be noted. Usually the patient's airway should be fully dilated at the time of the assessment. To this end the exercise can usefully follow the measurement of FEV_1 before and after inhalation of salbutamol; but neither bronchodilator nor cromoglycate should be given when it is proposed to assess exercise-induced airflow limitation. Next the subject partially undresses for measurement of skinfold thickness at the four sites described on page 56. The measurements are used to calculate the percentage of body mass which is fat and hence the fat free mass (page 57). The subject now lies down on a couch and if appropriate a 12 lead electrocardiogram is recorded. The three chest electrodes are then applied over the upper and lower sternum and in the 5th left intercostal space at the line of the nipple for recording the electrocardiogram in the CM 5 configuration. The subject now mounts the ergometer; if a treadmill is used the belt should be horizontal and stationary, if a cycle the saddle should be adjusted so that the leg is almost straight when the ball of the foot is on the pedal in the down position. The chest electrodes are connected to the electrocardiograph, and any other equipment, for example a control for the visual analogue scale of breathlessness, adjusted appropriately. In the case of a treadmill, instruction is given on how to stop or have the operator decelerate the belt. The mouthpiece is adjusted and the nose clip applied. Before or at this point the subject undertakes a short walk to get used to the treadmill and then sits or stands for recording the pre-exercise ventilation and other variables. Normally a 2 min period of recording is sufficient. The subject is now ready for exercise at the initial ergometer setting indicated by the protocol. In the case of a treadmill the subject is reminded how to walk correctly (page 418) and instruction is given on discontinuing exercise in the event of material symptoms.

During the exercise one operator should observe the subject, provide encouragement and monitor the electrocardiogram. If the exercise equipment is nearly or fully automated the observer can also attend to what still needs to be done manually; if there are instruments to be read a second observer will be required.

In subjects with a relatively normal capacity for exercise the endpoint for the submaximal test will normally be when the cardiac frequency has reached 85% of the maximum predicted from Table 14.9 (equivalent to 80% of the predicted maximal oxygen uptake), the respiratory exchange ratio has risen to unity (RER = 1.0) or the oxygen uptake has reached a specified level, for example, $67\,mmol\,min^{-1}$ ($1.5\,l\,min^{-1}$). These limits will also apply to those patients who do not stop earlier on account of symptoms. The exercise should then be discontinued. Either the treadmill is decelerated to zero speed or the subject stops pedalling. However, in the case of symptom-limited exercise, depending on how many data points have been obtained, there may be a case for encouraging the subject to complete the current 30 s period of observation. Subsequently, any symptoms which contributed to the subject discontinuing exercise should be described and recorded. To this end on disconnecting from the mouthpiece the subject should immediately be engaged in conversation or asked to read aloud; the degree of panting should be noted. The subject should be asked to describe the symptoms

Table 14.9 Linear regression equations which describe aspects of the physiological response to exercise of men and women in an erect posture

Aspects of function	Relationship	SD or c of v	Source
(a) *Healthy subjects*			
Ventilation on oxygen uptake	$\dot{V}_E$ $(l\,min^{-1})^* = 0.5\ \dot{n}o_2\dagger + 2$	5.4	Cotes, unpublished
	$\dot{V}_{E45}$ $(l\,min^{-1}) = 19.5 + 0.095$ age $+ 0.87$ if SM	2.81	Weller *et al.* (1988)
Tidal volume on vital capacity	Vt_{30} $(l) = 0.13$ VC(l) $+ 0.87$	0.22	Cotes, unpublished
	$Vtmax$ $(l) = 0.64$ VC(l) $- 0.64$	0.21	Jones, Rebuck (1979) (Fig. 15.30).
Oxygen uptake during steady state cycling	$\dot{n}o_2$ $(mmol\,min^{-1}) = 0.53$ W (watts) $+ 0.31$ BM $- 4.1$	4.0	Cotes (1969)
Cardiac frequency on oxygen uptake and fat free mass	fc $(min^{-1}) = (1590 + 58\dot{n}o_2\dagger)FFM^{-1} + 34$	12%	Cotes, Berry *et al.* (1973) (Fig. 14.9).
	fc_{45} $(min^{-1}) = 71.6 - 5.47$ AG $+ 1812$ FFM^{-1} $+ 0.35$ %fat	10.8	Weller *et al.* (1988)
Maximal cardiac frequency (*fc*max)	fc $(min^{-1}) = 210 - 0.65$ age (years) [85% fcmax $= 168 - 0.52$ age]	19	Åstrand *et al.* (1973)
Cardiac output on oxygen uptake	$\dot{Q}t$ $(l\,min^{-1}) = 0.37\dot{n}o_2\dagger + 3.4$	0.9	Reeves *et al.* (1961)
Maximal O_2 uptake			
(a)	$\dot{n}o_2$ max $(mmol\,min^{-1}) = 1.11$ St $+ 0.84$ BM $+ 6.7$ AS $- 1.03$ age $- 103$	18.5	Jones *et al.* (1985)
(b)	$\dot{n}o_2$ max $(mmol\,min^{-1}) = 70 + 1.43$ FFM $+ 6.3$ AS $- 0.95$ age -8.1 if SM	17.3	Weller *et al.* (1988)
(c)	$\dot{n}o_2$ max $(mmol\,min^{-1}) = 70.1 + 0.63(\dot{n}o_2$ at RER$_{1.0}$) $+ 0.78$ FFM $- 0.29$ $fc_{45} - 0.86$ %fat	12.1	Weller *et al.* (1988)
(b) *Subjects with respiratory impairment*			
Maximal exercise ventilation on FEV$_1$	$\dot{V}$Emax, ex $(l\,min^{-1}) = 33.1$ (FEV$_1$)$^{0.73}$	18%	Cotes, Posner, Reed (1982) (Fig. 14.8).
Maximal O_2 uptake on FEV$_1$ and $\dot{V}_{E45}$	$\dot{n}o_2$ max $(mmol\,min^{-1}) = 66.4 + 13.4$ FEV$_1$ (l) $- 0.94$ $\dot{V}_{E45}$ $(l\,min^{-1}) + 0.45$ FFM $- 0.31$ age (years)	11.6	Cotes, Zejda, King (1988)
Maximal O_2 uptake as % of predicted	% $\dot{n}o_2$ max $= 52.3 + 0.44$ %FEV$_1$ $- 0.78$ $\dot{V}_{E45}$ $+ 0.16$ %Tl.co $+ 52.3$	7.3%	Cotes, Zejda, King (1988)

* For female subjects the ventilation is about 10% higher.
† $\dot{n}o_2$ = uptake of oxygen (mmol min^{-1}). When uptake of oxygen is measured in l min^{-1} the coefficient for $\dot{n}o_2$ should be multiplied by 1000 and divided by 22.4.
FFM = fat free mass (kg); BM = body mass (kg); St = stature (m); SM = smoker. Activity scores: AS 1 inactive to 4 very active. AG 1 inactive to 3 very active. % FEV$_1$ % Tl,co = percentage of predicted value.

and the Borg scale for perceived exertion should be completed (Table 13.2, page 390). After this the subject should dismount from the ergometer and lie on a couch for 5 min during which time the electrocardiogram and the blood pressure should be recorded. The computer output can also be inspected with a view to providing tentative answers to any questions which the subject may ask about the test.

Interpreting results

The person reporting the response to exercise will normally be provided with the information indicated in Table 14.8. The graphs and the detailed print-outs on which they were based should be scrutinised and an opinion formed as to the quality of the data. Scatter or inappropriate trends between serial readings can be an indication for redoing the analysis or repeating the test (see e.g. Fig. 4.1, page 80).

The *submaximal exercise ventilation* will usually be reported as $\dot{V}_{E45}$ ($\dot{V}_E$ 1.0) and not ventilation equivalent for the reason given on page 60. The ventilation can be influenced by the subject hyperventilating or adopting an unusual respiratory frequency. Hyperventilation is associated with an increase in respiratory exchange ratio over the normal level of 0.83 (range 0.73–0.92); however, hyperventilation is more common at rest and during near maximal exercise than at the work level under consideration. Shallow breathing is accompanied by a reduction in Vt_{30} relative to its reference value (Table 14.9). A high respiratory exchange ratio or low value for Vt_{30} is an indication for caution in interpreting all the results.

Amongst 542 shipyard workers in one shipyard the $\dot{V}_{E45}$ was correlated positively with age and negatively with exercise tidal volume, body mass index and physiological evidence of airflow limitation (FEV% reduced or RV% increased). In another shipyard population after allowing for age $\dot{V}_{E45}$ was increased amongst smokers and those who gave a history of previous pneumonia or pleurisy or of having sprayed asbestos. The average increase associated with each of these conditions was $2.25 \, l \, min^{-1}$ (approximately 10%). Amongst patients larger increases can be observed. For example Cotes and King found that the average increase associated with moderate asbestosis (mean score for small opacities 5.63 ILO units) was $6.0 \, l \, min^{-1}$. Reed and colleagues found a mean increase of $10 \, l \, min^{-1}$ amongst women with mitral stenosis prior to valvotomy. In the latter instance the increase in ventilation was associated with an average reduction in Vt_{30} of 0.35 l. The tachypnoea was reversed by the operation and was attributed to stimulation of pulmonary J receptors. More marked increases can occur in individual patients (see illustrative cases in Chapter 16). In many instances the increases are associated with defective gas transfer leading to progressive hypoxaemia during exercise, and more normal levels of ventilation are observed while breathing oxygen. However, the association with hypoxaemia is not invariable. Thus in some patients with interstitial fibrosis the progressive hypoxaemia is due to the increased work of breathing depressing the ventilatory response to exercise hence giving relatively low values for $\dot{V}_{E45}$. In these circumstances the ventilatory response to hypoxic drive is reduced. Therefore, interpretation of the $\dot{V}_{E45}$ should take account of other features of the response to exercise. A high value for $\dot{V}_{E45}$ contributes to exercise limitation and is a guide to respiratory disability (page 443).

In a patient with respiratory impairment and in whom exercise is limited by symptoms, a value for *maximal exercise ventilation* which approaches that predicted from the FEV_1 indicates the presence of respiratory disability (page 441). However, if Owles' point is readily discernible there may possibly be circulatory limitation as well (page 404).

The *cardiac frequency during submaximal exercise* will usually be reported as fc_{45} (fc 1.0). The reference value is inversely related to stroke volume which is determined by the amount and tone of the cardiac muscle. These aspects are in turn related to fat-free mass and the level of habitual activity; both variables influence fc_{45} and should be taken into account when calculating the reference value (Table 14.9). For example in the shipyard population the effect of a sedentary life style was to increase the fc_{45} by an average of $11.9\,min^{-1}$ (Table 14.9); there were significant differences between trades. A value for fc_{45} which is high relative to the fat-free mass is usually evidence of anxiety, a low level of habitual activity (which could be a consequence of lung disease), hypoxaemia or cardiac failure. It can also be due to anaemia, hyperthermia, alcohol or the patient being on steriods or other drugs. A relatively low fc_{45} in a young subject often indicates athletic training, and in an older one, indicates a cardiac conduction defect or treatment with β blocking drugs. A high fc_{45} in a patient with uncomplicated respiratory disability can presage a favourable response to exercise training.

When exercise is limited by symptoms the *maximal exercise cardiac frequency* should be reported. A value for fcmax which approaches the reference value (Table 14.9) suggests that exercise was limited by circulatory and related factors. A relatively low fcmax can confirm a diagnosis of respiratory disability. These aspects are considered below.

Assessment of exercise capacity

The exercise capacity during ergometry can be obtained by direct measurement of the maximal oxygen uptake or maximal work rate. Alternatively it can be expressed in terms of indices obtained from the submaximal exercise test or other variables. The direct assessment entails maximal exercise; this is acceptable to most persons of an athletic disposition. It is also well tolerated by the majority of patients with respiratory disability for whom maximal exercise is often a familiar experience from which recovery is rapid (page 405). By contrast maximal exercise is not well tolerated by the majority of sedentary but otherwise healthy subjects; particularly amongst such persons the procedure can be hazardous in the presence of risk factors for myocardial ischaemia. Thus amongst relatively healthy subjects the direct measurement of exercise capacity is usually undertaken in relation to athletes, physical training and fitness, or for obtaining reference values. In patients with respiratory impairment the measurement is often obtained from the progressive exercise test when this is curtailed by the onset of symptoms (page 430). In other circumstances there should be a compelling reason for undertaking the test; this will often be in relation to compensation for some form of injury.

Direct assessment

The protocols for the cardiovascular stress test (Table 14.5) give a rough guide to the maximal oxygen uptake. The definitive measurement is the time for which the subject continues with the exercise, and the corresponding oxygen uptake given in Fig. 14.4 is that for an average subject. This has wide confidence limits because the method does not allow for variation in mechanical efficiency between subjects; the discrepancy is greatest for unfamiliar forms of exercise but is also apparent with treadmill walking (e.g. Table 14.2). Thus where possible the maximal oxygen uptake should be measured directly.

Definition of maximal oxygen uptake. This is currently undergoing a change. Strictly it is the highest value obtained during a progressive exercise test which is continued until a further increase in work rate fails to increase the oxygen uptake (see test procedure below). Alternatively it is the oxygen uptake at the predicted maximal heart rate. However, the values so obtained depend on the mass of muscle used during the test and therefore are not independent of the ergometer. Usually treadmill exercise is taken as the standard. In this event the result during cycling is on average 10% lower, except in experienced cyclists; the result can be increased by combining cycling with some hand cranking. However, when strenuous hand cranking is added or the subject performs maximally on a ladder mill the maximal oxygen uptake exceeds that during treadmill exercise. Thus the form of ergometry should be specified.

Test procedure. The assessment starts with a submaximal protocol such as one of those proposed for assessing the cardiorespiratory response to submaximal exercise (page 423 and Table 14.4). The procedure for that assessment, including the measures needed for quality control, should be followed closely. In patients with respiratory impairment the test will often be brought to a stop by symptoms. In the absence of symptoms the submaximal protocol is completed. The maximal performance can then be assessed either by going immediately to an estimated maximal work rate or by undertaking the protocol for maximal exercise. The latter can be performed after an interval of at least 30 minutes or in a separate session. If the former the second stage of the appropriate protocol in Table 14.4 should be used without modification. If a separate session is to be used the second stage of the protocol should be preceded by a period of submaximal exercise by way of 'warm up'.

The formal criteria for stopping the maximal test are that a plateau of oxygen uptake, defined as a minute-to-minute variation of less than $7 \, \text{mmol min}^{-1}$ ($150 \, \text{ml min}^{-1}$), has been reached, the predicted maximal cardiac frequency (Table 14.9) has been attained or there is circulatory insufficiency as indicated by one of the features listed in Table 14.6 (page 425). Alternatively the subject may stop on account of symptoms which are then usually musculo-skeletal in nature.

At the end point of maximal exercise the loading on the ergometer should be materially reduced whilst the subject continues to exercise against a diminishing load for 2 min; this gives time for the circulation to readjust. The subject should then transfer to a couch for 5 min in the manner described for the submaximal test.

The indices to be obtained from the maximal test are listed in Table 14.8.

Indirect assessment

As an alternative to direct measurement, the maximal oxygen uptake can be obtained by extrapolation or empirical equations using the results of the submaximal exercise test; the latter can be supplemented by other information about the subject including age and fat-free mass. In patients with respiratory impairment the additional information will include the FEV_1. In healthy subjects the maximal oxygen uptake can also be estimated using simple indices which are obtainable without recourse to a laboratory. The latter are less accurate but can be used to provide reference values with which the results of the maximal or submaximal assessment can be compared.

Extrapolation method. This method is used for healthy subjects and others in whom the capacity for exercise is limited mainly by the ability of the cardiovascular system to deliver oxygen to the active muscles. The method is based on the nearly linear relationship between cardiac frequency and oxygen uptake during exertion (Fig. 14.6). The relationship is obtained during submaximal exercise, either progressive using 1 or 3 min time increments or steady state with 4–6 min work periods; these can be separated by rest pauses. In the simplified procedure of Åstrand extrapolation is made from the cardiac frequency at one rate of work, but it is better to use at least four work loads, of which the highest should be within 20% of the maximum estimated from cardiac frequency (Table 14.9). The resulting relationship of cardiac frequency to oxygen uptake should be linear. Maximal oxygen uptake is obtained by extrapolating the relationship to the cardiac frequency which the equation in Table 14.9 predicts is the maximum for the subject's age. Although this is appropriate for Swedish people it appears to

435

over-estimate the maximal frequency of British people by on average $6\,min^{-1}$. Thus the maximal cardiac frequency should where possible be based on local reference values.

The method depends on the relative constancy between subjects of the relationship of cardiac output to oxygen uptake (page 397). Subjects with a low capacity for exercise have a low stroke volume hence high cardiac frequency compared with others who can take more exercise (e.g. Fig. 13.8, page 409). The measurement has an acceptable reproducibility but the accuracy of prediction of maximal oxygen uptake is poor. This is because the relationship of cardiac frequency to oxygen uptake often becomes curvilinear at near to the maximum and because the prediction formula for fcmax fails to take account of the fact that maximal frequency varies inversely with the quantity of cardiac muscle. Consequently this method is not recommended where an alternative is available.

Empirical method. This approach to estimating maximal oxygen uptake is based on the dimensional consistency of the components of the oxygen transport chain from the lungs to the mitochondria (e.g. Fig. 13.1, page 386). The method is appropriate for persons who are apparently healthy and any relevant index can be used.

The most informative is probably the maximal stroke volume; this can be measured non-invasively by the carbon dioxide rebreathing method (page 421) but the procedure requires a high level of co-operation and is liable to cause headache in some subjects. Alternatively, use can be made of the oxygen uptake associated with a specified level of lactacidaemia, for example $6\,mmol\,min^{-1}$. The relevant oxygen uptake is obtained by interpolation from the graph relating oxygen consumption to lactate concentration during successive periods of steady state or quasi-steady state exercise. For the latter a progressive protocol with 3 min increments of work can be used. The lactic acid concentrations are those for peripheral venous or capillary blood. However, the need for repeated blood sampling and the relatively high cost of the measurements of blood lactate concentration detract from the usefulness of the method. The ventilation or anaerobic thresholds, based respectively on Owles' point and Wasserman's point (page 427), can be used to estimate the maximal oxygen uptake but in many laboratories the thresholds have a poor reproducibility. A related index is the oxygen uptake at a respiratory exchange rate of unity ($\dot{n}o_2$ at $RER_{1.0}$). This is obtained during assessment of the cardiorespiratory response to exercise for which it is an appropriate end point. The index has been reported as providing an accurate prediction; this can be further improved upon by also including the cardiac frequency at an oxygen uptake of $45\,mmol\,min^{-1}$ in the regression equation (Table 14.9).

To obtain the reference values the maximal oxygen uptake is estimated from variables which can be obtained at rest. The optimal combination of reference variables has still to be determined but a reasonably good estimate can be obtained using age, fat-free mass, gender and level of habitual activity estimated on a four point scale (Table 14.9). The inclusion of smoking habit improves the accuracy of the description but depending on the application the use of smoking as a reference variable may not be appropriate (page 446).

In patients with lung disease the indirect assessment of maximal oxygen uptake should take into account the likely cause of exercise limitation. Where exercise is limited by ventilatory capacity the maximal oxygen uptake can be estimated from the forced expiratory volume (or forced vital capacity) together with ventilation during submaximal exercise, age and fat-free mass (Table 14.9). However, most persons in this category exercise up to their symptom-limited maximum so indirect assessment is irrelevant. It becomes useful if other features suggest that the subject may have discontinued exercise prematurely for any reason. Indirect assessment can also be useful for determining the respiratory component of disability in patients with some respiratory impairment but in whom the capacity for exercise is limited by myocardial ischaemia or other non-respiratory cause. These aspects are considered below.

Reporting the maximal oxygen uptake

Maximal oxygen uptake is best reported in absolute units together with the reference value; the difference provides an indication of the physical condition of the subject and takes into account the age and fat-free mass. Ways of expressing the difference are considered on page 59. Alternative practices are to express the maximal oxygen uptake per kg of body mass and as a multiple of the resting energy expenditure (METS, see e.g. Fig. 14.4, page 424). The former is inappropriate because the relationship of maximal oxygen uptake to body mass or fat-free mass is not a proportional one; indeed, the oxygen uptake per unit of mass is negatively correlated with mass. The use of metabolic equivalents (METS) can be helpful when considering residual ability (page 438) but not exercise capacity since an insufficient allowance is made for body mass.

Simplified tests

Simple tests of exercise performance. A simple test of performance alone is quick and does not require sophisticated facilities. It can be used to confirm that exercise is, indeed, limited by shortness of breath, provide information on exercise capacity and, in conjunction with tests of lung function, can illuminate the causes of exercise limitation. The *12 minute walking test* of McGavin and colleagues is appropriate for subjects with material respiratory disability and is often a better way of monitoring the effects of treatment than repetition of the lung function tests. The subject is asked to walk as far as possible in 12 min. Continuous walking is desirable but the subject can slow down or stop if this proves to be necessary. The main feature is that at the end of the test the subject should feel that he could not have gone further. The test is commonly performed on a level track, usually a hospital corridor, but a steady incline is acceptable. The patient is accompanied by an attendant who provides encouragement and records the time and distance walked. There is a strong learning effect so the test should be performed twice on separate days; the distance walked on the second occasion is definitive. It is likely to be in the range 100–600 m with a coefficient of variation of approximately 4.2%. Alternatively a 6 min distance can be used. The test assesses endurance and the result is correlated with the symptom-limited maximal oxygen uptake, but usually not with the FEV_1.

In a multi-storey building the exercise performance can be assessed using the stairs. In this form the test is suitable for persons with moderate disability. Alternatively exercise of progressively increasing intensity can be performed using a cycle, treadmill or motorised step test. The end point is usually dictated by symptoms so the electro-cardiogram should be monitored during the test (see ergocardiography, page 423). A treadmill can also be used for the 12 min walking test (the speed of the treadmill is controlled by the subject) and for assessing suitability for portable oxygen therapy (page 623).

The *Harvard pack test* is used to assess physical fitness for very strenuous work. The test is based on the observation that the rate of recovery of cardiac frequency after exercise is faster in well trained than in untrained subjects (Fig. 13.10, page 410).

The test requires a stop-watch, a metronome and a box of height 50 cm (20 in) for men and 43 cm (17 in) for women. A pack weighing one-third of body weight may be worn on the back in which case hand grips are provided to assist the subject. The test is performed by the subject stepping on and off the box at a rate of 30 steps per min for 5 min unless obliged to stop sooner. Each step up should be completed by the subject standing erect through the full height of the step. The time of exercise is recorded. In the simplest form of the test, the pulse is counted at the wrist for a period of 30 s starting 1 min after the end of exercise. The physical fitness index (PFI) is:

$$PFI = \frac{\text{duration of exercise in seconds} \times 100}{5.5 \times \text{number of heart beats}} \qquad (14.6)$$

In subjects of average physical ability the index is in the range 80–50. Higher and lower values are found respectively in 'fit' and 'unfit' subjects. The test is influenced by the manner of stepping, the breathing pattern and the ambient temperature. It has been reviewed by Sloan.

Assessing disability and residual exercise ability

Introduction

In patients with respiratory impairment the residual exercise ability is

438

the starting point for rehabilitation (page 644) and for decisions about life style. Residual ability is related to but not synonymous with the capacity for exercise (maximal oxygen uptake). Residual ability varies with the type of exercise, and in respiratory patients is even less for tasks which involve the arms and the accessory muscles of respiration than for exercise with the legs compared with healthy subjects.

Respiratory disability is not yet defined in a standard way. Most countries follow the World Health Organization in defining it as the loss of exercise capacity resulting from loss of lung function, i.e. from respiratory impairment. This usage is followed in the present account. However, in the USA a reduction in exercise capacity is considered to be part of respiratory impairment. The term 'respiratory disability' is used to describe the social hardship which results from the impairment. This usage is based on, and reinforces, the assumption that loss of lung function and loss of exercise capacity are highly correlated. Unfortunately this is not the case. The commonly used lung function tests can at best describe 20% of the variance in maximal oxygen uptake leaving at least 80% unexplained. The confusion generated by the unwarranted assumption of a high correlation has recently been clarified following an intervention from the European Society for Clinical Respiratory Physiology (SEPCR, now European Respiratory Society, ERS).

Grades of respiratory impairment

Loss of lung function is best described quantitatively in terms of the actual function, the reference values and the confidence limits of each. However, the terms mild, moderate and severe impairment are widely used so it is helpful that they should be defined for the commonly used tests. This has been attempted by the American Thoracic Society (ATS) and the SEPCR. The two classifications are broadly similar but differ in their definition of the lower limit of normal and of their treatment of FEV_1/FVC (Table 14.10). Both classifications imply that there is a fixed relationship between losses of forced expiratory volume, forced vital capacity and transfer factor and the consequent reduction in exercise capacity. Since this is not the case the classification needs to be used with discretion.

Table 14.10 Categories of respiratory impairment of the European Society for Clinical Respiratory Physiology (now European Respiratory Society). The categories relate to FVC, FEV_1, $FEV_1\%$ and Tl

Impairment category	Criterion — with respect to reference value
None (normal)	Within 1.64 SD*
Slight	Not normal but > 60%
Moderate	In range 59–40% (50% for FVC)
Severe	<40% (<50% for FVC)

* The American Thoracic Society's criterion is > 80% and for FEV > 75%.
(Sources: De Coster A. *Bull Eur Physiopathol Respir* 1983; **19**: 1P–3P; ATS. *Am Rev Respir Dis* 1986; **133**: 1205–1209.)

Rating scale for respiratory disability

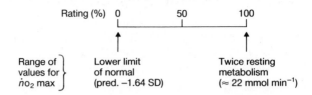

Fig. 14.7 Diagram indicating the derivation of the percentage disability. (Source: Cotes JE. *Eur Respir J* 1990; **3**: 1074–1077.)

Grades of disability

Disability is defined as reduction in exercise capacity. The starting point might therefore be the subject's performance before the onset of respiratory impairment with allowance made for the deterioration expected as a result of ageing. However, this information is not normally available. Instead the starting point is taken as the lower limit of normal which is 1.64 standard deviation units below the reference value. Disability is considered to be present when the exercise capacity is below this level. Thereafter it increases in severity up to a point where the person is considered to be 100% disabled. Using the SEPCR classification this point is reached when the subject is no longer able to double the resting energy expenditure, i.e. to reach an oxygen uptake of approximately 22 mmol min^{-1} (0.5 l min^{-1}). The percentage disability is expressed on a linear scale between zero which is the reference value minus 1.64 SD and 100% when the $\dot{n}o_2$ max is less than or equal to 22 mmol min^{-1} (Fig. 14.7). The percentages can be grouped into grades (Table 14.11). These are of the same form as those for respiratory impairment (Table 14.10) but it should be clearly understood that the two sets of grades are not interchangeable.

Assessing respiratory disability

Respiratory disability is present when a loss of exercise capacity is due to respiratory impairment, so the first step is the assessment of lung function. If the forced expiratory volume, vital capacity and transfer factor are within normal limits there is by definition no respiratory

Table 14.11 Grades of respiratory disability; distribution amongst 157 men who met the criteria for respiratory limitation of exercise

% Disability	Grade	Number
0	0 (none)	44
1–39	1 (slight)	59
40–59	2 (moderate)	40
60–100	3 (severe)	14

(Source: Cotes JE. *Eur Respir J* 1990; **3**: 1074–1077.)

disability. If one or more index is grossly impaired a rating of 100% disability is likely to be appropriate. In between these limits the assessment is made by having the subject perform a progressive exercise test up to the symptom-limited maximum and then interpreting the results. The procedure for the exercise test is described on page 425. The result can be used to place the subject into one of three categories; uncomplicated respiratory disability, exercise limitation which is clearly due to a non-respiratory cause, and ambiguous when more than one factor may be contributing.

Uncomplicated respiratory disability is present when the subject's exercise is limited by breathlessness, the exercise ventilation at the point of maximal breathlessness is the maximum which would be expected for the level of ventilatory capacity (i.e. the dyspnoeic index approaches 100%) (Fig. 14.8), the subject's pattern of breathing is appropriate for the lung function and the ventilation is not artificially increased by emotional or voluntary hyperventilation. The latter two criteria are met if the Vt_{30} is appropriate for the vital capacity and the respiratory exchange ratio is appropriate for the level of exercise (Table 14.9). In addition the maximal cardiac frequency should be below that expected for a healthy subject of similar age. The presence or absence of arterial desaturation on exercise is unimportant. Experience suggests that these criteria are met by approximately 20% of persons with respiratory impairment who attend for assessment.

Exercise limitation from a non-respiratory cause is relatively common. The cause may be cardiovascular (e.g. Table 14.6, page 425), musculo-skeletal, reduced erythropoiesis or other system disorder. The first and third of these conditions are often accompanied by hyperventilation and tachycardia. Alternatively, the limitation can be of the type observed in healthy subjects (Table 13.6, page 405). An ambiguous exercise

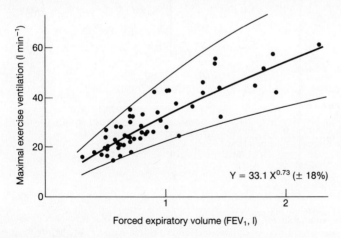

$$Y = 33.1 X^{0.73} (\pm 18\%)$$

Maximal exercise ventilation (l min^{-1})

Forced expiratory volume (FEV$_1$, l)

Fig. 14.8 Relationship of maximal exercise ventilation to forced expiratory volume for well-motivated patients with chronic lung disease. In patients not limited by breathlessness or in whom motivation is suspect the ventilation is often below the lower confidence limit. (Source: Cotes JE, Posner V, Reed JW. *Bull Eur Physiopathol Respir* 1982; **18**(Suppl. 4): 221–228.)

result is most likely to occur in a subject who is anxious; it can also be due to malingering but this is usually considered to be uncommon. The anxiety frequently arises from a mild respiratory disorder or other medical condition. It is usually accompanied by tachycardia which is present at rest and persists throughout the exercise. The tachycardia can also be evidence for the subject being unfit; in this event the increase in cardiac frequency relative to the expected value is more marked on exercise than at rest. Reference values for exercise cardiac frequency are given in Fig. 14.9. An anxious person often hyperventilates at rest; the hyperventilation usually decreases or disappears during submaximal exercise and may reappear when the exercise becomes

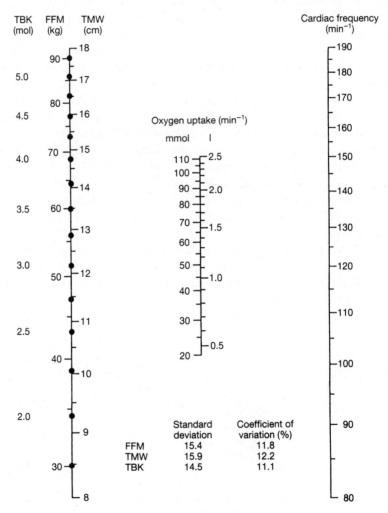

Fig. 14.9 Nomogram for deriving of the mean exercise cardiac frequency of young adults of both sexes from oxygen uptake and either fat-free mass (FFM, kg) or thigh muscles width (TMW, cm) or total body potassium (TBK, mol). The data are for cycling (ambient temperature 20°C); results for walking on a treadmill are similar (Table 14.3, page 422). To convert to other ambient temperatures a correction factor may be used (page 690). For children see Fig. 15.9, page 466 (Source: Cotes JE, Berry G, Burkinshaw L *et al. Q J Exp Physiol* 1973; **58**: 239–250, also Table 14.9, page 431.)

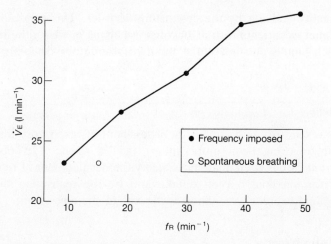

Fig. 14.10 Effect of a voluntary change in respiratory frequency upon the exercise ventilation of a healthy subject cycling at a constant rate of work. The respiratory exchange ratio and end tidal carbon dioxide tension were normal throughout.

strenuous. It is detected by its effect on respiratory exchange ratio which is increased relative to the reference value (e.g. Table 14.9). An increase in ventilation can also be due to tachypnoea without hyperventilation (i.e. fast, shallow breathing). In this event the respiratory exchange ratio is normal. An example of the effect of a change in respiratory frequency on the exercise ventilation of a healthy subject is given in Fig. 14.10.

Rating respiratory disability

In a subject who meets the criteria for uncomplicated respiratory disability, the percentage disability is given by:

$$\text{disability (\%)} = \frac{100[(\dot{n}\text{O}_2\text{max ref.} - 1.64 \text{ RSD}) - \dot{n}\text{O}_2\text{max obs}]}{[(\dot{n}\text{O}_2\text{max ref.} - 1.64 \text{ RSD}) - 22]} \quad (14.7)$$

where $\dot{n}\text{O}_2\text{max}$ and $\dot{n}\text{O}_2\text{max}$ ref. are the observed and expected maximal oxygen uptakes in mmol min^{-1} and 22 is twice the average resting oxygen uptake in the same units (cf. Fig. 14.7). The rating can be checked by using instead of the observed maximal oxygen uptake, the uptake calculated from FEV_1 and $\dot{V}_{E45}$ (see below). The two ratings should be similar. Persons with respiratory impairment usually present with breathlessness on exertion when the rating for respiratory disability is of the order of 30%.

When exercise is limited by a non-respiratory disorder any respiratory contribution to the disability cannot be assessed directly. However, it is possible to estimate from the lung function and ventilation during submaximal exercise (regression of maximal oxygen uptake on FEV_1 and $\dot{V}_{E45}$, Table 14.9) how seriously exercise might have been limited in the absence of that other disorder. The derivation assumes that the relevant variables are influenced only by the respiratory

443

abnormality and not by the co-existing disorder. This condition may not be met in patients with myocardial ischaemia in whom the indirect approach can overestimate the putative respiratory disability (page 605).

Comment

Unlike respiratory impairment the assessment of respiratory disability has for too long been more an art than a science. Its objective measurement has been made possible by the development of reference values for maximal oxygen uptake and by the realisation that the submaximal exercise ventilation is the key to the assessment.

Guide to references

The references (Chapter 18) are classified under subject headings of which the following are particularly relevant to the present chapter:

444

15: Lung Function Throughout Life: Determinants and Reference Values

Introduction

Determinants of normal function

Some of the tests of lung function are measurements of physical characteristics, such as volume or compliance, others are measures of performance. The results given by these tests are determined by the
volume of the lungs, the diameter of the airways, the profusion of
alveolar capillaries, the mobility of the lung, the chest wall and the
diaphragm, and the strengths of the respiratory muscles. These factors,
in turn, depend on the age and gender of the subject, his stature, body
mass and composition, his personal habits (such as smoking or athletic
pursuits), his genetic make up (including both racial and familial
characteristics) and the environment in which he lives and works. This
chapter considers these determinants and the ways in which they influence the lung function of normal subjects. Such results serve as reference
values with which the lung function of individuals can be compared.

Normality

Normal subjects are healthy people who have no respiratory symptoms,
e.g. they do not have a regular cough, phlegm production, wheeze or
undue breathlessness on exertion, and have no history of chest disease
in the past, or of acute chest illness in the last 6 weeks. Thus normality
is usually defined without reference to chest radiography or other
investigations, but in some studies subjects are not regarded as normal
unless their FEV_1 is more than 70% of the FVC.

Reference values

Reference values describe the lung function of healthy individuals in
terms of some features which influence it. The features are called

445

reference variables; they are usually age, stature, gender and ethnic group. In appropriate circumstances the level of habitual activity and the other determinants of function listed above can also be reference variables. Thus smoking can be a reference variable if the aim is to investigate the effect upon the lung of some factor other than smoking, for example, welding fumes or interstitial fibrosis. Smoking cannot be a reference variable when the aim is to assess the effects of smoking; the effects themselves are described on page 482.

In the context of reference values the *smoking history* is important because a number of interacting factors determine if a person is to start smoking and if and when smoking will be discontinued. On this account being an asymptomatic smoker or an asymptomatic non-smoker is the outcome of a complex selection process which is not independent of the lung function. The process can lead to bias in the *reference population*. The difficulty can be partly overcome by including in the reference population all smokers and non-smokers who meet the criteria for respiratory health; ex-smokers are excluded. The *reference variables* then include a term for smoking (yes or no). This approach is recommended by the European Coal and Steel Community amongst others. The principal alternative, recommended by the American Thoracic Society, is to confine the reference population to lifetime non-smokers. This could lead to error if, as is sometimes the case, above average lung function is a selection feature leading to a person taking up smoking, or below average function is a reason for refraining from smoking. However, the error is likely to be small. Alternatively the reference values can be based on communities where smoking is socially unacceptable, for example the Mormons. However, this approach limits the range of reference variables with respect to genetic constitution and environmental exposure.

The reference population should ideally number several hundred persons; they should be distributed uniformally across the range of ages in adults and of stature in children. In addition the exposure to other possible reference variables, for example habitual activity, should be appropriate for the proposed application. Ideally the reference population should be a random sample drawn from a defined population. In practise the use of a non-random population such as all eligible hospital staff and visitors appears not to introduce significant bias.

Types of reference values

Reference values are *cross-sectional* when they describe the lung function of a group of individuals at one point in time, *longitudinal* when they describe changes with time and *internal* when they relate to individuals. The type should be appropriate for its purpose. Thus for the study of overall deviation from normal at one point in time cross-sectional reference values for non-smokers would be appropriate. The information so obtained could be used to select for a particular occupation or to determine the risk category for life or medical insurance.

It could also be used to demonstrate the effects of smoking. However, in a smoker, to assess possible lung damage due to a condition which is itself unrelated to smoking, the appropriate reference values should be those for asymptomatic smokers.

The effects of an illness or occupational exposure are best assessed by comparison with previous results for the same individual, but such internal reference values are seldom available. Alternatively changes over time in an individual can be compared with those observed longitudinally in an appropriate reference population. Thus there is a need for both cross-sectional and longitudinal reference values. They differ because the lung functions of individuals develop and decay at different rates. The long-term changes are influenced by personal factors and by environmental factors which differ between individuals, between localities and from one decade to another. Environmental changes with time cause the lung function to be influenced by the year of birth; this results in a cohort effect which has been studied by Quanjer and colleagues amongst others. In addition longitudinal reference values are influenced by life expectancy since impaired lung function is a marker of increased mortality from respiratory, cardiovascular and other disorders. Thus a cross-sectional population includes some high risk individuals who will not be able to take part in a longitudinal study. The need for longitudinal reference values is greatest for persons in occupations which carry an increased risk of lung disease. For such persons the population reference values should ideally be those for the cohort that is being assessed. They should be supplemented by internal reference values obtained prior to employment.

Quality control

Reference values should be obtained using methods which are technically reliable. To this end the apparatus should meet the relevant criteria for overall characteristics, response time and accuracy, the observer should have been trained, the circumstances of the test should minimise biological variation, the procedure and performance of the test including the intermediate results should be technically satisfactory and the results should be calculated in the recommended manner. These aspects of quality control are discussed in Chapter 3 and in relation to the individual tests; they are summarised in Chapter 4.

Newborn babies and young infants

Introduction

Healthy newborn babies have made the transition from placental to pulmonary gas exchange with all the attendant changes. Other babies experience difficulties on account of developmental disorders, prematurity, placental insufficiency, atelectasis or other factors. In this event the principal need is usually to monitor the arterial blood gases and to

447

correct any material departure from normal. Measurement of neonatal lung function has seldom had a high priority. However, information about the neonatal lung is increasing rapidly and is progressively leading to clinical applications. Recent work has been reviewed by the paediatric working group of the European Society for Clinical Respiratory Physiology (now the European Respiratory Society) in their report *Standarisation of Lung Function Tests in Paediatrics*. Additional technical information is contained in the *Manual of Infant Lung Function Testing* recently produced by members of the Respiratory and Anaesthetics Units of the Institute of Child Health in London.

Summary of neonatal respiratory physiology

The architecture of the lung, including the airways and the pulmonary arteries and veins, is completed during intra-uterine life. The process of development is assisted by respiratory movements which occur *in utero*. Oligohydramnios or other abnormalities can impair fetal breathing and cause congential pulmonary hypoplasia. If the abnormality occurs before the 16th week of gestation the number of airway generations can be reduced. At the 21st to 24th week of gestation the cuboidal cells of the distal airspaces are replaced by pavement epithelium. This change is usually accompanied by the appearance of surface active material which has the effect of lowering the surface tension at the air to tissue interface in the manner described on page 96. The lung is now capable of normal expansion and of supporting life. True alveoli first appear at about 28 weeks of gestation and continue to multiply for up to 4 years after birth. Thereafter increases in lung volume are achieved primarily by increases in alveolar size.

The haemoglobin dissociation curve for oxygen of the fetus is to the left of that in the adult (Fig. 9.3, page 280) and the haemoglobin concentration is somewhat higher. The positions of the curves reflect the respective concentrations of blood electrolytes and the structure of fetal haemoglobin which leads to it taking up less 2,3-diphosphoglycerate than is the case for adult haemoglobin (page 281); the evidence is reviewed by Bartels. The displacement of the curve facilitates the absorption by the fetus of oxygen from the maternal blood; the process is assisted by the passage of acid substances across the placenta in the reverse direction (Bohr effect, page 280).

Before birth the external respiration of the fetus takes place across the placenta. Here the transfer of oxygen has been shown by Gurtner to be facilitated by cytochrome P450 in the placental cells. The function of this substance is impaired by carbon monoxide from tobacco smoke and by barbiturates, diphenhydramine and some other drugs. At birth the fall in skin temperature augments the drive to breathing and contributes to the baby taking its first breath of air (page 352). It may also increase the blood levels of adrenaline and arginine vasopressin which promote the reabsorption of fluid from the lungs. The expansion of the lung reduces the pulmonary vascular resistance. At the same time the interruption of blood flow to the placenta raises the resistance in the systemic circulation. These changes create a pressure gradient between the left and right atria, which leads to closure of the foramen ovale. Concurrently the muscle of the ductus arteriosus contracts to occlude its lumen. This diverts the entire right ventricular output through the lung.

Following the onset of respiration the functional residual capacity becomes stabilised within a few breaths; thereafter the ventilation minute volume, the alveolar ventilation and the work of breathing are comparable to those in adults when allowance is made for the difference in metabolic rate. The functional residual capacity is smaller than expected and is associated with a relatively high frequency of breathing. The ventilation and the consumption of oxygen are functions of the weight of the infant. In addition the consumption varies with age, being relatively less on the day of birth than on subsequent days; it diminishes when the baby is hypoxaemic and it exhibits variations with the ambient and the deep body temperatures.

In normal circumstances the lung of the baby adapts rapidly and completely to the conditions of extra-uterine life. In the rare instances when it fails to do so, it is often because the baby has failed to develop sufficient surfactant. The deficiency causes the condition of respiratory distress in the newborn (page 522).

Assessment of lung function

Methods for assessing lung function in newborn babies and infants up to 2 years old were pioneered by Cross, Cook, Karlberg and others; these have recently been reviewed by a joint committee of the American Thoracic and European Respiratory Societies (p. 695). Between the ages of 2 and 5 years assessments are more difficult: thereafter the procedures developed for adults can usually be applied. In the neonatal laboratory the principal measurements are of the mechanical function of the lungs and thoracic cage including forced partial expiratory flow–volume curves. The transfer factor can be measured using a steady state method (page 300) but the index is of limited usefulness in this age group. The flow–volume techniques can also be applied in the paediatric departments of general hospitals for the assessment and management of airflow obstruction in babies.

Basic methods. The laboratory should be warm (23–25°C) and equipped with appropriately miniaturised apparatus which can be sterilised. The characteristics of the analysers should be adequate with respect to linearity, frequency response and stability (page 33).

The assessment procedures are applied during quiet non-REM sleep either natural, as after a feed, or induced by an appropriate sedative. These can influence the responses. The infant is studied in a supine position. Body temperature is monitored using a probe in the axilla. The infant's oxygen saturation can also be monitored by a probe

449

applied to the lateral border of the foot or to the ear lobe. Connection with the recording instruments is made via an oronasal mask. This should fit snugly and not leak at the line of contact with the face. The connection should be tested for leaks. The basic measurements are of pressure, volume and flow. Pleural pressure can be measured in the lower third of the oesophagus (page 160). However, gradients of pleural pressure often occur; these can be associated with paradoxical chest movements, rapid breathing ($f_R > 60\,min^{-1}$) or airflow obstruction. The reliability of the oesophageal pressure should be checked by comparing it with the pressure within a closed face mask over two or three breaths. The two should agree to within 10%. Tidal volume can be measured using a spirometer but is commonly obtained by integration of a flow signal from a pneumotachograph. Functional residual capacity is usually measured in a body plethysmograph (Fig. 15.1); it can also be obtained by the helium dilution method (cf. page 150). In either case the baby is breathing spontaneously and the flow rates are those during tidal breathing. However, maximal flows can be generated by external compression of the thorax; this is best done in a controlled way using an inflatable jacket connected to a pressure reservoir (Fig. 15.3, page 452). Maximal flows are not developed consistently during crying.

Lung and chest wall compliance. The stiffness of the lung is increased in respiratory distress syndrome so the measurement of lung compliance can contribute to the management of this condition. The measurement is made in one of three ways. The traditional method is that of Mead and Whittenberger which is applied during tidal breathing (page 171). The dynamic lung compliance is then the tidal volume divided by the difference in pleural pressure between the start and end of inspiration. The pleural pressure is measured via a catheter placed in the oesophagus and checked in the manner described above. Second, the measurement can be made during closed circuit spirometry. A weight is applied to the spirometer bell and the resulting increase in pressure within the circuit raises the resting respiratory level. The compliance is then the

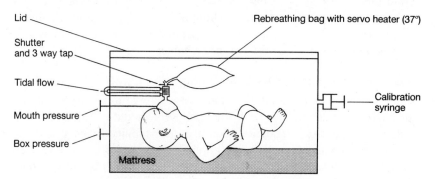

Fig. 15.1 Whole body plethysmograph for the measurement of lung volumes and airway resistance in babies. The method is described on page 156. (Source: Milner AD. *Arch Dis Child* 1990; **65**: 548–552.)

volume change divided by the mean increase in pressure within the circuit. Using a series of weights a volume pressure curve can be constructed. In young infants the compliance measured in this way is effectively that of the lung since the compliance of the thoracic cage is relatively high. The chest wall compliance decreases as the infant gets older and after the age of 6 months it makes a more significant contribution to the total respiratory compliance. Third, the compliance can be measured during multiple interruption of airflow (page 161). The method is suitable for infants due to their normally having a well-developed Hering−Breuer reflex; on this account the respiratory muscles relax when occlusion is made at a lung volume in excess of functional residual capacity. The linear part of the relationship of mouth pressure to lung volume is then the total respiratory compliance. Stocks and colleagues have validated the method for older infants using some 20 occlusions over the tidal range. However, in newborn babies the interruption, as well as initiating the Hering−Breuer reflex may cause adduction of the larynx. This prevents the attainment of pressure equilibrium within the thorax during occlusion unless the airway is held open by intubation of the trachea.

The occlusion technique can be extended by monitoring the passive expiratory flow−volume curve following the release of the occlusion. In the absence of muscular contraction the slope of the linear part of the curve is the time constant of the respiratory system; this is the product of total thoracic resistance and compliance (page 183). The compliance is measured so the resistance can be obtained by division. In practice the passive flow−volume curve which is obtained may not be linear and the resistance is best obtained in other ways.

Airway and chest wall resistance. Airflow limitation in babies can be assessed by measurement of airway resistance using whole body plethysmography (page 167). The pneumotachograph should be supplied with air at body temperature saturated with water vapour. The equipment is illustrated in Fig. 15.1. The result is expressed as specific airway conductance. The procedure has been described by Dezateux and colleagues from the Hospital for Sick Children at Great Ormond Street. It is technically demanding. The alternative of measuring total thoracic resistance by the forced oscillation technique (page 169) is more practicable. The method can be of use for serial observations; single observations cannot easily be interpreted as the results in healthy infants extend over a wide range.

Indices of forced expiratory flow. The techniques of external thoracic compression can be used to produce forced expiratory flow−volume curves (Fig. 15.2). The curves provide qualitative information on the site of any airflow limitation. A quantitative index is provided by the forced expiratory flow rate at FRC. The equipment comprises a pneumotachograph attached to an oronasal mask, an integrator, a compression jacket, a gas reservoir with pressure relief valve (range

451

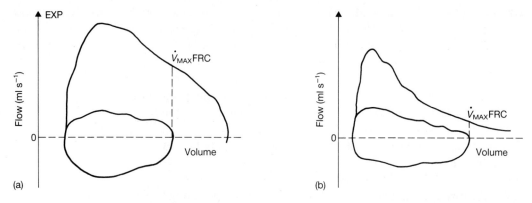

(a)

(b)

Fig. 15.2 Forced partial expiratory flow–volume curves superimposed on that for tidal breathing. (a) Result for a healthy infant. (b) Curve showing airflow limitation. (Source: Tepper RS, Morgan WJ, Cota K, Taussig LM. *J Pediat* 1986; **109**: 1040–1046.)

$0-5\,kPa$, $0-50\,cmH_2O$), and a three way tap with wide bore connections (Fig. 15.3). The tubing should be rigid to prevent kinking. The pneumotachograph should be linear over the range $0-30\,l\,min^{-1}$ (e.g. Fleish No. 1) and coupled both to an oscilloscope for monitoring tidal breathing and to a recorder. The jacket should cover the thorax and abdomen; when the airway is occluded at least 60% of the applied jacket pressure should be transmitted to the mouth. The inflation time should be less than $0.1\,s$. Pressure is applied by opening the tap at end inspiration during a period of regular breathing. The pressure is released when the lung volume has returned to the resting respiratory level. The initial inflation pressure is $1\,kPa$ and is increased in subsequent compressions up to $5\,kPa$. The maximal flow is usually obtained at a pressure of approximately $3.5\,kPa$. Ten readings are made at this pressure and the highest flow rate at FRC is reported.

Reference values. Information about the lung function of healthy neonates and infants is available from many laboratories but relates to

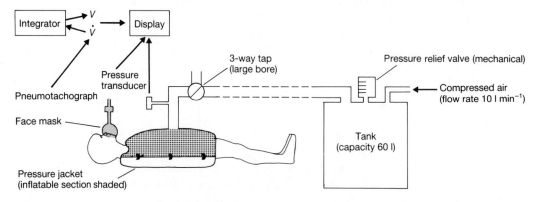

Fig. 15.3 Equipment for measuring partial expiratory flow–volume curves in infants. (Source: Beardsmore CS, Godfrey S, Silverman M. *Eur Respir J* 1989; **2**: Suppl. 4, 154S–159S.)

452

Table 15.1 Approximate values for some indices of lung function in newborn babies

Index		Body weight (kg)		
		2	3	4
$\dot{V}_E$	ml min^{-1}	450	550	650
f_R	min^{-1}		25−40	
V_t	ml	14	17	20
V_d	ml	7	9	10
$\dot{n}_{O_2}$	mmol min^{-1}	0.85	1.03	1.25
$(\dot{V}_{O_2})$	(ml min^{-1})	(19)	(23)	(28)
FRC	ml	58	87	116
Raw	kPa l^{-1} s (cmH$_2$O l^{-1} s)		4.0 (40)	
Pa,$_{O_2}$	kPa (mmHg)		9.0 (68)	
Pa,$_{CO_2}$	kPa (mmHg)		4.5 (34)	
$\dot{Q}$va/$\dot{Q}$t	%		20	
$\dot{Q}$s/$\dot{Q}$t	%		10	
$\dot{Q}$c	l min^{-1} kg^{-1}		0.15	
a-AD_{N_2}	kPa (mmHg)		0.8 (6.0)	

relatively few subjects; the methods have usually been to some extent unique to the laboratory and of variable technical quality so the present reference values are provisional. The principal reference variables are body mass and length or stature. The mass is usually obtained by difference from weighing the mother with and without her baby who should be in dry nappies; the measurement should be made before a feed. The length is measured in the supine position by two persons using an infant stadiometer. One observer positions and holds the head whilst the other positions the trunk and depresses the knees against the table. The stature is measured using the method described on page 54. Approximate reference values for newborn babies are given in Table 15.1.

For healthy infants the lung volumes and ventilatory capacity can be described by reference equations based on stature which are given in Table 15.2. After allowing for size the values are similar to those in older children. The main difference from other age groups is in indices

Table 15.2 Lung function in healthy infants and young children

	n	r^2	Source
FRC = 0.0052St$^{2.44}$	41	0.837	(a)
= 5.39St − 209.6	129	0.83	(b)
$\dot{V}$max, FRC			
= 0.0114St$^{2.47}$	25	0.93	(a)
= 9.67St − 399.8	148	0.51	(b)

FRC = functional residual capacity (ml); St = stature (cm); $\dot{V}$max FRC = maximal forced expiratory flow at FRC (ml s^{-1}).
(Sources: (a) Shulman DL, Bar-Yishay E, Beardsmore CS *et al. J Appl Physiol* 1987; **63**: 44−50; (b) Hanrahan JP, Tager IB, Castile RG *et al. Am Rev Respir Dis* 1990; **141**: 1127−1135.)

which reflect the calibre of the smaller lung airways which is relatively low and the compliance of the chest wall which is relatively increased.

Children aged 8–16 years

From about the age of 7 years children can perform most tests of lung function. Many data are available for school populations of children aged 8–16 years; there are fewer for random samples from whole populations and for adolescents older than 16 years. Most studies have been cross-sectional but longitudinal studies are more informative. Comparisons between studies have been hindered by the use of several different models to describe the relationship of lung size and function to body size. After allowing for size the lung volumes and volume-dependent indices in boys are in general superior to those in girls; indices of forced expiratory flow standardised for lung volume are superior in girls. Both within and between the sexes the lung function is greatly influenced by genetic factors; these have been investigated through study of twins. Other factors which influence the lung function of children are ethnic group, air pollution (including parental smoking), the level of habitual activity and for those exposed to it, a reduced ambient pressure associated with living at high altitude.

Cross-sectional models of lung function during growth

The rate of growth of the lung resembles that of stature in being maximal in infancy and having a secondary peak during adolescence. However, the onset of adolescence does not materially influence the relationship of lung function to overall body size; thus the coefficients of variation about the regression relationships for children aged 6–11 years are not appreciably smaller than those for children up to age 16 years. The wider age range is used in the present account.

The relationship of lung function to body size is best expressed in terms of stature; this is slightly more accurate than using sitting height (e.g. Table 15.6, page 460) and considerably more convenient (page 54). Sitting height has been used to investigate differences between the sexes and in relation to ethnic group and should be borne in mind for such circumstances. For most indices of lung function the relationship to stature is curvilinear (e.g. Fig. 15.4). The relationship can be made linear by subdividing it into segments which are effectively linear or by using an appropriate mathematical transformation (non-linear model). The use of subdivision has the disadvantage that the new relationships seldom match up at the points where they should join. In the proportional model the lung function is a proportion of stature raised to an appropriate power (i.e. $y = c.x^m$). The logarithm of the lung function index is then linearly related to the logarithm of stature (i.e. $\ln y = m.\ln x + c$). This relationship is widely used for describing the lung function of children. It can be extended to include the contributions of other variables, for example gender, ethnic group,

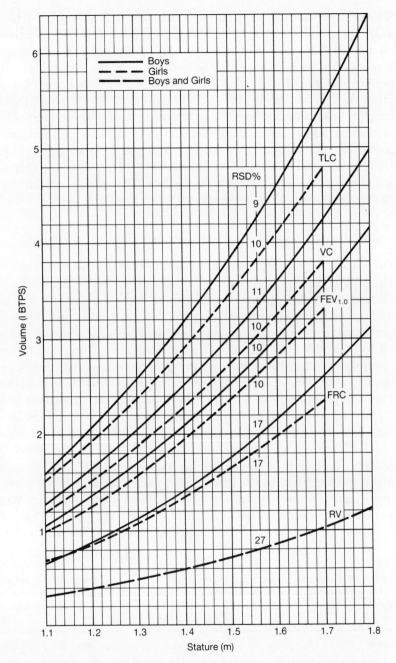

Children aged
8–16 years

Fig. 15.4 Relationship of total lung capacity (TLC), vital capacity and forced vital capacity (VC), forced expiratory volume (FEV$_1$), functional residual capacity (FRC) and residual volume (RV) to stature in healthy boys and girls of European descent (for additional information see Table 15.6).

fat-free mass/stature^2, percentage body fat and thoracic dimensions standardised for stature. The model has been used to show that indices of lung function which influence inspiratory capacity are both larger in boys than girls and influenced by the proportion of body muscle. The functional residual capacity and residual volume are inversely related to the proportion of body fat. The proportional model is sometimes referred to as the power relationship; it is used in the present account. Some of its properties are described on page 60. An alternative exponential model which has the form $y = a.e^{kx}$ has been used by Michaelson *et al.* and by Weng and Levison. Over the physiological range of heights the two models yield similar results. However, neither of them is adequate for describing the lung function of young men during late adolescence. For youths up to age 17 years a hyperbolic model of the form $(k + \text{stature})/(k - \text{stature})$ has been shown by Quanjer and colleagues to give a good fit to the data. Thereafter a model which includes age is likely to be required (Table 15.8, page 467).

Which reference values?

There have been many studies of lung function in children, some of which have included a wide range of tests; examples are the studies by Michaelson, Weng, Zapletal with their respective colleagues and the studies cited below. Some of the published reference equations have been condensed into summary equations by Polgar and Promadhat and by Polgar and Weng. The equations illustrate the relationships of lung function indices to stature. However, the several equations are not of equal quality. The equations are widely used, particularly in the USA. They are given in Table 15.3 and the values calculated for individual heights are listed in Table 15.4. Additional reference equations up to 1989 have been tabulated by Quanjer and colleagues in *Standardised Lung Function Tests in Paediatrics* (page 696). Thus the choice of reference equations is wide and laboratories should select those in which the methods and average values match their own experience (page 494). The present account relies mainly on the results for some 300 Cardiff children (Table 15.6 and Figs 15.6–15.9). This group has the advantages of having been studied in depth by standard methods

Table 15.3 Regression relationships for the prediction of lung function of boys and girls of European descent computed by Polgar and Promadhat from data in the literature. Stature is in metres and gas volumes in l BTPS. Numerical values at different statures are given in Table 15.4. c of v is coefficient of variation (page 64)

Index	Gender	Relationship	c of v (%)
Total lung capacity (l)	M	$1.226St^{2.67}$	11.6
	F	$1.153St^{2.73}$	
Vital capacity (l)	M	$0.963St^{2.67}$	13.0
	F	$0.909St^{2.72}$	
Functional residual capacity (l)	M	$0.496St^{2.92}$	18.0
	F	$0.538St^{2.74}$	
Residual volume (l)	M + F	$0.291St^{2.41}$	22.8
Forced expiratory volume ($FEV_{1.0}$ l)	M + F	$0.796St^{2.80}$	9.0

Table 15.4 Reference values for lung function of healthy boys and girls of European descent compiled by Polgar and Promadhat. Residual standard deviations (%) are in parentheses. The regression equations are given in Table 15.3

St		Boys			Boys + girls		Girls		
		TLC	VC	FRC	FEV$_1$	RV	TLC	VC	FRC
(m)	(in)	(11.6)	(13.0)	(18.0)	(9.0)	(22.8)	(11.6)	(13.0)	(18.0)
1.10	43.3	1.58	1.24	0.66	1.04	0.37	1.50	1.18	0.70
1.12	44.0	1.66	1.30	0.69	1.09	0.38	1.57	1.24	0.73
1.14	44.9	1.74	1.37	0.73	1.15	0.40	1.65	1.30	0.77
1.16	45.7	1.82	1.43	0.77	1.21	0.42	1.73	1.36	0.81
1.18	46.5	1.91	1.50	0.80	1.27	0.43	1.81	1.43	0.85
1.20	47.2	1.99	1.57	0.84	1.33	0.45	1.90	1.49	0.89
1.22	48.0	2.08	1.64	0.89	1.39	0.47	1.99	1.56	0.93
1.24	48.8	2.18	1.71	0.93	1.45	0.49	2.08	1.63	0.97
1.26	49.6	2.27	1.78	0.97	1.52	0.51	2.17	1.70	1.01
1.28	50.4	2.37	1.86	1.02	1.59	0.53	2.26	1.78	1.06
1.30	51.2	2.47	1.94	1.07	1.66	0.55	2.36	1.86	1.10
1.32	52.0	2.57	2.02	1.12	1.73	0.57	2.46	1.93	1.15
1.34	52.8	2.68	2.10	1.17	1.81	0.59	2.56	2.01	1.20
1.36	53.5	2.78	2.19	1.22	1.88	0.61	2.67	2.10	1.25
1.38	54.3	2.90	2.27	1.27	1.96	0.63	2.78	2.18	1.30
1.40	55.1	3.01	2.36	1.32	2.04	0.66	2.89	2.27	1.35
1.42	55.9	3.12	2.46	1.38	2.12	0.68	3.00	2.36	1.41
1.44	56.7	3.24	2.55	1.44	2.21	0.70	3.12	2.45	1.46
1.46	57.5	3.37	2.64	1.50	2.30	0.73	3.24	2.54	1.52
1.48	58.3	3.49	2.74	1.56	2.39	0.75	3.36	2.64	1.57
1.50	59.1	3.62	2.84	1.62	2.48	0.77	3.49	2.74	1.63
1.52	59.8	3.75	2.94	1.68	2.57	0.80	3.62	2.84	1.69
1.54	60.6	3.88	3.05	1.75	2.67	0.82	3.75	2.94	1.75
1.56	61.4	4.02	3.16	1.82	2.76	0.85	3.88	3.05	1.82
1.58	62.2	4.16	3.26	1.89	2.87	0.88	4.02	3.15	1.88
1.60	63.0	4.30	3.38	1.96	2.97	0.90	4.16	3.26	1.95
1.62	63.8	4.44	3.49	2.03	3.07	0.93	4.31	3.38	2.02
1.64	64.6	4.59	3.61	2.10	3.18	0.96	4.45	3.49	2.08
1.66	65.4	4.74	3.73	2.18	3.29	0.99	4.60	3.61	2.16
1.68	66.1	4.90	3.85	2.26	3.40	1.02	4.75	3.73	2.23
1.70	66.9	5.05	3.97	2.34	3.52	1.05	4.91	3.85	2.30

based on spirometry; the stature and body mass of the subjects were representative of UK children of the same ages and their lung function was on average very similar to that described in Polgar's summary equations.

A reference equation describes the overall relationship of a lung function test to the reference variables. When applied to a reference population the results for half the individuals will fall on or below the regression line and half above it. Thus the regression is the 50th percentile. The spread of results above and below the regression is given by the residual standard deviation (RSD) which for the power model is also the coefficient of variation (c of v). Five per cent of results are more than 1.64 RSD below the mean line; hence the mean minus 1.64 RSD is described as the 5th percentile. Other percentiles are given in Table 15.24 (page 512). For the proportional model the percentiles are constructed using the form:

$$\ln y(a) = (m \ln x + c) \pm Z_{a,\text{RSD}} \qquad (15.1)$$

where $y(a)$ is the value of y at the percentile 'a' and Z_a, RSD is the standardised deviate associated with that percentile (Table 15.24). An example is given in Fig. 15.5.

Longitudinal models. As a first approximation individual children who initially have small or large lungs relative to stature continue to do so; such differences are reflected in the percentiles about the reference equations. The percentiles constitute a simple longitudinal model. The lungs of young children tend to grow along their own percentiles which can be used to monitor progress and identify trends in response to treatment or from progression of disease. More complex longitudinal models are needed to describe the changes which occur during adolescence. Thus the use of percentiles is best confined to a limited age range (Fig. 15.5).

Reference values in children

Indices which are independent of body size. After allowing for body size the lung function of children is nearly independent of age; thus those indices which are independent of size can mostly be described by a mean value with its standard deviation. This is the case for the

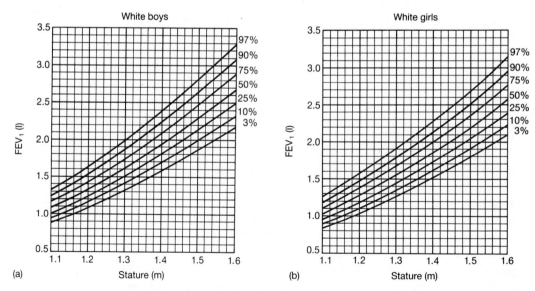

Fig. 15.5 Percentiles describing the development of forced expiratory volume in White children aged 6–11 years in six US cities. The charts can be used for Black children in this age group (stature 1.15–1.55 m) after multiplying their results by 1.13 (but see page 476). Similar charts are available for FVC. (Source: Dockery DW, Berkey CS, Ware JH *et al. Am Rev Respir Dis* 1983; **128**: 405–412.)

indices of uneven distribution of lung ventilation and perfusion, and for the tensions of oxygen and carbon dioxide in the arterial blood. It is also the case for ratios of volumes, for example the ratio of the residual volume or of the functional residual capacity to the total lung capacity and the ratio of the forced expiratory volume to the vital capacity. For the latter index the results using FEV_1 and $FEV_{0.75}$ are very similar (Table 15.5). The former is used routinely in adults and there is little advantage in using the shorter time interval for children. However, for those who wish to do so the conversion factor from the one to the other is given in the table. For some indices the effects of lung size can be eliminated by expressing the result per litre of lung volume: such indices are nearly constant throughout childhood. Thus as a first approximation the specific conductance, i.e. (airway resistance $\times$ lung volume)$^{-1}$, can be described by a single number as can, over most of its range, the specific compliance, i.e. compliance ÷ lung volume. The static recoil pressure, for example that at 90% of total lung capacity, is related to stature but the retraction coefficient, which is the maximal recoil pressure ÷ total lung capacity, is independent of it. The constancy of these indices throughout childhood is due to the airway conductance and the static compliance both increasing as the lung gets larger. These changes are illustrated in Fig. 15.8 (page 464).

Table 15.5 Lung function in healthy children: mean values and residual standard deviations (RSD) or coefficients of variation (C of V) for indices which are effectively independent of age and body size

	Mean values			Source
Lung volumes and ventilatory capacity				
$FEV_{0.75}\%$ ($FEV_{0.75}$/VC)	81♀	78♂	RSD 5	Cotes *et al.* (1973)
$FEV_1\%$ (FEV_1/VC)	88♀	84♂		Strang (1959)
$FEV_{0.75}\%/FEV_1$ (%)	93		RSD 2.7	Cotes *et al.* (1973)
RV% (RV/TLC)	24		RSD 2.4	Helliesen *et al.* (1958)
FRC% (FRC/TLC)	47		RSD 5	Cotes *et al.* (1973)
$MEF_{50\% VC}$/TLC (s^{-1})	0.95		RSD 0.15	
$MEF_{60\% TLC}$/TLC (s^{-1})	0.91		RSD 0.14	Zapletal, Motoyama *et al.* (1969)
PEF/TLC (s^{-1})	1.32		RSD 0.22	
Lung mechanics				
sGaw (*Gaw*/TGV) (s^{-1}kPa^{-1})	1.7		1.4−3.0	Zapletal, Motoyama *et al.* (1969)
(s^{-1}cmH$_2$O^{-1})	0.17		0.14−0.30	
sC (*Cst*/FRC) (kPa^{-1})	0.57		C of V ≈ 10%	Cook *et al.* (1958)
(cmH$_2$O^{-1})	0.057		C of V ≈ 10%	
Indices of gas distribution				
Vd/Vt (rest) (%)	26		RSD 7	Beaudry *et al.* (1967)
Lung clearance index	7.8		RSD 0.9	Kjellman (1969)

Indices of gas exchange (boys & girls)	(kPa)	(mmHg)	
P_{A,O_2}	14.0, RSD 0.2	104.9, RSD 1.7	
P_{a,O_2}	12.7, RSD 0.5	95.5, RSD 3.7	Levison *et al.* (1970)
A-aD_{O_2}	1.3, RSD 0.6	9.4, RSD 4.8	
P_{a,CO_2}	4.9, RSD 0.2	37.1, RSD 1.6	
pH	7.39	RSD 0.01	

Lung function indices which vary with body size. The individual regression equations which best describe the lung volumes and ventilatory capacity of healthy boys and girls are given in Table 15.6. Here the equations are in terms of both stature and sitting height; the former are likely to be the more useful (see models of lung function above). Virtually identical results can be obtained by using a common power for stature (stature$^{2.68}$) with appropriate coefficients, or by using common equations for boys and girls with a percentage adjustment for the boy−girl difference. The extent of the difference is indicated in Table 15.6. For some of the indices slightly greater precision can be secured by also including in the equations fat-free mass standardised for stature (FFM/St^2) or percentage body fat (see models of lung function above).

Table 15.6 Reference equations for lung function in healthy boys and girls of European descent. Stature (St) and sitting height (SH) are in metres. Gas volumes are in l BTPS

Index	Gender	Stature* Relationship	Diff (%)†	RSD%	Sitting height Relationship	RSD%
TLC (l)	M	$1.227St^{2.80}$	9	9	$7.242 \times SH^{2.90}$	11
	F	$1.189St^{2.64}$		10	$6.554 \times SH^{2.90}$	
VC and FVC (l)	M	$1.004St^{2.72}$	10	11	$5.641 \times SH^{2.80}$	11
	F	$0.946St^{2.61}$		10	$5.053 \times SH^{2.80}$	
IC (l)	M	$0.720St^{2.55}$	11	15	$3.363 \times SH^{2.62}$	15
	F	$0.657St^{2.47}$		14	$3.190 \times SH^{2.62}$	
ERV (l)	M	$0.264St^{3.37}$	6	24	$2.054 \times SH^{3.28}$	24
	F	$0.283St^{2.90}$		19	$1.916 \times SH^{3.28}$	
FRC (l)	M	$0.500St^{3.12}$	4	17	$3.597 \times SH^{3.20}$	19
	F	$0.528St^{2.81}$		17	$3.387 \times SH^{3.20}$	
RV (l)	M + F	$0.237St^{2.77}$	—	27	$1.448 \times SH^{3.12}$	31
FEV$_{(0.75)}$ (l)	M	$0.780St^{2.67}$	5	11	$4.437 \times SH^{2.88}$	12
	F	$0.744St^{2.66}$		11	$4.137 \times SH^{2.88}$	
FEV$_{(1)}$ (l)‖	M	$0.812St^{2.77}$	6	10	$4.807 \times SH^{2.93}$	12
	F	$0.788St^{2.73}$		10	$4.527 \times SH^{2.93}$	
PEF (l s^{-1})	M + F	$7.59St - 5.53$	—	13	$15.94 \times SH - 6.87$	13
*T*l (SI)‡	M	$2.695St^{2.46}$	10	14	$12.55 \times SH^{2.49}$	14
	F	$2.536St^{2.33}$		13	$11.24 \times SH^{2.49}$	
*D*m (SI)‡§	M	$5.161St^{2.07}$	12	21	$20.29 \times SH^{2.37}$	23
	F	$4.023St^{2.41}$		21	$17.81 \times SH^{2.37}$	
*V*c (l)	M	$0.0177St^{2.91}$	7	22	$0.100 \times SH^{2.69}$	24
	F	$0.0199St^{2.40}$		24	$0.093 \times SH^{2.69}$	
*K*co (SI)‡ (*T*l/*V*A)	M + F	$2.359St^{-0.4}$	—	12	$1.751 \times SH^{-0.53}$	12

* These relationships are illustrated in Figs 15.4, 15.6 and 15.7.
† Boy−girl difference (%).
‡ mmol min^{-1} kPa^{-1} and (in the case of *T*l/*V*A) l^{-1}; to convert to ml min^{-1} mm Hg^{-1} multiply by 2.99.
§ The values for *D*m are influenced by assumptions made about the reaction rate θ (page 317).
(Source: Cotes JE, Dabbs JM, Hall AM *et al. Thorax* 1973; **28**: 709−715 and *Ann Hum Biol* 1979; **6**: 307−314.)
‖ Measured without backward extrapolation; if this practice is adopted add 2.5% (page 138).

However, at best the effect of the additional terms is to reduce the standard deviation by about one-tenth of the value given in the table; this order of improvement is unlikely to justify the additional complexity except in special circumstances. The equations based on stature are illustrated in Figs 15.4, 15.6, 15.7 and 15.8.

The slopes of the relationships of lung function to stature are positive except in the case of K_{co} which diminishes with increasing body size. The decrease does not extend to the ratio of diffusing capacity of the alveolar capillary membrane to the volume of blood in the alveolar capillaries (Dm/Vc ratio); instead the ratio during childhood is the same as in adult life. This suggests that the reduction in the K_{co} which occurs during childhood could reflect an expansion of the interstices between the alveolar capillaries rather than a change in the dimensions of the capillaries themselves.

Relationships which describe some indices of forced expiratory flow, lung mechanics and closing volume are given in Table 15.7. Some of these relationships are illustrated in Figs 15.6 and 15.8. The peak expiratory flows for very young children (stature $<$ 1.1 m, Fig. 15.6) were obtained by voluntary effort after a full inspiration; they were higher than those obtained by the external compression method at functional residual capacity during sleep (Table 15.2). Additional relationships are given in *Standardisation of Lung Function Tests in Paediatrics*.

Physiological response to exercise. Due to differences in body size, the tidal volume and stroke volume of children are smaller than those of adults. Thus to achieve the same ventilation or cardiac output the respiratory or cardiac frequency must be greater. The difference from adults is most marked in small children and diminishes with growth. However, the tidal volume bears the same relationship to vital capacity as in adults (Table 14.9, page 431) and this also appears to be the case for the relationship of cardiac frequency to indices of body muscle (Figs 15.9 and 14.9, page 442).

The relationship of cardiac output to uptake of oxygen (Table 14.9) is similar in children and adults and across the sexes. However, the stroke volume is in general larger in boys than girls and the cardiac frequency is lower. The differences persist after standardising for body muscle (Fig. 15.9). The intrinsic and environmental components of the difference in cardiac frequency have been investigated by Kagaminori and colleagues amongst others.

The maximal cardiac frequency in children is similar to that in young adults. The relationship of alveolar ventilation to uptake of oxygen in children is also similar to that in adults. However, due to the higher respiratory frequency the deadspace ventilation and hence the minute volume relative to uptake of oxygen are somewhat greater. The physiological deadspace has been described by Godfrey and Davies:

$$Vd = 1.54 \, BM + 0.049 \, Vt + 2 \, (RSD \, 22 \, ml) \qquad (15.2)$$

461

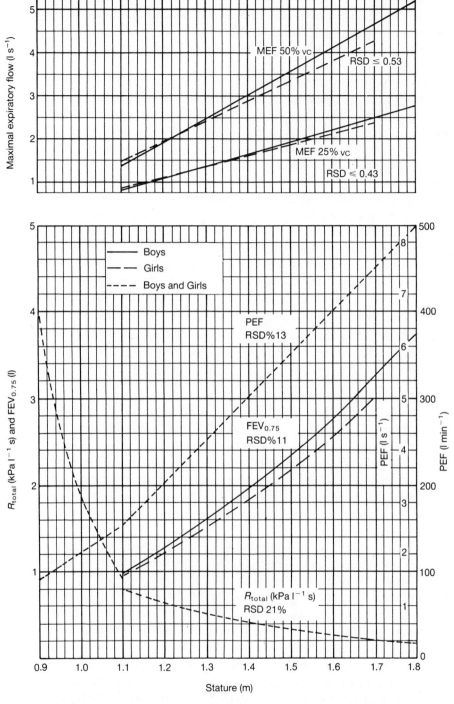

Fig. 15.6 Maximal expiratory flow when 50% and 25% of vital capacity remain to be expired (MEF$_{50\% \text{ vc}}$ and MEF$_{25\% \text{ vc}}$, total thoracic resistance (Rtotal), peak expiratory flow (PEF) and forced expiratory volume (FEV$_{0.75}$) in healthy boys and girls of European descent (for sources see Tables 15.6 and 15.7).

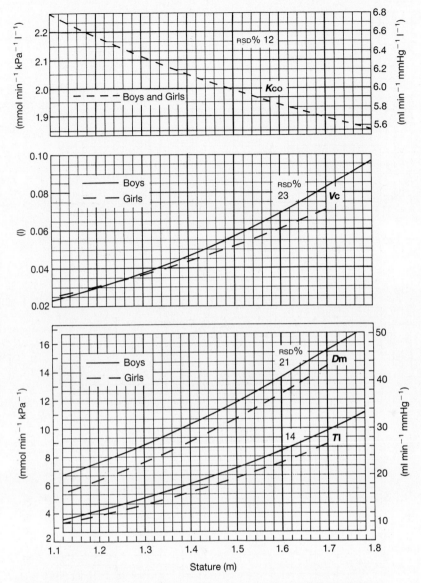

Fig. 15.7 Relationship of transfer factor (diffusing capacity) for the lung (*T*l), its subdivisions (*D*m and *V*c) and the diffusion constant (*K*co, i.e. *T*l/*V*A) to stature in healthy boys and girls (for source see Table 15.6). The values for *D*m are influenced by assumptions made about the reaction rate θ (page 317).

where *V*d and *V*t are physiological deadspace and tidal volume (ml) and BM is body mass (kg). The maximal tidal volume as a fraction of vital capacity has been found by Jones and Rebuck to resemble that of adults (Table 14.9). Thus the physiological response to exercise in children is a scaled down version of that in adults. However, the potential for physical training appears to be greater in children (page 472).

463

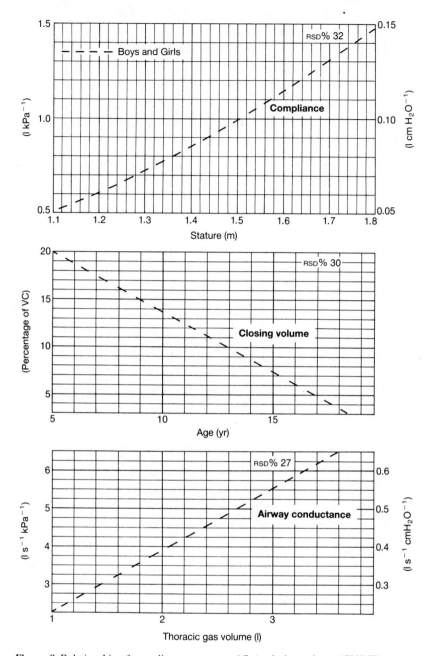

Fig. 15.8 Relationship of compliance to stature (*C*st), closing volume (CV/VE) to age, and airway conductance (Gaw) to thoracic gas volume in healthy boys and girls of European descent (for sources see Table 15.7).

Adolescence

Before puberty the function of the lungs is nearly identical in boys and girls of equal size though the vital capacity of boys is on average 8% larger than that of girls and indices which relate to vital capacity also differ by this amount. At puberty the rate of growth of stature increases

Table 15.7 Regression relationships describing aspects of lung function not included in Tables 15.3 or 15.6. Most are for boys and girls of stature > 1.1 m but those of Robinson are for infants (stature $0.9-1.1$ m). The abbreviations are explained in Table 2.2 (page 13). The units are as in Table 15.6

Index	Units	Relationship	RSD%	Fig.	Source
Cst	$1\,kPa^{-1}$*	$0.418St^{2.18}$	32	15.8	Helliesen *et al.* (1958)
Gaw	$1s^{-1}kPa^{-1}$*	$1.63TGV + 0.71$	27	15.8	Zapletal *et al.* (1972)
CV/VC	%	$26.12 - 1.25$ age	30	15.8	Mansell *et al.* (1972)
Rtotal	$kPa\,l^{-1}s$*	$7.39/antilog_{10}(0.89St)$	21	15.6	Mansell, Levison *et al.* (1972)
Rtotal (St $\leqslant 1.1$ m)	$kPa\,l^{-1}s$*	$1.81St^{-7.39}$	35	15.6	Robinson (unpubl.)
PEF (St $\leqslant 1.1$ m)	$1s^{-1}$	$4.93St - 2.9$	14	15.6	Robinson (unpubl.)
Pst 90% TLC	kPa	$2.04St - 0.0018St^2$	78.6	—	Zapletal *et al.* (1976)
MEF$_{50\%}$ VC					
M	$1s^{-1}$	$5.43St - 4.58$	0.47†	15.6	Zapletal *et al.* (1969)
F	$1s^{-1}$	$4.48St - 3.37$	0.49†	15.6	Zapletal *et al.* (1969)
MEF$_{25\%}$ VC					
M	$1s^{-1}$	$2.82St - 2.31$	0.40†	15.6	Zapletal *et al.* (1969)
F	$1s^{-1}$	$2.48St - 1.86$	0.40†	15.6	Zapletal *et al.* (1969)

* For conversion to traditional units see Table 2.5 (page 17).
† At stature 1.5 m.

and the lung grows concurrently. DeGroodt and others have shown that the growth affects the length more than the width of the thorax which becomes elongated in consequence. In girls the maximal rate of lung growth occurs at about age 11 years. Subsequently skeletal growth ceases due to fusion of epiphyses throughout the body. At almost the same time the growth of lung stops. Thus young women usually attain their adult lung size at approximately age 16 years. Thereafter in non-smokers the lung function usually remains nearly constant for at least a decade and then starts to decline. However, the vital capacity can decline earlier in young women who put on weight in their late teens.

In adolescent boys the maximal rate of growth of the lungs occurs at about age 13 years. Thereafter the growth in stature continues for 5 years on average. Longitudinal growth then ceases but lateral growth of the rib cage and clavicles continues up to about age 24 years. In addition respiratory muscle strength continues to increase (e.g. Fig. 5.4, page 91). These features lead to young men who do not

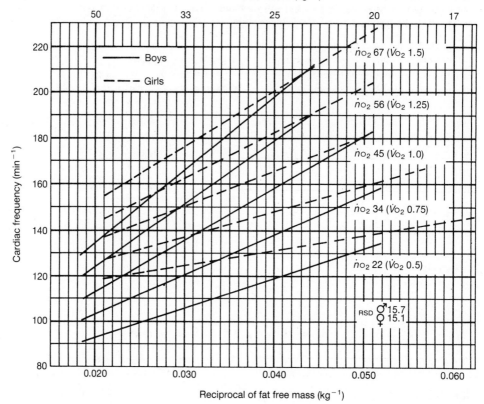

Fig. 15.9 Exercise cardiac frequency in relation to the reciprocal of fat-free mass for boys and girls ages 8–16 years at different levels of oxygen uptake ($\dot{n}o_2$ in mmol min^{-1}, $\dot{V}o_2$ in l min^{-1}). See also Fig. 14.9, page 442. (Source: Kagamimori S, Robson JM, Heywood C, Cotes JE. *Ann Hum Biol* 1984; **11**: 29–38.)

smoke attaining maximal lung function after skeletal growth has apparently ceased. On average the forced expiratory volume and transfer factor reach their peak at age 20–23 years, the forced vital capacity at about age 25 years and the peak expiratory flow at age 30, but with wide individual variations. Subsequently the lung function declines (page 485). In smokers the decline is brought forward by damage to the lungs from the cigarette fumes so the last phase of lung growth is curtailed.

The continued growth of the male lung after attainment of adult stature leads to a dissociation between lung volume and stature and probably also between lung volume and the calibre of extra-thoracic airways. Hence the relationship between lung function and stature in male children and teenagers underestimates the lung size in young adults. Several factors probably contribute to the difference of which some are given above. However, there is as yet no satisfactory model which can link the lung function of adolescent males with that in children and young adults (page 456). Instead the lung function of the

466

adolescent male is best described empirically. Some reference values for this age group are given in Table 15.8.

The third phase of lung growth which occurs in young men but not women is possibly atypical in that the increase in lung weight appears not to keep pace with the increase in lung volume (Fig. 15.10). This is consistent with the male lung being relatively more expanded than the female lung and with the observation of Pearce and colleagues that per

Table 15.8 Regression equations describing the lung function of 701 asymptomatic young men aged 16–25 years studied cross-sectionally

	Regression coefficients			
	Age (years)	Stature (m)	Constant	RSD
Forced expiratory volume (l)	—	5.03	−4.48	0.48
Forced vital capacity (l)	0.024	6.72	−6.96	0.51
$FEV_1\%$ (of FVC)	−0.61	−7.41	107.2	6.3
Peak expiratory flow ($1s^{-1}$)	0.044	7.90	−5.17	1.37
Total lung capacity (l)	0.098	8.83	−10.91	0.65
Inspiratory vital capacity (l)	0.060	6.90	−8.02	0.55
Residual volume (l)	0.032	1.96	−2.97	0.30
RV% (of TLC)	0.25	6.65	0.28	4.0
Transfer factor (SI)	0.13	12.7	−13.1	1.58
Kco (Tl/alv. volume)	−0.006*	−0.59	3.00	0.23

* In smokers; in non-smokers the term was not significant. Smoking did not affect the other indices.
(Source: Chinn DJ, Bridges N, Cotes JE. Unpublished.)

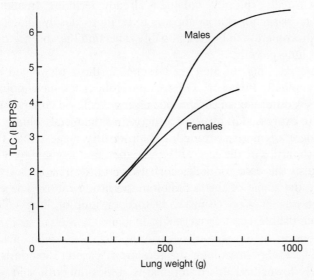

Fig. 15.10 Relationship of the total lung capacity to the lung weight in children and adolescents of both sexes. In females the relationship is relatively linear; in males at the time of puberty the increase in the weight of the lung fails to keep pace with the increase in lung size. The data are from the *Handbook of Respiration*; for lung weight and lung volume in males and females they were obtained respectively by Scammon and by Robinson and Morse.

litre of lung volume the adult male lung contains less collagen. The difference may have implications for the ageing of the lung (page 488). The consequences for lung function are considered below.

Young adults

Differences in lung function between men and women

Differences between the sexes in the size of the lungs relative to stature appear during childhood and enlarge during adolescence. In young adults the average difference was found by Amrein and his colleagues to be approximately 900 ml for the vital capacity and approximately 460 ml for the functional residual capacity. However, the magnitude of the difference appears to vary with the respective levels of habitual activity of members of the two sexes and is probably in part culturally determined. The residual volume of young adults after standardising for body size, is nearly identical in each sex.

The greater size of the lungs of young men compared with young women appears to extend to all its component parts, including the airsacs, the alveoli and the air passages from respiratory bronchioles to trachea; the airway resistance of men is somewhat less in consequence. This factor combines with the greater muscle strength and the larger vital capacity of men to give them the larger ventilatory capacity. However, the proportion of the forced vital capacity (FVC) which can be expired in 1 s is less for men than for women; this is partly due to the FVC in men but not in women, continuing to enlarge at a time when the forced expiratory volume is already declining. In addition the tracheal cross-sectional area appears to be more closely related to lung volume in women than in men possibly reflecting the absence of a third phase in lung growth.

Because the lungs of men are larger than those of women they are more compliant; however, Gibson and colleagues have pointed out that the sex difference in compliance disappears if the volume−pressure curves are expressed in terms of a theoretical maximal volume which is independent of muscle strength. Their results suggest that the bulk elastic properties of the lungs of young men and women are identical. This is also the case for indices of the intrinsic function of the lung including the range of the ventilation−perfusion ratios. The evidence on the levels of Kco (transfer factor per unit of lung volume) is conflicting (Table 15.21, page 509).

The tension of oxygen in the arterial blood is similar in men and women; however, in women the tension of carbon dioxide is usually marginally lower and this difference is associated with a lower value for the constant term B of the ventilatory response to breathing carbon dioxide (page 346). The further change in this index during pregnancy is discussed below. The ventilation during moderate exercise when standardised for the consumption of oxygen is slightly greater in women than in men; this is because a smaller tidal volume and greater frequency of breathing wastes more of the ventilation in the deadspace. In addition because women are less muscular they have a smaller cardiac stroke volume than is the case for men; the difference largely disappears when fat-free mass is used as the reference variable (Fig. 14.9, page 442). But in absolute terms women have a lower maximal cardiac output and utilise rapid glycolysis as a source of energy at lower levels of oxygen uptake. Their ventilation is then further increased relative to that of men for the reasons which are discussed on page 356.

With advancing years, the lungs of men deteriorate to a greater extent than those of women, so the initial male superiority diminishes. The deterioration is accentuated by exposure to tobacco smoke and other atmospheric pollution which is usually greater in men than women. However, it occurs in the absence of these factors so is primarily biological in origin. The changes with age are considered on page 487.

Menstrual cycle and pregnancy

In adult women the *luteal phase of the menstrual cycle* is accompanied by increases in basal metabolism and body temperature. The rise in body temperature is on average approximately 0.5°C and is associated with comparable increases in the temperature thresholds for cutaneous vasodilatation, shivering and chest sweating. The consequent redistribution of blood volume leads to an increased quantity in the lung capillaries and hence to a rise in the transfer factor. The thermoregulatory changes are at least partly due to the production of progesterone from the corpus luteum. The progesterone stimulates breathing, lowers the arterial tension of carbon dioxide, increases the ventilatory sensitivities to hypoxia and hypercapnia and raises the ventilation during exercise. Breathlessness during exercise is increased and the maximal oxygen uptake is usually reduced in consequence. The changes are accompanied by an increase in inspiratory muscle endurance.

Women with asthma may experience exacerbation of their symptoms in the premenstrual period. The additional symptoms are sometimes accompanied by a reduction in peak expiratory flow. No change in forced expiratory volume has been reported and the airway reactivity to histamine and to acetylcholine is not increased. The mechanism is unclear.

Pregnancy enhances the ventilatory changes which occur during the luteal phase of the menstrual cycle described above. The changes are due to the increased blood level of progesterone supplemented by an increase in metabolic rate. The hyperventilation increases progressively throughout pregnancy and causes a nearly linear decline in the tension of carbon dioxide in the arterial blood. The tension is on average 4.5 kPa (35.5 mmHg) at the 8th week and 3.7 kPa (28 mmHg) at term but with wide individual variations. Breathlessness varies proportionately.

The cardiac output is increased to supply the pregnant uterus. The increase has been reported by Sady and colleagues to be approximately $2.5 \, l \, min^{-1}$ at the 28th week of gestation independent of the level of activity. The increase is effected by rises in both cardiac frequency and stroke volume. The adaptations are usually adequate for normal activity but to the extent that they are incomplete there may be insufficient blood flow to the active muscles. The muscle metabolism is then sustained by rapid glycolysis and the associated lactacidaemia can contribute to fatigue, hyperventilation and breathlessness (page 356).

The airway resistance is reduced during pregnancy and this change together with elevation of the diaphragm reduces the residual volume and expiratory reserve volume and hence the functional residual capacity. The inspiratory capacity increases possibly due to an increase in the excursion of the ribs. The total lung capacity, ventilatory capacity and closing volume are usually unaffected by pregnancy.

Cyclical variation in lung function

The function of the lung exhibits seasonal and diurnal variations about a mean which itself changes with age; in women additional changes occur in phase with the menstrual cycle. The variations have a complex origin and whilst they relate to the pattern of sleep, posture, meals, ambient temperature, and, in females the levels of hormone production, other factors, including the hours of daylight, may also be involved.

Normal sleep, but not rapid eye movement sleep (REM sleep), reduces the central drive to respiration; the accompanying reduction in alveolar ventilation raises the tension of carbon dioxide and reduces the tension of oxygen in the arterial blood (page 350). Earlier reports of diurnal change in the control of respiration in awake subjects have not been confirmed.

The posture of the subject influences the position of the diaphragm and hence functional residual capacity (page 104). The axis of the thorax with respect to gravity affects the volume and the distribution of blood in the alveolar capillaries (page 187). The distribution of blood also varies in relation to meals and with the ambient temperature. The ingestion of food and a rise in the skin temperature are associated with diversion of blood to the organs concerned and a reduction in the volume of blood in the alveolar capillaries; the transfer factor (diffusing capacity) for the lung is then reduced (page 294).

The ambient temperature contributes to the regulation of respiration and the inhalation of cold air causes bronchoconstriction in subjects with reactive airways. These and other factors interact with cyclical changes in blood cortisol and adrenaline levels to cause diurnal variations in lung function (Fig. 16.5, page 548). The airway resistance is higher by night than by day and causes lower values for the forced expiratory volume, a larger functional residual capacity and less uniform distribution of inspired gas. Differences between the morning and the afternoon have also been demonstrated by McDermott and her colleagues for the airway resistance (mean fall 2.5% per hour) and by Cinkotai and Thomson for the transfer factor (mean fall 1.2% per hour); these findings have been confirmed by others. They lead to subjects with airflow limitation often experiencing symptoms at night and to their exhibiting enhanced circadian variation in peak expiratory flow (Fig. 16.8, page 556).

Seasonal variation has been observed by McKerrow and others. The forced expiratory volume exhibits cyclical variations with an amplitude in healthy subjects of about 0.1 l. The values are correlated with the hours of daylight which, in the northern hemisphere, are minimal in mid-December and maximal in mid-June. Converse changes have been demonstrated by Spodnik and others for the airway resistance which is highest in January.

The effects upon the measurements of lung function of sleep, the ingestion of food and other cyclical factors can be avoided by adopting standard conditions for the tests. In particular the measurement of transfer factor and the cardiorespiratory responses to exercise should not be attempted after a main meal and a period of at least 1 h should be allowed to elapse after a light one. In addition, any differences which are observed between measurements made when the subject is awake and during sleep, between night and day and, for the airway resistance and transfer factor, between the morning and the afternoon, should be interpreted with care. These factors are of particular importance when comparing subjects before and after exposure to pollutants or drugs. Comparisons should always be done at the same time of day and in the same season of the year. In other respects, the occurrence of cyclical variations is of interest rather than of practical importance and need not interfere with the assessment of pulmonary function in the laboratory.

High altitude

Ascent to altitude or to simulated altitude in a decompression chamber is associated with a reduction in barometric pressure; this causes hypoxia by lowering the inspired oxygen pressure. The hypobaria also lowers the density and kinematic viscosity of the respired gas; the effects on ventilatory capacity are described on page 124 and some long-term effects on page 617. Permanent residents at high altitudes in excess of 3000 m (10 000 ft) usually have larger lungs than dwellers of comparable stature at lower altitudes. The change appears to be a consequence of hypoxaemia during childhood influencing the growth of the lung since a similar change occurs in experimental animals; however, most animal studies relate to simulated altitudes of the order of 5500 m (18 000 ft) so are not strictly comparable. The increase in size of the lung, when it occurs, does so during adolescence and some evidence suggests that it may reflect interaction between hypoxaemia and another factor which could be genetic but is possibly a high level of habitual activity. The interaction could explain the relatively large lungs of the Quecha Indians of Peru and the mountain people of the Himalayas including the Bods of Ladak in Kashmir, the high altitude natives of Nepal and the inhabitants of the Lumana region of Bhutan.

Residents at the intermediate altitude of approximately 1800 m (6000 ft) can also have relatively large lungs. This is the case for the highlanders of New Guinea and people who live in the foothills of the Himalayas. However, similar changes have not been seen in Denver, Colorado or in the high Veldt of the Transvaal in South Africa, so the mechanism is uncertain. It could reflect the relatively higher level of habitual activity during childhood of the former subjects or be a consequence of warfare in previous generations leading to the selective elimination of subjects with small ventilatory capacities. Further comparative studies are needed to illuminate these aspects. The mountain dwellers also have an increased potential for gas exchange. This is reflected in an increased transfer factor for carbon monoxide (Table 15.9, below). The change is partly due to the hypoxaemia both increasing the reaction rate (θ) of carbon monoxide with haemoglobin and causing polycythaemia with its attendant rise in blood haemoglobin concentration (cf. equation 10.19, page 316). Structural changes associated with the increase in lung size can also contribute.

Thus if a period of time has been spent at high altitude, it should be taken into account when considering what are the appropriate reference values for lung function in an individual or group of subjects. The pathological effects of high altitude including pulmonary oedema and chronic mountain sickness are considered on page 617.

Physical activity and training

A high level of habitual activity is a feature of people living at high altitude and in hill country, many agriculturalists, nomads and those who participate in gymnastics, ball games, athletics and active outdoor recreations. These conditions can be subdivided into those where the high level of activity is mandatory from an early age, and where it is acquired during adolescence or in adult life. The former, in particular, is associated with an increase in the size of the lung and its capacity to transfer gas. The changes are partly due to the release of growth hormone which activates several insulin growth factors, including IGF-1 and 2, to stimulate tissue growth. A low level of habitual activity is a common feature of urban life, particularly for children living in tall buildings with lifts, amongst whom the vital capacity relative to stature is some 7% less than in children who are physically active. These effects of habitual activity should be taken into account when considering reference values for individuals and groups of subjects. The differences are well documented for athletes compared with non-athletes and for persons who have taken part in a training programme for one or more groups of muscles. However, equally large differences occur in other circumstances. Some examples are given in Tables 15.9 and 15.10. Some effects of physical training upon factors which underlie the capacity for exercise are given on page 408.

Table 15.9 Relation of lung function and the cardiorespiratory response to exercise to ethnic group and level of habitual activity in young women. The lung function has been standardised for age, stature and, in the case of Tl haemoglobin concentration (hence Tls,st). The exercise ventilation ($\dot{V}_{E45}$) has been standardised for oxygen uptake ($45\,mmol\,l^{-1}$, $1.0\,l\,min^{-1}$) and the cardiac frequency also for body muscle ($fc_{,45}$,st). The data suggest that the transfer factor is influenced by previous habitual activity and the exercise tidal volume standardised for vital capacity (Vt_{30},st) by ethnic group. The lung volume and probably the exercise ventilation are influenced by both factors

	Activity			
	High	Medium		Low
	New Guinea highlanders	New Guinea coastal people	UK housewives	Jamaican housewives
fc_{45},st (min^{-1})	122*	135	134	145*
Tls,st ($mmol\,min^{-1}\,kPa^{-1}$)†	11.0*	9.6	9.4	7.7*
Vt_{30},st (l)	1.07*	1.01*	1.34	1.11*
TLCst (l)	4.82	4.12*	4.97	4.22*
$\dot{V}_{E45}$ ($l\,min^{-1}$)	24.6*	27.6	26.9	29.5*

* Significant difference compared with UK housewives ($p < 0.05$).
† For conversion to traditional units see Table 2.5 (page 17).
(Source: Cotes JE, Anderson HR, Patrick JM. *Phil Trans R Soc B* 1974; **268**: 349–361.)

Table 15.10 Lung function and the response to exercise in 35 amateur racing cyclists compared with the average for healthy young men of the same age (22 years) and stature (1.75 m). All the differences are significant ($p < 0.05$)

	Observed	Expected
Forced expiratory volume (l) (FEV_1)	4.60	4.38
Inspiratory capacity (l)	3.75	3.40
Expiratory reserve volume (l)	2.08	1.83
Residual volume (l)	1.37	1.54
Transfer factor* ($mmol\,min^{-1}\,kPa^{-1}$)	13.4 (39.9)	12.3 (36.6)
Kco* ($mmol\,min^{-1}\,kPa^{-1}\,l^{-1}$)	2.01 (5.99)	1.83 (5.46)
Exercise cardiac frequency† (min^{-1})	109	122
Maximal O_2 uptake ($mmol\,min^{-1}$) ($l\,min^{-1}$)	196 (4.39)	158 (3.53)
Maximal exercise ventilation ($l\,min^{-1}$)	161	127

* Traditional units ($ml\,min^{-1}$ and $mmHg^{-1}$ are in parentheses).
† At consumption of oxygen $67\,mmol\,min^{-1}$ ($1.5\,l\,min^{-1}$).
(Source: as for Table 15.9.)

Athletes do not comprise a homogenous group. They include middle-distance runners who have long legs, often are lightly built and have high aerobic capacities, sprinters and weight lifters who have great muscle strength, also well-developed shoulder girdles, and long-distance swimmers who usually have a thick layer of subcutaneous fat. After age and stature have been taken into account, the findings on assessment of pulmonary function in individual athletes usually lie within the accepted normal range. However, for participants in middle-distance running, cycling or swimming events the transfer factor is often large in relation to stature. The vital capacity is often increased as well and in this event the Kco (transfer factor per unit of lung volume) can be relatively normal (cf. page 293).

Training of the muscles of the shoulder girdle increases the inspiratory capacity, and hence the total lung capacity, by increasing the strength of the accessory muscles of inspiration. This is a feature of oarsmen, weight lifters and participants in archery and other sports in which these muscles are employed. The change is not accompanied by a corresponding increase in the forced expiratory volume, so the $FEV_1\%$ (i.e. the proportion of the forced vital capacity which these subjects can expire in 1 s) tends to be relatively low. A similar pattern of lung function is observed in deep sea divers. The increase in vital capacity is then associated with a reduction in forced expiratory flow at small lung volumes ($MEF_{25\%}$ FVC, pages 124 and 700). Denison and colleagues have observed a comparable change in some athletes. The mechanism is unclear. In short- and middle-distance swimmers the increase in vital capacity due to muscle training is superimposed on that associated with a long trunk length which probably also confers a competitive advantage.

In divers, underwater swimmers and persons who undertake periods of breathing against a resistance, the ventilatory response to carbon dioxide is often reduced; the tolerance to carbon dioxide of such subjects can be said to be increased. The phenomenon appears to be an adaptation to an increase in the work of breathing. It also occurs with athletic training (cf. page 349). However, in the swimmers it may be due in part to their having a high proportion of body fat which can increase the work of breathing; other such subjects have a similar response. Thus the association could be an example of the process whereby individuals participate in events in which they have a natural advantage. For a similar reason, individuals with long legs take up middle-distance running, whilst forwards in a rugby football team are recruited from amongst those who are sturdily built. As well as affecting lung function physical activity and training influence the cardiorespiratory response to exercise and the exercise capacity. This aspect is considered on page 408.

Differences between ethnic groups

What is ethnic group?

Ethnic group is used to describe the subgroup of *Homo sapiens* to which a person belongs. The principal groups are listed in Table 15.11; they reflect differences in geographical origin, appearance and skin colour which presumably have a genetic basis. Other genetic features which have an ethnic connotation are known but they are uncommon (Table 15.12). In general the identified genetic differences between typical members of the several groups have proved to be smaller than those within the groups so the classification of ethnic groups has no clear genetic basis. The groups are subdivided by cultural differences which reflect the effects of geography, migration, emigration, wars,

Table 15.11 Principal ethnic groups

Table 15.11 Principal ethnic groups

Group	Origin	Other regions
Caucasian	Europe	World-wide (Whites)
Negroid	Africa	North America (Blacks)
Mongoloid	Asia	Eskimo, American Indians
Indian	India	Plantations world-wide
Aboriginal	Australia	—
Polynesian	Pacific islands	New Zealand
Hispanic	Central and South America	North America

Table 15.12 Examples of genetic abnormalities with ethnic affiliations

Abnormality	Condition	Affiliation
HbS formation	Sickle cell anaemia	Negroid people
HbA deficiency	β-Thalassaemia	East Mediterranean
Hbα chain abnormal	α-Thalassaemia	South-east Asia
G6PD deficiency	Haemolytic anaemia	Negroid people
Cystic fibrosis	Dysfunction of exocrine glands	North Europeans
Retrovirus HTLV-1	Spastic paraparesis	Afro-Caribbeans Japanese
HLA BW 46	Antigenic variant	Cantonese
HLA BW 42	Antigenic variant	Negroid people

Hb = haemoglobin; HLA = human leucocyte antigen; G6PD = glucose 6-phosphate dehydrogenase.
(Source: *Ethnic Factors in Health and Disease.* Cruickshank, Beevers, eds. London: Wright, 1989.)

and other influences; these have led to differences in diet, religion and life style which contribute to the ethnic identities.

Variables which can relate to ethnic group

Geographical location. Traditional ethnic groups have a strong geographical association in which some related environmental factors, especially the level of habitual activity, and the diet can contribute to the lung function. A high level of habitual activity stimulates the growth of the lungs during childhood and the associated increase in muscle strength enlarges the vital capacity. This factor can operate more for people living in temperate rather than tropical climates, but the effect is small. It is greater for high altitude populations but some of the increase is then due to hypoxia which provides an additional stimulus to lung growth (page 471).

Diet. The calorific value and protein content of the diet has in the past been linked to ethnic group. An inadequate diet has been the main cause of the generally short stature of the traditional Japanese, New Guineans and other people. The leg length has been affected more than trunk length but the deficiency has contributed to the relatively small size of their lungs. The change to a western style higher protein diet has led to a material increase in body size. There is evidence that it has also improved the size of the lungs relative to stature. Thus the extent of acculturation should be taken into account when considering the lung function of mongoloid people. It should also be considered for New Guineans, Polynesians and people from the Indian subcontinent who eat a traditional diet. Whether or not a western diet can bring the lung size of such people up to the Caucasian level is at present uncertain. It appears to have done so in the case of Chinese people living in Hong Kong and some others, but Buist and colleagues found lung volumes to be lower than those of Caucasians amongst ethnic Chinese born in the USA.

Ethnic variation in lung function

Total lung capacity. The principal difference in lung function between ethnic groups is in total lung capacity and indices dependent on it. The lung volumes of people of African descent are smaller than those of Caucasians and the difference persists after standardising for stature. The difference is independent of geographical location, culture and social status. It is, however, affected by cross-breeding. The work of Reed suggests that the Caucasian admixture in the average black urban American is now in excess of 22% and a similar trend is occurring in other countries. In the Caribbean the descendants of mixed marriages have been shown by Miller and colleagues to have lung volumes which are intermediate between those for genetically pure blacks and whites. Thus amongst negroid and Caucasian people there is at present an association between skin colour and lung size but this could be disrupted by further cross-breeding. This association is also apparent amongst people from the Indian subcontinent and is independent of their present domicile. People from south India have smaller lungs than those from northern India some of whose ancestors were Caucasians.

The picture in northern India is further complicated by a mongoloid component and this also contributes to ethnic differences in South East Asia and elsewhere. Mongoloid people have mainly been found to have lung volumes which are (relative to stature) intermediate between those of Caucasians on the one hand and negroes and south Indians on the other. These intermediate levels have been observed in many parts of the world; however, recent observations suggest that they may be at least partially determined by environmental factors.

Mechanism for ethnic variation. The ethnic factor affects principally the total lung capacity and indices which depend on lung volume. Smaller differences obtain for the forced expiratory flow rates and, in some studies, the transfer factor. In other studies the transfer factor has been found to be independent of ethnic group. The total lung capacity reflects the size of the thoracic cage, the strength of the inspiratory muscles and the compliance of the lungs and chest wall. The lung compliance appears to be independent of ethnic group and an ethnic factor in respiratory muscle strength would seem unlikely. The volume enclosed by the rib cage was shown by Paul to be smaller in East African negroes than in Caucasians; this was associated with the Africans having shorter bodies and longer legs than Caucasians. Thus expressing the total lung capacity in terms of sitting height instead of stature reduces the ethnic difference in lung volume between black and white people. However, Miller, Schwartz and others have found that it does not eliminate the difference. In addition the use of sitting height as a reference variable does not affect the ethnic difference between Caucasians and Indians in whom the average trunk/leg length ratio is similar. The trunk length of mongoloid people is increased and the leg length is shorter compared with Caucasians of comparable stature, so for comparison between these ethnic groups the use of sitting height as a reference variable increases the ethnic difference. Thus the anthropometric basis for ethnic variation in lung size cannot be explained in terms of a single body measurement. Instead a three-dimensional approach is needed. The topic is worth pursuing since expressed in terms of stature the ethnic variation in lung size is of the order of 30% (Fig. 15.11).

Pattern of breathing and respiratory control. During exercise, or the breathing of carbon dioxide in air, the size of the lung influences the pattern of breathing; subjects having a relatively small vital capacity use a relatively high respiratory frequency but small tidal volume to

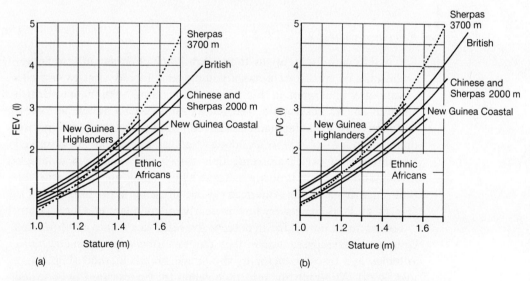

Fig. 15.11 Forced expiratory volume and forced vital capacity as a function of stature in boys of various ethnic groups studied in their traditional environments during the International Biological Programme. Values for girls are on average lower by approximately 10% (Table 15.6, page 460). The values for children of pure African descent (rural Jamaicans) can also be applied to children brought up in the ways traditional of the sub-continent of India. The relationships have been recalculated using where practicable a common exponent on stature; the resulting proportional differences between the groups are given overleaf. The sources are given in the references.

achieve a given minute volume. The effect can be expressed in terms of the tidal volume at a minute volume of $30 \, \text{l} \, \text{min}^{-1}$ (Vt_{30}); this is related to the vital capacity (Table 14.9, page 431). Ethnic variation in vital capacity affects the Vt_{30}. However, relative to the vital capacity the Vt_{30} exhibits ethnic variation; the tidal volume during progressive exercise or during rebreathing carbon dioxide in oxygen is less in non-Europeans (e.g. Table 15.9). Similar differences have been observed by Patrick, Reed and others for the ventilatory response to carbon dioxide. The implications of these observations for the physiological response to exercise and for clinical respiratory medicine have still to be worked out.

Response to exercise. Ethnic variation in the pattern of breathing during exercise is described above. The relationships of ventilation and cardiac frequency to uptake of oxygen appear to be independent of ethnic group except to the extent that this influences habitual activity and other environmental factors. The relationship of exercise cardiac frequency to fat-free mass (Fig. 14.9, page 442) is itself independent of ethnic group. Ethnic group likewise does not appear to affect the maximal oxygen uptake. However, anthropometric features which are associated with ethnic group can influence ability at particular events. For example, the relatively long limbs of the African confer an advantage in running and boxing. The large lungs of the Caucasian are of benefit during swimming (page 474). However, similar anthropometric variations also occur within ethnic groups.

Reference values

For children brought up in their traditional environments some relationships of forced expiratory volume and forced vital capacity to stature are illustrated in Fig. 15.11. Compared with native British children the values for negroid (rural Jamaican), Chinese and New Guinean coastal and highland children differed respectively by approximately -23%, -9%, -16% and 5%. Smaller differences are observed for children of mixed descent; thus for 'black' American children, amongst whom there is now a material white admixture (page 476), the difference from white Americans is, at present, approximately 13% (Fig.15.5). Peak expiratory flow is nearly independent of ethnic group.

For adults of pure African descent the reference values of Miller and colleagues are representative; they embrace dynamic spirometry, lung volumes and transfer factor by the single breath method (Figs 15.12 and 15.13). Alternatively, reference values for Caucasians can be scaled down by appropriate factors (Table 15.13). This approach was pioneered by Rossiter and Weill. However, in many studies the ethnic factor is independent of stature and nearly independent of age. In these circumstances the reference value for a non-Caucasian can be obtained by subtracting from the Caucasian value the mean ethnic difference for forced expiratory volume and vital capacity in negroes; this is given in

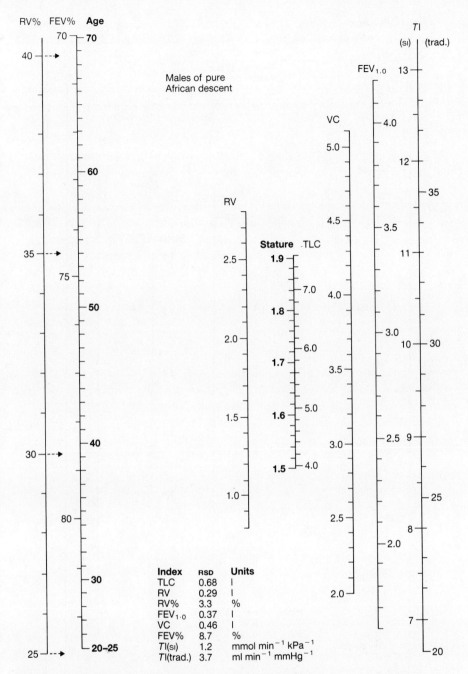

Fig. 15.12 Nomogram relating indices of lung function to stature and age for healthy adult males of African descent. The RV% and FEV% are related only to age and the TLC only to stature. (Source: Miller GJ, Cotes JE, Hall AM *et al. Q J Exp Physiol* 1972; **57**: 325–341.)

Table 15.13. For people in or from the Indian sub-continent the spread of reference values is wide (Table 15.14) so local values should be used where possible. Representative values for men from the north of the subcontinent including the Punjab and Pakistan are given in Fig. 15.14.

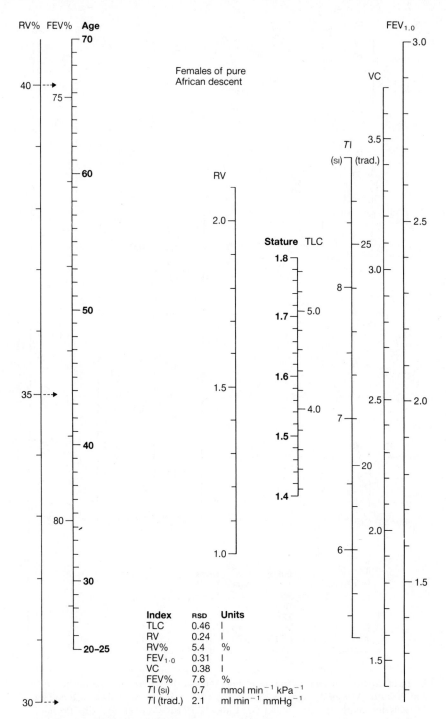

Fig. 15.13 Nomogram relating indices of lung function to stature and age for healthy adult females of African descent. The RV% and FEV% are related only to age and the TLC only to stature. (Source: as for Fig. 15.12.)

The corresponding levels in women mostly resemble those for south Indians (Fig. 15.15). However, with acculturation the situation is likely to change. Alternatively for south Indians and people from Bangladesh the values for Negroes can be used instead (Figs 15.12 and 15.13).

For mongoloid people reared on a westernised diet reference values for Europeans are unlikely to mislead, though local values should be used where possible. Reference values are also available for many pacific peoples including New Guineans and Maoris (see references). Those for Latin Americans resemble Europeans. This is also the case for many peoples living in the eastern and southern shores of the Mediterranean sea and in the Middle East. The extent of the deviation from values for Europeans reflects both the negro admixture which is higher in some countries than others, and the levels of habitual activity which have a large cultural component. In these circumstances the confidence limits are wide. It should be possible to improve the estimates by including both additional anthropometric indices and scores for habitual activity, and possibly other environmental factors.

Comment on further work. The compilation of local reference values is likely to continue. If possible, it should be broadly based on a range of

Table 15.13 Approximate conversion factors for adjusting European reference values for application to men of other ethnic groups. Factors for children are given in the text (page 478). For persons of mixed race the factor should be adjusted according to the ethnic origins of the grandparents

	FEV$_1$	FVC	Source
Orientals			
Hong Kong Chinese	×1.0*	×1.0*	Lam *et al.* (1982)
Japanese Americans	×0.89	—	Marcus *et al.* (1988)
Polynesians	×0.9	×0.9	de Hamel, Welford (1983)
N. Indians and Pakistanis	×0.9	×0.9	Malik *et al.* (1972)
S. Indians, as for Negroes			Kamet *et al.* (1982)
Blacks (USA)	×0.87*†	×0.87*†	Rossiter, Weill (1974)
			Dockery *et al.* (1985)
Negroes	−0.45‡	−0.70‡	Cotes (1979)

* Factor can also be used for women.
† Also for TLC. Other factors were for RV% and *K*co 1.05 and for *T*l 0.93.
‡ The corresponding factors for women are 0.4 and 0.61.

Table 15.14 Mean ventilatory capacity at age 35 years and height 1.65 m for men from different parts of the Indian subcontinent: comparison with other ethnic groups

Origin	Domicile	FEV$_1$ (l)	FVC (l)	Source
Calcutta	India	3.03	3.68	Chatterjee *et al.* (1988)
W. Pakistan	UK	3.20	3.72	Malik *et al.* (1972)
Uttar Pradesh	Guiana	2.79	3.42	Miller *et al.* (1970)
Madras (city)	India	2.66	3.34	Kamet *et al.* (1977)
Madras (rural)	India	2.51	3.15	Milledge (1966)
Negroes	Guiana	2.95	3.59	Miller *et al.* (1970)
Caucasians	Various	3.48	4.21	Table 15.16

Other studies from the subcontinent have given comparable results despite having, in many instances, a predominance of younger subjects.

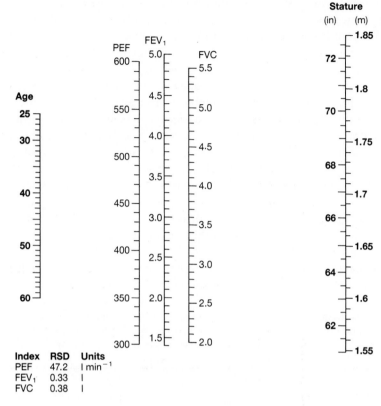

Stature
(in)   (m)

Index	RSD	Units
PEF	47.2	l min^{-1}
FEV$_1$	0.33	l
FVC	0.38	l

Fig. 15.14 Nomogram relating FEV$_1$, FVC and PEF (Wright peak flow meter) to age and stature for men from Pakistan working in the UK. (Source: Malik MA, Moss E, Lee WR. *Thorax* 1972; **27**: 611–619.)

anthropometric variables and embrace genetic and local environmental factors, for example the ethnic groups of grandparents, skin pigmentation and habitual activity. Objective evidence on the technical quality of the measurements should be supplied. The smoking habits should be recorded (cf. page 63). Publication is likely to be mainly in local medical journals but papers which develop unifying hypotheses should continue to attract general interest.

Tobacco smoke

Tobacco smoke contains a number of substances which can damage the lungs and cardiovascular system. Some of the substances form aggregates or droplet nuclei which stimulate receptors in the airways (page 88). The carbon monoxide impairs the respiratory function of the blood (page 291) and can damage the myocardium. The tar, superoxides, ozone and oxides of sulphur and nitrogen exert an irritant effect upon the bronchial epithelium, affect adversely the cilia and alveolar macrophages and can cause emphysema. The tar can cause lung cancer. The nicotine is addictive; its effects include increases in the cardiac frequency and systemic blood pressure. The magnitude of the effects varies with

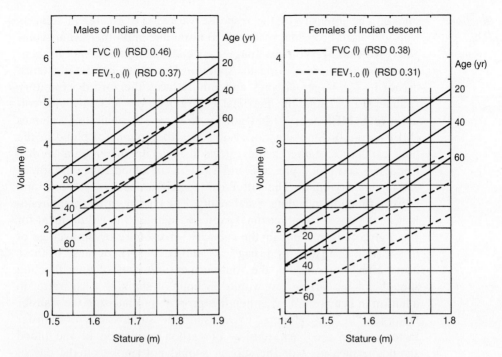

Fig. 15.15 Ventilatory capacity in Indian men and women; these results are applicable to south Indians. (Source: Miller GJ, Ashcroft MT, Swan AV, Beadnell HMSG. *Am Rev Respir Dis* 1970; **102**: 979–981.)

the type of tobacco and the manner of its preparation and use. The response is dose dependent, so heavy and long-term smokers and those who inhale their tobacco smoke incur more damage than subjects whose exposure is less. However, whilst for lung cancer the association with dose is fairly strong, for changes in the airways the association is weaker, with light and short-term smoking exerting a disproportionate effect. Persons who do not smoke but are exposed to tobacco smoke can also be affected. Passive smoking occurs in the home, on public transport, at work and in places of recreation, especially clubs. Maternal smoking is particularly damaging to young children, especially those who are constitutionally predisposed to develop asthma. Amongst persons who smoke but do not inhale, the practice of smoking a pipe or cigars is less damaging than smoking cigarettes. The effects of marijuana are similar to those of tobacco which have been reviewed by the Royal College of Physicians of London amongst others. Smoking history as its affects reference values is discussed on page 446.

Acute effects

The inhalation of tobacco smoke causes an immediate rise in the airway resistance which persists for at least an hour. The change is a reflex response to the deposition of particles upon the epithelium of the larynx, trachea and larger bronchi, and is not specific to tobacco

483

smoke. The intensity of the response varies; it is greater in subjects with increased bronchial reactivity to histamine and other agents compared with non-responders (page 174) and amongst smokers it is enhanced in those who bring up sputum. The acute rise in resistance occurs in the larger airways and this reduces the forced expiratory volume (FEV_1) and the maximal expiratory flow at large lung volumes (e.g. $MEF_{50\% FVC}$) but not the flow rate at small lung volumes ($MEF_{25\% FVC}$). Smoking can also reduce the volume of blood in the lung capillaries. Other acute effects include an increase in cardiac frequency and blood pressure and a rise in the blood concentration of carboxyhaemoglobin. The latter can impair aspects of cerebral and sensory function including visual acuity. The changes affect the physiological responses to submaximal exercise, increase the requirement for rapid glycolysis and impair the capacity for exercise by an average of $8 \, mmol \, min^{-1}$. (Table 14.9, page 431 and page 395). Because of these acute effects of smoking the routine measurements of lung function should not be carried out within an hour of smoking a cigarette; in addition in heavy smokers, when it is proposed to measure the transfer factor or, in any smokers, to measure the subdivisions of transfer factor, either the back tension of carbon monoxide in the blood should be measured or the subject should not smoke on the day of the test. Abstinence is also desirable prior to the performance of an exercise test.

Subacute effects

In many smokers the regular inhalation of an irritant aerosol causes damage to the walls of airways and alveoli leading to chronic bronchitis, emphysema and variable airflow limitation. These conditions impair the function of the lungs and are described subsequently (page 528). Less marked changes in function occur in asymptomatic smokers; they need to be recognised because such subjects are usually regarded as normal. However, there is on average slight narrowing of large airways so the forced expiratory volume and peak expiratory flow are reduced. Narrowing of small airways occurs as a result of bronchiolitis which can be asymptomatic; it is none the less associated with a reduction in maximal expiratory flow at small lung volumes ($MEF_{25\% FVC}$), premature closure of airways during expiration (hence increases in residual and closing volume), and uneven distribution of inspired gas. Consequently the single breath nitrogen index is increased and the distribution of ventilation–perfusion ratios is widened. There is then some degree of hypoxaemia. The distensibility of the lung is increased and there is an increase in the permeability of the alveolar capillary membrane as measured using ^{99m}Tc-DTPA (page 705). The transfer factor is reduced by an average of $1.0 \, mmol \, min^{-1} \, kPa^{-1}$ ($3 \, ml \, min^{-1} \, mmHg^{-1}$), and on exercise the pulmonary arterial pressure is somewhat increased. Some examples of the effects of smoking on widely used lung function indices are summarised in Table 15.15 and Fig. 15.16.

Table 15.15 Lung function of middle aged subjects who habitually smoked 20 cigarettes per day (s) compared with non-smokers of the same age (n-s). In the case of each index the lung function of the smokers was significantly inferior to that of the non-smokers ($p < 0.05$)

	Men		Women	
	n-s ($n = 136$)	s ($n = 91$)	n-s ($n = 97$)	s ($n = 84$)
FEV_1 (l)	3.80	3.42	2.65	2.45
VC (l)	5.11	4.80	3.07	2.91
FEV_1/VC (%)	77	74	87	84
RV/TLC (%)	36	38	—	—
MVV ($l\,min^{-1}$)	153	141	—	—
MMF ($l\,s^{-1}$)	3.86	3.12	3.43	3.01
Raw ($kPa\,l^{-1}\,s$)	0.20	0.23	0.21	0.24
($cmH_2O\,l^{-1}\,s$)	2.0	2.3	2.1	2.4
Tl ($mmol\,min^{-1}\,kPa^{-1}$)	11.7	10.0	8.8	7.8
($ml\,min^{-1}\,mmHg^{-1}$)	34.9	29.9	26.2	23.2
Pa,o_2 (kPa)	—	—	12.0	11.6
(mmHg)	—	—	90.2	86.9

(Sources: *for men*: Krumholz RA, Hedrick EC. *Am Rev Respir Dis* 1973; **107**: 225−230; *for women*: Woolf CR, Suero JT, *Am Rev Respir Dis* 1971; **103**: 26−37.)

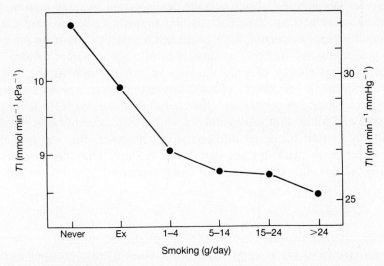

Fig. 15.16 Relationship of the transfer factor to smoking category in male dockyard workers. (Source: Harries PG. See Fig. 16.18, page 594.)

Longitudinal changes

The subacute and chronic effects of cigarette smoke upon lung function have been confirmed by longitudinal studies. These have shown that in young adult males the third phase of development of the lung is curtailed. Thus for example the peak expiratory flow reaches a maximum at a younger age in a smoker than a non-smoker so the maximal value is on average reduced. The age at which the lung function starts to

Table 15.16 Mean age at start of lung function decline in 488 young shipyard workers analysed by smoking categories

	Smokers* (years)	Non-smokers (years)	Difference
FEV$_1$	18.5	25.1	$p < 0.05$
FVC	25.8	35.6	$p < 0.05$
PEF	35.0	45.2	$p < 0.05$

* At any time during period of follow up (7.2 years).
(Source: Chinn DJ, Cotes JE. Unpublished.)

decline is also brought forward (e.g. Table 15.16). The change can be represented as an increase in the rate of decline of lung function with age (Fig. 15.17). It can also be represented as a loss of function per pack year of smoking.* Thus Dockery and colleagues observed an average reduction in FEV$_1$ of 7.4 ml per pack year in men and 4.4 ml in women. The rate of decline of transfer factor with age is similarly increased by smoking whilst the rate of increase of lung distensibility with age (exponent k of Colebatch, page 100) is enhanced. The changes are cumulative and over a period of years can lead to material respiratory impairment and disability. If repeated measurements of FEV$_1$ or transfer factor reveal above average deterioration in an asymptomatic individual or a group of individuals, this suggests a poor prognosis and should prompt the search for a cause and a remedy. The main physiological feature of subacute as distinct from acute exposure to tobacco smoke is narrowing of small airways so indices such as the single breath nitrogen test which reflected this change were *a priori* assumed to have predictive properties. Stanescu and colleagues were amongst those who found that most smokers whose FEV$_1$ deteriorated rapidly initially had an increased nitrogen slope; however, this was also the case for many who did not deteriorate unduly. Thus the predictive value of this class of test has still to be confirmed.

Discontinuing smoking

Discontinuing smoking lowers the alveolar concentration of carbon monoxide from 50–100 ppm (in a heavy smoker) to 2–10 ppm within 24 h. Giving up smoking also has a nearly immediate beneficial effect on lung function; this is most marked in young adults and children in whom both the ventilatory capacity and the transfer factor increase. The age at which the lung function starts to decline can be postponed in consequence. In older subjects who abandon smoking an improvement in ventilatory capacity is not invariable and is usually more marked in persons with respiratory symptoms than in those who are asymptomatic. The average improvement in FEV$_1$ has been reported by Dockery and

* The number of pack years is the product of the number of packs each containing 20 cigarettes which are smoked per day and the years of smoking.

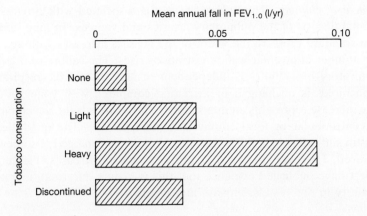

Fig. 15.17 Effect of smoking upon the mean annual decline in forced expiratory volume of men followed for 5 years. The light and heavy smokers consumed respectively 1 to 14 and more than 14 cigarettes per day. (Source: Higgins ITT, Oldham PD. *Br J Ind Med* 1962; **19**: 65–76.)

colleagues as 123 ml for a typical man and 107 ml for a typical woman. Alternatively when expressed as rate of change per year the effect of giving up smoking is to slow the functional decline (Fig. 15.17). The long-term benefits of giving up smoking also include amelioration of respiratory symptoms and diminished mortality from respiratory failure, lung cancer and ischaemic heart disease; however, the improved life expectancy is not apparent until some 10–15 years have elapsed.

Changes with increasing age

Underlying factors

Mechanisms. During adult life the function of the lung declines. The causes include a deterioration in the tissues of which the lung is composed, a reduction in the strength of the respiratory muscles (Fig. 5.4, page 91) and an increase in stiffness of the thoracic cage. Analogy with other tissues suggests that the intrapulmonary changes are due in part to an impaired nutrient blood supply from the bronchial arteries. They are also due to superoxides and proteolytic enzymes from the blood and alveolar macrophages. These and other agents diminish the permeability of cell membranes and alter the molecular structure of collagen and other tissues. The changes have the effect of increasing the rigidity and reducing the tensile strength of the lung tissue; they also reduce the viability of the epithelial cells and the ability to recuperate after injury. The rate of deterioration varies from one individual to another and can be slowed down by a diet rich in antioxidants. For the lung, the effects of ageing are aggravated by exposure to polluted atmospheres, including local pollution by tobacco smoke. Single episodes of acute chest illness do not have a deleterious effect unless recovery is incomplete.

Structural changes. The ageing process is associated with progressive intimal fibrosis of the pulmonary arteries and venules. In lung inflated to a standard pressure the width of the air sacs increases with age and the number of alveolar wall fenestrations rises. The calibre of the non-respiratory bronchioles is independent of age; that of the respiratory bronchioles is unchanged or increased compared with young adults. The increase represents an intermediate stage towards the development of centrilobular or focal emphysema (Chapter 16). The quantities of elastin and collagen in the lung parenchyma are unchanged or somewhat reduced. However, the total quantity of elastin increases. Pierce and Ebert have published evidence that this is mainly due to an increased quantity in the vessels, airways and pleura.

Lung elasticity. The elastic recoil pressure decreases with age and the static lung compliance probably increases, though this has not been found in all studies. Hence, the volume–pressure curve is mainly displaced upwards. The change reduces the traction on the walls of bronchioles which normally preserve their patency (page 97). Hence, during expiration closure of airways occurs at progressively larger lung volumes as age advances. On this account, in men, the residual volume increases from an average value of about 1.3 l at age 20 to about 2.2 l at age 60. The closing volume is similarly increased over the same period from about 10% VC to 23% VC (Fig. 15.24, page 502). By contrast, the total lung capacity does not increase to an important extent since the diminution in the elastic recoil is offset by a reduction in the strength of the respiratory muscles and in the compliance of the thoracic cage. In women the total lung capacity tends to diminish. In both sexes the residual volume as a percentage of total lung capacity rises from about 25% at age 20 to about 37% at age 60. The vital capacity decreases in consequence (Fig. 15.18).

Lung function

Ventilatory capacity. All the indices of ventilatory capacity decline with age. The process begins in early adult life and starts at a younger age for indices which depend solely on lung elasticity compared with those which are to some extent effort dependent (Table 15.16). The onset of decline is brought forward by smoking (page 485). The subsequent rate of decline is mainly a manifestation of reduced lung recoil pressure. Thus assuming a linear decline the reductions between the ages of 25 and 65 years in men are on average 85% for $MEF_{25\% \ FVC}$ and 54% for $MEF_{50\% \ FVC}$ compared with only 18% for the peak expiratory flow (data from Table 15.18, pages 496 and 497, reductions expressed as $\Delta x / \bar{x}$, page 59). In reality the rate of decline probably accelerates with age. It is also increased in association with respiratory symptoms. When expressed in absolute units the rate of decline is positively correlated with the initial size of the lung; the association appears to apply within and between the sexes and between ethnic groups but

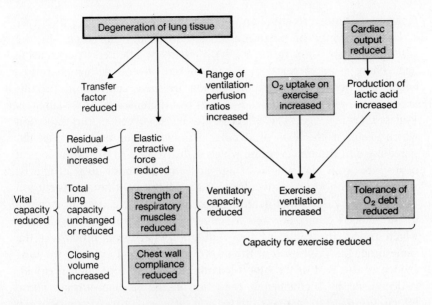

Fig. 15.18 Effects of age upon lung function and the capacity for exercise.

further confirmation would be helpful. The concept is due to Cole. Numerous values for the apparent decline with age of the several indices of lung function are given in other parts of this chapter.

The decline in ventilatory capacity with age is independent of the airway resistance which, at a lung volume of about 1 l in excess of the functional residual capacity, shows no significant upward trend with age. The change with age in the resistance to movement of the chest wall is poorly documented but it is probably increased since both the total pulmonary resistance and the oxygen cost of breathing rise with age. In addition, the strength of the respiratory muscles declines with age, but the contribution of this factor to the reduction in the ventilatory capacity has still to be assessed.

Comment. In terms of lung mechanics, there are apparent inconsistencies between the indices which show deterioration with age and those which are unaffected. For example, the loss of elastic recoil of the lung is more marked than the increase in the compliance; similarly, the reduction in the ventilatory capacity and the increase in the residual volume with respect to the total lung capacity are not associated with a rise in the airway resistance. Hence there is a dissociation between the calibre of the bronchioles and their resistance to deformation. These observations indicate a need for further research into the effects of age upon the function of the human lung.

Ventilation—perfusion inequality. With increasing age, the range of expansion ratios of the alveoli widens; the indices of uneven ventilation show deterioration in consequence. For example, in men between the ages of 33 and 66 years the Fowler nitrogen index was observed by

489

Cohn and Donoso to show an average change of from 1.34 to 2.3%.

The uniformity of perfusion of the lung and the range of the ventilation−perfusion ratios are both adversely affected by increasing age. There is an increase in the number of alveoli with high ratios, which are poorly perfused in relation to their ventilation; on this account, the physiological deadspace at rest increases by approximately 1 ml per year of age. The effect of the increase and of the reduction which occurs in the level of alveolar ventilation (see below) raises the percentage of the tidal volume which is distributed to the physiological deadspace from about 20% at age 20 years to about 40% at age 60 years. The proportion of alveoli which have a low ventilation−perfusion ratio also increases with advancing age. This change causes an increase in the venous admixture and a similar deterioration in other indices which reflect the range of the ventilation−perfusion ratios. At the same time, the saturation of the mixed venous blood entering the lung (which is also that of the blood leaving the poorly ventilated regions), is decreased by a concurrent reduction in the cardiac output. These effects summate to increase the tension difference for oxygen between mean alveolar gas and the systemic arterial blood from about 1 kPa (8 mmHg) at age 20 years to about 2.7 kPa (20 mmHg) at age 60 years. Over this period, for a subject breathing air at sea level, there is little change in the average tension of oxygen in the alveolar gas; the increase in the gradient is, therefore, due to a reduction in the tension of oxygen in the arterial blood. The reduction can be described by the relationship of Raine and Bishop which is representative of the published data; it is given in Table 15.22 (page 511). Concurrently the arterial oxygen saturation falls from about 97% to about 94%.

The exchange of gas across the alveolar capillary membrane is affected by the loss of lung tissue which is one facet of ageing. The loss reduces the area of surface which is available for the exchange of gas. At the same time the volume of blood in the alveolar capillaries diminishes but to a smaller extent. These changes give rise to a reduction in the transfer factor (diffusing capacity) for the lung between the ages of 20 and 60 years of about 25%.

Ventilation and exercise. The level of exercise ventilation is determined by the responsiveness of the respiratory system, the extent of the ventilation−perfusion inequality and the uptake of oxygen. The respiratory responses to hypoxia and to hypercapnia decline with age; at least part of the changes are accounted for by the concomitant reduction in vital capacity (cf. page 349). The overall effect is small since the tension of carbon dioxide in the arterial blood is independent of age as is the alveolar ventilation standardised for the consumption of oxygen. By contrast the minute volume relative to the consumption of oxygen increases with age because the physiological deadspace is enlarged (Fig. 15.19). The oxygen uptake also changes. When the subject is at rest, the requirement for oxygen decreases with age because the metabolism of body tissues is reduced. The alveolar ventilation at rest therefore

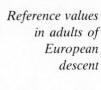

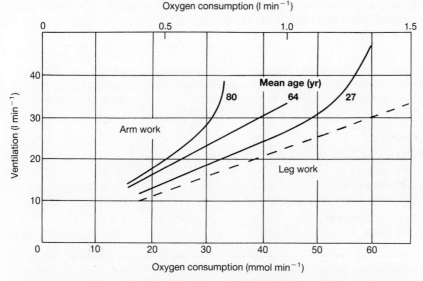

Fig. 15.19 Effect of age on the relationship of ventilation minute volume to consumption of oxygen for men performing work with the arms, obtained by Norris, Shock and Yiengst. The ages are expressed as the mid-points of their ranges for the three groups of subjects. The ventilation is higher than when exercise is performed with the legs (dashed line, from Fig. 12.4, page 371).

decreases with age; this change almost exactly compensates for the increase in the ventilation of the deadspace with the result that, under quiet resting conditions, the ventilation minute volume shows no significant change with age despite material alterations in its component variables. However, during standardised exercise, on account of poor motor co-ordination, the elderly subject expends more energy in overcoming friction in muscles and joints and in preserving the balance; the consumption of oxygen, and the exercise ventilation are therefore increased. At the same time, as a result of reductions with age in both the maximal cardiac output and the size of the peripheral vascular bed, the need for rapid glycolysis becomes apparent at lower levels of energy expenditure in elderly than in young subjects; the exercise ventilation is then somewhat increased and the capacity for exercise is reduced (Fig. 15.19). The reduced cardiac output is due mainly to a diminution in cardiac frequency; the reduction extends from rest to maximal exercise (equation 13.4, page 397). The change is associated with a reduced sympathetic tone and an increase in the response of the blood pressure to isometric work.

Reference values in adults of European descent

Underlying considerations

Physiological anthropometry. The principal factor determining the magnitude of individual indices of lung function is the overall size of the

Table 15.17 Effects upon lung function and the response to exercise of a gain in body-weight of 4 kg in men of mean age 44 years

	Treatment group		Control group	
	Initial	3 months	Initial	3 months
Body weight (kg)	69.5	73.6*	69.1	69.0
FEV_1 (l)	2.69	2.60*	2.71	2.70
FVC (l)	3.98	3.89*	4.00	4.04
FRC (l)	3.25	3.10*	3.67	3.85
Walking 2.5 mph, 10% incline				
$\dot{V}E$ (l min^{-1})	40.7	43.3*	41.9	39.7
$\dot{n}O_2$ (mmol min^{-1})	72.8	79.9*	73.2	71.9
fc (min^{-1})	116	123*	117	113
At $\dot{n}O_2$ 67 mmol min^{-1}				
$\dot{V}E$ (l min^{-1})	37.5	36.6	38.5	37.8
fc (min^{-1})	112	113	113	111

* Indicates a significant change ($p < 0.05$).
(Source: Cotes JE, Gilson JC. *Ann Occup Hyg* 1967; **10**: 327–335.)

lung. This is related to body size, particularly stature which is a slightly better descriptor than sitting height (cf. page 454) and much better than body mass. The stature can if necessary be replaced by the arm span though few reference values have been expressed in this form. After allowing for stature the body muscle, expressed independent of stature as fat-free mass divided by stature squared, contributes to the description of indices which include inspiratory capacity (page 106). In adolescent boys the width of the thorax can help to describe the transition to adult lung function (page 465). However, in adults the chest width does not contribute usefully to the description. The quantity of body fat influences the lung volumes by occupying space within the thoracic cage and contributing to the position of the diaphragm. The effect is mainly on the functional residual capacity which summates reductions in both the residual and expiratory reserve volumes. However, the distribution of body fat varies with age and between the sexes and not all changes in total body fat have equal effects upon lung function. In working men the effect of a small increase in body mass due to inactivity is illustrated in Table 15.17. Larger increases can contribute to hypoventilation (page 579). For purposes of reference values the physical dimensions of the subject are usually represented in terms of stature.

Models of adult lung function. Reference values summarise the lung function of healthy persons and provide a basis for interpreting the results in individuals†. The criteria for health and the different types of reference values are discussed on page 445. There are at present few longitudinal reference values (page 703), and more are needed. Cross-

† This implies that the two data sets are technically comparable, see e.g. page 48 and Fig. 3.14, page 58.

sectional reference values are considered in this section. The reference equation is usually in terms of age, stature and gender and is for persons of a specified ethnic group. This has not always been so: thus the reference values of Kory and colleagues for US veterans comprised both Caucasians and Negroes. The lung function is usually described in terms of a linear model (cf. page 63). Thus:

$$y = a.\text{stature} + b.\text{age} + c.\text{if smoker} + z \ (\pm \text{RSD}) \qquad (15.3)$$

where y is an index of lung function, a, b and c are regression coefficients and z is a constant. The model implies that the increment of lung function per unit of stature is the same for short and tall people; this appears to be the case. The model also implies that the decline in lung function which occurs throughout adult life is the same at all ages and is independent of stature and smoking habits. This is incorrect. The decline with age increases with age; in absolute units it is also greater for tall than for short people and it can be represented as occurring at a greater rate in smokers than in non-smokers. Thus the model is an oversimplification but it has none the less been of great practical use. Greater precision can be achieved by including quadratic and inter-active terms in the regression equation; thus

$$y = a.\text{stature} + b.\text{age} + c.\text{if smoker} + d.\text{age}^2$$
$$+ \ e.\text{age}.\text{smoking} \ldots \text{etc.} \ (\pm \text{RSD}) \qquad (15.4)$$

For most indices of lung function the coefficients a and b are respectively positive and negative. The smoking term is included as a categorical variable, one if a smoker and zero if a non-smoker so the term does not appear in reference values for non-smokers. RSD is the residual standard derivation about the regression equation. It is usually nearly independent of the value of y and can be used to describe the distribution of results about the regression equation provided the distribution is a 'normal' one (Table 15.24, page 512). The 5th percentile is usually taken as the dividing line between normal and abnormal. This is given by $(y \pm 1.64 \text{ RSD})$. If the distribution about the regression line is not normal the limits should be calculated separately for different values of y.

The linear model slightly overpredicts the lung function of young and old persons but is used in the present account because of its simplicity. The non-linear models are likely to be more accurate but this has not always been found to be the case. An interesting model is that proposed by Cole which has the form:

$$y.\text{St}^{-2} = k_1.k_2(a + b.\text{age}) \qquad (15.5)$$

where k_1 and k_2 are coefficient terms for gender and for ethnic group. The full potential of the model has still to be ascertained.

Choice of reference equations

Representative equations which were compiled for previous editions of this book are widely used and are given in Table 15.18; some of the equations are displayed as nomograms in Figs 15.20 and 15.21. Others are presented as charts (Figs 15.22−15.24). Values for forced expiratory volume and vital capacity in old people are given in Fig. 15.25. Linear regression equations published prior to 1983 have been reviewed for the European Coal and Steel Community (ECSC) by Quanjer in *Standardised Lung Function Testing*. The review also contains summary equations. They are given in Table 15.19 and some of the equations are displayed as nomograms in Figs 15.26 and 15.27. Equations in the format recommended by the American Thoracic Society (ATS) are given in their report *Lung Function Testing: Selection of Reference Values and Interpretative Strategies*. Of the recent equations listed in that report those for dynamic spirometry by Crapo, Miller and their respective collaborators, are complete and nearly identical. Both groups give results for the transfer factor but those of Crapo and colleagues were obtained at an altitude of 1400 m; the associated hypoxia increased the values above those observed at sea level. Relatively high values for the transfer factor were also reported by Knudson, Paoletti and their respective colleagues; these groups used a definition of breath holding time proposed by the ATS Epidemiology Standardization Project which is not now considered satisfactory. The transfer results of Miller and colleagues were matched by those of Roca *et al.* in Barcelona and appear to be representative. Crapo's group reported values for the total lung capacity and its subdivisions and these too appear to be representative. These selected United States reference values are given in Table 15.20 and displayed as nomograms in Figs 15.28 and 15.29. Mean values for some widely used lung function indices given by the equations from Lung Function, the European Coal and Steel Community and selected from the ATS report are listed in Table 15.21. Reference values for other lung function indices are given in Table 15.22. Reference equations which describe the physiological response to exercise are given in Table 14.9 (page 431). Exercise tidal volume is further illustrated in Fig. 15.30 and exercise cardiac frequency in Fig. 14.9 (page 442).

A laboratory planning to use published reference equations should check that the methods are compatible; this is usually the case except possibly for the transfer factor. For this test the alveolar oxygen tension during breath holding can vary depending on whether a European or US protocol is used. Having standardised for method the laboratory should then make measurements on a homogenous group of 10−20 persons whose ages are within the limits 25−65 years and who meet the selection criteria (cf. page 72). The mean results for the subjects should match those given by the chosen reference equations. In practice there is little to choose between the equations, and experience in interpretation is gained through the consistent use of a single set.

Using reference values. The reference values given in this chapter are almost all cross-sectional ones and are subject to a cohort effect (page 447). They provide average values for healthy persons with

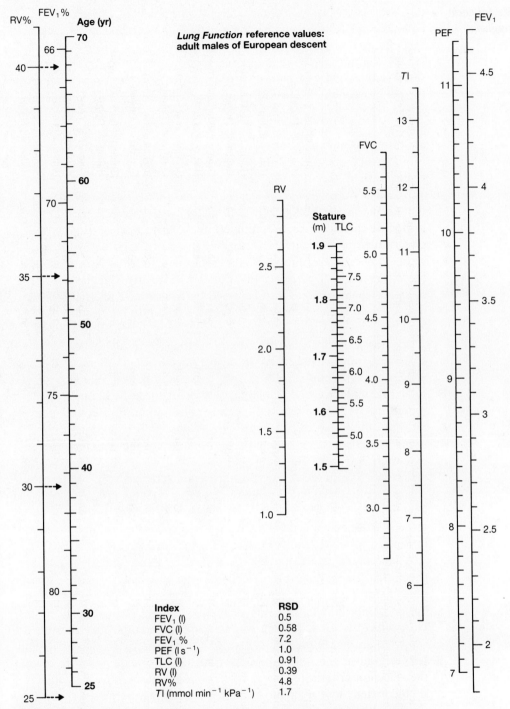

Fig. 15.20 Nomogram relating indices of lung function to stature and age for healthy adult males of European descent (for sources see Table 15.18). To use the nomogram a ruler is placed to overlie the age and stature of the subject: the lung function is then given by the intersections with the vertical lines. However, RV% and the FEV% are related only to age and TLC only to stature so these indices should be read directly from the respective columns. When stature is measured in inches these should be converted to metres by dividing by 39.4.

495

Table 15.18 Regression relationships (with residual standard deviations) for the prediction of indices of lung function from age (years), stature (st, m) and in some instances weight (kg) in asymptomatic adult male and female subjects of European descent. Gas volumes are expressed at BTPS. Equations which were originally quoted in other units have been modified

	Sex	Regression coefficients			Constant term	RSD	Figure	Source
		Stature	Age	Weight				
Total lung capacity (TLC, l)	M	8.67			−8.49	0.91	15.20	Cotes, Meade (unpubl.)
	F	7.46	−0.013		−6.42	0.51	15.21	Hall et al. (1979)
Expiratory and forced vital capacity (FVC, l)	M	5.20	−0.022		−3.60	0.58	15.20	Kory et al. (1961)
	F	4.66	−0.029		−2.88	0.44	15.21	Hall et al. (1979)
Residual volume (RV, l)	M	2.7	+0.017		−3.45	0.39	15.20	Goldman, Becklake (1959)
	F	2.8	+0.016		−3.54	0.31	15.21	Hall et al. (1979)
Functional residual capacity (FRC, l)	M	5.78	+0.016	−0.04	−4.24	0.61	15.22	Grimby, Söderholm (1963)
	F	6.60		−0.03	−5.76	0.43	15.22	Hall et al. (1979)
Inspiratory capacity (IC, l)	M	2.35	−0.020	+0.017	−1.40	0.47	—	Becklake et al. (1970)
	F	2.88		+0.014	−3.09	0.40	—	Cotes et al. (unpubl.)
Expiratory reserve volume (ERV, l)	M	3.50	−0.012	−0.018	−2.84	0.38	—	Becklake et al. (1970)
	F	3.35	−0.018	−0.019	−2.12	0.33	—	Cotes et al. (unpubl.)
(RV/TLC) (%)	M		+0.343		+16.7	4.8	15.20	Goldman, Becklake (1959)
	F		+0.43		+14.33	5.7	15.21	Hall et al. (1979)
Forced expiratory volume* (FEV$_1$, l)	M	3.62	−0.031		−1.41	≈0.5	15.20	Cotes et al. (1965)
	M	3.7	−0.028		−1.59	0.52	—	Kory et al. (1961)
	F	3.29	−0.029		−1.42	0.36	15.21	Hall et al. (1979)
FEV$_1$/FVC (%)*	M		−0.373		+91.8	7.19	15.20	Berglund et al. (1963)
	F		−0.222		+86.5	6.2	15.21	Hall et al. (1979)

Measurement	Sex						Fig.	Reference
Maximal voluntary ventilation (MVV, $l\,min^{-1}$)	M	134	−1.26		−21.4	29.0	—	Kory et al. (1961)
	F	81	−0.57		−5.5	10.7	—	Lindall et al. (1967)
Peak expiratory flow (PEF $l\,s^{-1}$)	M	st x	(−0.025)	...	(+6.58)	1.0	15.20¶	Leiner et al. (1963)
	F	6.23	−0.035		−1.88	1.1	15.21	Pelzer, Thomson (1964)
Max. mid-expiratory flow ($FEF_{25-75}.\ l\,s^{-1}$)	M		−0.057		+6.38	1.09	—	Birath et al. (1963)
	F		−0.063		+6.14	0.77	—	Birath et al. (1963)
Max. expiratory flow ($MEF_{50\% FVC}.\ l\,s^{-1}$)	M	2.72	−0.061	+0.04‡	+1.52	1.38	—	Chinn, Cotes (unpubl.)§
	F	3.28	−0.049	+0.04‡	−0.17	1.04	—	Chinn, Cotes (unpubl.)§
Max. expiratory flow ($MEF_{25\% FVC}.\ l\,s^{-1}$)	M	1.00	−0.033		+1.28	0.55	—	Chinn, Cotes (unpubl.)§
	F	1.11	−0.032		+0.94	0.49	—	Chinn, Cotes (unpubl.)§
Combined obstruction index	M (? and F)		0.312	−0.221‡	17.2	4.1	—	Chinn, Cotes (unpubl.)
Compliance, exponent $k \times 10^2$ ($pressure^{-1}$, page 100)	M and F		9.29×10^{-2}		+9.71	2.84	—	Colebatch et al. (1979)
Transfer factor (Tco,sb, SI†)	M	10.9	−0.067		−5.89	1.71	15.20	Cotes et al. (unpubl.)
	F	7.1	−0.054		−0.89	1.20	15.21	Billiet et al. (1963)
Kco (Tl/V_A) (SI†)	M		−0.013		2.20	0.27	15.23	Cotes, Hall (1970)
	F		−0.007		2.07	0.20	15.23	Cotes, Hall (1970)
$1/Dm$ (SI†)	M and F	−0.054	+0.00036		+0.135	0.062	15.23	Cotes et al. (unpubl.)
$1/Vc$ (ml^{-1})	M	−0.0201			+0.047	0.003	15.23	Frans (1971)
	F	−0.0274			+0.061	0.006	15.23	Cotes et al. (unpubl.)

* Measured without backward extrapolation. For use where this practice has been adopted add 2.5% (page 138).
† SI units $mmol\,min^{-1}\,kPa^{-1}$ and their reciprocal; for conversion of Tl, Dm and Kco to traditional units (ml, min and mmHg) multiply throughout by 2.99, see Table 2.5 (page 17).
‡ wt/st².
§ These equations replace those of Cherniack and Raber.
¶ Fig. 15.20 includes the linear form of this equation (PEF = 5.455 St − 0.0437 Age + 1.9687); the two equations give very similar results.

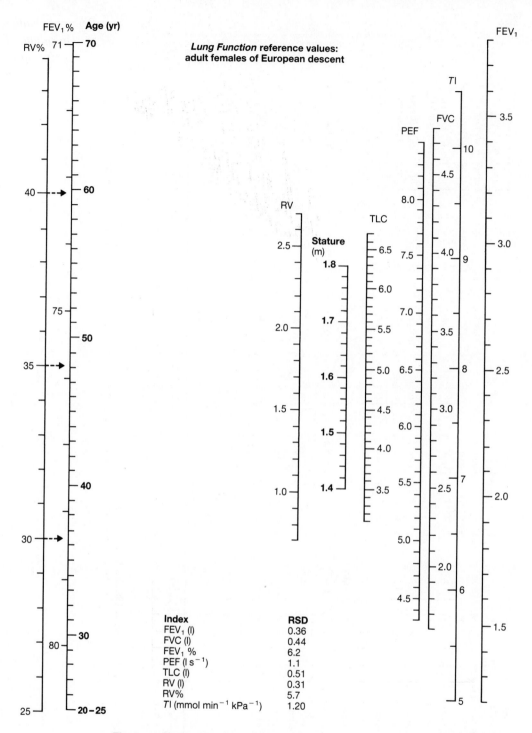

Fig. 15.21 Nomogram relating indices of lung function to stature and age for healthy adult females of European descent. (For sources see Table 15.18 and for other details see the caption to Fig. 15.20.)

498

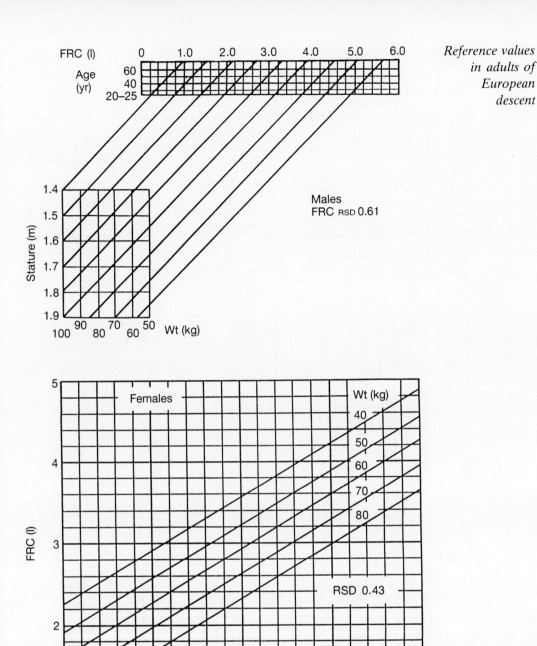

Fig. 15.22 Functional residual capacity (FRC) in healthy adult males and females. (Sources: see Table 15.18.)

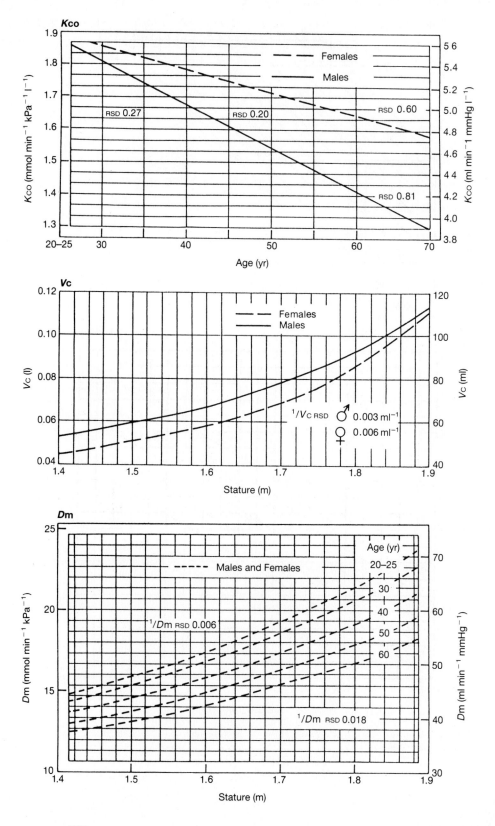

Table 15.19 The European Coal and Steel Community summary equations describing the lung function of healthy adults.

	Men	Women
TLC (l)	$7.99 \text{ St} - 7.08 \ (0.7)$	$6.60 \text{ St} - 5.79 \ (0.60)$
FVC (l)	$5.76 \text{ St} - 0.026 \text{ A} - 4.34 \ (0.61)$	$4.43 \text{ St} - 0.026 \text{ A} - 2.89 \ (0.43)$
RV (l)	$1.31 \text{ St} + 0.022 \text{ A} - 1.23 \ (0.41)$	$1.81 \text{ St} + 0.016 \text{ A} - 2.00 \ (0.35)$
FRC (l)	$2.34 \text{ St} + 0.009 \text{ A} - 1.09 \ (0.60)$	$2.24 \text{ St} + 0.001 \text{ A} - 1.00 \ (0.50)$
RV/TLC (%)	$0.39 \text{ A} + 13.96 \ (5.46)$	$0.34 \text{ A} + 18.96 \ (5.83)$
FEV_1 (l)	$4.30 \text{ St} - 0.029 \text{ A} - 2.49 \ (0.51)$	$3.95 \text{ St} - 0.025 \text{ A} - 2.60 \ (0.38)$
$FEV_1/VC(\%)$*	$87.21 - 0.18 \text{ A} \ (7.17)$	$89.10 - 0.19 \text{ A} \ (6.51)$
PEF (l s^{-1})	$6.14 \text{ St} - 0.043 \text{ A} + 0.15 \ (1.21)$	$5.50 \text{ St} - 0.030 \text{ A} - 1.11 \ (0.90)$
FEF_{25-75} (l s^{-1})	$1.94 \text{ St} - 0.043 \text{ A} + 2.70 \ (1.04)$	$1.25 \text{ St} - 0.034 \text{ A} + 2.92 \ (0.85)$
Tlco (SI)	$11.11 \text{ St} - 0.066 \text{ A} - 6.03 \ (1.41)$	$8.18 \text{ St} - 0.049 \text{ A} - 2.74 \ (1.17)$
Kco (SI)*		

* See footnotes to Table 15.21.
St is stature (m), A is age (years), RSD is in parentheses. Abbreviations are as in Table 15.18. The equations are given as nomograms in Figs 15.26 and 15.27. (Source: Quanjer PhH. *Bull Eur Physiopathol Respir* 1983; **19**:Suppl. 5.)

which the lung function results for individuals can be compared. The reference equations apply to a particular gender and ethnic group and enable adjustments to be made for age and stature which for this purpose are assumed to be independent of each other. This is not strictly correct since the stature declines with age, particularly in elderly women. The *allowance for age* is usually made on a linear basis. This is valid over a range which is commonly 25–70 years. Older subjects are included in some reference equations (e.g. Table 15.23). Alternatively the values can be obtained by linear extrapolation from age 70. This is usually acceptable even though the annual decline in lung function in individuals increases as they get older. The relatively high accuracy of the extrapolated results is due to persons with above average lung function having a below average mortality from many causes (page 606). The differential mortality raises the average lung function of the survivors compared with what would be expected from averaging the age-related deterioration of individuals. However, equations for the aged should be used when they are available (e.g. Fig. 15.25).

Reference values for children often apply only up to age of 16 years whilst those for adults are usually considered to be acceptable only beyond the age of 25 years. Between these ages the lung is either still developing, as in most young men, or at a plateau, as in young women.

Fig. 15.23 Diffusion constant ($k$co or $[Tl/V_A]$), volume of blood in the alveolar capillaries (Vc) and the diffusing capacity of the alveolar capillary membrane (Dm) in healthy adults of European descent. (Sources: see Table 15.18.)

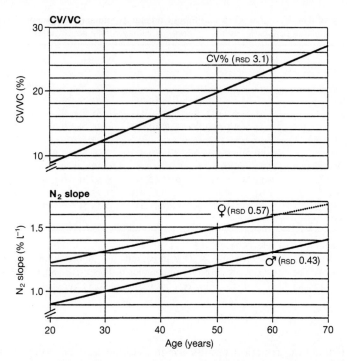

Fig. 15.24 Closing volume as a percentage of vital capacity and nitrogren slope for non-smokers. The values for smokers are on average twice those for non-smokers but with a wide scatter. (Sources: McCarthy DS, Spencer R, Greene R, Milic-Emili J. *Am J Med* 1972; **52**: 747–753; Buist AS, Ross BB. *Am Rev Respir Dis* 1973; **108**: 1078–1087.)

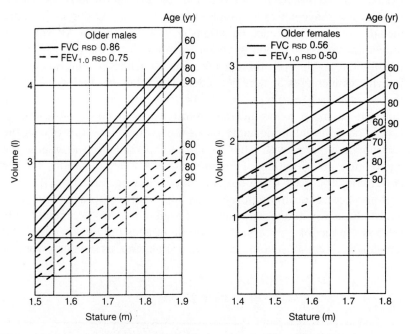

Fig. 15.25 Forced vital capacity (FVC) and forced expiratory volume (FEV$_1$) in healthy older adult males and females. (Source: Milne JS, Williamson J. *Clin Sci* 1972; **42**: 371–381). Alternatively equations in Table 15.18 can be used (see text).

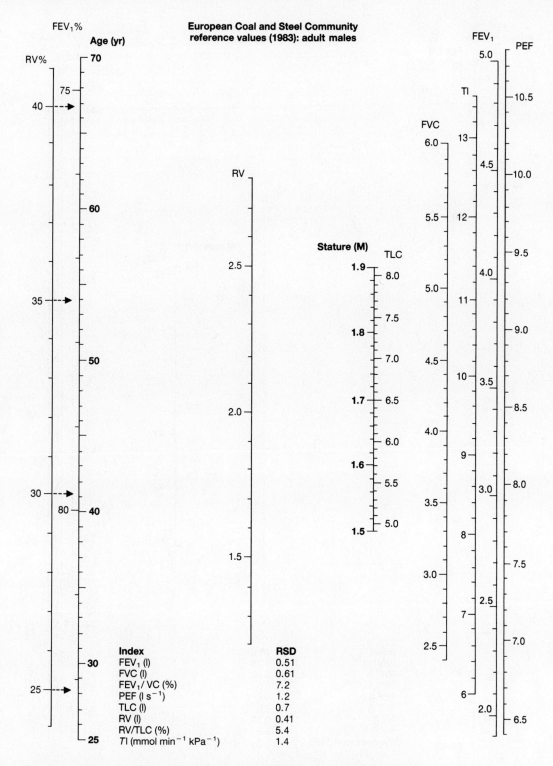

Fig. 15.26 Nomogram relating the lung function of adult males to age and stature using the summary equations of the European Coal and Steel Community (Table 15.19). The method for reading the nomogram is given in the caption to Fig. 15.20.

503

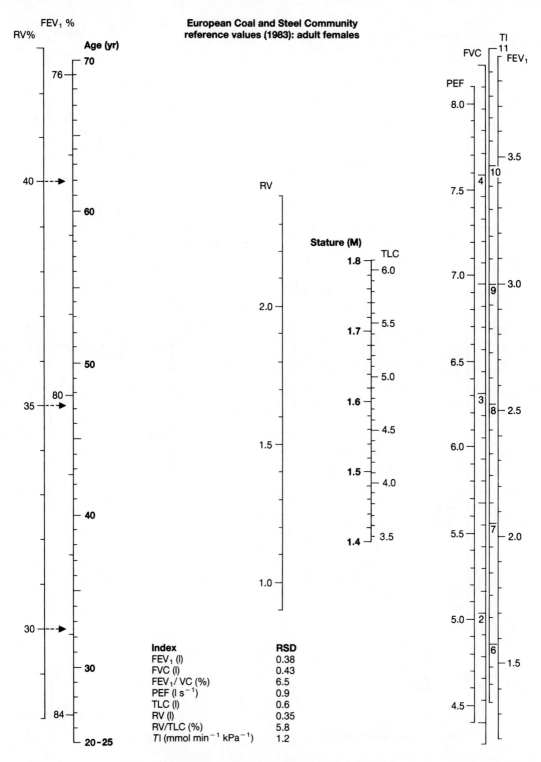

Fig. 15.27 Nomogram relating the lung function of adult females to age and stature using the summary equations of the European Coal and Steel Community (Table 15.19). The method for reading the nomogram is given in the caption to Fig. 15.20.

Table 15.20 Selected reference equations describing lung function in white adults (non-smokers) in USA

	Men	Women	Source
TLC (l)	$7.95 \text{ St} + 0.003 \text{ A} - 7.33$ (0.79)	$5.90 \text{ St} - 4.54$ (0.54)	Crapo et al. (1982)
FVC (l)	$7.74 \text{ St} - 0.021 \text{ A} - 7.75$ (0.51)	$4.14 \text{ St} - 0.023 \text{ A} - 2.20$ (0.44)	Miller et al. (1986)*
RV (l)	$2.16 \text{ St} + 0.021 \text{ A} - 2.84$ (0.37)	$1.97 \text{ St} + 0.020 \text{ A} - 2.42$ (0.38)	Crapo et al. (1982)
FRC (l)	$4.72 \text{ St} + 0.009 \text{ A} - 5.29$ (0.72)	$3.60 \text{ St} + 0.003 \text{ A} - 3.18$ (0.52)	Crapo et al. (1982)
RV/TLC (%)	$0.309 \text{ A} + 14.1$ (4.38)	$0.416 \text{ A} + 14.35$ (5.46)	Crapo et al. (1982)
FEV_1 (l)	$5.66 \text{ St} - 0.023 \text{ A} - 4.91$ (0.41)	$2.68 \text{ St} - 0.025 \text{ A} - 0.38$ (0.33)	Miller et al. (1986)*
FEV_1/FVC (%)	$110.2 - 13.1 \text{ St}^\dagger - 0.15 \text{ A}$ (5.58)	$124.4 - 21.4 \text{ St} - 0.15 \text{ A}$ (6.75)	Miller et al. (1986)*
FEF_{25-75} ($1\,s^{-1}$)	$5.79 \text{ St} - 0.036 \text{ A} - 4.52$ (1.08)	$3.00 \text{ St} - 0.031 \text{ A} - 0.41$ (0.85)	Knudson et al. (1983)
$MEF_{50\% \text{ FVC}}$ ($1\,s^{-1}$)	$6.84 \text{ St} - 0.037 \text{ A} - 5.54$ (1.29)	$3.21 \text{ St} - 0.024 \text{ A} - 0.44$ (0.98)	Knudson et al. (1983)
$MEF_{25\% \text{ FVC}}$ ($1\,s^{-1}$)	$3.10 \text{ St} - 0.023 \text{ A} - 2.48$ (0.69)	$1.74 \text{ St} - 0.025 \text{ A} - 0.18$ (0.66)	Knudson et al. (1983)
Dl ($ml\,min^{-1}\,mmHg^{-1}$)	$16.4 \text{ St} - 0.229 \text{ A} + 12.9$ (4.84)	$16.0 \text{ St} - 0.111 \text{ A} + 2.24$ (3.95)	Miller et al. (1983)
Dl/V_A	$10.09 - 2.24 \text{ St} - 0.031 \text{ A}$ (0.73)	$8.33 - 1.81 \text{ St} - 0.016 \text{ A}$ (0.80)	Miller et al. (1983)

* The regression equations of Crapo et al. (1981) are virtually identical.

† Coefficient on stature is not significant.

St is stature (m), A is age (years), RSD is in brackets. Abbreviations are as in Table 15.18. The equations are given as nomograms in Figs 15.28 and 15.29.

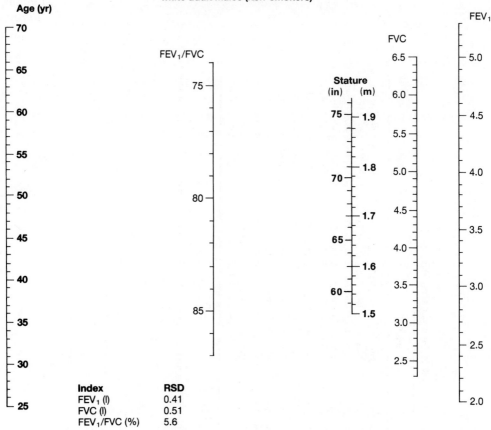

**US reference values for dynamic spirometry
white adult males (non-smokers)**

Age (yr)

FEV$_1$

FVC

FEV$_1$/FVC

Stature
(in)   (m)

Index	RSD
FEV$_1$ (l)	0.41
FVC (l)	0.51
FEV$_1$/FVC (%)	5.6

Fig. 15.28 Nomograms (above and facing page) relating the lung function of adult US males to age and stature. The regression equations are given in Table 15.20 and the method for reading the nomograms in the caption to Fig. 15.20.

Hence backward extrapolation from older age groups can lead to the prediction of higher results than those actually observed. Reference values for adolescents should be used instead (page 468). The *allowance for stature* is also made on a linear basis. This is acceptable over a wide range of statures from pituitary giants to pygmies. The curvilinear model of Cole which expresses the lung function per unit of stature squared does not improve the adjustment for stature though it does improve that for age (page 493).

Reference equations describe the test results of groups of people with apparently healthy lungs. Their use for an individual requires that person to be effectively part of the group. Whether or not this condition is met depends on the criteria used for selecting the group and the accuracy of prediction which is required; the latter is determined in part by the purpose for which the assessment is made (page 446). For *clinical assessment* of a patient who presents with respiratory symptoms the reference values will be those for asymptomatic individuals (e.g. Tables 15.18 and 15.19); the prediction need not be very precise so the

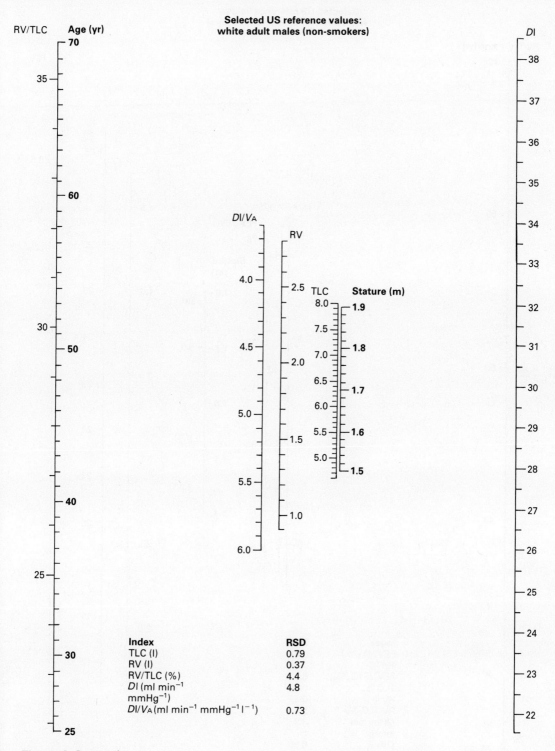

Fig. **15.28** *Continued*

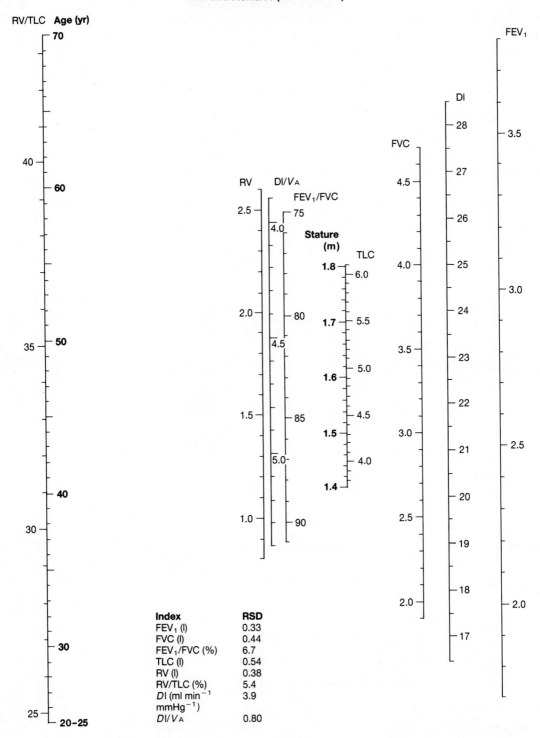

Fig. 15.29 Nomogram relating the lung function of adult US females to age and stature. The regression equations are given in Table 15.20 and the method for reading the nomogram in the caption to Fig. 15.20.

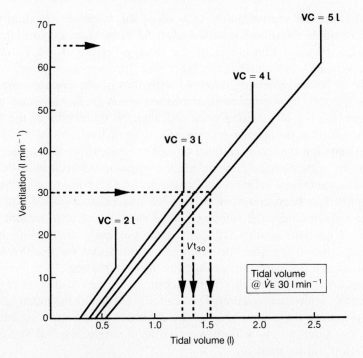

Fig. 15.30 Average relationships of exercise ventilation to tidal volume and vital capacity for men and women of European descent. The chart incorporates the values for Vt_{30} and Vtmax relative to vital capacity given in Table 14.9 (page 431).

Table 15.21 Mean values for lung function indices in adults aged 45 years given by reference equations from *Lung Function* (LF, Table 15.18), European Coal and Steel Community (ECSC, Table 15.19), and USA (Table 15.20)

	Men (mean stature 1.75 m)			Women (mean stature 1.65 m)		
	LF	ECSC	USA	LF	ECSC	USA
FEV_1 (l)	3.53*	3.73	3.94	2.70*	2.79	2.91
FVC (l)	4.51	4.57	4.84	3.50	3.24	3.59
FEV_1/FVC (%)	75.0*	79.1†	80.5	76.5*	80.5†	82.3
TLC (l)	6.68	6.90	6.72	5.30	5.10	5.20
RV (l)	2.04	2.05	1.87	1.80	1.71	1.73
RV/TLC (%)	32.1	31.5	28.0	33.7	34.3	33.1
Tlco (SI)	10.2	10.4	10.5	8.39	8.55	7.91
(trad.)	30.3	31.1	31.4	25.1	25.6	23.7
Kco (SI)	1.61	(1.51)‡	1.60	1.75	(1.68)‡	1.54
(trad.)	4.83	(4.51)‡	4.77	5.23	(5.01)‡	4.62
PEF (ls^{-1})	9.54	8.96	NA	6.82	6.61	NA
$MEF_{50\%}$ FVC (ls^{-1})	4.51	4.89†	4.78	3.99	4.08†	3.78
$MEF_{25\%}$ FVC (ls^{-1})	1.55	2.06†	1.91	1.33	1.72†	1.56
FEF_{25-75} (ls^{-1})	3.81	4.16†	3.98	3.30	3.45	3.15

* Measured without backward extrapolation (Table 15.18).
† Other evidence suggests that the equation gives results which are too high.
‡ Tlco/TLC is given as the equation published for Kco is incorrect.
SI units are mmol min^{-1} kPa^{-1} (and l^{-1}); trad. units are ml min^{-1} mmHg^{-1} (and l^{-1}).

usual scatter of approximately 15% about the reference equation will be acceptable. Attribution of some of the respiratory impairment to smoking requires knowledge of the average effect of the habit in asymptomatic individuals; however, the healthy smoker effect is likely to be unimportant compared with that of the disease process. Subsequently, to *monitor clinical progress* much greater accuracy may be needed, but the starting point will then be the results of the first assessment (i.e. the internal reference value which has narrow confidence limits) and not the cross-sectional reference value where the confidence limits are wide because they include the variation between individuals. The cross-sectional values would again become relevant to ascertain if recovery had been complete or if there was *residual impairment*. In these circumstances the reference value should take into account the level of habitual activity (cf. page 472). For *early detection* of lung damage due to smoking the reference value is that for healthy non-smokers and accurate measurement is again important.

The *criteria of normality* are determined by the scatter of results about the reference equation. The scatter is smaller at the mean age of the reference population than at the extremes of the age distribution but the difference is seldom material so a single residual standard deviation can be used.

The properties of the standard deviation are such that the mean plus and minus one standard deviation embrace 68% of the observations. Of the remainder, 16% exceed the mean by more than one standard deviation and 16% are less than the mean by at least a similar amount. The corresponding figures for 1.64 SD and for 1.96 SD are 5% and 2.5% (Table 15.24). A result which deviates by more than one standard deviation from the mean in the direction of abnormality merits scrutiny if other factors are suggestive of lung disease. A result which deviates by more than 1.64 SD is usually considered as outside the normal range (page 493). This will be true in 95% of cases but in 5% the result will be just within the normal range. Thus using this criterion there is a 5% risk of getting a false positive result. But the statistical approach assumes that subjects who are to be investigated were selected at random from the reference population. This condition can be met in respiratory surveys. In other circumstances selection for investigation is often biased towards those at the abnormal end of the normal distribution; such persons are more likely to develop symptoms and be referred for assessment compared with others whose lung function was initially above average. Thus the false positive rate of 5% is an under-estimate. The borderline group is likely to contain a disproportionate number of heavy smokers, the obese, persons who take little exercise, the anxious, and women whose lung function has been underestimated on account of their foundation garments (page 134).

The accuracy of the reference values for an individual subject would be improved if the position of that subject in the normal range could be estimated more precisely. Theoretically this could be done by introducing more variables into the reference equation. In practice the

Table 15.22 Approximate values in healthy men at rest for some indices of pulmonary function which are not included in Tables 15.18–15.20; in most instances they also apply to women. For sources see references. SI units are given first; traditional units are in brackets

Index	Units	Age 20	Age 60
Ventilation and metabolism			
$\dot{V}_E$	$l\,min^{-1}$		6.0–10.0
$\dot{V}_A$	$l\,min^{-1}$		4.0–7.5
f_R	min^{-1}		12–20
Vd	ml	100	200
$\dot{n}_{O_2}$ ($\dot{V}_{O_2}$)	$mmol\,min^{-1}$		11–13 (250–300)
$\dot{n}_{CO_2}$ ($\dot{V}_{CO_2}$)	$(ml\,min^{-1})$		9–11 (200–240)
R			0.8 (0.7–0.9)
Gas exchange			
P_{A,CO_2}	kPa (mmHg)		4.7–6.1 (35–46)
P_{a,CO_2}	kPa (mmHg)		4.8–6.3 (36–47)
C_{CO_2}	$mmol\,l^{-1}$		24–34
P_{A,O_2}	kPa (mmHg)		13–15 (100–110)
P_{a,O_2}*	kPa (mmHg)	13.2 (99)	11.9 (89)
S_{a,O_2}	%	95–97.5	93–96
pH (arterial blood)	$-log_{10}\,cH$		7.45–7.35
cH	$nmol\,l^{-1}$		36–44
$\dot{V}_A/\dot{Q}$ relationships			
N_2 slope	$\%\,l^{-1}$		See Fig. 15.24
Closing volume	% of VC		See Fig. 15.24
F_{A,N_2} after 7 min of O_2	%	1.5	2.5
Lung clearance index	—	5–10	
$V_A\,eff/V_A$	—	0.9–1.0	0.85–0.95
$\dot{Q}va/\dot{Q}t$	%	2	4
$\dot{Q}s/\dot{Q}t$	%	1	2
Lung mechanics			
R total (Table 5.4)†	$kPa\,l^{-1}\,s$ ($cmH_2O\,l^{-1}\,s$)		0.12–0.44 (1.3–4.4)
Raw‡	$kPa\,l^{-1}\,s$ ($cmH_2O\,l^{-1}\,s$)		0.05–0.2 (0.5–2.0)
sGaw	$s^{-1}\,kPa^{-1}$ ($s^{-1}\,cmH_2O^{-1}$)		1.3–3.5 (0.13–0.35)
Cst§	$l\,kPa^{-1}$ ($l\,cmH_2O^{-1}$)		0.9–4.0 (0.09–0.40)
sC	kPa^{-1} (cmH_2O^{-1})		0.3–1.4 (0.03–0.14)
Recoil pr. (max)	kPa (cmH_2O)		1.2–3.7 (12–37)
(TLC-20% VC)¶		1.4 (14)	0.9 (9)
Cth	$l\,kPa^{-1}$ ($l\,cmH_2O^{-1}$)		1.0–3.5 (0.1–0.35)

* Pao_2 (SI) = 0.133 (104 – 0.24 age, RSD 7.9). Data of Raine & Bishop.
† The ECSC gives R total in SI units as < 0.3 and sGaw > 0.85 and > 1.04 in man and women respectively.
‡ Raw (SI) = (4.2/TGV: range (2.9–7.7)/TGV) ÷ 9.8. Data of Briscoe & DuBois.
§ Cst (SI) = 9.8 (0.353 St (m) – 0.347, RSD 0.081). Data of Bevan & McKerrow (unpublished), see also Frank *et al.*
¶ Pstat (TLC –20% VC) (SI) = (16.67 – 0.13 age, RSD 2.13) ÷ 9.8.
To convert the equations to traditional unity the term outside the parentheses should be omitted.

increase in accuracy which can be achieved is very small except where a previous result is available; this is particularly useful in children. Nor is it valid, except where the indices are highly correlated, to use the position of one index as a guide to the position of another; a value in the middle of the range for the one can be associated with a value at the limit of variability for another. Williams and others have pointed out that this is inevitable whenever an individual is described in terms

Table 15.23 Reference equations for predicting $\log_e$ peak expiratory flow measured by Wright peak flow meter (designated y, $l\,min^{-1}$) in Caucasian male and female non-smokers aged 15–85 years

$$
\left.
\begin{aligned}
y \text{ (males)} &= 0.544 \log_e A - 0.0151A - 74.7Ht^{-1} + 5.48 \\[4pt]
y \text{ (females)} &= 0.376 \log_e A - 0.012A - 58.8Ht^{-1} + 5.63
\end{aligned}
\right\} \text{RSD} \approx 46\,l\,min^{-1*}
$$

* Lower limit of normal $= (y - 75\,l\,min^{-1})$.
A is age in years, Ht is height in cm.
(Source: Nunn AJ, Gregg I. *Br Med J* 1989; **298**: 1068–1070.)

Table 15.24 Values for the standardised deviate (z) associated with different cumulative frequencies (percentiles) in a normal (Gaussian) distribution

	Percentile (%)	
z value*	z negative	z positive
1.960	2.5	97.5
1.645	5	95
1.282	10	90
1.036	15	85
0.842	20	80
0.674	25	75
0.524	30	70
0.385	35	65
0.253	40	60
0.126	45	55
0	50	50

* $z = (x - H)\,\sigma$, where x and H are respectively the observed and expected values: σ is residual standard deviation.

of a number of indices. Indeed, on account of bias which is introduced by averaging, it is virtually impossible for a subject to have average values for all the indices at one time! For this reason the accuracy of prediction is greatest when the mean value for a group of subjects is required. For individual subjects the accuracy of prediction is inevitably much less. Sobol has shown that it is least for subjects whose reference values lie at the lower end of the physiological range. This is because both the reference population will have contained relatively few of such subjects and the variability is usually of relatively constant magnitude over the range. The variability then represents a larger proportion of the total for the subjects with the lower than with the higher values. Thus, particularly at the ends of the normal distribution only limited importance should be attached to a single comparison of an observed with an expected value.

Greater reliance can be placed on a comparison involving several indices, especially when the differences between them comprise one of the characteristic syndromes of lung function, such as those for healthy subjects which are described in this chapter or for subjects with abnormal lungs in Chapter 16. However, even in such cases it is wise to consider the interpretation of each index in terms of only three categories, probably normal, borderline or slightly abnormal, and definitely abnormal. Greater precision than this is hardly justifiable when, at best, only 60% of the variability of the index can be accounted for in terms of the variables which are used for prediction. On this account the practice of reporting the results of tests of lung function as percentages of the predicted values conveys a spurious precision. It is preferable that the absolute values should themselves be reported together with a commentary of the type indicated. Any conclusion which is based solely upon the use of predicted values should, so far as possible, be confirmed by clinical, radiographic or other means. In addition, because of the bias in selection described above, an abnormal lung function result should not be the principal indication for medical or surgical treatment. Thus careful consideration should be given to the relevance of any predicted values before taking action based upon them.

Guide to references

The references (Chapter 18) are classified under subject headings of which the following are particularly relevant to the present chapter:

16: Lung Function in Disease

Introduction

Numerous medical conditions affect the lungs either directly or by involving the pulmonary circulation. The responses usually conform to one of a limited number of syndromes of disordered lung function (Table 16.1); the syndromes can usually be identified by measurement of the ventilatory capacity, lung volumes and transfer factor, but in some instances the mechanical function of the lung or the physiological response to exercise must also be assessed.

The presence of a particular syndrome constitutes a functional diagnosis; this will reflect, and in some instances indicate precisely, the underlying changes in structure. The lung function tests can provide information on causation only if there is a unique feature such as a

Table 16.1 Syndromes of disordered lung function (after Scadding)

Ventilatory defect*		
(a) Obstructive	(i)	Reversible
	(ii)	Fixed
	(iii)	Small airway syndrome
(b) Non-obstructive	(i)	Restrictive
	(ii)	Hypodynamic
Defect of gas transfer		
Alveolar hypoventilation		
(sleep apnoea syndrome)		
Bronchial hyper-responsiveness	(i)	Non-specific
	(ii)	Specific

* FEV_1 is reduced except in case of (a)(iii).

bronchoconstrictor response to a specific allergen. The tests can be used to measure disability, monitor the course of the condition and its response to treatment, assess residual exercise capacity, and indicate prognosis. In these ways the lung function laboratory makes an important contribution to respiratory medicine. The contribution is most effective when there is full exchange of information between the clinician and the laboratory on why assessments have been requested and, subsequently, on their contribution to the clinical outcome. This information should include any morbid anatomical findings which may influence lung function.

Classification of conditions

Classification of conditions

Referral to the lung function laboratory will usually be for a suspected condition of the airways or parenchyma of the lung (Table 16.2). Less often the main point of interest will be the chest wall, respiratory control system or pulmonary circulation. Patients with acute infections are seldom referred. Diseases of the airways can be localised — e.g. a tumour or polyp — or generalised (Table 5.6, page 113). Generalised conditions of the airways can present with cough and expectoration of phlegm, with wheeze which may be episodic, or with breathlessness on exertion. The classical causes are then chronic bronchitis, asthma and emphysema; their typical features are described in subsequent sections. However, the conditions may co-exist and all can be associated with airflow limitation so the distinction between them is not always clear cut. This has led to use of the terms CNLD (chronic non-specific lung disease), COLD (chronic obstruction lung disease), COPD (chronic

Table 16.2 General conditions of the lung which often lead to a patient being referred to the lung function laboratory: other conditions are given in the text

Condition	Common presentation	Features
Chronic bronchitis	Chronic cough and phlegm (e.g. on most days for ≥3 months in the year)	Mucous gland hyperplasia, inflammation of bronchial wall
Asthma	Episodic airflow limitation	Chronic eosinophilic bronchiolitis
Emphysema*	Progressive exercise dyspnoea	Alveolar destruction, enlarged airspaces
COLD and related conditions†	Progressive airflow limitation (often partly reversible)	Reflect aetiology
Diseases of lung parenchyma	Breathlessness with shallow breathing	See page 558
Restrictive disorders	Chest illness, swelling of ankles	See page 574
Disorders of pulmonary circulation‡	Dyspnoea, syncope, chest pain, right heart failure	See text
Pneumoconiosis	Cough, breathlessness on exertion	See text

* Usually gives rise to COLD; is included in COPD (see text).
† See Table 16.3.
‡ Including cardiac, hepatic, renal and vascular disorders.

515

Table 16.3 Diseases of airways which have features in common with chronic obstructive lung disease (COLD)

Bronchi involved	Mainly bronchiolitis
Asthma	Chemical injury
Cystic fibrosis	Virus infections
(bronchiectasis)	Graft-versus-host disease
Byssinosis	Following lung transplantation

(Modified from Pride NB. *Eur Respir J* 1990; **3**: 1078–1080.)

obstructive pulmonary disease) and CAO (chronic airways obstruction). CNLD describes chronic airflow limitation associated with chronic bronchitis, emphysema or asthma and carries the implication that one or more host factors (for example, atopic status) may contribute to the flow limitation. COLD describes airflow limitation which is progressive, mainly irreversible and yet is clearly not due to bronchiolitis or asthma of defined aetiology. Conditions related to COLD are listed in Table 16.3. COPD is nearly interchangeable with COLD but can also describe emphysema without airflow limitation. CAO describes airflow limitation associated with partial bronchial obstruction and should strictly exclude flow limitation due to a reduced elastic recoil pressure as occurs in emphysema. However, the terms are of limited usefulness because they are seldom used in a precise sense.

Grades of disordered lung function

Respiratory impairment

Respiratory function is impaired when it is demonstrably inferior to that of control subjects at one point in time or when observed longitudinally (Chapter 15). Impairment can be present without symptoms and it is then difficult to diagnose. The likelihood of the condition being recognised is increased if the subject is habitually more breathless on exertion than others of the same age and sex. For a subject who is accustomed to walking out of doors the clinical grade of breathlessness can be assessed using the four-point scale of Fletcher, or an extended version of it (Table 16.4). The questionnaire can be supplemented by the subject taking a walk (cf. page 437). For a subject who is not accustomed to walking, the degree of respiratory insufficiency can be assessed in terms of whether or not breathlessness is experienced during sport, when mounting stairs, carrying a basket, bucket or chair, parking a car not equipped with power-assisted steering, bathing, washing, shaving, singing, dressing and undressing, or during meals or conversation. The ability with respect to some of these activities is encapsulated in the oxygen cost diagram of McGavin and colleagues (Fig. 13.2, page 388). To make a more precise assessment the capacity for exercise should be determined in the manner described on page 433.

Table 16.4 Clinical grades of breathlessness of Fletcher and related ability scores proposed by Cotes. The grades are assessed using the MRC Questionnaire on Respiratory Symptoms* where comparison is made with a healthy man of the same age. The levels of forced expiratory volume (FEV_1) are for men aged 50–75 years from Welsh mining valleys; they are approximate and the ranges are wide. The ability to take exercise is affected adversely by increasing age and by increasing body mass

Description	Clinical grade	Ability score	FEV_1
Is living: needs help with feeding	–	8	0.3
With help can dress and sit out of bed	–	7	0.5
Can converse, walk 10 m, bath with help	–	6	0.7
Can walk 100 m, sing, climb 8 stairs	–	5	1.1
Can walk 400 m	4	4	1.6
Can walk unlimited distance at slow pace	3	3	2.1
Can walk at normal pace on level ground without becoming breathless	2	2	2.6
Can hurry on level ground and walk uphill without undue breathlessness	1	1	3.1

* Obtained from the Medical Research Council, 20 Park Crescent, London W1N 4AL, UK.

Respiratory insufficiency

A subject with respiratory impairment is in a state of respiratory insufficiency if the tensions of oxygen and carbon dioxide in the arterial blood lie outside the range of normal variation. In the case of carbon dioxide, a tension at sea level which is consistently more than 6.3 kPa (47 mmHg) is regarded as abnormal. However, the definition does not apply to subjects breathing oxygen during strenuous exercise when the tension of carbon dioxide is normally increased (page 344). While breathing air the lower limits of oxygen tension are the same at rest and on exercise. At age 20 years a tension of oxygen of slightly less than 11 kPa (83 mmHg) and at age 60 years of less than 10 kPa (76 mmHg) indicates mild respiratory failure. The corresponding oxygen saturations are 95% and 93%. The tension of oxygen which indicates a serious derangement of lung function varies with circumstances; at sea level a reduction on account of lung disease to less than 8 kPa (60 mmHg) is always a cause for concern.

Syndromes of abnormal lung function

An *obstructive type of ventilatory defect* is usually diagnosed from a reduced $FEV_1\%$ (FEV_1/FVC) or from a reduced peak expiratory flow associated with a prolonged forced expiratory time. The condition is associated with premature closure of airways during expiration: this has implications for other aspects of lung function (page 529). Since the expiration is forced the airway closure is accentuated by dynamic compression which reduces the forced vital capacity relative to the inspiratory vital capacity (IVC). On this account the $FEV_1\%$ is reduced to a lesser extent than the Tiffeneau index (FEV_1/IVC) which is widely

517

used for diagnosis of airflow limitation in some western European countries.

The obstructive type of ventilatory defect can be described as reversible or irreversible. The criterion for reversibility is a meaningful increase in FEV_1 or PEF following inhalation of a bronchodilator aerosol which for FEV_1 has been defined by Tweeddale and colleagues as 190 ml. An increase of at least 12% is also accepted (e.g. by the American Thoracic Society, page 148). However, airflow limitation which does not initially respond to a bronchodilator aerosol can do so following steroid therapy; thus the distinction between reversibility and irreversibility is often not clear cut. Reversibility originally served to distinguish asthma from other types of airflow limitation; it is now mainly used in relation to bronchodilator therapy.

A *non-obstructive ventilatory defect* is a diminution in ventilatory capacity which is not due to limitation of airflow. It can be restrictive or hypodynamic in type and due to changes within the lung or chest wall, including weakness of the respiratory muscles. The principal diagnostic feature is reduction of both FEV_1 and FVC: hence the $FEV_1\%$ is normal or increased. These features are usually unambiguous. However, in patients with airflow limitation they can be mimicked if the forced vital capacity is disproportionately reduced by breathlessness or by predominant narrowing of small airways. The ambiguity is avoided by including as an additional criterion that the total lung capacity is reduced; TLC should be measured by plethysmography or a radiographic method to take account of non-ventilated airspaces.

A *restrictive ventilatory defect* of pulmonary origin is usually due to a decrease in the distensibility of the lung (i.e. the lung compliance is reduced). The reduction can be due to an increase in the quantity of interstitial tissue in the lung, for example interstitial pneumonitis, fibrosis, infiltration or oedema. Alternatively, the reduced lung compliance can be due to fibrosis of the visceral pleura and sub-pleural tissue. Any of these changes can increase the retractive force exerted on the walls of lung airways; the retraction reduces the airways resistance and increases the $FEV_1\%$. The peak expiratory flow and maximal breathing capacity are then well preserved (Fig. 16.1) so these indices cannot be used to make the diagnosis. Other changes are described on page 559.

A restrictive defect of intrapulmonary origin can be mimicked by a space-occupying lesion of the lung or pleura including pneumothorax; this reduces the lung volumes and FEV_1. It can also reduce the ventilation and perfusion of the affected part of the lung. Other aspects of lung function are often normal.

When the restrictive defect arises in the chest wall, the compliance of the lung is normal, but the compliance of the chest wall is decreased. This change can be a consequence of severe obesity, or a disease process affecting the ribs or the vertebral column, for example ankylosing spondylitis or kyphoscoliosis (page 575).

In the *hypodynamic type*, the ventilatory defect is due to a reduction in the maximal force that can be exerted by the respiratory muscles and this reduces the vital capacity (page 577). The principal diagnostic feature is then a low maximal inspiratory pressure (page 578).

The *syndrome of defective gas transfer* is characterised by a reduced transfer factor. In the absence of complicating factors the ventilatory response to exercise is increased. There may also be exercise hypoxaemia. The syndrome is associated with abnormalities of the lung parenchyma including interstitial pneumonitis, interstitial fibrosis and emphysema. In the former conditions there is also likely to be a restrictive type of ventilatory defect whilst with emphysema the other features of that condition will coexist (page 535).

The prominence of hyperventilation on exercise first attracted notice to the condition, which was then thought to be psychogenic in origin. Subsequently, Riley and others demonstrated the presence of hypoxaemia on exercise, and showed that the diffusing capacity of the lung for oxygen was reduced. This led to the theory that the syndrome was due to insufficient diffusion of oxygen across the thickened alveolar membranes, hence to *alveolar capillary block*. Later, Finley and others pointed out that oxygen had a high diffusivity so this aspect of gas exchange was unlikely to be seriously impaired except with pulmonary oedema; thus the term alveolar capillary block syndrome appeared to be inappropriate. Instead, the reduction of transfer factor and the associated hypoxaemia on exercise were believed to be due to other factors, for example included splinting or enlargement of respiratory

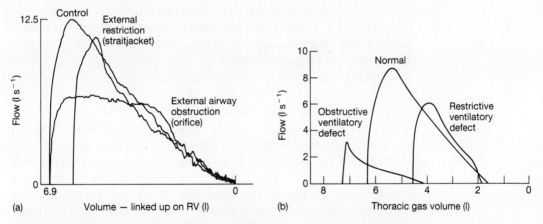

Fig. 16.1 Maximal expiratory flow–volume curves showing the changes associated with external and internal airway obstruction and restriction to lung expansion. (a) Normal subject breathing through a 6 mm orifice and wearing a strait jacket. The effect of the orifice resembled that of narrowing of the trachea (Fig. 5.13b, page 116) and the effect of the restriction resembled that of an incomplete inspiration. (b) Patients with COPD and pleural plus diffuse interstitial fibrosis. COPD was associated with an obstructive type of ventilatory defect (curve concave upwards); residual volume was increased but FEV_1, FVC, $FEV_1\%$, and all maximal flow rates were reduced. Extensive lung fibrosis (due to asbestos) reduced the total lung capacity and FEV_1, but compared with the healthy subject the $FEV_1\%$ was increased; relative to the absolute lung volume the maximal flow rates were apparently increased as well. (See also Figs 5.13a and 5.17, pages 115 and 125.)

bronchioles increasing the path length for diffusion in the airspaces (cf. Fig. 7.3, page 185), and the destruction of some alveolar capillaries increasing the rate of flow of blood through the remainder. The time for which the red cells were in contact with the alveolar gas might then be too short for gas exchange to continue to equilibrium (Fig. 9.4, page 284). Thus the exercise hypoxaemia was attributed to imperfect distribution of the surface which was available for the exchange of gas with respect to lung volume (Tl/V_A inequality), to blood flow (Tl/Qc inequality) and to lung capillary blood volume (Tl/Vc inequality, see also page 322). Hypoxaemia from these causes occurs principally on exercise. In addition the structural changes were believed to cause maldistribution of ventilation with respect to perfusion and hence to hypoxaemia at rest by mechanisms which are given in Chapter 7. Recent work from several sources including Rodriguez-Roisin and his colleagues in Barcelona and Hughes and his colleagues in London have largely confirmed this dual explanation for the hypoxaemia; however, the relative contributions of the distributive and diffusive components are still in doubt.

The features of defective gas transfer can be obscured by any coexisting mechanical derangement of the lung. Where this is minimal, as in some pulmonary infiltrations, the hypoxaemia and possibly other factors increase the drive to respiration causing marked hyperventilation at rest as well as on exercise. The hyperventilation partly corrects the hypoxaemia; it also leads to hypocapnia and to a compensatory re-adjustment to the acid−base balance of the body which is described below. In other patients there is a material restrictive, obstructive or hypodynamic type of ventilatory defect; these reduce the ventilatory response to exercise and accentuate the ventilation perfusion inequality. The degree of exercise desaturation is then increased. Thus the effects of defective gas transfer upon exercise ventilation and the arterial oxygen tension can be represented by a continuum with the ventilatory and blood gas components being to some extent negatively correlated.

The *syndrome of primary alveolar hypoventilation* is characterised by an overall reduction in the level of alveolar ventilation in the absence of disease of the lungs. The hypoventilation causes hypercapnia both directly (e.g. Fig. 9.1, page 266) and by increasing the proportion of alveoli which are poorly ventilated relative to their perfusion (page 205). The commonest cause is sleep apnoea syndrome. This and other types of alveolar hypoventilation are considered on page 579.

Acid−base balance of the blood and cerebrospinal fluid

The acid−base balance of the body is affected by any alteration in the balance between total alveolar ventilation and perfusion, and to a lesser extent by local inequalities of ventilation−perfusion ratios. An increase in alveolar ventilation augments the excretion of carbon dioxide and reduces the amounts of both carbon dioxide and the products of dissociation of carbonic acid which remain in the blood; this process is described as *respiratory alkalosis*. Some causes are given in Table 16.5.

Table 16.5 Some causes of respiratory alkalosis

Stimulus to hyperventilation	Circumstances	Page
Cerebral cortex	Voluntary or psychogenic over-breathing, anxiety	586
Hypoxaemia	Hypoxic gas mixture, ascent to altitude, acute asthma attack	612
Pulmonary J receptor stimulation	Mitral stenosis, left ventricular failure, pulmonary oedema, pulmonary embolism	334, 599
Multiple causes	Syndrome of defective gas transfer*	558
Increased central drive to respiration	Hyperthermia, salicylate poisoning	338
Over-ventilation	Respirator therapy	647

* Especially in absence of restrictive ventilatory defect.

A decrease in alveolar ventilation has the opposite effect of increasing the amounts of carbon dioxide and its derivatives which are present in the blood; this process is described as a *respiratory acidosis*. It has many causes of which some are listed in Table 16.18 (page 580). Other causes include chronic mountain sickness and breathing a gas containing carbon dioxide.

The process of respiratory alkalosis, when it is of sudden onset, is associated with an initial fall in the concentrations of carbonic acid and hydrogen ions and a rise in the pH of the blood (Fig. 16.2). There is then a fall in the blood concentration of ionised calcium which may give rise to tetany. However, the kidneys immediately compensate for the alkalaemia by increasing the excretion of sodium bicarbonate. The effects of this are detectable within a few hours and in 2 or 3 days the pH is restored to very near to the initial value. For a subject who has travelled to live at high altitude the blood pH returns to normal more slowly, taking about a month; the longer time is due to interaction with other effects of hypoxaemia (page 358). Respiratory alkalosis occurring as a result of medical conditions (Table 16.5) is seldom completely compensated.

Respiratory acidosis of sudden origin has the converse effect of causing an initial rise in the concentrations of carbonic acid and hydrogen ions and a fall in the pH of the blood. However, due to buffering by constituents of blood, the changes in pH are small in relation to the quantities of hydrogen ions which are involved; the important buffer systems based on carbon dioxide and bicarbonate are illustrated in Fig. 9.5 (page 287). The acidaemia also sets in motion compensatory adjustments which further reduce the imbalance; of these the most important is an increase in the excretion by the kidney of hydrogen ions combined as ammonium salts and as acid phosphates:

$$NH_3 + H^+ \rightleftharpoons NH_4^+ \qquad (16.1)$$

521

$$HPO_4^- + 2H^+ \rightleftharpoons H_2 + PO_4^- \qquad (16.2)$$

These reactions replace urinary sodium ions by hydrogen ions. The changes lower the pH of the urine and increase the concentration of sodium in the blood where it is associated with an increase in the concentration of bicarbonate. Other tissues also contribute to the changes; these come into effect rapidly at first and subsequently more slowly, until the blood hydrogen ion concentration is restored to near to its initial value. However, in respiratory acidosis, unlike respiratory alkalosis occurring at high altitude, the compensation for the change in cH is seldom complete; instead the cH usually remains somewhat below the initial value (Fig. 16.2).

A change in the tension of carbon dioxide in the jugular venous blood leads to an equivalent movement of the gas into or out of the

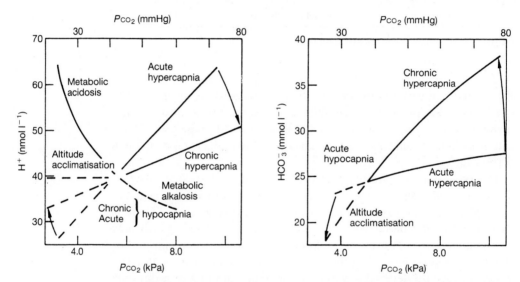

Fig. 16.2 Adaptation of the buffering capacity of the blood to a change in the tension of carbon dioxide. The diagrams show steady state values for the blood hydrogen ion concentration and plasma bicarbonate at a range of tensions of carbon dioxide produced by breathing mixtures of CO_2 in air. The relationships are given below in SI units. (For P_{CO_2} in mmHg the conversion factor 7.5 should be omitted). The data for acute hypercapnia were obtained in healthy subjects by Brackett, Cohen and Schwartz:

$$H^+ = 0.77 \times 7.5 P_{CO_2} + 8.0$$
$$HCO_3^- = 24.7 \times 7.5 P_{CO_2} \div (0.77 \times 7.5 P_{CO_2} + 8.0)$$

The data for chronic hypercapnia were obtained in patients with chronic lung disease by Van Ypersele de Strihou, Brasseur and de Coninck:

$$H^+ = 0.3 \times 7.5 P_{CO_2} + 26.8$$
$$HCO_3^- = 24.7 \times 7.5 P_{CO_2} \div (0.3 \times 7.5 P_{CO_2} + 26.8)$$

The relationship for primary metabolic acidosis was obtained by Bone, Cowie, Lambie and Robson:

$$P_{CO_2} = 962 \div (7.5 \times ([H^+] - 12))$$

The data for hypocapnia before and after acclimatization to high altitude (in healthy subjects), and for chronic hypocapnia at sea level (in patients with lung disease) are based on measurements made by Lambertsen, Dill and Dulfano and their respective collaborators.

522

cerebrospinal fluid, but the area of surface across which the exchange takes place is relatively small. Thus, although a change in the cerebrospinal fluid is detectable within 1 min of an alteration of the tension in the blood, the time for equilibrium is probably materially longer. Buffering in the cerebrospinal fluid is dependent on electrolytes rather than on proteins, which buffer the blood. Consequently, at equilibrium, the tension of carbon dioxide is on average higher than that in the arterial blood by about 1 kPa (8 mmHg) and the pH is correspondingly lower (mean value approximately 7.33). In addition a change in the tension of carbon dioxide produces a somewhat larger change in pH. However, as in the case of blood, the deviation from the normal pH is reduced over a period of days. The compensation is achieved by the active transport of ions across the blood-to-CSF barrier. Before the compensation is complete, the brain is particularly vulnerable to a change in the tension of carbon dioxide. For this reason, the condition of carbon dioxide narcosis is more likely to occur following a rise in P_{CO_2} which is of moderate size but rapid onset, than a larger rise which occurs more slowly.

The acid—base balance of the blood is influenced not only by CO_2 but also by the levels of other proton donors and bases (i.e. proton acceptors). The levels are affected by the ingestion, metabolism and excretion of substances with acid—base properties. The respective processes are described as metabolic acidosis, or metabolic alkalosis, depending on whether they tend to increase or to decrease the accumulation of acid in the body.

Metabolic acidosis is caused by accumulation of acids other than carbonic acid or depletion of bicarbonate. The acids include β-hydroxybutyric acid and acetoacetic acid; these substances are produced from fatty acids when carbohydrate metabolism is impaired, as in diabetic keto-acidosis, or the quantity of carbohydrate is reduced by starvation or persistent vomiting. However, vomiting is associated with loss of gastric acid so the net effect on the blood hydrogen ion concentration is unpredictable. Renal failure is associated with acidosis because of a reduced ability to conserve bicarbonate and to excrete an acid urine. Bicarbonate can also be lost from the gastro-intestinal tract as a result of diarrhoea, intestinal fistula or intestinal aspiration.

Increased production of lactic acid is an important cause of metabolic acidosis. The site of production is either generalised or mainly in the liver which can change from being a net consumer of lactic acid, converting it to carbohydrate, to being a producer. These two groups of disorders have been called type A and type B by Cohen and Woods. Increased hepatic production (type B) can occur in diabetes mellitus, liver disease, acute alcoholic intoxication and treatment with oral hypoglycaemic biguanides such as phenformin. The type A lactacidaemia can occur transiently when exercise is limited by the capacity of the circulation (Chapter 13); it can occur over a longer period following a reduction in cardiac output due to shock, or as a result of hypoxaemia due to acute respiratory failure or cardiac arrest.

Acidaemia increases the level of ventilation (Chapter 11); this enhances the excretion of carbonic acid as carbon dioxide which in turn increases the capacity of the buffer systems of the blood to neutralise the invading acid. The compensation is not complete since, whilst the pH of the blood is lowered by the production of acid, that of the cerebrospinal fluid, because of the relative impermeability of the blood-to-CSF barrier, is initially unaffected. Subsequently, following the blowing off of carbon dioxide (described as compensatory respiratory alkalosis), the pH of the cerebrospinal fluid rises temporarily, and this has the effect of limiting the rise in the overall drive to respiration. However, the increase in ventilation is usually sufficient to secure time for the kidney to correct the acidaemia in other ways.

Metabolic alkalosis is characterised by a reduction in blood hydrogen ion concentration from loss of fixed acids or accumulation of bicarbonate. The commonest cause is loss of hydrochloric acid from vomiting, as with pyloric stenosis, or gastric aspiration. The loss of acid is then accompanied by loss of chloride which promotes the reabsorption and retention of bicarbonate by the renal tubules. Chloride depletion can occur during treatment with diuretic drugs including thiazides and frusemide. Metabolic alkalosis can also be due to ingestion of basic substances including sodium bicarbonate.

Depletion of intracellular potassium is an important cause of metabolic alkalosis. This occurs from the potassium ions being replaced by hydrogen ions which migrate into the cells from the extracellular fluid; the concentration of hydrogen ions in extracellular fluid falls in consequence and the blood pH rises. Potassium deficiency can be due to an inadequate diet, loss from the gastro-intestinal tract, or increased excretion in the urine. Increased renal loss of potassium occurs in a number of conditions including diuretic therapy, primary aldosteronism, Cushing's syndrome and treatment with corticosteroid drugs or carbenoxolone. Potassium excretion is also increased in acidosis when it is secondary to migration of potassium ions from the intracellular to extracellular compartments.

Depletion of hydrogen ions reduces the drive to respiration; this can lead to hypercapnia which, when it occurs, usually corrects the acidaemia. However, if the patient is taking depressant drugs or has some condition which predisposes to chronic respiratory acidosis (page 579) the superimposition of a metabolic alkalosis can precipitate carbon dioxide narcosis (page 580). The changes in the blood can be represented in terms of the arterial blood concentration of plasma bicarbonate, and tension of carbon dioxide (Fig. 16.3). Alternatively the changes can be analysed in terms of the relationship of the hydrogen ion concentration to the tension of carbon dioxide as in the left hand part of Fig. 16.2.

Respiratory distress in the newborn

Almost all babies make a successful transition from the conditions of intra-uterine to those of extra-uterine life; the associated physiological

524

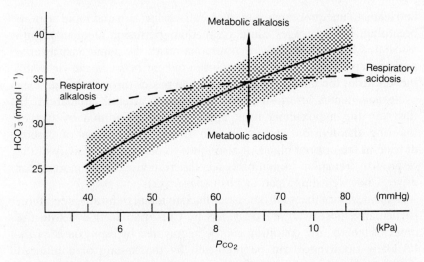

Fig. 16.3 Diagram illustrating the acid–base equilibrium in chronic hypercapnia. The broad line is the relationship of the plasma bicarbonate to the tension of carbon dioxide during chronic hypercapnia (from Fig. 16.2): the shaded area provides an estimate of the 95% confidence limits (these were obtained on dogs). The upward vertical arrow shows metabolic alkalosis, as may occur after vomiting or ingestion of sodium bicarbonate; the associated rise in blood pH can reduce the drive to respiration. The downward vertical arrow shows metabolic acidosis, as may occur after administration of a carbonic anhydrase inhibitor. The effects of recent improvement in alveolar ventilation and of acute hypercapnia from any cause are shown by the interrupted lines; these are based on the carbon dioxide titration curves for healthy men breathing mixtures of CO_2 in air shown as the lower line in the right hand half of Fig. 16.2. The corresponding blood hydrogen ion concentrations can be obtained by reference to the left hand half of Fig. 16.2. (Source: Cohen JJ, Schwartz WB. *Am J Med* 1966; **41**: 163–167.)

changes are described on page 448. However, a very small minority (about 1%) have difficulty in breathing either at birth or within the first 2 h thereafter. The condition usually occurs amongst babies who are premature; in some it is transient, whilst in others it progresses. The depth of respiration then decreases and the respiratory rate rises to between 60 and 100 breaths per min; the chest wall appears to be drawn in during inspiration and the infant makes a grunting noise during expiration. Cyanosis develops and, in the absence of ventilatory support, often is not corrected by the administration of oxygen; the hypoxaemia is associated with hypercapnia. The duration of the illness is usually less than 3 days. The more premature the baby the worse the prognosis; in treated cases it is excellent for babies of more than 28 weeks gestation. At post-mortem some respiratory bronchioles, alveolar ducts and atria are found to be lined with hyaline eosinophilic material and many air-sacs and alveoli contain no air; there may be numerous haemorrhages. Avery, Mead and Pattle were the first to show that fluid extracted from the lung does not have the property of lowering the surface tension at an air-to-water interface. The deficiency of surface-active material is due mainly to immaturity affecting its synthesis by the type II alveolar pneumonocytes (page 96). The high surface tension reduces the lung compliance and the functional residual capacity, and leads to unequal expansion of alveoli, atelectases and rapid shallow breathing; these changes cause ventilation–perfusion inequality, with associated hypoxaemia. The hypoxaemia raises the pulmonary arterial pressure and hence alters the pressure gradient between the right and the left atria; the mixed venous blood then passes through the foramen ovale and ductus arteriosus into the systemic arterial circulation. In this way the hypoxaemia itself aggravates the condition by further lowering the tension of oxygen and raising the tension of carbon dioxide in the arterial blood. It also tends to depress the activity of the respiratory reticular formation since the response to chemoreceptor drive is not well developed at birth (page 354).

In the newborn the syndrome is confined to infants who are premature, particularly those who are delivered by Caesarian section before the onset of labour; the condition can be aggravated by asphyxia at birth. Its likely occurrence can be predicted by the finding of a reduced concentration of lecithin relative to sphingomyelin in the amniotic fluid immediately prior to parturition. It can be prevented by measures to avoid prematurity, and by administration to the mother of a glucocorticoid drug 48 h before birth to stimulate surfactant production in the fetus. Once developed, the condition usually resolves spontaneously through the reversal of the lung pathology on the third to fifth day and the long-term prognosis is excellent. In the acute stages before this change takes place the life of the baby can usually be preserved by the administration of oxygen; this may need supplementing by assisted ventilation using continuous positive airway pressure or controlled ventilation with positive end expiratory pressure (page 649). Alternatively, if the lungs prove difficult to ventilate, extra-corporeal gas exchange can be used instead. The condition is likely to be eliminated by the use of genetically engineered exogenous surfactant when this becomes generally available.

Respiratory distress syndrome in adults is described on page 569.

Acute respiratory infections

The common cold or an infection with influenza virus can precipitate acute bronchitis; those most at risk are young children, the elderly and patients with chronic bronchitis (page 529). In addition, an uncomplicated viral infection is often associated with changes in the lung, including a reduction in the transfer factor as measured by the steady state method and evidence of narrowing of the small airways, but the forced expiratory volume, vital capacity and maximal expiratory flow rate ($MEF_{50\% \ FVC}$) are not usually affected. An acute infection of the lower respiratory tract or lung parenchyma can cause gross impairment of lung function both directly and through its secondary effects. Narrowing of the airways by inflammation and secretions increases the airway resistance and reduces the ventilatory capacity. Changes in the lung parenchyma, including congestion of the alveolar capillaries, interstitial oedema and exudation into the alveoli, reduce the lung compliance and the transfer factor; the changes also causes uneven distribution of pulmonary ventilation and perfusion. This gives rise to hypoxaemia and sometimes hypercapnia (page 204). The effects can be aggravated by the infection causing weakness of the respiratory muscles (page 577) or by inflammation of the pleura. The latter then leads to shallow breathing, impairs coughing and further reduces the vital capacity. Other facets of lung function are impaired to a variable extent, including the drive to respiration; this may be reduced either as a direct result of the pneumonia or as a side effect of the treatment. The management of oxygen therapy and the possible role of assisted ventilation in these circumstances are discussed in Chapter 17.

Borderline between health and disease

Respiratory symptom questionnaires

In healthy persons transient productive cough, wheeze or breathlessness on moderate exertion can occur during acute infections of the upper or lower respiratory tract. Persistence of the symptoms is usually evidence of chronic disease which in most instances will be in the lungs. The presence and severity of the symptom is explored using the Medical Research Council Questionnaire of Respiratory Symptoms (page 517). The questionnaire was designed for use in respiratory surveys of chronic bronchitis and emphysema in conjunction with measurement of ventilatory capacity. To this end the questions were about cough, phlegm production, wheeze, breathlessness on exertion, previous chest illness and smoking history. Additional questions can be added which are relevant for investigation of asthma, angina of effort and occupational lung disorders. The intensity of coughing can be assessed using a scoring technique developed by Field. A persistent productive cough is evidence of *chronic bronchitis*; this condition is characterised by increased secretion of mucus, hypertrophy of mucous secretory glands and often bronchial inflammation. The condition is compatible with normal lung function and life expectancy. However, airflow obstruction often coexists. Conversely the lung function can be impaired in subjects who are asymptomatic. Thus the symptoms and the lung function should both be considered.

Tests of lung function

The ventilatory capacity represented by the forced expiratory volume and vital capacity is the principal screening test for the presence of airflow limitation. It is used in respiratory surveys for investigating the contribution of genetic and environmental factors to respiratory impairment. The result is expressed by the parameters of multiple regression equations in which the FEV_1 is described by terms for age, stature, other nuisance variables and the factors under consideration (page 63). Other ventilatory tests can also be used but the variability about

527

the equation is usually greater than for the FEV_1 (page 132) so the description of airflow limitation in the population being investigated is less complete.

The FEV_1 is insensitive to narrowing of small lung airways so this condition is likely to be missed unless appropriate tests are used. The choice then includes the residual volume and the closing capacity both of which are increased relative to the total lung capacity, i.e. the ratio indices RV/TLC and CC/TLC are increased. In addition the airway narrowing impairs intrapulmonary mixing, so the slope of the alveolar plateau for nitrogen following a breath of oxygen is increased (page 214) and the alveolar volume measured by a single breath method (V_A eff) is less than that by other methods (V_A eff/V_A is reduced). The indices $FEV_1\%$, RV% and V_A eff/V_A are combined in the obstruction index (page 222). In the presence of a normal FEV_1 an abnormal result for one of these indices may be associated with a slightly increased risk that the FEV_1 will decline in the future. But the association is not always present and the concept of sensitive tests of small airway disease which will supplement the FEV_1 has not stood the test of time. Recent evidence based on comparison with lung histology by Paiva and colleagues suggested that of a number of such tests, the difference in slope of the single breath alveolar plateaus for helium and sulphur hexafluoride is most closely related to small airway disease (page 221). The slope of the single breath nitrogen plateau was not correlated with the anatomical changes.

Risk factors for chronic obstructive lung disease

Exposure to risk factors often produces symptoms and the advent of symptoms often modifies exposure. In addition the different risk factors may interact. Thus any description of their effects is inevitably approximate. The problem is greatest in the case of smoking, which is the principal cause of airway narrowing that is not due to asthma. The decision whether or not to take up regular smoking is influenced by other risk factors for COLD including social class, atopy and bronchial hyperreactivity (page 174). Thus a person is likely to take up smoking and subsequently to smoke heavily if the parents smoke, the working environment is one where smoking is usual, for example some shipyards, and the person does not have bronchial hyperreactivity. Conversely the development of symptoms may prevent a person from taking up regular smoking or cause him or her to cut down on the amount smoked or to give up altogether. The existence of these interactions leads to populations of non-smokers differing from smokers in a number of respects, and not just in their use of tobacco. They are a reason for obtaining reference values on whole populations including smokers and not just on non-smokers (page 446). This strategy involves the investigator in making an appropriate allowance for the amount smoked; the allowance should take into account both short-term and long-term effects (page 482). Some risk factors which have been shown to impair lung function in populations though not necessarily in individuals are

Table 16.6 Risk factor for chronic airflow limitation (for sources, see page 707)

Positive factors	Neutral factors
Smoking, active or passive*	Acute bronchitis†
	Whooping cough†
Air pollution,*	
Domestic (e.g. coal fires)	Altitude‡
Environmental (e.g. SO_2, NO_2, O_3)	Ambient temperature‡
Occupational	
Constitutional	
Factors related to atopy§	
α_1 antitrypsin deficiency	
Ethnic group (esp. Caucasians)	
Gender (men > women)	
Other*	
Low socio-economic status, low birth weight	
Damp house	

* Also contributes to chronic bronchitis.
† From childhood onwards; in infancy the lung is more vulnerable.
‡ Extreme cold can be harmful.
§ Especially eosinophilia and bronchial hyperreactivity.

given in Table 16.6. Some Dutch workers have evidence that the most important is atopic status which is a feature of approximately 20% of most populations (page 547); nearly half such subjects exhibit bronchial hyperreactivity in response to an appropriate stimulus (Table 16.12, page 555).

Chronic obstructive pulmonary disease (COPD)

Predominant airway disease

Chronic obstructive pulmonary disease (COPD) describes the patient with narrowing of lung airways which is not due to asthma or the other conditions listed in Table 16.3. Some contributory causes are given in Table 16.6. The narrowing can involve the large airways from the start of the illness in which case the forced expiratory volume is reduced throughout the course. Alternatively the narrowing can start in the small airways. In the latter circumstances the maximal expiratory flow rate ($MEF_{25\%\ FVC}$) is reduced but the FEV_1 is initially normal (cf. Between Health and Disease, page 527). Subsequently all classes of airway are likely to be affected. At this stage further deterioration is probable unless the cause is removed. The progressive narrowing of airways has structural and functional components (Table 5.6, page 113). These interact, as already shown for the structural support that normally contributes to the patency of lung airways (page 97).

Ventilatory capacity and lung volume. The patient will usually have respiratory symptoms and these can be recorded using the MRC questionnaire (Table 16.4, page 517). The course of the disease is best monitored using the FEV_1 which should be measured each time the patient is seen. Where possible this should be done before and after administration of a bronchodilator aerosol (page 145) as part of the obstruction is usually reversible. An example is given in Case Study 16.1. The maximal mid-expiratory flow (MMEF) can also be used to monitor the early stages but this test is insensitive when the condition is advanced (page 140).

The calibre of the airways decreases during expiration on account of reduced traction from the lung parenchyma. This effect is superimposed on the narrowing due to disease. It leads to closure of airways at larger lung volumes than would otherwise be the case. Thus the residual volume and the closing volume are increased (Fig. 16.4) whilst the relaxed expiratory vital capacity (EVC) and inspiratory vital capacity (IVC) are reduced. During forced expiration the closure of airways is enhanced by dynamic compression; this reduces the forced vital capacity (FVC) relative to the EVC and IVC. The effect is maximal with emphysema (page 537) but also occurs without it. The narrowing and

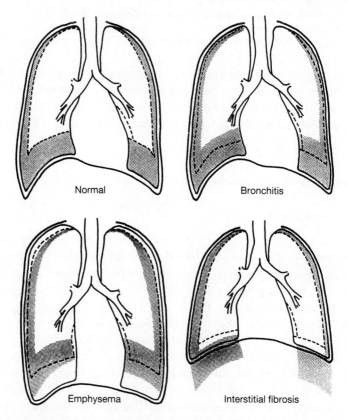

Normal

Bronchitis

Emphysema

Interstitial fibrosis

Fig. 16.4 Outlines of chest radiographs taken on inspiration and expiration. They show the relationships of lung expansion to lung size in patients with predominant airway disease, emphysema and interstitial fibrosis. The area inside the dashed line reflects the residual volume and that outside it the vital capacity. The relationship in healthy subjects, shown in the top left hand quadrant, is reproduced as the shaded areas in the other quadrants.

530

Case Study 16.1 Lung function in patients with COPD

Mild

Mr A. was a machine fitter aged 51 years, who, 18 months before the consultation, developed a head cold which went to his chest. Before this he coughed occasionally but was otherwise in good health; subsequently he had a persistent cough with morning sputum and episodes of wheeze and tightness of the chest. He smoked 20 cigarettes per day. The remaining medical history was unexceptional, as was the physical examination, the chest X-ray and the electrocardiogram. On assessment of lung function the FEV_1 was reduced and represented a smaller proportion than normal of the forced vital capacity (FEV_1% reduced). The FVC was less than the IVC; this was evidence for dynamic compression during forced expiration. The FEV_1 was increased following the inhalation of a bronchodilator aerosol. The dynamic lung compliance was less than the static measurement. The other indices of lung function were within normal limits. The findings were typical of moderate airway obstruction in a patient with bronchitis. In this instance the sputum and wheeze disappeared and the FEV_1 increased from 1.8l to 2.4l after a course of antibiotic drugs; the patient was advised to give up smoking.

Advanced

Mr B. entered the coal-mines at the age of 13 years. He was a light smoker. At the age of 23 he had the first of many episodes of bronchitis and at 34 he moved from the mines into light employment. He gave up work at the age of 49. Two years later during an acute chest illness Mr B. was observed to have a severe productive cough, an audible wheeze and coarse rhonchi and crepitations over both lung bases. His chest radiograph did not show specific changes; bronchograms were negative for bronchiestasis. The cardiac outline, the ECG and the haemoglobin concentration were within normal limits. Assessment of lung function showed evidence of gross obstruction to the lung airways but with a normal transfer factor. Five years later, at the age of 56, Mr B. developed congestive cardiac failure during an acute chest illness. The ECG then showed the features of pulmonary heart disease and the mean pressure in the pulmonary artery at rest was 39mmHg. The haemoglobin concentration was increased. These conditions responded to treatment which included long-term oxygen therapy. Oxygen from a portable apparatus and later from an oxygen line improved the capacity for exercise.

For the last 4 years of his life Mr B. had marked hypoxaemia

Continued on p. 532

Case Study 16.1 *Continued*

and hypercapnia $Pa,o_2 < 5.3$ kPa (<40 mmHg), $Pa,co_2 > 8.0$ kPa (>60 mmHg) and frequent acute exacerbations of his respiratory and cardiac failure; in several of these he required assisted ventilation for the treatment of carbon dioxide narcosis. He died suddenly at the age of 65 following an injury sustained at home.

At post-mortem the bronchi exhibited evidence of chronic inflammation and the pulmonary arteries showed atheroma and thickening of their walls; an old thrombus partly occluded the left main pulmonary artery. The lung contained emphysematous bullae at the apices and along the fissures, but the parenchyma was relatively intact.

Emphysema

Mr C., aged 48 years, was a Civil Servant, who presented with breathlessness on exertion (Grade 3) and recurrent episodes of cough and sputum of 7 years' duration. He gave a history of being chesty as a child, but his symptoms cleared up completely during adolescence. As a young man he passed the medical examination for the RAF as Grade 1 and he lost only a very few days from work prior to the onset of breathlessness. It was after this that he developed bronchitis. He smoked 14 cigarettes per day, reducing to six per day during periods of chest illness. On examination he was breathless, cyanosed and underweight; his chest was held in an inspiratory position and the percussion note was hyper-resonant. The breath sounds were faint, expiration was prolonged and soft sibilant rhonchi were present at both bases posteriorly. The chest X-ray showed increased transradiancy and the vascular markings in the periphery of the lung fields were reduced. The ECG showed deep S waves in V_6 but was otherwise normal.

On assessment of lung function the FEV_1 was greatly reduced, but increased in response to a bronchodilator aerosol; the FVC was within normal limits. The total lung capacity was enlarged in association with a very high static lung compliance and low recoil pressure. The residual volume was increased proportionally more than the TLC so the RV% was increased as well. The airway resistance was high especially during expiration reflecting the low static recoil pressure. The transfer factor (diffusing capacity) for the lung was much reduced despite the enlarged total lung capacity. The reduction was due to a very low Kco. The arterial carbon dioxide tension was low on account of hyperventilation and the oxygen tension was low at rest, falling further during exercise.

The patient was diagnosed as having emphysema together with chronic airflow limitation, which was partly reversible. He was

Continued on p. 533

Case Study 16.1 *Continued*

treated with bronchodilator and antibiotic drugs and was able to increase his capacity for exercise by use of portable oxygen equipment.

Over the next 3 years there was little alteration in the indices of lung function, apart from the transfer factor which fell to a low level. This change was associated with an increase in breathlessness and a reduction in the capacity for exercise; the patient was then confined to bed. He died from respiratory failure 12 years after the onset of his symptoms. At post-mortem the lung was large with peripheral bullae and did not deflate when the chest was opened. The large lung sections showed gross panacinar emphysema with extensive loss of lung tissue, including the vascular bed. The features were those of deficiency of $\alpha 1$ antitrypsin with additional reversible airflow limitation.

Table B16.1 Case study measurements

Subject:	Mr A.	Mr B.	Mr C.
Condition:	Mild airway disease	Advanced airway disease	Emphysema
Age (yrs)	51	$57^* \rightarrow 65$	$48 \rightarrow 51$
Stature (m)	1.70	1.64	1.83
Body mass (kg)	77	50	53
FEV_1 (l)	1.8	0.7	0.8
Response to bronchodilator (%)	+17	+10	+45
FVC (and IVC) (l)	3.4 (3.95)	1.55	4.7
FEV%	53	45	17
TLC (l)	6.30	6.18	9.81
RV (l)	2.35	3.86	5.09
RV%	37	62	52
Cstat§	3.1 (0.31)	1.4 (0.14)	6.0 (0.6)
Cdyn§	1.6 (0.16)	—	3.4 (0.34)
Raw (inspiration)§	0.082 (0.82)	—	0.54 (5.4)
(expiration)§	—	—	0.78 (7.8)
Tlco§	7.9 (24)	$7.7 (23) \rightarrow 4.7 (14)$	$5.8 (23) \rightarrow 3.0 (9)$
Pa,o_2§	12.8 (96)	$8.0 (60) \rightarrow 4.9 (37)$	8.0 (60)†
Pa,co_2§	5.1 (38)	$5.3 (40) \rightarrow 10.7 (80)$	4.5 (34)
$\dot{V}E$, ex air ($l\,min^{-1}$)‡	36.5	23	33
O_2 ($l\,min^{-1}$)	31.1	16	21
Dyspnoeic index (air)	—	107	125
Hb concentration ($g\,dl^{-1}$)	—	$14.7 \rightarrow 18.7$	$- \rightarrow 17.3$

* 1 year after onset of cardiac failure. Arrow indicates passage of time.
† On exercise the Pa,o_2 fell to 5.7 kPa (43).
‡ Walking at 2.5 mph up incline of 1 in 10.
§ The data are given in SI units with traditional units in brackets, e.g. for Pa,o_2 kPa (mmHg), Tl mmol $min^{-1}kPa^{-1}$ ($ml\,min^{-1}mmHg^{-1}$), for Cstat and Cdyn $l\,kPa^{-1}$ ($l\,cmH_2O^{-1}$) and for Raw $kPa\,l^{-1}$ s ($cmH_2O\,l^{-1}s$). The conversion factors are given in Table 2.5 (page 17)

the dynamic compression also reduce the maximal flow rates which can be developed during expiration. Thus the FEV_1 and related indices are reduced as are the $FEV_1\%$ (FEV_1/FVC) and Tiffeneau index (FEV_1/IVC). These aspects are discussed above under 'obstructive type of ventilatory defect' (page 517).

The total lung capacity is normally unaffected by airway narrowing but the accuracy of the measurement can be impaired. The gas dilution methods can fail to record gas spaces which are poorly ventilated whilst the plethysmograph method can result in overestimation (page 157).

Lung mechanics and transfer factor. The airway narrowing is reflected in the airway resistance (*R*aw) which is increased. The increase is due mainly to narrowing of large numbers of small airways (diameter 2−4 mm). The resistance of the large airways is much less affected despite the airway walls being thickened by the enlarged subepethelial mucous glands. The resistance is inversely related to the lung volume at which the measurement is made, hence the reciprocal of the resistance, which is airway conductance, is nearly proportional to lung volume (Fig. 5.12, page 111). Consequently the resistance can be expressed by the conductance per litre of lung volume which is the specific conductance (s*G*aw).

The lung compliance, and in most circumstances the transfer factor, are unaffected by chronic airway obstruction without emphysema. However, depending on how the measurements are made, both indices can show reduction. The lung compliance is reduced if it is obtained as dynamic compliance (*C*dyn) during rapid breathing (page 165). This source of confusion is avoided by measuring the static compliance of the lung (page 161). The transfer factor is reduced if the lung volume during breath holding is underestimated by its being calculated from the dilution in the lung of the single breath of test gas (hence *T*l eff is reduced, page 302). This error is avoided if the residual volume is measured by the closed circuit helium dilution method or by plethysmography (hence *T*l), but there remains some unquantifiable inaccuracy because the alveolar sample obtained in the presence of airways obstruction is probably not a true representation of mixed alveolar air.

Uneven lung function. The airway narrowing is not uniform throughout the lung but varies in the different parts. This leads to a wide range of distribution of expansion ratios, temporal inequality of ventilation and ventilation−perfusion inequality. The abnormality is detected as impaired intrapulmonary mixing, a wide range of ventilation−perfusion ratios and hypoxaemia which is present at rest and is often not much affected by exertion. The indices which can be used to document these changes include the single breath nitrogen test of intrapulmonary mixing (page 214), the physiological deadspace as a percentage of tidal volume (*V*d/*V*t, page 251), the intrabreath respiratory exchange ratio (intrabreath *R*), the distribution of ventilation−perfusion ratios (page 255) and the alveolar–arterial tension differences for oxygen and carbon dioxide. The uneven distribution of ventilation increases the ventilatory cost of exercise. This contributes to exercise limitation (page 392). In the most affected parts of the lung the local hypoxaemia causes pulmonary arterial vasoconstriction. This reduces the ventilation–perfusion imbalance but at the cost of increasing the pulmonary arterial pressure and the pulmonary vascular resistance. The pulmonary hypertension is most marked during exercise. Some consequences of the uneven lung function are considered under 'advanced disease' below.

Emphysema

Definitions and mechanisms

Emphysema is a condition of the lung characterised by an increase beyond the normal in the size of air spaces distal to the terminal bronchioles. The expansion commonly affects the second order of respiratory bronchioles. That due to destruction of the walls of the airways is known as centriacinar (or centrilobular) emphysema (page 84); when it is due to dilatation which is secondary to the accumulation of inert dust in the lung it is called focal emphysema. Compensatory and senile types of emphysema also occur. Panacinar emphysema refers to the condition in which there is destruction and expansion of more than one order of airway within the acinus, i.e. that portion of the lung which is distal to each terminal bronchiole; the condition can then arise in the air-sacs and alveolar ducts (Fig. 5.3, page 85). Bullous emphysema may be said to be present when, in the inflated lung, the diameter of one or more of the emphysematous spaces exceeds 1 cm. Emphysema was first described in detail by Laennec, and Dr Samuel Johnson was one of the first recorded victims. The distinction between centriacinar and panacinar emphysema was first made using whole tissue slices (large lung sections) from lungs fixed in the inflated position. The technique for doing this was introduced by Gough and Wentworth. The functional implications have been clarified by Eidelman and his colleagues including Kim amongst others.

Diffuse emphysema that is not focal in character is usually due to autodigestion by proteolytic enzymes which are released into the lung. The extent of the emphysema is then the resultant of the actions of elastases and elastase inhibitors present in the fluid lining. The fluid can be sampled by bronchoalveolar lavage. In *centriacinar emphysema* the process of autodigestion is usually initiated by inhaled tobacco smoke. On this account the topographical distribution within the lung is uneven and narrowing of small airways often coexists. The aerosol enters the second order of respiratory bronchioles where the particles attract and are ingested by macrophages. The macrophages in turn attract polymorphonuclear leukocytes; these cells are activated by the tobacco smoke to release the proteolytic enzyme human neutrophil elastase. The elastase both causes local destruction which leads to emphysema (but also some local fibrosis) and it inhibits the naturally occurring protective enzyme α_1 protease inhibitor (also called α_1 anti-trypsin). The latter enzyme is also inactivated by oxygen radicals present in tobacco smoke. In *panacinar emphysema* the proteolytic enzymes come from the circulating blood. Either the blood concentration of enzymes is increased, as occurs in chronic pancreatitis, or the body's mechanism for inactivating the enzyme is impaired. This occurs from hereditary deficiency of the protective enzyme α_1 antitrypsin. The association of emphysema with the homozygous state of α_1 antitrypsin deficiency was first demonstrated by Eriksson. In addition there is now limited evidence that some subjects who are both heterozygous and heavy smokers are also at greater risk than members of the general population. In panacinar emphysema the distribution is predominantly basal reflecting the distribution of blood flow. There is little fibrosis or structural narrowing of small airways.

Clinical features

The clinical features of emphysema are relatively independent of the underlying pathology, except in the case of large bullae when the symptoms and signs of a space-occupying lesion can be superimposed. In this event surgical excision can lead to clinical improvement. Some degree of centriacinar emphysema is present in the lungs of most smokers. The tobacco smoke can also cause chronic bronchitis and narrowing of lung airways and the features of the latter condition usually predominate. The proportion of smokers who present with primary emphysema is relatively small. In most countries the patient is then typically an elderly male of linear physique. However, in some parts of India and other countries where there is a tradition of heavy smoking in childhood, the condition can present much earlier. When the condition is due to deficiency of α_1 antitrypsin the presentation is usually in the 4th or 5th decades of life. Both sexes are affected but because the enzyme deficiency acts synergistically with tobacco smoke the condition occurs earlier in smokers than in non-smokers. The clinical history is of progresssively increasing breathlessness, whilst cough and expectoration can be mild and of late onset. Wheeze is common and there is sometimes a useful clinical response to broncho-dilator aerosol. On clinical examination the chest is held in an inflated position. The chest radiograph typically shows over-inflation and loss of lung tissue (Fig. 16.4). On the posterio-anterior film one diagnostic feature is an increase in transradiancy which is associated with a paucity and narrowing of the pulmonary arteries, especially in the middle zone and in the outer third of the lung fields. On the lateral film the presence of a wide retrosternal space between the sternum and the anterior margin of the ascending aorta (width < 3 cm) is usually a reliable guide.

However, these are features of advanced disease. At an earlier stage the diagnosis can be made by computer-assisted tomography (CT).

This can identify both bullae and areas of reduced density where lung tissue has been destroyed. The areas of low density can be highlighted in the CT display. In centriacinar emphysema the distribution of lesions is mainly in the upper lobes and the apical segments of the lower lobes reflecting a role for gravitational force (page 182). By contrast in panacinar emphysema the distribution is predominantly basal reflecting the distribution of blood flow. The clinical course of emphysema is usually progressive and is considered below. However, for patients with deficiency of α_1 antitrypsin, the course may be ameliorated by replacement therapy. In addition, where there are large bullae which are compressing the adjoining lungs, and are not associated with severe generalised emphysema, their excision can lead to clinical improvement.

Lung function

The physiological features of diffuse emphysema are secondary to the loss of lung tissue; this affects both the elastic recoil of the lung and the surface area which is available for the exchange of gas. The elastic recoil is reduced to its greatest extent in panacinar emphysema whilst the loss of surface occurs equally in centriacinar and panacinar emphysema. The loss of elastic recoil leads to characteristic changes in the volume−pressure curve of the lung. At all lung volumes the elastic recoil pressure is reduced and on this account the total lung capacity is usually increased (see Fig. 16.4, page 530). There is also an increase in the static lung compliance. The loss of lung elasticity decreases the traction which normally tends to expand the intrapulmonary airways. This causes premature closure of the airways during expiration but not during inspiration, hence indices of forced inspiratory flow can be relatively normal. These features are reflected in the pattern of breathing. Inspiration is achieved at a high rate of flow over a short period of time. Expiration is slow and preferably effected in a relaxed manner as this avoids dynamic compression. The compression is reduced by the tidal breathing starting from an increased functional residual capacity; this maximises the expansive traction on the airways. The increase in FRC is achieved by contraction of inspiratory muscles. During expiration their role can be partly replaced by the subject voluntarily raising the pressure in the lung airways, either by pursing the lips or by intermittently closing the larynx to produce a jerky grunting expiration. The raised FRC has the disadvantage of reducing the inspiratory capacity and hence the increase in tidal volume which can be achieved during exercise. Thus the final breathing pattern is a compromise between different factors. During expiration the airways obstruction increases the airway resistance, while air-trapping increases the residual volume; some of the trapped gas is not detected when the volume is measured by helium dilution but it is measured by plethysmography. The difficulties in measuring the volumes are referred to under 'predominant airways disease' above. Closure of airways eliminates ventilation by bulk flow to some parts of the lung; the aeration of these regions is then maintained by collateral ventilation. Some of the ventilation goes to lung units with a high compliance which are poorly perfused with blood and hence constitute an enlarged physiological deadspace (see page 192). The airflow obstruction also reduces the ventilatory capacity; this aspect is described on pages 110 and 119.

The increase in total lung capacity causes a related reduction in Kco (i.e. transfer factor per litre of lung volume, Tl/Va) (page 293). With emphysema a further reduction can occur on account of loss of lung tissue, and at this stage the transfer factor is diminished. Both the diffusing capacity of the alveolar capillary membrane and the volume of blood in the lung capillaries are reduced. In addition, due to the destruction of the alveolar capillary bed, the normal increase which occurs during exercise in the volume of blood in the lung capillaries is greatly attenuated. These changes give rise to some of the features of the syndrome of defective gas transfer including an undue increase in the level of ventilation during exercise. At rest the tension of carbon dioxide in the arterial blood is usually normal or slightly below normal whilst the tension of oxygen is often maintained at about 8 kPa (60 mmHg). The arterial oxygen tension usually falls during exercise. The capacity for exercise can then be increased by the use of portable oxygen therapy (page 623). In the late stages of the disease the blood oxygen tension at rest diminishes and the tension of carbon dioxide rises. Death can then be due to failure of the lung, failure of the right heart or cardiac arrest precipitated by hypoxia.

Diagnosis

The diagnosis of emphysema is suspected on the basis of the clinical features and the chest radiograph. The diagnosis is confirmed by the findings on computer-assisted tomography and the assessment of lung function. The changes in lung function typically include a reduced Kco(Tl/Va) relative to total lung capacity, evidence for increased lung distensibility and a well-marked reduction in FEV_1 related to FVC (hence $FEV_1\%$ is reduced) and to maximal inspiratory flow. This pattern of change in the bellows and mechanical function of the lungs is characteristic of panacinar emphysema but less so of centriacinar emphysema where much of the respiratory impairment is due to primary narrowing of small airways whilst the loss of elastic recoil is a less prominent feature.

The diagnosis of emphysema in the presence of predominant airway disease can be made using the Kco (Tl/Va) which is low relative to the total lung capacity in emphysema but not in airway disease. The transfer factor is usually also reduced in emphysema but may be normal in the early stages. The diagnosis of emphysema in these circumstances is of limited importance when the lesions are of the centriacinar type since the treatment is then that of the associated airway disease. It becomes important with panacinar emphysema on account of the availability of specific treatment.

538

Emphysema and interstitial fibrosis typically have in common a reduced transfer factor and other features of defective gas transfer (page 519). The distinction between them is not always clear cut. It can usually be made using the total lung capacity and the static volume−pressure curve. A large total lung capacity, a maximal recoil pressure of less than $1.0\,kPa$ ($10\,cmH_2O$) and a static compliance on expiration in excess of $4.01\,kPa^{-1}$ ($0.41\,cmH_2O^{-1}$), or a value for the exponent k in excess of the reference value (page 497), are strong presumptive evidence of emphysema. Where the volume−pressure curve is intermediate, it may be because the two conditions coexist. The features are then likely to include some degree of airflow limitation, a reduced transfer factor and Kco and a *relatively normal* total lung capacity. The diagnosis can often be confirmed by computer-assisted tomography.

The lung function in panacinar emphysema is illustrated by the case of Mr C. in Table B16.1.

Localised emphysema

Localised transradiancy (*Macleod's syndrome*) or the presence of bullae can cause uneven lung function in the absence of generalised airflow limitation. The impairment may be amenable to thoracic surgery provided that generalised emphysema does not coexist. In borderline cases surgery is most likely to be beneficial when the elastic recoil pressure at total lung capacity is not less than $1\,kPa$ ($10\,cmH_2O$) and the lesions are mainly confined to the lung bases.

Consequences of irreversible obstruction to airflow

Chronic lung disease with relatively irreversible airflow limitation is the commonest cause of respiratory impairment and of death from respiratory disease. The condition can occur secondary to chronic bronchitis and with emphysema, cystic fibrosis and asthma. It can also occur as a complication of interstitial fibrosis and other generalised diseases of the lung. These conditions usually present with characteristic patterns of lung function summarised in Table 16.7, and other characteristic features, but subsequently the features can merge to form a common pathway to premature death from respiratory failure. This outcome reflects deterioration of lung function which proper management can often slow down.

Uneven ventilation

The airway narrowing, and changes in compliance associated with emphysema or pulmonary fibrosis, are not uniform throughout the lung, so the distribution of the inspired gas is uneven. The maldistribution is reflected in indices of uneven lung function of which some are listed on page 213. The changes range from relative overventilation (high $\dot{V}A/\dot{Q}$ ratios) to underventilation (low $\dot{V}A/\dot{Q}$ ratio) in different

Table 16.7 Lung function in well-developed cases of chronic obstructive pulmonary disease and disease of the lung parenchyma with interstitial fibrosis compared with normal function at the same age using a 5-point scale $(-,-,N,+,++)$

	Chronic obstructive pulmonary disease			Disease of lung parenchyma
	Airway disease	Common features	Primary emphysema	
FEV_1		− −		−
Response change to bronchodilator		+		N
FVC		−		−
$FEV_1\%$		−		N (or +)
TLC	N		+	− (or N)
IVC	−		− (or N)	−
FRC	N (or +)		+	−
RV		++		−
RV/TLC%		++		N (or −)
Air-trapping	+		++	No
Tl,co (and Dm)	N (or −)		− −	−
Vc		N (or −)		N (or −)
VA eff/VA		−		N
Pa,O_2		− −	−	N (or −)
Pa,CO_2	N (or +)		N	− (or N)
$\dot{V}A/\dot{Q}$ ratios‡	−		+	+
Pulmonary vascular resistance	++		+	+
$\dot{V}E,ex$ − air		+		++
− oxygen†		− −		− −
Pst	N (or −)			+
Cst	N (or −)		+	− −
$Cdyn$		−		− −
Raw (expir)		+		−

* Standardised for consumption of oxygen.
† Compared with breathing air.
‡ Predominant abnormality.

parts of the lung. Wagner and colleagues have found that in some patients the regions of hyperventilation predominate; these patients appear to fall into the category described by Donhorst as *pink puffers* (type A). The regions of high $\dot{V}A/\dot{Q}$ ratio are probably located centrally in the lung and are associated with a large physiological deadspace; many of the patients have panacinar emphysema. At the other extreme are the patients described as *blue bloaters* (type B). These patients have predominant regions of lung in which the $\dot{V}A/\dot{Q}$ ratio is reduced. The local hypoventilation leads to a compensatory reduction in pulmonary blood flow; this is achieved by constriction and hypertrophy of the walls of small pulmonary arteries supplying the affected region. The mechanism is related to hypoxaemia and has a constitutional component (page 204). The response has the effect of minimising the ventilation− perfusion inequality at the expense of a rise in the resistance to the flow of blood through the pulmonary circulation. Compensation for the uneven distribution of the inspired gas is never complete; instead the range of the ventilation−perfusion ratios widens as the disease

540

advances. There are then further increases in the physiological deadspace and in the venous admixture effect. The slope of the intra-breath R and the tension differences for oxygen, carbon dioxide and nitrogen between the mixed alveolar gas and the systemic arterial blood are increased; the tension and the saturation of oxygen in the systemic arterial blood are reduced in consequence (Chapter 7).

Pulmonary hypertension

Compensatory vasoconstriction of small pulmonary arteries raises the pulmonary arterial pressure. The pulmonary hypertension is first detectable on exercise and can occur at an early stage in the illness, when the ventilatory capacity is only reduced to a small extent and the arterial oxygen saturation is virtually normal (e.g. Fig. 7.11, page 201). Subsequently pulmonary hypertension occurs at rest, and the work of the right heart is increased. The resulting changes include enlargement of the main pulmonary artery which can be seen on the chest radiograph. Thickening of the right ventricular wall and tricuspid regurgitation can be detected by echocardiography and used to estimate the pulmonary systolic blood pressure. The electrocardiogram exhibits pulmonary P waves, right-axis deviation, a q-R pattern in aVR and other evidence of right ventricular strain, and later of right ventricular hypertrophy. The right ventricular end-diastolic pressure rises and this raises the pressure in the systemic veins. The patient is now vulnerable to episodes of congestive cardiac failure. Some contributory factors are given in Fig. 16.14 (page 577). The failure becomes manifest as a rise in jugular venous pressure in the neck, engorgement and enlargement of the liver and oedema of dependent parts of the body, starting with the ankles. If untreated, the oedema can extend to the abdomen and sacrum. The hepatic engorgement can progress to cirrhosis of the liver. These complications of airways obstruction affect particularly the patients with predominant airway disease (type B) rather than those with predominant emphysema. The pulmonary hypertension is reduced by breathing oxygen which is sometimes an effective treatment (page 623). The ways in which the intra-vascular pressure can be increased by the associated changes in the airway resistance are discussed by Harris and by Lockhart amongst others.

Haematocrit and blood volume

The hypoxaemia stimulates the production of erythropoietin; this hormone increases the rate at which iron from the plasma is incorporated in haemoglobin and hence increases red cell production. The change usually increases the haematocrit and the blood haemoglobin and red cell concentrations, but these features can be partly concealed by a rise in the plasma volume. Segal, Bishop, Harvey and others have evidence that the hypervolaemia is usually associated with an increase in the central (pulmonary) blood volume. The change, especially when it is accompanied by acidaemia, engorges the pulmonary vascular bed and this reduces its distensibility. It also increases the pulmonary wedge pressure; the risk of the patient developing congestive cardiac failure or vascular thrombosis is increased in consequence. The enhanced erythropoiesis resembles that which occurs during acclimatisation to high altitudes but, for a given level of hypoxaemia, it seldom develops to the same extent; it occurs mainly in type B patients in whom hypoxaemia is a prominent feature at rest. The hypoxaemia is usually accompanied by hypercapnia. The carotid bodies are enlarged. Increased erythropoiesis is not a feature of type A patients in whom the hypoxaemia occurs mainly on exercise and is due in part to impaired gas transfer (page 538).

Control of respiration and response to exercise

The presence of a wide range of ventilation–perfusion ratios increases the tension difference for carbon dioxide between mixed alveolar gas and the arterial blood (page 204). This predisposes to a rise in the tension of carbon dioxide which would normally stimulate respiration. However, particularly in patients with advanced airway disease, the ventilatory response to carbon dioxide is reduced by the high airway resistance and the increase in the work of breathing to which it gives rise (cf. Fig. 12.6, page 375). Instead, the patient adapts to the hypercapnia in the manner described on page 521 (see also Fig. 16.2). During acute chest illnesses both the ventilation–perfusion inequality and the airway resistance are further impaired; the patient is then liable to develop acute hypoventilation while breathing oxygen and, in unfavourable circumstances, the condition can progress to carbon dioxide narcosis (page 585). The hypercapnia, unlike that associated with sleep apnoea syndrome, is observed only when the ventilatory impairment is severe ($FEV_1 < 1.3$ l). It can be aggravated by a reduced responsiveness of the respiratory system to the factors which normally stimulate breathing. The reduction has both inherited and acquired components, the latter including a heavy build which further augments the work of breathing (page 128). The hypoventilation can be exacerbated by respiratory depressant drugs, both therapeutic and self-administered (page 580).

By reducing the maximal breathing capacity the limitation of airflow can cause intense breathlessness during mild exercise. The underlying factors are discussed on page 392. The ventilatory cost of submaximal exercise depends on the extents to which the deadspace and the alveolar ventilation are abnormal. The deadspace, on account of the wide range of ventilation–perfusion ratios, is invariably increased. The alveolar ventilation is often within normal limits, but may be increased in type A patients and reduced in type B patients or when the condition is advanced.

Many patients with COPD experience a disproportionate reduction in exercise ventilation while breathing oxygen; this response can occur at a stage in the disease when no similar reduction occurs with oxygen at rest. It is an indication that the subject's capacity for exercise can be increased by the use of portable oxygen equipment (page 407) and when it occurs to a marked extent it is associated with a poor prognosis.

A less reliable guide to the possibility that breathing oxygen will increase exercise tolerance is provided by comparing the arterial oxygen saturation at rest with that during exercise breathing air. In many subjects, the arterial oxygen tension remains at its resting level during exercise; in some, as a result of more even distribution of ventilation, the arterial oxygen tension rises, whilst in others it falls progressively. The latter response is a feature of patients with emphysema who can often increase their exercise capacity by breathing oxygen. However, a reduction in oxygen saturation can occur independent of whether or not the ventilation during exercise is reduced by breathing oxygen.

Breathlessness in patients with chronic lung disease can be reduced by measures which increase the ventilatory capacity, reduce the ventilatory cost of exercise or reduce the sensation of breathlessness. Some examples are given in Table 16.8: the remedies include correction of either obesity or undernutrition. The latter occurs in some patients with emphysema, and is due to the combined effects of breathlessness reducing the food intake and the increased energy cost of breathing increasing the metabolic rate. The suggestion that a high fat diet could be used to reduce the output of carbon dioxide and hence the ventilatory cost of exercise has not been confirmed.

Consequences of irreversible obstruction to airflow

Table 16.8 Ways of improving the exercise capacity of patients in the chronic obstructive pulmonary disease (COPD), see also Table 16.13 (page 559)

Aspect	Procedure	Mechanism
$\dot{V}_E$ max ex ↑	Bronchodilator therapy	Raw reduced
	Training the diaphragm	Pdi max increased
	Better nutrition	P max increased
	Continuous positive airway pressure*	Respiratory work reduced
$\dot{V}_E$ submax. ex ↓	Physical training	f_R.ex reduced‡
	Breathing oxygen	Hypoxic drive eliminated
	Venesection (if polycythaemic)	$\dot{V}_A/\dot{Q}$ improved
$\dot{n}_{O_2}$ sub max ↓	Weight reduction (if obese)	Work done reduced
Breathless ↓ (and coughing)	Controlled coughing (if hypersecretion)	Secretions cleared
	Postural drainage (if hypersecretion)	
	Morphine and other drugs†	Various
Pulmonary hypertension	Long-term oxygen therapy	
	Diuretics (short term)	
	Vasodilator drugs	

* During weaning from a ventilator.
† In experimental studies.
‡ Also improves tolerance of breathlessness.

543

Gas transfer

The hypoxaemia which occurs at rest in patients with chronic airways obstruction is almost entirely due to ventilation−perfusion inequality. By contrast, the transfer of oxygen across the alveolar capillary membrane is unaffected by airways obstruction. Thus when measured by the single breath method with a separate measurement of residual volume, the transfer factor is normal or increased in patients with asthma and usually normal in patients with predominant airway disease, or even increased, in the presence of polycythaemia (page 294). Gas transfer is impaired by the loss of alveolar surface and by the destruction of the alveolar capillaries which occur with panacinar emphysema, and by the increase in the path length for diffusion in the gas phase which occurs with centriacinar emphysema. For these reasons the Kco is reduced early in the course of emphysema and the transfer factor decreases progressively as the disease advances. The reduction in the transfer factor in type A patients is associated with an increase in the difference in oxygen tension between alveolar gas and blood leaving the alveolar capillaries (Fig. 9.4, page 284) and hence with hypoxaemia during exertion.

Assessment of life expectancy

Life expectancy in patients with chronic obstructive lung disease is determined by a number of factors; they include the home conditions, the extent to which effective use is made of medical services and aggravating factors such as smoking and atmospheric pollution. It is also related to the respiratory symptoms and the severity of the underlying changes in the lung. On this account any index of function that is impaired by the disease processes provides a guide to prognosis. The application of a battery of tests yields additional information but much of it is duplicated because many indices are intercorrelated. The results of longitudinal studies suggest that the value of a test for prognosis depends upon the stage of the disease at which it is applied. In addition some indices such as the total lung capacity and the lung compliance are of predictive value when they are abnormal but a normal result can occur despite life-threatening airway obstruction. Findings which are of prognostic value in the early and the intermediate stages of the disease include the clinical grade of breathlessness, the forced expiratory volume and the airway resistance, the proportion of the forced vital capacity which can be expired in 1 s ($FEV_1\%$) and the residual volume in absolute units or as a percentage of the total lung capacity. Tests of uneven lung function can probably be of use but the evidence is incomplete. With advanced disease the tests that predict prognosis include the capacity for exercise, the tension of oxygen in the arterial blood, the transfer factor (diffusing capacity) for carbon monoxide and the presence or absence of pulmonary heart disease and disproportionate hypoventilation when oxygen is breathed during exercise. Loss of weight is also informative. In addition, when the haematocrit or the CO_2 tension in arterial blood are increased the outlook is poor, but normal values do not necessarily imply a good prognosis.

Bronchiectasis

Bronchiectasis is a chronic dilatation of one or more bronchi; the cause can be congenital but the condition is usually acquired as a result of infection for which there is usually a predisposing cause. This can be local obstruction by a foreign body, a mechanical abnormality or malfunction of cilia, cystic fibrosis or an immunological disorder, for example, hypogammaglobulinaemia. The condition can be associated with allergic bronchopulmonary aspergillosis. It can also be due to a mechanical abnormality or malfunction of cilia. The clinical features include production of copious purulent sputum, haemoptysis and lassitude. Recurrent fever and/or pleuritic pain can also occur. The predominant change in lung function is irreversible airways obstruction; there may also be evidence of generalised narrowing of the small airways. When the bronchiectasis complicates interstitial fibrosis the lung function exhibits the features of this condition also (page 558). The changes are usually the same for the cylindrical as for the saccular type of bronchiectasis; they are influenced by the aetiology, the extent of the condition (including the number of segments which are involved) and the severity of the associated bronchitis. The abnormal bronchi can usually be visualised by computer-assisted tomography (CT). The condition is often alleviated by energetic physiotherapy (page 646) and chemotherapy; it can be aggravated temporarily by bronchography.

Cystic fibrosis

Cystic fibrosis is an inherited defect of epithelial secretory cells which affects those 0.04% of children who are homozygous for the condition. The permeability of cell membranes to chloride ions is impaired by abnormal control of the chloride channels. The abnormality reduces the ability to reabsorb chloride ions from the sweat and respiratory epithelium and also probably the other organs which can be involved; these include the pancreas, the small intestine and the seminal vesicles. In the lung the airway fluid is rich in chloride ions and relatively deficient in sodium ions; the electrical potential across the airway epithelium is increased above its normal level of $<30\,\text{mV}$.

The changes increase the viscosity of pulmonary secretions and interfere with their clearance by the action of cilia. This results in bacterial colonisation and infection of the respiratory tract by *Pseudomonas*, *Staphylococcus aureus* and other organisms. The infections can lead to bronchiectasis. The principal change in lung function is an obstructive type of ventilatory defect which involves all classes of airways (page 517). Thus the forced expiratory volume is reduced and there is evidence of narrowing of small airways with an increase in residual volume and

545

ventilation−perfusion inequality; the latter can cause hypoxaemia. Non-specific bronchial hyperreactivity is a common feature. The reduced ventilatory capacity impairs the capacity for exercise. The late stages can include gross bronchiectasis, carbon dioxide retention and right heart failure. Suitable patients can be treated by lung transplantation. The advent of complications can be postponed by properly managed treatment (Table 16.8). The missing gene has been identified so it may soon be possible to prevent the condition by genetic counselling or replacement therapy.

Asthma (reversible obstruction to lung airway)

Clinical definition and features

Asthma refers to the condition of subjects in whom there is widespread airflow limitation which changes in intensity over short periods of time either spontaneously or with treatment and is not due to cardiovascular disease. The airflow limitation is frequently worse at night or first thing in the morning, can usually be provoked by non-specific, and sometimes by specific, stimuli and is responsive to treatment. The symptoms include periodic wheeze, chest tightness, cough and breathlessness. The condition affects some 8% of children aged 7 years in a proportion of whom it is mis-diagnosed as 'wheezy bronchitis'. In most children the symptoms disappear during adolescence but in approximately one-third they persist into adult life. Thereafter, if uncontrolled by treatment, the airway obstruction can become progressively less reversible until it comes to resemble the predominantly obstructive type of chronic obstructive pulmonary disease (COPD, type B). The initial mechanics and the underlying pathological changes for the two groups of conditions are different but the late stages can be the same. Thus in most patients with COPD the airway obstruction is to some extent reversible with bronchodilator drugs and the incidence of non-specific bronchial hyper-reactivity is increased. On account of this overlap the diagnosis of asthma is best made on the basis of the clinical and related features in the early stages of the illness; these are summarised in Table 16.9.

Mechanisms and pathology

The mechanisms of asthma are incompletely understood but the condition is believed to develop along the following lines. The underlying lesion is a chronic inflammation of bronchioles; this is due to the local release of inflammatory mediators from mast cells, from eosinophils and from other cells which are attracted to the affected bronchioles. The process of attraction begins with the activation of alveolar macro-phages and mast cells. The activation is usually effected by an inhaled antigen combining with a specific circulating immunoglobulin E (IgE) which in turn combines with receptors on the surface of the cell. The

546

Table 16.9 Principal features of asthma (for details, see text)

Feature	Likely mechanism
Inflammation of small airways (ISA) (evident at post-mortem)	Platelet activating factor from alveolar macrophages*
Episodic symptoms of airflow limitation	Mediators cause bronchoconstriction and secretion of mucus
Nocturnal aggravation	Defences against bronchoconstriction weakest at night (Fig. 16.5)
Increased response to provocation	Secondary to ISA (Table 16.13)
Vulnerable to specific antigens	Sensitisation via IgE (if atopic), or IgG or other pathway

* Inflammation aggravated by exposure to ozone or sulphur dioxide; these two substances potentiate each other.

reactions are facilitated if the level of circulating IgE is high, which is the case for some 20% of persons; they are said to be atopic. Atopy is an inherited condition which appears to be due to a single abnormal gene. Diagnosis is supported by a positive response to skin prick tests using saline suspensions of house dust, animal danders, pollens and other antigens. The response is a raised bleb (weal) of diameter more than 2 mm occurring at 15 min after the innoculation. The weal may be accompanied by transient redness (flair). The activated mast cells secrete histamine and other substances. The alveolar macrophages secrete chemotactic substances including a platelet activating factor (PAF). This substance attracts eosinophils which in turn secrete leukotriene C4 (LTC4) and other substances. The LTC4 causes bronchoconstriction and stimulates the secretion of mucus. The constriction is due to mediators acting on receptors in the surface of the smooth muscle cells. This leads to hydrolysis of phosphoinositide (PI) to inositol triphosphate (IP$_3$) which releases calcium from the intracellular stores. The calcium triggers the contractile response (page 401). As well as acting on eosinophils, the PAF attracts platelets which release another bronchoconstrictor substance (spasmogen). PAF also causes local vasoconstriction and an increase in permeability of blood vessels. This leads to oedema of the walls of bronchioles. The resulting narrowing of the lumina of small airways predisposes to non-specific bronchial hyperreactivity.

Other cells which contribute to the pathological features of asthma include macrophages, monocytes and neutrophils. The pharmacologically active substances include the constrictors histamine and prostaglandin D2 (mainly from mast cells), prostaglandin F2α, the prostanoid substance thromboxane A2, the bradykinin precursor kininogen, adenosine and other substances. These substances interact. In addition the neural control of the smooth muscle in the walls of airways is disturbed and this can contribute to bronchial hyper-reactivity. Both the autonomic and the non-adrenergic, non-cholinergic nervous systems appear to be affected. Understanding of the contribution of all these components of the asthmatic syndrome has been advanced by the development of specific inhibitory substances and this process is continuing. The subject has been reviewed by Barnes and Holgate. Their summaries of the likely mechanisms for noctural aggravation of asthma and for exercise-induced asthma are reproduced in Figs 16.5 and 16.6.

On histological examination the bronchi show hypertrophy of the smooth muscle, hyperplasia of the mucous glands and goblet cells and thickening of the epithelial basement membrane. The epethelium is permeated with eosinophils. Following acute episodes of asthma there may be areas of epithelial desquamation. The resulting debris can contribute to mucous plugging of all classes of airways proximal to the respiratory bronchioles. The main ingredients of the plugs are viscid mucus, epithelial cells, eosinophils and a proteinaceous exudate. The plugs contribute to uneven lung function.

Agents causing asthma

Asthma is not synonymous with non-specific hyper-responsiveness but the latter condition usually coexists. The asthma is extrinsic when it is due to a specific substance and cryptogenic when no specific cause can be discovered. Extrinsic asthma in the general population is usually associated with atopy; it is then commonly due to sensitisation to residues of the house-dust mite or one of the other antigens mentioned

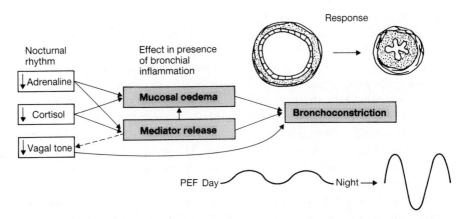

Fig. 16.5 Nocturnal aggravation of asthma. Circulating adrenaline and cortisol normally prevent airway inflammation but the blood levels oscillate and are low at night. There is then increased release of mediators from inflammatory cells and increased microvascular leakage leading to swelling of the airway sub-epithelium. Concurrently the vagal cholinergic tone is increased at night. The resulting bronchoconstriction, superimposed on the swelling, greatly reduces the airway calibre. (Source: Barnes PJ, Holgate ST. In Brewis RAL, Gibson GJ, and Geddes D, eds. *Respiratory Medicine*. London: Ballière Tindall, 1990, 591.)

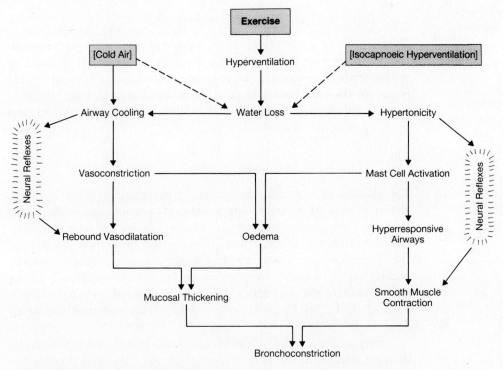

Fig. 16.6 Pathogenesis of exercise-induced asthma. (Source: as for Fig. 16.5.)

above in relation to skin tests. Many other IgE-related antigens occur and can cause asthma of occupational origin. Non-atopic extrinsic asthma can occur from sensitisation involving other immunoglobulins (IgD, IgG and IgM). Small chemical molecules can also bind with receptor sites through the mediation of larger carrier molecules; in this role they act as haptens. Some causes of asthma are given in Table 16.10.

Table 16.10 Some causes of asthma

Atopic (domestic)	*Atopic (occupational)*
House-dust mite	Platinum salts*
Danders from domestic animals	Gum acacia
Grass pollen	Ipecacuanha
Flour dust (often occupational)	Western red cedar
Other Ig mechanisms	*Other mechanisms*
Avian residues (IgG)	Toluene di-isocyanates*†
Epoxy curing agents (IgG)*	Plicatic acid*†
Pine resin (colophony) (IgM)*†	Ethanol
Tartrazine (IgD)*	Aspirin

* Acts as hapten.
† Can also cause non-specific irritation.
(Source: Cotes JE, Steel J. *Work-Related Lung Disorders.* Oxford: Blackwell Scientific Publications, 1987.)

Lung function – underlying mechanisms

During acute episodes of asthma the calibre of most airways is reduced; the change extends from the glottis, through the large airways down to the small airways including the respiratory bronchioles. The narrowing is due to the combined effects of acute inflammation which thickens the subepithelium, contraction of bronchial smooth muscle and mucous plugging of some airways.

Lung volumes and ventilatory capacity

The changes described in the preceding paragraph combine to cause airway closure at a larger lung volume than would normally be the case, thus the residual volume and closing volume are increased. The airflow obstruction affects expiration more than inspiration due to both the dependence of elastic recoil pressure on lung volume and the occurrence of dynamic compression during expiration. Hence during tidal breathing the expiratory flow rate is reduced and expiration is prolonged; the brief inspirations are made at an increased rate of air flow.

During acute attacks of asthma the static elastic recoil pressure is reduced relative to the lung volume (Fig. 16.7) and concurrently the functional residual capacity (FRC) rises (Case Study 16.2).

The new FRC can reflect the static equilibrium between the elastic recoils of the lungs and chest wall (cf. page 104); however, more often the FRC is increased by a need to maintain traction on the lung

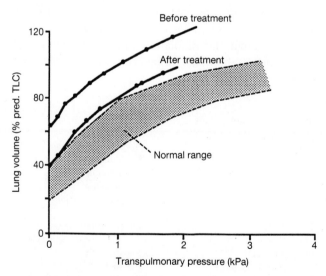

Fig. 16.7 Static volume-pressure curves for a patient with acute asthma before and after treatment. During the attack the total lung capacity was increased both in absolute terms and relative to the transpulmonary pressure. (Source: Gold WM, Kaufman HS, Nadel JA. *J Appl Physiol* 1967; **23**: 433–438.)

Case Study 16.2 Lung function in a patient with asthma

Asthma

Mr D., a non-smoker aged 57 years, had left the police force after 25 years service on account of late onset asthma. There was a past history of nasal polyps and a strong family history of asthma. The patient was admitted to hospital on the 10th day of his third significant exacerbation at which time he was severely ill with marked hypercapnia and respiratory acidosis. The sputum contained eosinophils and hyperinflation was evident on the chest radiograph. Treatment was with intravenous hydrocortisone, aminophylline and oxygen in controlled amounts. Lung function measurements were made on the third day of admission at which time there was a gross obstructive type of ventilatory defect with very material air trapping. The physiological deadspace and the alveolar–arterial tension difference for oxygen were increased and there was a small intrapulmonary shunt. This was evidence that some acini were perfused but not ventilated. However, the transfer factor was normal. The measurements were repeated 8 days later at which time most had reverted to normal.

The findings were considered to be typical of status asthmaticus.

Table B16.2 Case study measurements

Subject:	Mr D.	
	Asthma	
Condition:		
	Relapse	Remission
Age (yrs)	57	
Stature (m)	1.85	
Body mass (kg)	83	
FEV_1 (l)	0.6	2.7
FVC (l)	2.6	5.3
FEV_1%	23	51
TLC (l)	8.97	6.72
FRC (l)	5.63	3.83
RV (l)	4.31	1.58
RV/TLC%	48	23.5
Tl (single breath)*	11.4 (34)	11.4 (34)
Vd/Vt (%)	52	32
A-aDo_2*	6.7 (50)	1.2 (9)
$\dot{Q}s/\dot{Q}t$ (%)	5.7	3.4
Pa,o_2*	8.0 (60)	13.1 (98)
Pa,co_2*	4.9 (37)	4.7 (35.5)
$\dot{V}E$, rest air (l min^{-1})	17.5	12.7
fR (min^{-1})	19.7	14.3

* For units see footnote to Table B16.1 (page 533).

airways and exceeds the equilibrium position. The loss of elastic recoil is associated with an increase in the total lung capacity (TLC, Fig. 16.7). This is a real event which is demonstrable by chest radiography but it can be overestimated when measured by the plethysmographic method (page 160). However, the increase in TLC is less than that for the residual volume so the vital capacity can be greatly reduced. The changes in lung volumes combine with the airway obstruction to reduce the ventilatory capacity. The features are those of an obstructive type of ventilatory defect (page 517). Reductions occur in the forced expiratory volume, the $FEV_1\%$ (FEV_1/FVC) and in the maximal expiratory flow rates at all lung volumes. The changes can be partly or completely reversed by inhalation of a bronchodilator aerosol (Fig. 6.8, page 146).

The changes in *lung mechanics* include an increase in the airways resistance hence a reduction in airways conductance (page 112). The static lung volume−pressure curve is displaced upwards in the manner described above (Fig. 16.7). The change has the effect that the recoil pressure is reduced at all lung volumes below TLC but the static compliance is relatively unaffected. The dynamic compliance is reduced by the coexisting airways obstruction (cf. page 165). The mechanism for the reduction in recoil pressure is not known but it appears to be a dynamic and not a structural phenomenon since it is also observed when an external resistance is imposed experimentally.

Uneven lung function

The narrowing of airways is uneven. This leads to uneven distribution of inspired gas which is aggravated by mucous plugging of some airways. The changes are reflected in indices of distribution of inspired gas (page 213). The maldistribution of ventilation leads to a compensatory redistribution of blood flow (page 200). However, the latter is incomplete so indices of ventilation−perfusion inequality show evidence of impairment; thus the alveolar−arterial tension difference for oxygen is increased as is the slope of the intrabreath R. The distribution of ventilation−perfusion ratios shows the presence of lung units having a low but finite $\dot{V}A/\dot{Q}$ ratio. Wagner and colleagues found that when breathing air these poorly ventilated units were on average perfused by approximately 20% of cardiac output. The proportion was nearly doubled while breathing 100% oxygen. The change indicated the extent of hypoxic vasoconstriction. However, there was no blood shunt compartment; this suggested that the lung tissue behind any plugged airways was supplied by collateral ventilation. During expiration the hypoxic vasoconstriction of those arterioles which supply poorly ventilated regions can be supplemented by a rise in intrathoracic pressure and a reduced elastic recoil pressure. The changes increase the pulmonary arterial pressure and hence the load on the right ventricle; the patter can be reflected in the electrocardiogram (page 541).

Gas exchange and control of ventilation

The transfer factor for the lung (Tlco) is not reduced by acute asthma except to the extent that in some forms of the test the uneven distribution and the reduced expiratory flow rate can lead to error (page 302). The hypoxaemia is due solely to ventilation−perfusion inequality. However, it is often ameliorated by an increase in cardiac output raising the pulmonary venous oxygen tension. The hypoxaemia in turn increases the chemoreceptor drive to respiration; this raises the level of alveolar ventilation and hence the alveolar oxygen tension whilst at the same time inducing mild hypocapnia. The changes interact with the increase in resting respiratory level described above to increase the work of breathing and to cause fatigue in the inspiratory muscles. When the airway obstruction is severe the hyperventilation cannot be sustained. The patient then develops respiratory acidosis with hypercapnia. The hypercapnia can be aggravated by the ventilation−perfusion inequality (page 204) and the acidosis by lactic acid produced in the inspiratory muscles. McFadden and Lyons have evidence that the critical level of ventilatory capacity for development of hypercapnia is a reduction in FEV_1 to approximately 20% of the reference value.

Chronic childhood asthma

A person who develops mild asthma during childhood often acquires a large total lung capacity and high transfer factor relative to the reference values. The change could reflect increased growth of the lungs secondary to training of the respiratory muscles. With the prolonged systemic steroid therapy which is required for more severe asthma there is a risk of stunted growth; the risk is small when the steroids are given by inhalation.

Chronic severe asthma

Patients with episodic asthma can progress to show the features of chronic airflow limitation which is, at best, incompletely reversible. In addition there is persistence of the ventilation−perfusion imbalance but, whilst this is often variable from week to week, it is often partly corrected by hypoxic vasoconstriction in poorly ventilated areas. The arterial blood gases can then be relatively normal. Rodriguez-Roisin and colleagues observed only relatively mild $\dot{V}$A/$\dot{Q}$ imbalance; they attributed this to mucous plugging being an inconsistent feature of their patients and to the airflow limitation affecting mainly the larger airways. However, in some chronic asthmatics the hypoxic and haemo-dynamic aspects can be more conspicuous. The features then resemble those of the advanced airway type of chronic obstructive pulmonary disease (COPD, page 539).

Diagnosis of asthma

The diagnosis is made on the basis of the clinical history and other features of the condition and not the lung function alone (page 546). In clinical practice the physiological aspects include an episodic reduction in FEV_1 or peak expiratory flow which exhibits material reversibility, and a normal or slightly increased total lung capacity and transfer factor. The findings are compared with those of chronic obstructive pulmonary disease (COPD) in Table 16.11.

In epidemiological surveys the diagnosis of asthma is usually made on the basis of answers to questions such as those in the MRC questionnaire of respiratory symptoms with additional questions. The questionnaire is frequently supplemented by spirometry or measurement of peak expiratory flow which should preferably be carried out before and after administration of a bronchodilator aerosol (page 145). In addition the survey may include a screening test for atopy, bronchial hyperreactivity, circadian variation or specific sensitisation (Table 16.12). The first two of these procedures provide evidence of increased susceptibility to asthma. The third and fourth can provide evidence of sensitisation to specific agents; this information opens the way to preventing further acute episodes or progressive lung damage. In an occupational context the information can also have important preventive and medicolegal implications. However, challenge with an antigen to which the subject is sensitive is not without risk, so if the context is not primarily a medical one the case for obtaining the information should be reviewed impartially before the test is performed. Ways of making the assessments are listed in Table 16.12.

Table 16.11 Typical physiological features of asthma contrasted with those of chronic obstructive pulmonary disease (COPD)

	Asthma	Predominant airway type of COPD	Emphysema
Obstructive ventilatory defect	Episodic	Persistent	Persistent
Reversibility	Marked	Often present	Can be material
Total lung capacity	Normal or increased	Normal	Often increased
Transfer factor	Normal or increased	Normal	Reduced
$K_{CO}(Tl/V_A)$	Normal*	Normal	Reduced*
Static compliance	Normal	Normal	Reduced
Recoil pressure (below TLC)	Reduced†	Normal	Reduced
Hypoxaemia	Present	Often marked	Present

* After allowing for total lung capacity with which K_{CO} is negatively correlated (page 293).
† During acute episodes.

Table 16.12 Techniques for assessing susceptibility or sensitisation to inhaled allergens

Atopy	Skin prick tests (page 547) (weal diameter > 2 mm), serum IgE (>350 µg/ml)	Approximately 20% of normal persons are positive
Bronchial hyperreactivity	Histamine (Fig. 16.18) Methacholine Exercise (Fig. 16.6 and page 176) Cold air ($-10°C$)	Approximately 10% of normal persons are positive
Circadian variation in peak expiratory flow rate	Morning dip pattern (Fig. 16.8) Decline over shift and working week (Fig. 16.9)	Measurements should extend over whole weeks, weekends and on return from a holiday
Specific	Radio-allergosorbent (RAS) test	Tests for specific IgE in serum
	Inhalation challenge test (Fig. 16.10)	Can cause acute symptoms or sensitisation

The presence of *non-specific bronchial hyperreactivity* is usually assessed in terms of the dose of histamine or methacholine which reduces the forced expiratory volume (FEV_1) by 20% (designated provocation concentration 20% or PC_{20, FEV_1}) or the specific airway conductance by 35% ($PC_{35, sGAw}$). The test procedure is described on page 174. It is given in more detail by Sterk and colleagues who have recently reviewed non-specific bronchial hyperreactivity and specific airway responsiveness for the European Coal and Steel Community.

The occurrence of *exercise-induced airflow limitation* can give rise to disability in children and in physically active adults. Its assessment can therefore contribute to the management of individual patients. The procedure can also be used as an alternative to inhalation challenge with histamine. The method of assessment is described on page 176.

Testing for *circadian variation* can be used to identify patients in whom airflow limitation is more likely to be due to asthma than to chronic bronchitis. For this purpose the patient records the peak expiratory flow in the morning and evening. A morning dip pattern is then suggestive of asthma (Fig. 16.8). Alternatively, measurements made every 2 h throughout the day can be used to investigate a possible occupational cause for the symptoms. Asthma of the immediate onset occurs soon after the exposure so the association with exposure is usually made by the patient. Challenge testing is most likely to be of diagnostic value if the occupational exposure is of low intensity or if the asthma is of the delayed onset type (Fig. 16.9).

The response to *challenge using a specific antigen* should only be assessed if the information obtained up to this point is incomplete and the need to make a positive diagnosis outweighs the possible risk. The test is undertaken when the patient is in a stable state with no material airflow obstruction (e.g. $FEV_1 > 80\%$ predicted when off drugs) and not within a week of previous exposure to the suspected antigen or to histamine. It should preferably be carried out in a manner which

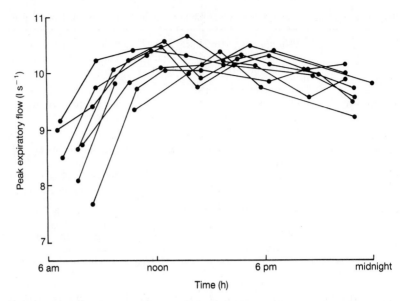

Fig. 16.8 Circadian measurements of peak expiratory flow in a pigeon fancier (precipitin positive) with exercise induced airflow limitation. There was a morning dip pattern which was reproducible from day to day. The morning dip was not reduced following 2 weeks without exposure; this suggested that the airflow limitation was not related to exposure. (Source: Cotes JE, Steel J. *Work-Related Lung Disorders*. Oxford: Blackwell Scientific Publications, 1987.)

mimics exposure at work such as painting, welding, soldering, sifting or mixing. The manoeuvre should be performed within the hospital complex in a booth or small chamber ventilated to outside air. Full safety precautions should be available, including nebulised and intravenous bronchodilator drugs, intravenous hydrocortisone, oxygen and facilities for respiratory and cardiac resuscitation. The inhaled concentration of test substance should not exceed the hygiene standard and should be less than that experienced at work. The subject should not be taking bronchoactive drugs at the time.

Challenge can also be undertaken using a nebulised aerosol. This should be prepared as a 10% weight-for-volume suspension in phosphate buffered saline. The suspension is agitated for 24h at 4°C, filtered, dialysed against phosphate buffered saline, freeze-dried, re-suspended at an appropriate concentration (which might be in the range $0.01-10\,\text{mg}\,\text{ml}^{-1}$) and sterilised using a multipore filter. The concentration for inhalation should initially be less than that which causes a positive prick test.

When an immediate response to challenge is expected the FEV_1 or peak expiratory flow should be monitored. A delayed response can also reduce the FEV_1 but this is not invariable. It may affect only the flow rate in small airways, in which case the $MEF_{25\%\ FVC}$ obtained from the expiratory flow volume curve is the index of choice. The procedure should normally start at 9.00 a.m. so that measurements of lung function can be made throughout the day, initially at 5 min intervals

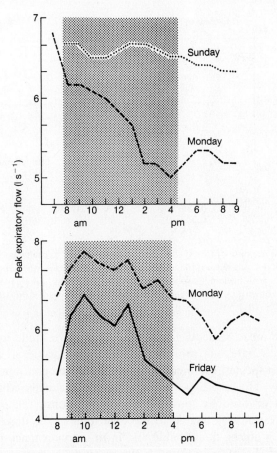

Fig. 16.9 Circadian measurements of peak expiratory flow (PEF) in two electrical workers with occupational asthma resulting from exposure to colophony (indicated by stippling). Subject A (upper record) gave a normal response on the Sunday. On the Monday he went to work and developed an initial followed by a delayed reaction. The result for the Friday (not included) showed a morning dip which masked the initial fall in PEF. Subject B (lower record) showed a morning dip followed by a delayed reaction. This became progressively more pronounced and occurred from a progressively lower level of PEF as the week advanced. The result for Sunday (not illustrated) was similar to that for Friday but recovery occurred by the following Monday. (Source: Burge PS, Harries MG, O'Brien I, Pepys J, *et al. Clin Allergy* 1980; **10**: 137–149.)

and subsequently every hour. On day 1 the subject is instructed in the procedure and control measurements are made. On day 2, and if necessary on subsequent days, graded exposures are given and later these are repeated using a refined extract or after administration of sodium cromoglycate or other protective agent. Thus in a study of the effects of colophony (pine resin) Burge, Pepys and colleagues initially had their subjects inhale one natural breath of soldering fume, followed by three and six breaths at 15 min intervals if no reaction had occurred by then. If there was still no response the exposure was increased on subsequent days (up to a total of 4) by the subject using the soldering iron once every 30 s for three periods of respectively 1 and 2 min, 5 min, 20 min and 60 min. In the case of an uncomplicated immediate

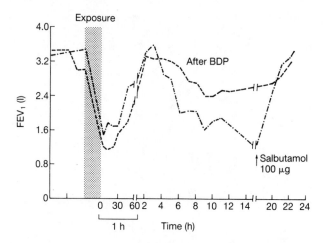

Fig. 16.10 Dual response of forced expiratory volume (FEV₁) to challenge with rye flour in a baker. The delayed but not the immediate asthmatic reaction was largely prevented by pretreatment with beclomethasone diproprionate (BDP) but not by placebo treatment (not shown). (Source: Hendrick DJ, Davies RJ, Pepys J. *Clin Allergy* 1976; **6**: 241−250.)

response the measurements can be discontinued or made infrequently once the flow rate has returned to the initial value. If a delayed response is suspected the measurements should be continued into the following day. The results of the challenge tests are analysed graphically (Fig. 16.10) or used to construct a dose−response relationship; an immediate response is related to the logarithm of the dose but a late response may not be quantifiable and in this circumstance is reported as present or absent or in terms of the mean peak expiratory flow for the 12 h following challenge.

Management of airflow limitation

The principles of management apply equally to patients with chronic obstructive pulmonary disease (COPD) with or without emphysema, asthmatics and patients with cystic fibrosis; however, the emphasis is different depending on the condition. The principles of management are summarised in Table 16.13. Some aspects of treatment are discussed in Chapter 17.

Interstitial lung disease

The quantity of interstitial tissue is increased in many disorders of the lung. Usually reticulum is laid down and there is proliferation of cubical type II cells in the walls of the alveoli, sometimes with desquamation into the lumen, hyperplasia of the bronchiolar epithelium and arteritis of the small pulmonary arteries. These disorders are associated with diffuse nodular and/or irregular opacities on the chest radiograph. They are sometimes accompanied by dry cough and vague chest pains, and usually by breathlessness which is due to characteristic

Table 16.13 Management of airflow limitation

Interstitial lung disease

Remove aggravating factors	Smoke from cigarettes
	Environmental pollution (SO_2, O_3, passive smoking etc.)
	Specific antigens (in home, e.g. aspirin; at work, hobbies)
	Bronchoconstrictor drugs (e.g. β blockers)
Active prophylaxis	Against influenza—immunisation
	Against asthmatic attacks—sodium cromoglycate, corticosteroids*
Bronchodilator therapy	β receptor agonists (e.g. salbutamol), Anticholinergic drugs (e.g. ipratropium bromide), Methylxanthines (e.g. theophylline). See page 642
For severe attacks	Oral prednisolone or intravenous hydrocortisone in high dosage, oxygen etc.
Treat infections	Antibiotics (e.g. amoxycillin)
Clear secretions	See page 646 (incl. Table 17.6)
Rehabilitation	See table 16.8 (page 543)

* These substances respectively can prevent the immediate and delayed responses to an inhaled antigen (e.g. Fig. 16.10).

changes in lung function. In many of the conditions the lesions are initially reversible, either by removal of the cause or in response to treatment by steroid or immunosuppressant drugs; subsequently they can progress via interalveolar and peribronchial fibrosis to diffuse interstitial fibrosis. This may be further complicated by infection, by diffuse dilatation of airways, by emphysematous distortion of parts of the lung and by extensive destruction of the pulmonary vascular bed leading to pulmonary hypertension and right heart failure.

The conditions have been classified by Turner Warwick under five headings.

1 Widespread granulomas; these include sarcoidosis, beryllium disease, extrinsic allergic alveolitis caused by various organic dusts, tuberculosis and other granulomas. In these conditions widespread crepitations are unusual except when there is extensive bronchial damage (see separate sub-headings below).

2 Interstitial exudates; these are non-inflammatory when due to uraemia (page 573) or to a raised left atrial pressure as in mitral stenosis (page 603), or to failure of the left ventricle (page 605). Inflammatory exudates occur with infections, cryptogenic fibrosing alveolitis (Hamman Rich syndrome) and systemic connective tissue disease. The associated changes in lung function are described below.

3 Disorders caused by inhaled inorganic particulates; these conditions are mainly of occupational origin (page 587).

4, 5 Tumours and congenital dysplasias. Some of the conditions are listed in Table 16.14.

The lung function of patients with interstitial lung disease usually combines the features of a restrictive ventilatory defect and a defect of

Table 16.14 Interstitial lung diseases which give rise to characteristic findings on
assessment of lung function

(a) *Systemic diseases which can involve the lung*:
Sarcoidosis, beryllium disease
Disorders of connective tissue, including:
  progressive systemic sclerosis, rheumatoid arthritis, lupus erythematosus, polyarteritis
  nodosa
Coeliac disease
Schistosomiasis (bilharzia)
Xanthomatoses, including eosinophilic granuloma
Disseminated tuberculosis, carcinomatosis, neurofibromatosis and other conditions
Chronic interstitial oedema (from left ventricular failure, hexamethonium, uraemia etc.)

(b) *Diseases which primarily involve the lung*:
Interstitial pneumonitis, including Hamman Rich Syndrome (diffuse fibrosing alveolitis)
Extrinsic allergic alveolitis (Table 16.23, page 596)
Nitrous fume exposure (e.g. silo-filler's disease)
Virus pneumonia
Drug sensitivity (e.g. to nitrofurantoin, bleomycin, busulphan)
Chronic interstitial fibrosis, including: cases of interstitial pneumonitis, asbestosis,
  talcosis, hard metal disease, acute silicosis, radiation fibrosis
Bronchiolar or alveolar cell carcinoma, lymphomatous infiltrate
Alveolar proteinosis and micro-lithiasis; pulmonary muscular hyperplasia
  leiomyomatosis and other conditions

---

gas transfer. However, one or other may predominate depending on
the lung pathology. In the late stages the typical features may be
obscured by airflow obstruction. The changes are summarised in
Fig. 16.11, illustrated by two examples in Case Study 16.3 and described

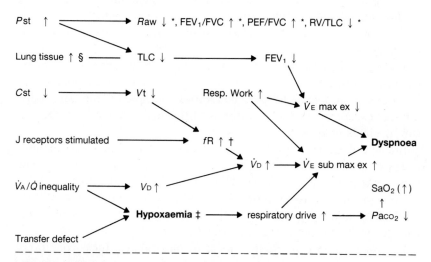

* direction of change can be reversed by secondary infection.
† can be associated with anxiety.
‡ at rest due to uneven $\dot{V}_A/\dot{Q}$ distribution and on exercise partly to the transfer defect.
  Can contribute to dyspnoea.
§ can narrow small airways (hence RV% ↑).

Fig. 16.11 Lung function in interstitial lung diseases (for details see text).

below. Interstitial lung diseases of occupational origin are described subsequently (page 595).

Interstitial lung disease

Case Study 16.3 Lung function in two patients with diffuse fibrosing alveolitis

Uncomplicated disease

Mr E., aged 42 years, presented with breathlessness on exertion of 3 months' duration which was rapidly getting worse. He had a dry, unproductive cough. He gave a history of apparently trivial exposure to a number of noxious chemicals and of a recent nervous break-down. On examination he was overweight. There were a few coarse crackels at the right base. The blood pressure was 150/110 mmHg. The chest X-ray showed mottled opacities throughout both lung fields and elevation of the right diaphragm. The ECG showed left axis deviation. The Mantoux reaction was positive at 1/1000; the serum proteins were normal. The physical signs were consistent with fibrosing alveolitis affecting particularly the right lung. However, in view of the history of psychosomatic illness, the patient was referred for assessment of lung function with a view to obtaining confirmatory evidence for the diagnosis.

On assessment of lung function the forced expiratory volume and forced vital capacity were both reduced, as were all the components of the total lung capacity. The ratios FEV_1/FVC and RV/TLC were within normal limits. The transfer factor (diffusing capacity) for the lung was diminished due to a reduction in the membrane component. The lung volume index of uneven ventilation was within normal limits. The tensions of oxygen and carbon dioxide in the arterial blood when breathing air at rest were on the low side of normal. The ventilation on exercise was increased both when breathing air and when breathing oxygen. The lung compliance was greatly reduced and the airway resistance was low. The findings were considered typical of interstitial pulmonary fibrosis and this diagnosis was confirmed at lung biopsy. The low compliance was also noted by the anaesthetist who experienced difficulty in maintaining the ventilation of the lung by manual compression of the anaesthetic bag. The patient subsequently received steroid therapy which improved his symptoms but the transfer factor and total lung capacity continued to deteriorate.

Complicated by airways obstruction

Mr F., aged 51 years, was charge-hand in a flour mill where he had worked for 16 years. Before that he worked as a cleaner on

Continued on p. 562

Case Study 16.3 *Continued*

the railways and served in the army, but did not go outside the continent of Europe. He presented with breathlessness of recent origin and a history of recurrent winter bronchitis; he was otherwise in good health and had no sputum at the time of investigation. He smoked 10–20 cigarettes per day. On examination he was overweight; coarse crackles and rhonchi were heard on auscultation of the chest. The Mantoux reaction was strongly positive and the sputum contained *Aspergillus*; no tubercle bacilli were detected. The plasma proteins were normal. The precipitin reaction for aspergillia and the Casoni test were both negative. The chest X-ray showed an enlarged heart, prominent pulmonary arteries, diffuse mottling in both lung bases and what appeared to be a small pleuropericardial cyst in the left cardiophrenic angle. The ECG was within normal limits. The patient was referred for assessment of lung function, as a case of obstructive lung disease with some atypical features.

The findings on assessment of lung function included reductions in the forced expiratory volume and $FEV_1\%$; the total lung capacity

Table B16.3 Case study measurements

Subject:	Mr E.	Mr F.	Reference values
Diffuse fibrosing alveolitis:	Uncomplicated†	Mixed	
Age (yrs)	42	51	
Height (m)	1.72	1.69	
Weight (kg)	92	75	
FEV_1 (l)	1.78	1.20	3.1
Change with bronchodilator (%)	0	0	<10
FVC (l)	2.18	2.50	4.1
FEV%	82	48	73
TLC (l)	2.80	5.08	6.2
IVC (l)	1.94	3.25	4.1
FRC (l)	1.68	2.72	3.8
RV (l)	0.86	1.83	2.0
RV%	31	36	34
Air trapping	No	Yes	No
Tl (single breath)*	4.7 (14)	5.5 (17)	9.0
V_A eff/V_A	0.95	0.85	> 0.85
Pa,o_2*	11 (82)	9.3 (70)	12
Pa,co_2*	4.7 (35)	4.8 (36)	4.8–6.3
$\dot{V}_E$, ex air (l min^{-1})	44.8	44.7	37
O_2 (l min^{-1})	34.6	30.9	35
Cst (inspn)*	0.5 (0.05)	2.6 (0.26)	2.4
$Cdyn$*	0.4 (0.04)	1.6 (0.16)	2.4
Raw (plethysmograph)*	0.076 (0.76)	0.30 (3.0)	0.11

* For units see footnote to Table B16.1 (page 533).
† Reference values were not very different from those for Mr F.

Continued on p. 563

Case Study 16.3 *Continued*

was somewhat reduced but the residual volume as a percentage of total lung capacity was normal. Some air trapping was evident on the spirogram. The transfer factor (diffusing capacity) for the lung was reduced as were both its components. The tension of oxygen in the arterial blood was reduced and that of carbon dioxide was on the low side of normal. The ventilation during exercise was increased when breathing air and markedly reduced when breathing oxygen. The dynamic compliance was less than the static compliance and the airway resistance was increased.

The changes in the ventilatory capacity, airway resistance and dynamic lung compliance were evidence for airways obstruction, but the combination of a low transfer factor with a small total lung capacity and a normal residual volume was not typical of this condition. These latter observations were interpreted as evidence for associated fibrosing alveolitis and this diagnosis was confirmed at lung biopsy. The patient was treated with corticosteroid drugs and his symptoms improved.

Lung volumes and ventilatory capacity

In the interstitial lung diseases the lung volumes can be reduced by an increase in volume of interstitial tissue, replacement of ventilated lung units by fibrous tissue and diffuse interstitial fibrosis which reduces the distensibility of those units which remain. An increased quantity of interstitial tissue can encroach on the lumen of small airways. In the early stages of the condition the residual volume is then affected to a variable extent depending on the balance between displacement of gas by interstitial tissue which reduces the residual volume and the narrowing of small airways which increases it by causing premature airway closure during expiration. The narrowing reduces the maximal expiratory flow rate at small lung volumes and leads to pronounced frequency dependence of the dynamic lung compliance. Later in the course of the disease the fibrous tissue may exert traction on the small airways delaying their closure during expiration and reducing the residual volume. If the patient develops chronic bronchitis with airflow obstruction later in his illness, the associated closure of airways can lead to the residual volume increasing again.

Loss of lung units and diffuse interstitial fibrosis both reduce the distensibility of the lung, hence the static lung compliance is reduced and the recoil pressure at total lung capacity is increased. These changes progressively reduce the inspiratory capacity and alter the indices to which inspiratory capacity contributes, for example, total lung capacity, vital capacity, transfer factor, forced expiratory volume and radiographic lung volume (Fig. 16.12). However, the maximal expiratory flow rates are also influenced by the fibrous tissue because the traction exerted on

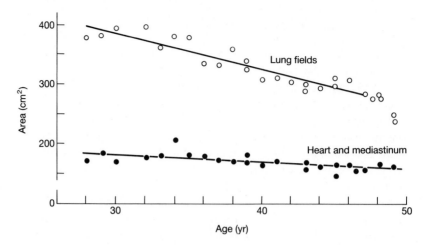

Fig. 16.12 Area of the chest radiographs showing a progressive reduction in the patient's lung area between first exposure to asbestos at the age of 26 years and death at the age of 49 years; very little change was observed in the area of the mediastinum.

the walls of airways tends to lower the airway resistance and the specific conductance is increased. There is little dynamic compression during expiration. The FEV_1 is high relative to the vital capacity ($FEV_1\%$ increased) and the peak expiratory flow can be virtually normal. Possibly on account of these opposing effects of lung fibrosis Turner Warwick and colleagues found the FEV_1 to be a poor guide to prognosis in this condition. However, the beneficial effects on airway calibre are partially offset by an increase in lung tissue resistance. In addition the reduction in lung volume reduces the initial length of the fibres in the respiratory muscles at the start of expiration. The applied force is reduced in consequence. In the early stages of interstitial lung disease the resultant of these and other factors is to cause a moderate reduction in the maximal breathing capacity, but the ability to increase the ventilation on exercise is seldom seriously impaired. Later in the course of the disease, as a result of peribronchial fibrosis or in the presence of complications including infection or sarcoid granuloma of the epithelium, there is superimposed obstruction of the airways; the airway resistance then tends to rise and the ventilatory capacity is further reduced.

Ventilation–perfusion relationships and exchange of gas in the lung (see also page 519)

The distribution of inspired gas in patients with disease of the lung parenchyma is affected by the increase in the elastic recoil and by the presence of interstitial fibrosis both of which limit the expansion of some alveolar units. The former expands the anatomical deadspace relative to the thoracic gas volume and, by securing the patency of the airways, ensures that the times of filling and emptying of the alveoli are relatively uniform; there is then little temporal inequality of ventilation and tests of the distribution of inspired gas which reflect this attribute of the lung can be normal. The variability of the expansion ratios leads to a widening of the range of the ventilation–perfusion ratios, especially when the condition is advanced. The indices which reflect this change therefore show evidence of abnormality (Chapter 8). In particular the physiological deadspace is increased and the tension of oxygen in the arterial blood is lower than the mean alveolar tension (A-aDo_2 is increased). The $\dot{V}A/\dot{Q}$ inequality is probably compensated by hypoxic pulmonary vasoconstriction which mitigates the hypoxaemia both at rest and during exercise. The hypoxaemia is aggravated by defective gas transfer on exertion even if (as sometimes happens early in the disease) the transfer factor is normal at rest. The ways in which the transfer defect contributes to hypoxaemia are discussed on page 284.

The transfer defect reflects both of diminution in lung expansion (page 294) and loss of alveolar capillaries. In a healthy person the former can be simulated by a submaximal inspiration which on average reduces the transfer factor by one SI unit ($3\,ml\,min^{-1}\,mmHg^{-1}$) per litre of lung volume. Thus the lung volume should be taken into account when interpreting the result. This can be done using the above correction factor. Alternatively the Kco (transfer factor/alveolar volume) can be interpreted instead. This index is normally reported at total lung capacity and higher values are observed when the measurement is made at a submaximal lung volume. Thus if the lung volume is subnormal the Kco should be high relative to the reference value. In the presence of a reduced total lung capacity a normal or reduced Kco is evidence for a transfer defect; a relatively high Kco is evidence that the restriction is due to changes in the pleura or chest wall and not the lungs (page 574).

A low transfer factor seldom occurs in isolation but can do so in some circumstances including treated pulmonary eosinophilia, progressive systemic sclerosis and lupus erythematosus, and also after high dosage radiation therapy to the lung.

The hypoxic pulmonary vasoconstriction is initially beneficial for the reasons given above. However, the pulmonary vascular resistance can be further increased by the occurrence of obliterative endarteritis secondary to the disease process. The two mechanisms summate and may eventually cause right heart failure (see Fig. 16.14, page 577).

Control of respiration and response to exercise

A prominent feature of patients with disease of the lung parenchyma is breathlessness on exertion. This is due mainly to an increase in the ventilation for which there are a number of contributory causes summarised in Fig. 16.13.

The increase in elastic recoil alters the pattern of breathing and increases the basal metabolism. The ventilation–perfusion imbalance and shallow breathing increase the proportion of ventilation which does not contribute to gas exchange. The hypoxaemia increases the

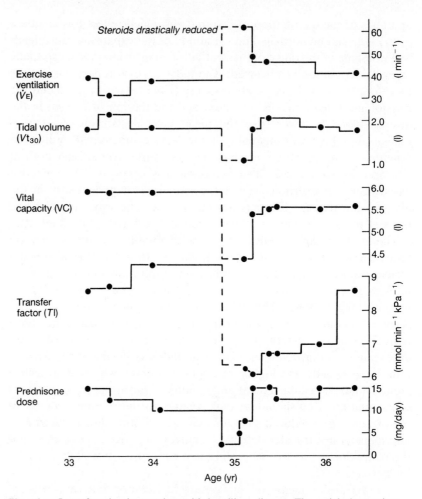

Fig. 16.13 Lung function in a patient with beryllium disease. The serial observations illustrate an acute episode precipitated by a reduction in the dosage of prednisone. The patient became hypoxaemic at rest (due probably to $\dot{V}_A/\dot{Q}$ inequality), the exercise ventilation (at $\dot{n}_{O_2}$ 67 mmol min^{-1}) and respiratory frequency increased whilst the tidal volume at ventilation 30 l min^{-1} (Vt_{30}) diminished. The patient experienced breathlessness on exertion. At other times normal values were observed for most of the indices including the arterial oxygen tension at rest. However, the transfer factor was reduced and, probably on this account, the arterial oxygen tension decreased during exercise:

		Relapse	Remission
Pa_{O_2}*	Rest	8.9 (67)	11.9 (89)
	Exercise	6.1 (46)	8.3 (62)
Pa_{CO_2}*	Rest	5.3 (40)	4.7 (35)
	Exercise	4.1 (31)	4.7 (35)

* For units see footnote to Table B16.1, page 533.

chemoreceptor drive to breathing. In addition, in some conditions, J receptors are stimulated to cause tachypnoea and subjective anxiety; the latter can aggravate the tachypnoea and associated breathlessness. Each of these changes contributes to pulmonary ventilation by increasing either the deadspace or the alveolar components ($\dot{V}_D$ and

$\dot{V}_A$ respectively). The latter increases the excretion of carbon dioxide from the lung and causes respiratory alkalosis. This is compensated by renal and other changes (page 520). There is both a reduction in the tension of carbon dioxide in the arterial blood and an increase in the ventilatory response to gas mixtures containing carbon dioxide (page 346). Once this adaptation has taken place the inhalation of oxygen instead of air during exercise, whilst it causes an immediate decrease in ventilation does not at once restore it to a normal level. Instead the hyperventilation persists because the buffering capacity of the blood and the cerebrospinal fluid are reduced. However, the breathlessness improves while breathing oxygen. In one patient Guz and colleagues found that it could be eliminated by blocking the vagus nerves in the neck. Thus in this patient the breathlessness was due to sensory information from the lungs. In other subjects the tachypnoea was significantly ameliorated during non-REM sleep; this suggested that the cerebral cortex was contributing to this abnormality.

In interstitial lung disease the extent of the disturbance to ventilation varies with the nature and the severity of the underlying pathological changes. When there are parenchymal lesions with little fibrosis the hyperventilation and/or the tachypnoea are often prominent features at rest as well as on exercise; the changes are usually readily ameliorated by corticosteroid drugs (Fig. 16.13); when there is fibrosis the hyperventilation may occur only on exercise. With marked fibrosis the ventilatory capacity is greatly reduced; the exercise ventilation standardised for the consumption of oxygen may then be within or below the accepted normal range.

Sarcoidosis, relation to radiographic appearance

In sarcoidosis showing radiographic hilar adenopathy the lung fields may appear normal; however, a high proportion of biopsy specimens obtained at fibreoptic bronchoscopy show involvement of the lung parenchyma. There may then be breathlessness on exertion which is due to impared lung function. The changes include reductions in vital capacity, compliance and transfer factor (diffusing capacity) and an increase in elastic recoil pressure. The alveolar epithelium becomes more permeable to fluid. There is often narrowing of small lung airways. In the event of clinical and radiographic improvement, the vital capacity usually enlarges, but the transfer factor may continue to deteriorate.

When there are nodular pulmonary infiltrations which have been present for less than 2 years the lung function is often normal, or it may revert to normal following treatment with corticosteroid drugs; in this event, if the drug is discontinued the function can deteriorate (cf. Fig. 16.13). When the infiltration is suggestive of interstitial fibrosis, or when the lesions are known to have been present for 2 years or longer, the function of the lung is usually impaired and seldom improves to a material extent with treatment. Thus any treatment is best given early in the course of illness. The severity of the transfer defect is, in general, related to the duration of the disease and the extent of the pulmonary fibrosis; in addition, Young and colleagues have shown that the increase in ventilation is related to the prevalence of granulomas, whilst the tachypnoea and the reduction in the vital capacity are related to the increase in thickness of the alveolar walls.

Summary

The pattern of abnormal function due to interstitial lung disease is easily recognised when the syndrome is fully developed (Fig. 16.11). Diagnosis is more difficult in the early stages when the findings often lie within the limits of normal variation or resemble hyperventilation of psychogenic origin (cf. Fig. 16.13). In the late stage, the pattern can be obscured by secondary changes due to chronic obstructive pulmonary disease. This was the case of Mr F. whose findings are summarised in Case Study 16.3 (see also Fig. 16.11).

The cardinal features of fibrosing alveolitis are hyperventilation on exercise and reductions in transfer factor, lung volumes and static lung compliance; the proportion of the forced vital capacity which can be expired in 1 s is normal or increased. These changes are associated with normal values for the residual volume as a percentage of the total lung capacity and relatively normal values for indices of distribution of inspired gas. However, indices which reflect the range of the ventilation−perfusion ratios show evidence of abnormality. The tension of carbon dioxide in the arterial blood in the early and intermediate stages of the disease is usually reduced, especially during exercise. In the terminal stages the tension can be increased. The tension of oxygen in arterial blood is often normal in the early stages and declines as the condition progresses; it usually falls further during exercise. The breathlessness can then be ameliorated by the use of portable oxygen apparatus (page 639).

For monitoring the progress of patients the use of vital capacity and transfer factor is usually sufficient. For making a physiological diagnosis these tests should be supplemented by an exercise test. The static lung compliance should preferably also be measured, particularly if there is a possibility that emphysema may coexist. The pathological diagnosis may need to be substantiated by lung biopsy.

Liver disease

In liver disease a number of factors can contribute to impaired function of the lungs. The presence of ascitic fluid can reduce the total lung capacity and its subdivisions. It can also lead to treatment with thiazide diuretic drugs which can cause hyperventilation and hypocapnia. Peri-bronchial oedema at the lung bases can reduce the ventilation of the lower zones of the lung and increase the closing volume. The closure of airways can result in shunting of blood through the non-ventilated areas; this gives rise to hypoxaemia which may be ameliorated by inspiration to total lung capacity. Other causes of hypoxaemia include intrapulmonary arterio-venous anastomoses and portapulmonary shunts which are secondary to portal hypertension; the anastomoses can be of considerable magnitude but the shunts are usually small. These vascular shunts differ from those due to lung disease in being associated with a low pulmonary vascular resistance which is not much increased by hypoxia. Hypoxaemia occurs mainly as a result of ventilation–perfusion inequality, due to the presence in the lung of dilated precapillary vessels. The transit time for blood perfusing such vessels is relatively short but not sufficient to cause a diffusion defect. The vasodilatation appears to be due to a vasoactive polypeptide which is normally removed from the blood on its passage through the liver (page 203). The resulting hypoxaemia contributes to an increase in ventilation during exercise which can cause incapacitating breathlessness on exertion; the hyperventilation is reduced by portable oxygen therapy. The hyperventilation can be preceded by a reduction in the transfer factor for which the cause is not known. The lung volumes and ventilatory capacity are completely normal except when there is a restrictive type of ventilatory defect on account of coexisting fibrosing alveolitis; however, this condition occurs infrequently. Other features are a high cardiac output and a shift to the right of the haemoglobin dissociation curve. The condition has been studied by Stanley, Reeves, and Rodriguez-Roisin with their respective colleagues amongst others; it is illustrated by the case of Mr G. (Case Study 16.4).

Adult respiratory distress syndrome

The adult respiratory distress syndrome occurs in response to acute injury to the lung from any of a number of causes which can be local or arise outside the lung (Table 16.15). The condition is characterised by interstitial and alveolar oedema without a hydrostatic cause (the pulmonary venous and wedge pressures, and the plasma osmotic pressure, remain normal), there is hypoxaemia which shows little response to oxygen therapy, and the lungs are stiff with a very low compliance. The hypoxaemia is a consequence of ventilation–perfusion inequality; this is aggravated by a diminution in the normal pulmonary vasoconstrictor response to hypoxia. The syndrome is believed to be caused by superoxide radicals which increase the permeability of the alveolar capillary membrane. The capillaries become congested and neutrophils, platelets and other components of an inflammatory reaction are attracted to the site. Fibrin is laid down, blood vessels and lymphatics become thrombosed and hyaline membranes appear in the alveoli. The alveolar type II cells diminish in number and there is then deficiency of lung surfactant; this leads to atelectases which further reduce the lung compliance. The changes are maximal at about the 5th day from the onset. Thereafter fibrous tissue is laid down in the lung interstitial tissue and alveolar type I cells proliferate.

Recovery can be complete but many patients subsequently exhibit

Case Study 16.4 Lung function in liver disease

Mr G. aged 30 was a building constructor who gave a 9-month history of shortness of breath which started during a holiday in Mexico; the breathlessness disappeared on return to sea level but recurred following a head cold: he was anorexic, had lost 5 kg in weight and experienced night sweats. His symptoms had led to his discontinuing playing rugby. In the past he had regularly drunk 12 pints of beer a night but did not smoke. On examination he was cyanosed, had gross finger clubbing, a flapping tremor, numerous spider naevi and palpable liver and spleen. Assessment of lung function revealed a low transfer factor, exercise hyperventilation and hypoxaemia. The latter was only partly corrected by breathing oxygen, indicating that the patient also had a large right to left shunt across the lungs. The lung volumes and ventilatory capacity were normal. Studies of regional lung function using Xe^{-133} showed that the perfusion was normally distributed. The ventilation was reduced at the lung bases but this could not account for the hypoxaemia which was not improved by inspiration to total lung capacity. At rest breathing air the pulmonary arterial pressure was $15/7$ mmHg despite the cardiac output being $14 \, l \, min^{-1}$.

The patient's breathlessness was ameliorated by the use of portable oxygen apparatus but he became progressively more disabled. Death was due to an overwhelming haemoptysis. The findings at post-mortem were of portal cirrhosis and of a highly vascular lung, including arterio-venous anastomoses particularly at the lung bases.

Table B16.4 Case study measurements

Subject:	Mr G.		
Condition:	Portal cirrhosis		
Age (yrs)	30	Tl co,sb*	4.8 (14.4)
Stature (m)	1.83	Kco*	0.8 (2.3)
Weight (kg)	76	Pao_2*	5.5 (41)
FEV_1 (l)	4.2	$Paco_2$*	2.3 (31)
FVC (l)	5.17	$\dot{Q}s/\dot{Q}t$ (%)	50
TLC (l)	6.28	Ve, ex air† ($l \, min^{-1}$)	62
RV%	17	O_2 ($l \, min^{-1}$)	51

* For units see footnote to Table B16.1 (page 533).
† At O_2 uptake 45 mmol min^{-1}.

features of diffuse interstitial fibrosis (see preceding section). The likelihood of this occurring is related to the duration of the acute phase of the illness rather than to the severity in the first few days. Thus early treatment and avoidance of secondary infection are important.

Table **16.15** Some causes of adult respiratory distress syndrome   *Surgery*

Local trauma	Pulmonary contusion
Pneumonia	Bacterial, viral or drug-induced
Via airways	Aspiration (e.g. gastric contents)
	Inhaled toxic fumes
	Breathing oxygen (>40%)
Embolic	Fat, amniotic fluid, multiple thrombi
Other	Extensive trauma or burns, endotoxins secondary to septicaemia,* pancreatitis
	Pre-eclampsia
	Raised cerebral pressure
	Cardio-pulmonary by-pass

*Especially from Gram-negative organisms.

The treatment includes oxygen in moderate dosage and, in mild cases continuous airway pressure. In more severe cases the patient should be treated by assisted or controlled ventilation (page 647); when this is done the inspiratory phase should be followed by a prolonged post-inspiratory pause. Positive end-expiratory pressure can reduce the extent of the atelectases. If the ventilation should be inadequate the elimination of carbon dioxide can be increased using the technique of partial extracorporeal carbon dioxide removal. Steps can also be taken to reduce the fluid accumulated in the lung and to provide cardiac, circulatory and renal support. However, the mortality from the condition is high, so strenuous efforts should be directed towards prevention.

Surgery

Non-thoracic surgery

If lung function is already impaired this can contribute to the development of complications following non-thoracic surgery, or it can detract from the final outcome. Thus the lung function should be considered pre-operatively. Normally it will not be a contraindication to surgery. However, an obstructive type of ventilatory defect or a low peak expiratory flow rate might indicate a chronic chest infection; this could be aggravated by the pre-operative medication (atropine) increasing the viscosity of bronchial secretions, by the anaesthetic impairing ciliary action or by post-operative pain reducing the effectiveness of coughing. A reduced lung compliance could lead to difficulty in providing assisted or controlled ventilation (e.g. Mr E., page 561). The presence of pre-operative hypercapnia could increase the ill-effects of post-operative hypoventilation. The risk is greatest when oxygen therapy is required during recovery from the anaesthetic (page 619). The hazards associated with impaired lung function formerly led to the practice of limiting surgical intervention in such patients to emergency procedures. However, advances in anaesthesia have changed the perspective. Severe

Table 16.16 Levels of respiratory impairment at which post-operative assisted ventilation may be needed

Index	Level
Forced expiratory volume (l)	<1.0
Arterial O_2 tension (kPa and mmHg)	
If patient breathless at rest	<9.5 (70)
If not breathless at rest	<6.0 (40)
Arterial CO_2 tension	not contributory

(Source: Milledge JS, Nunn JF. *Anaesthesia* 1988; **43**: 543–551.)

respiratory impairment can be an indication for post-operative assisted ventilation (Table 16.16) but only rarely for the abandonment of a necessary surgical procedure.

Non-thoracic surgery can occasionally cause respiratory impairment. This can arise from infection or trauma to the lung or pleura or pulmonary embolism secondary to venous thrombosis. Damage can also occur as a result of immuno-suppression for transplantation of another organ or as part of the process of organ rejection. Any resulting infection should be treated energetically.

Thoracic surgery

Thoracic surgery is usually directed to the removal of diseased lung tissue which does not contribute to lung function. Where this objective is achieved the function of the lung is unlikely to be impaired by the operation. Hence the considerations discussed for non-thoracic surgery also apply. Difficulty arises when much functioning lung tissue is removed as can occur with pneumonectomy for lung cancer, or when the remaining tissue is emphysematous; it is then at risk of becoming overdistended. In the case of pneumonectomy for lung cancer Corris has found that the forced expiratory volume (FEV_1) is on average reduced by approximately 20%. However, the proportion varies depending on the condition of the affected lung. A successful post-operative result is likely if the estimated post-operative FEV_1 (i.e. observed FEV_1 less 20%) exceeds 40% of the reference value. In addition the pre-operative arterial oxygen tension should preferably exceed 8.0 kPa and the arterial carbon dioxide tension be less than 5.9 kPa. If the proposed operation is a bullectomy or lung plication for relief of emphysema the criteria for surgery are mainly clinical; however, severe respiratory impairment with much ventilation–perfusion inequality is usually a contraindication.

Lung transplantation

Heart–lung transplantation uncomplicated by features of rejection can produce an excellent functional result with normal lung function. The loss of pulmonary innervation appears not to be a disadvantage. Thus at rest and during sleep the gas exchange and the pattern of breathing are essentially normal when breathing air. The ventilatory response to hypoxia is normal. The ventilatory response to carbon dioxide and the $P_{0.1}$ are usually normal except when the vital capacity is low. The pulmonary denervation can be associated with an increased broncho-constrictor response to methacholine but this is not invariable; the bronchoconstriction is not attenuated by a subsequent full inspiration as occurs in normal subjects. The denervation of the heart is associated with a raised resting cardiac frequency. During submaximal exercise the ventilation is somewhat increased due to increases in both tidal volume and respiratory frequency; the arterial carbon dioxide tension is reduced in consequence. These changes appear to be due to the loss of afferent information from pulmonary stretch receptors; but the ventilatory transients at the start and end of exercise and the sensation of breathlessness are unaffected (pages 354 and 387). By contrast the changes in cardiac frequency at the start and at the end of exercise are delayed. In addition rapid glycolysis occurs at a relatively low rate of energy expenditure and the capacity for exercise is reduced. These changes could be due in part to cardiac denervation but they are also due to lack of physical fitness and are improved by physical training.

Acute lung rejection is caused by damage from activated lymphocytes infiltrating the walls of bronchioles and small blood vessels. The resulting bronchiolitis can be aggravated by infection. The condition is associated with impaired lung mixing and with reductions in forced expiratory volume (FEV_1) and transfer factor and can occur without radiographic abnormality. The FEV_1 is sometimes used to indicate a need for transbronchial biopsy with a view to treatment but a more sensitive index is needed. The diagnosis should be made early as otherwise the condition can progress to chronic obliterative bronchiolitis and to severe respiratory failure.

Renal disease

Renal failure leading to uraemia arises from diseases of the kidneys and conditions which obstruct the urinary tract. The causes include prostatic obstruction and pyelonephritis with hypertension. The lungs can be affected secondarily. In addition glomerulonephritis can involve the lungs directly by extension of the immunological disorder from the glomerular capillaries or basement membrane to the lung parenchyma.

In acute glomerulonephritis the number of functioning glomeruli and hence the urinary output are reduced but the capillary permeability is increased and this depletes the plasma albumin. These changes cause fluid retention and reduce the plasma osmotic pressure; they lead to an increase in the volume of interstitial fluid in the lungs and other tissues. The condition can progress to acute pulmonary oedema with pleural effusions. The increase in interstitial fluid stimulates the pulmonary J receptors to cause breathlessness; it also reduces the vital capacity, and hence the ventilatory capacity, and transfer factor. The residual volume and closing volume are increased secondary to narrowing of the lumina of bronchioles by the interstitial fluid. The changes cause ventilation−perfusion inequality and this increases the alveolar-to-arterial tension difference for oxygen (A-aDo_2). Most of the changes regress following treatment. However, the A-aDo_2 often remains elevated, indicating that the recovery is incomplete.

Acute proliferative glomerulonephritis affecting the glomerular basement membrane can be accompanied by similar changes in the alveolar basement membrane. The condition can give rise to *Goodpasture's syndrome* in which the features of acute renal failure are accompanied by intrapulmonary haemorrhage with haemoptysis; however, the renal consequences of the disease are often relatively slight. The haemorrhages displace gas from the lungs and thereby reduce the total lung capacity and its subdivisions; they also result in ventilation−perfusion inequality which causes hypoxaemia. These changes can progress to a stage where the patient is in need of assisted ventilation. However, the blood accumulated in the alveoli is able to combine with carbon monoxide so the transfer factor and Kco (Tl/Va) are increased. On this account the measurement of Kco can be used to monitor the response to treatment; this is by plasmapheresis to remove the circulating antibody, and by immunosuppressant drugs.

Chronic renal failure affects the chemical composition of the blood and causes a metabolic acidosis. This stimulates respiration to cause breathlessness which is often associated with an increase in tidal volume (Kussmaul respiration). There is then a compensatory respiratory alkalosis (page 524).

Haemodialysis for the temporary correction of uraemia is accompanied by hypoxaemia. There may also be carbon dioxide retention and a fall in transfer factor. The latter appears to be a consequence of activation of leucocytes by complement on the membrane used for dialysis; the activated leucocytes accumulate in the lung. The carbon dioxide retention is secondary to hypoventilation reflecting a reduction in ventilatory drive. The drive is influenced by the composition of the dialysate fluid. The hypoxaemia is accompanied by an increased alveolar-to-arterial tension difference for oxygen and, therefore, it is probably due to ventilation−perfusion inequality. The changes are not of clinical significance in persons with healthy lungs but could become so in patients with lung disease, particularly those in whom the glomerular disease process also affects the lung.

Restricted lung expansion

In the absence of lung disease (already considered on page 558), restriction of the lung can occur from abnormality of the thoracic skeleton, the pleura or the soft tissues of the chest wall. The causes include ankylosing spondylitis, kyphoscoliosis, diffuse pleural fibrosis, muscle disease, and scarring of the skin. The condition can be simulated

574

by the application to the chest of a strait-jacket or binder. In all of these circumstances the function of the lung is either normal throughout or is affected as a secondary consequence of the primary disorder. By contrast, *pectus excavatum* (funnel-chest deformity) seldom restricts the movement of the lung. The condition may however interfere with the diastolic filling of the heart during exercise or cause psychological disturbance on account of the unusual appearance of the chest; it may then give rise to lassitude or to breathlessness of psychogenic origin.

Diffuse pleural fibrosis

This condition usually affects both the parietal and the visceral pleura. It can be primary as following exposure to asbestos or secondary to pleural effusion or haemothorax. The presence of fibrous tissue reduces the lung compliance and increases the recoil pressure. These changes in turn reduce the inspiratory capacity and the forced expiratory volume, the vital capacity and the maximal tidal volume during exercise. The transfer factor is reduced but the Kco is increased; the physiological basis for these changes is discussed on page 293. In addition the fibrous thickening of the pleura is not uniform and this distorts the pattern of lung expansion. The resulting uneven lung function appears to contribute to hypoxaemia occurring during exercise.

Ankylosing spondylitis

In this condition the ribs are often held in a position which is rather closer to full inspiration than in healthy subjects; thus the functional residual capacity is increased and the inspiratory reserve volume is reduced. Zorab has pointed out that the change takes place at an early stage in the disease when it may have the effect of minimising the pain which is a prominent symptom. However, the compliance of the chest wall is reduced and this could affect the position of pressure equilibrium across the chest wall (Fig. 5.7, page 96). The total lung capacity is usually within normal limits but the residual volume is increased, possibly because the ribs tend to become fixed in their new position. The vital capacity is somewhat reduced in consequence. These changes resemble those in chronic non-specific lung disease. However, whereas in the latter condition the changes are secondary to narrowing of airways, in ankylosing spondylitis the airways are unaffected; the indices of uneven distribution of the inspired gas are therefore within normal limits as are the tensions of oxygen and carbon dioxide in the arterial blood. The ventilatory capacity, including the forced expiratory volume, is well maintained in the early stages of the disease; thus the proportion of forced vital capacity which can be expired in 1 s ($FEV_1\%$) is greater than in healthy subjects. In the late stages, partly as a result of progressive fibrosis of the upper lobes, the vital capacity and the ventilatory capacity are diminished. The change seldom progresses to a stage where the subject is seriously disabled or liable to hypoventilation.

In the absence of other disease processes, the prospect for lung function is reasonably good.

Kyphoscoliosis

Deformation of the dorsal region of the vertebral column can distort the thoracic cage. This then causes a restrictive type of ventilatory defect. Similar changes can follow cervical cordotomy for the relief of pain. An important feature is straightening of the ribs and paradoxical movement on inspiration. The changes decrease the mechanical advantage of the respiratory muscles and hence their effectiveness in expanding the thorax; they also progressively reduce the compliance of the deformed tissue and this further decreases the range of movement of the chest wall. The changes have the effect of reducing the vital capacity and hence the total lung capacity; the diminution is proportional to the degree of curvature. Scoliosis in young children impairs the development of the lung and this further reduces the subdivisions of total lung capacity including the residual volume. The residual volume as a proportion of total lung capacity is usually normal; however, the RV% can be increased by the deformity limiting expiration. The subject exhibits the features of a restrictive ventilatory defect including a normal or raised $FEV_1\%$, a reduced transfer factor and raised Kco (page 293).

The reduced size of the lung is associated with closure of alveolar units particularly at the lung bases; the perfusion of the lower zones and the compliance of the lung are reduced in consequence. At the same time the work of breathing, which is already high on account of the deformation of the chest wall, is further increased. The increase is to some extent mitigated by an increase in the rate and a decrease in the depth of breathing, but these compensatory changes also increase the proportion of the tidal volume which is expended in ventilating the physiological deadspace. The alveolar component of the tidal volume is then reduced, but the minute volume is not increased proportionately. The resulting hypoventilation raises the tension of carbon dioxide in the arterial blood. The associated acidaemia raises the pressure in the pulmonary circulation, both directly by causing pulmonary vasoconstriction and indirectly via an increase in the central blood volume. At the same time the wide range of ventilation−perfusion ratios and the hypoventilation give rise to hypoxaemia; this interacts with the acidaemia to aggravate the pulmonary hypertension. The pulmonary vascular resistance can be further increased by a rise in the blood viscosity, due to secondary polycythaemia induced by the hypoxaemia. The polycythaemia can be complicated by intravascular thromboses which aggravate the pulmonary hypertension. These events can progress to congestive cardiac failure (Fig. 16.14).

The pattern of lung function in the late stage of restrictive lung disease due to kyphoscoliosis resembles that of chronic obstructive pulmonary disease. However, whereas in COPD the narrowing of the

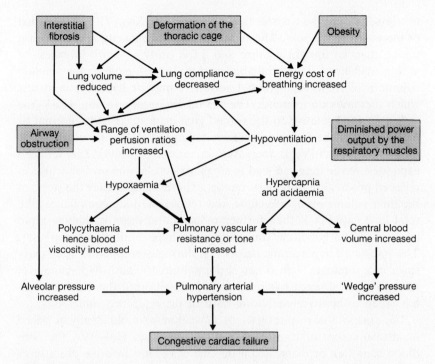

Fig. 16.14 Sequence of changes leading to congestive cardiac failure. In kyphoscoliosis the effects are aggravated by an increased susceptibility to intercurrent infection.

airways is the principal abnormality, in restrictive lung disease the airways are involved secondarily to intercurrent chest infection.

Respiratory muscle weakness

Many conditions which can give rise to hypoventilation are associated with a reduction in the strength of the diaphragm; depending on the mechanism and the site of the lesion the strengths of the intercostal and accessory muscles can also be reduced. The conditions are amongst those listed in Table 16.18 (page 580).

Localised lesions affecting one phrenic nerve can cause unilateral paralysis of one hemidiaphragm; this can cause breathlessness at the outset but seldom gives rise to notable symptoms. However, Green and colleagues have noted that breathlessness can be experienced during singing. The paralysis can aggravate a ventilatory defect from other causes. The principal symptom of respiratory muscle weakness is breathlessness on exertion. This can be associated with orthopnoea and with intolerance of restraints to breathing from tight clothing, carrying a rucksack or immersion in water. The muscle weakness is accentuated at night during REM sleep when it can cause the syndrome of sleep apnoea/hypopnoea (page 352).

The muscle weakness causes a hypodynamic type of ventilatory defect; this affects the inspiratory capacity which is reduced. There are corresponding reductions in the vital capacity, total lung capacity and to a lesser extent the transfer factor ($Tl\text{co}$). The $K\text{co}$ ($Tl/V\text{A}$) is normal or increased (page 293). The reduction in vital capacity is greater in a supine than an upright posture and a fall on lying down in excess of 30% is evidence for material abnormality. In such patients the residual volume is likely to be increased and there may be hypoxaemia at rest which increases on exercise. The forced expiratory volume (FEV_1) is well preserved relative to the forced vital capacity ($FEV\%$ normal or increased) but the forced inspiratory volume (FIV_1) is reduced, hence the ratio FEV_1/FIV_1 is increased in excess of unity. The reduced expansion of the lung can lead to small atelectases and probably also to reduced production of lung surfactant. These changes alter the slope of the lung volume–pressure curve and reduce the lung compliance; the total lung capacity is then further reduced and there is shallow rapid breathing. The condition can progress to hypoventilation (page 581). The associated hypercapnia occurs first during exercise, and at an early stage can summate with other abnormalities to cause hypercapnia at rest. In their absence hypercapnia is unlikely until the vital capacity has fallen to approximately one-third of the reference value.

The diagnosis of respiratory muscle weakness should ideally be based on measurement of transdiaphragmatic pressure. However, the condition can often be diagnosed using one of the less invasive procedures summarised in Table 16.17. The maximal transdiaphragmatic pressure is the maximal pressure difference between oesphageal and intragastric pressure; the measurement is made by inspiration from functional residual capacity against a closed airway, or in response to a sniff. The lower limits of normal have been given by Green and colleagues as approximately -10 and $-8\,kPa$ in men and women respectively. The cause of the muscle weakness can sometimes be identified by measurement of the conduction time in the phrenic nerve, electromyography or muscle biopsy. The treatment is that of the cause. Additional help can

Table 16.17 Stages in the diagnosis of notable weaknesses of the respiratory muscles.

Measurement	Technique	Positive result
Vital capacity: change from sitting to supine	Spirometry	$>30\%$
Maximal inspiratory pressure at mouth ($P\text{i.max}$)	Suction against shutter (cf. Table 5.4, page 109)	<-6 to $-8\,kPa$
Nasopharyngeal pressure (sniff $P\text{i,np}$ max)	Nasal probe	$<-6\,kPa$
Oesophageal pressure (sniff $P\text{i,oes}$ max)	Oesophageal catheter (cf. page 160)	$<-6\,kPa$
Transdiaphragmatic pressure (sniff $\Delta\,Pdi$) (twitch $\Delta\,Pdi$)	Oesophageal and gastric catheters, stimulation of phrenic nerve	$<-10\,kPa$ in men $<-7\,kPa$ in women

(Adapted from Moxham J. *Prob Resp* 1990; **3**: 312–329.)

sometimes be given by training the respiratory muscles (page 645) or reducing their work load temporarily by assisted ventilation (page 647). The response to treatment can most conveniently by monitored by serial measurements of peak expiratory flow.

Hypoventilation

Hypoventilation is a diminution in alveolar ventilation sufficient to reduce the elimination of carbon dioxide and raise the tension of this gas throughout the body. In the early stages the hypercapnia can cause a respiratory acidosis (page 521), but later a new equilibrium is achieved between CO_2 production and excretion. The cardinal feature is a raised $Paco_2$. Its extent is determined by the alveolar ventilation (defined on page 194) and the rate of production of carbon dioxide by metabolism. The relationship between the $Paco_2$ and the alveolar ventilation for a healthy subject under quiet resting conditions is illustrated in Fig. 9.1 (page 266). Some causes of hypoventilation are given in Table 16.18. In the majority of instances the condition arises from two or more of these processes acting in combination. In addition the hypoventilation itself initiates a sequence of events which aggravates the patient's difficulties.

Ondine's curse (Table 16.18) describes cases of alveolar hypoventilation in which the dominant lesion is loss of central respiratory drive. The subject can often perform voluntary respiratory manoeuvres and the lung function is initially normal. *Pickwickian syndrome* strictly describes cases of sleep apnoea/hypopnoea syndrome which are associated with obesity and evidence for hypoplasia of the anterior pituitary gland; however, the term is often applied in a more general sense and on this account has probably outlived its usefulness. *Obstructive sleep apnoea syndrome* (OSAS) should be used instead and an indication given of the aetiology (Table 11.5, page 352). The commonest cause is obesity in association with some predisposing anatomical features. This condition is illustrated by the case of Mr I. in Case Study 16.5. The patient experienced daytime somnolence and hypoxaemia during sleep; these features were an indication for detailed study of the nocturnal cardiorespiratory function. Other indications for sleep studies are given in Table 16.19. The conditions are frequently accompanied by snoring but this symptom by itself is not a sufficient reason for intervention. The techniques for studying sleep disorders are described on page 366.

Effects of hypoventilation

The syndrome of hypoventilation may develop insidiously during the course of another illness or be presaged by hyperventilation which is due to anxiety arising from the underlying condition. The features of a hypodynamic type of ventilatory defect can coexist. The hypoventilation often occurs first at night when it is associated with poor sleep and morning headache; there may also be nocturnal bradycardia, urinary

Table 16.18 Some conditions associated with hypoventilation

Central alveolar hypoventilation (Ondine's curse)
  Primary in new born babies
  Secondary to lesions in brain stem (consciousness often impaired)
    Poliomyelitis
    Infarction
    Haemorrhage
    Atherosclerosis
    Multiple sclerosis
    Encephalitis
    Syringobulbia
    Tumour

Drug-induced respiratory depression
  Morphine, pethidine, codeine, barbiturates, tranquillising and anaesthetic agents

Lesions of spinal cord or peripheral nerves*
  (Tractotomy)
  Ablation of ventral ascending tracts
  Acute anterior poliomyelitis
  Motor neurone disease (progressive muscular atrophy)†
  Polyneuritis (infective, toxic, metabolic etc.)

Myoneural block*
  Myasthenia gravis, carcinomatous myasthenia, poisoning by curare,
    antichlolinesterases (nerve gas)

Disorders of muscles*
  Progressive muscular dystrophy
  Myopathy, metabolic (thyrotoxic, potassium depletion, e.g. from diuretics or familial),
    drug-induced (corticosteroid, alcohol etc), carcinomatous

Skeletal disorders including kyphoscoliosis (page 576)

Obstruction to upper airways (Table 11.5, page 352, also page 126)
  Associated with sleep apnoea/hypopnoea (page 350)

Secondary to respiratory impairment†
  Increased work of breathing,
  Loss of chemoreceptor drive (acquired or with O_2 therapy).

* See also respiratory muscle weakness (page 577).
† Example given in Case Study 16.5.

incontinence and fits. These features can be an indicator for undertaking sleep studies (Table 16.19). Alternatively the condition can present with cyanosis, lassitude and sometimes breathlessness on exertion, or with the symptoms and signs of congestive cardiac failure. The sequence of events which lead up to the latter condition is summarised in Fig. 16.14 (page 577). The breathlessness is due either to the increased effort which is required to ventilate the lung or to a disproportion between the drive to respiration and the relatively small ventilation minute volume to which it gives rise.

The principal effects of hypovention are due to the raised tension of carbon dioxide. This is associated with cutaneous vasodilatation and a full pulse. The accompanying respiratory acidosis is compensated by the excretion of an acid urine and by increases in the buffering capacity of the blood and cerebrospinal fluid (page 521). Once these changes

Case Study 16.5 Lung function in three patients with hypoventilation

Chronic hypoventilation

Mr H. was a motor engineer, aged 57 years, who developed severe breathlessness on exertion as a result of progressive muscular atrophy (motor neurone disease). He was referred for assessment with a view to the relief of breathlessness by portable oxygen therapy.

On examination he was weak, anxious and restless. He was cyanosed when breathing air and his respiration was shallow and rapid. His maximal breathing capacity was only $15\,l\,min^{-1}$. The tension of oxygen in his arterial blood was $6.8\,kPa$ ($51\,mmHg$) and the tension of carbon dioxide was $8\,kPa$ ($60\,mmHg$). The alveolar ventilation was only $2.2\,l\,min^{-1}$. He was given oxygen to breathe for a trial period of $8\,min$, during which time he became drowsy and his speech unintelligible; his depth of respiration diminished to a level which was less than the normal physiological deadspace. The tension of carbon dioxide rose to $10.4\,kPa$ ($78\,mmHg$) and he became hot and sweaty, although he was in a relatively cool environment. A diagnosis was made of hypoventilation syndrome with incipient carbon dioxide narcosis when breathing oxygen. Portable oxygen therapy was therefore out of the question. Instead the patient was in urgent need of mechanical assistance to his breathing.

Table B16.5 Observations on Mr H., a patient with progressive muscular atrophy

Inspired gas		Air	Oxygen
MVV	$l\,min^{-1}$	15.4	—
$\dot{V}_E$ (rest)	$l\,min^{-1}$	10.4	5.2
$\dot{V}_A$	$l\,min^{-1}$	2.2	0.86
Vt	l	0.24	0.14
f_R	per min	43	36
$Pa,_{O_2}$	kPa (mmHg)	6.8 (51)	—
$Pa,_{CO_2}$	kPa (mmHg)	8 (60)	10.4 (78)
$Sa,_{O_2}$	%	84	100

Obstructive sleep apnoea syndrome

Mr I. was a 53 year old taxi driver. He presented with a history of excessive daytime somnolence and episodes of falling asleep whilst driving his 'cab'. His wife reported that he snored excessively and 'thrashed around' at night, so much so that on occasions she moved into the spare bedroom to 'get some sleep'.

On examination his weight was $105\,kg$ and his height $1.75\,m$.

Continued on p. 582

Case Study 16.5 *Continued*

His collar size was 18. The only abnormal physical finding was an elevated systemic blood pressure of 160/105 mmHg. There was no evidence of pulmonary hypertension. Assessment of lung function showed a mild restrictive ventilatory defect in keeping with obesity. In the clinic the arterial blood gases were normal.

The history and examination were suggestive of obstructive sleep apnoea syndrome (OSAS). Accordingly the patient was submitted to overnight sleep studies starting with recording the oxygen saturation using an oximeter. Analysis of the result showed numerous brief reductions in saturation of greater than 4% (Fig. 16.15) in keeping with OSAS. Subsequently a full overnight polysomnographic study was carried out with monitoring of airflow at the mouth, oxygen saturation and chest and abdominal wall movements. The electro-cardiogram and electro-encephalogram were recorded together with the electro-occulogram which indicated the stage of sleep.

Analysis of the record showed that over a 1 h period the patient experienced over 20 episodes of apnoea of greater than 10 s duration each associated with a fall in oxygen saturation of greater than 4%. The chest and abdomen moved paradoxically during the apnoeas indicating their obstructive origin. These changes were associated with rapid eye movement sleep.

Analysis of the relative time spent at each oxygen saturation showed that the saturation was less than 90% for 37% of the time. Treatment was by weight reduction and overnight continuous positive airway pressure (CPAP via nasal mask). This completely abolished the episodes of obstructive sleep apnoea. There was a clear and significant improvement in overnight oxygen saturation (Fig. 16.16) and the patient's symptoms of daytime sleepiness resolved rapidly.

Acute hypoventilation

Mr J., aged 60 years, developed breathlessness due to progressive massive fibrosis of coal-workers' pneumoconiosis with recent deterioration. On admission to hospital he gave a history of increased cough, sputum and breathlessness and of some pleuritic pain on coughing. He had also noticed recent hoarseness in his voice and twitching of his hands; this was so severe that he had difficulty in drinking from a cup. On examination the patient was pale, agitated and tremulous. The eyes were prominent and there was bilateral lid lag. The breathing was shallow, the respiratory frequency was 50 per min and the cardiac frequency 132 per min. The skin was moist with sweat and the temperature was subnormal. No cyanosis

Continued on p. 583

Case Study 16.5 *Continued*

was detected. The thyroid gland was just palpable in the neck. On auscultation of the chest a few fine râles were heard at the lung bases but the remaining findings were unexceptional.

The patient was considered to have acute thyrotoxicosis precipitated by an episode of chest illness; he was treated with antibiotics and a sedative in low dosage whilst further investigations were arranged. The patient became drowsy and he was referred for a second opinion on this account. On examination the tongue and the mucous membranes were now grossly cyanosed; the tension of oxygen in the arterial blood was 3.9 kPa (29 mmHg) and the tension of carbon dioxide was 9.5 kPa (71 mmHg). The blood pH was not measured but was almost certainly reduced. A diagnosis was made of acute hypoventilation during an episode of chest illness in a patient with chronic lung disease. The signs of thyrotoxicosis were attributed to hypoxaemia. The patient was given oxygen at a flow rate of 2 l min^{-1} though nasal cannulae and the sedative was discontinued. No active stimulation of respiration was necessary and the patient made a relatively uneventful recovery. Prior to discharge, when breathing air, the tension of oxygen in the arterial blood had improved to 8.7 kPa (65 mmHg) and the tension of carbon dioxide to 6.1 kPa (46 mmHg).

Table 16.19 Indications for polysomnography i.e. sleep studies which relate the disturbed cardiopulmonary function to the stage of sleep

Chronic airflow limitation complicated by:
  pulmonary hypertension, right heart failure, secondary polycythaemia, daytime hypoxaemia ($Pa,o_2 < 7.3$ kPa, 55 mmHg)

A restrictive ventilatory disorder complicated by:
  hypoventilation and hypercapnia plus disturbed sleep, morning headache, fatigue or any feature given above

Deranged respiratory control associated with:
  hypercapnia ($Paco_2 > 6$ kPa, 45 mmHg) plus any feature given above

Excessive daytime sleepiness

Nocturnal cardiac abnormalities:
  pronounced periodic bradycardia, A-V conduction defects, ventricular extra systoles occurring during sleep

(Based on recommendations of American Thoracic Society. *Am Rev Respir Dis* 1989; **139**: 559–568). The stages of sleep are given on page 350 and the ways of performing sleep studies on pages 364–367.

have begun to take place a further increase in the tension of carbon dioxide causes a smaller rise in the concentration of hydrogen ions in the blood and hence a smaller incremental stimulus to respiration than

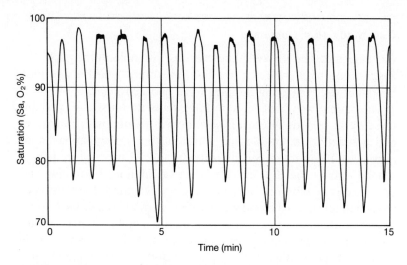

Fig. 16.15 A record of Mr I.'s oxygen saturation measured by pulse oximetry during sleep showing numerous brief periods of desaturation. Other information is given in Case Study 16.5 and Fig. 16.16.

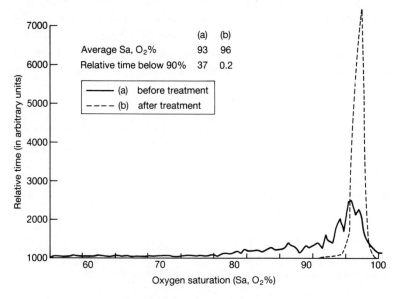

	(a)	(b)
Average Sa, O_2%	93	96
Relative time below 90%	37	0.2

(a) before treatment
(b) after treatment

Fig. 16.16 Graphs showing the relative times for which Mr I.'s oxygen saturation was at different levels during a 6 h period of sleep. The measurements were made before and after treatment for obstructive sleep apnoea syndrome. Other information is given in Fig. 16.15.

before the onset of hypoventilation.* The drive to respiration by carbon dioxide is now reduced and no longer protects the subject from further hypercapnia. When the tension of carbon dioxide exceeds about 9.3 kPa (70 mmHg) the hypercapnia itself exerts a depressant effect upon the respiratory centre. The depression is most marked when it occurs

---

* This is very obvious when measuring mixed venous P_{CO_2} by the rebreathing method.

acutely and is ameliorated by the increase which then occurs in the buffering capacity of the cerebrospinal fluid (page 523). The drive to respiration is usually maintained by hypoxaemia which is present as a result of both the reduction in alveolar ventilation and the increase in the range of the ventilation−perfusion ratios to which it gives rise (page 204). The position of equilibrium between the chemoreceptor drive which is increased by hypoxaemia, and the central drive, which is depressed by hypercapnia, is unstable; it is easily disturbed by any deterioration in the condition which was the primary cause of the hypoventilation. In this event the exchange of gas takes place on the steep part of the oxygen dissociation curve where a small reduction in ventilation causes a profound fall in the arterial oxygen saturation; this has serious consequences unless the condition is improved by treatment. The blood gas tensions in patients with respiratory failure are illustrated in Fig. 7.13 (page 208).

Aggravation of hypoventilation can occur as a result of acute chest illness or treatment with a drug which depresses respiration (e.g. Mr J., Case Study 16.5). However, the most catastrophic change takes place following the uncontrolled administration of oxygen; this procedure, by depriving the subject of the hypoxic drive to respiration, greatly reduces the activity of the respiratory centre and can lead to the tension of carbon dioxide rising to a level where it causes narcosis. The sequence of events is illustrated in Fig. 16.17. The recognition and the treatment of the condition are described on pages 629 and 647.

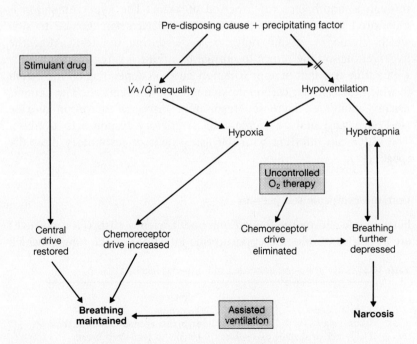

Fig. 16.17 Carbon dioxide narcosis secondary to uncontrolled oxygen therapy: causes and means of correction. Interventions and outcomes are respectively in boxes and bold type.

Table 16.20 Some conditions which can be associated with hyperventilation

Physiological	Ascent to high altitudes, pregnancy
Psychological	Anxiety, agoraphobia, anorexia nervosa, Da Costa's syndrome etc.
Pathological, lungs	Emphysema, interstitial lung disease, asthma
Pulmonary circulation	Pulmonary embolism Raised pulmonary capillary pressure, mitral stenosis, left ventricular failure
Brain (pontine disease)	Cerebral vascular disease, tumours
Other	Thyrotoxicosis, renal failure, diabetic ketosis

Hyperventilation syndrome

Hyperventilation with hypocapnia can be persistent or episodic. The former is a component of the physiological adaptation to high altitude. At sea level hyperventilation is usually associated with an identifiable medical condition (Table 16.20). Alternatively it can be of psychogenic origin when it is called hyperventilation syndrome. The syndrome is associated with symptoms of which the most impressive but least common is tetany; this is due to the respiratory alkalosis lowering the level of ionised calcium in the plasma. Some more common symptoms are listed in Table 16.21. The symptoms can often be precipitated by a medical consultation or by attendance at the lung function laboratory. The symptoms can usually be provoked by the patient hyperventilating through a mouthpiece for a period of 3 min. The hyperventilation is monitored by measurement of the end tidal carbon dioxide tension which should be in the range 2–2.5% during the test. After the hyperventilation the return to normal breathing is often relatively slow with a time constant of approximately 20–60 s depending on the extent to which the alveolar carbon dioxide tension was reduced. The patients usually exhibit an increased respiratory response to carbon dioxide (see page 346) and an increase of ventilatory response to exercise. The latter can interfere with the assessment of respiratory disability (page 442).

Immuno-compromised persons

Persons infected by the human immunodeficiency virus (HIV positive) are at risk of developing opportunistic infections of the lung of which

Table 16.21 Some symptoms associated with hyperventilation

Anxiety	Palpitations
Breathlessness	Tenseness
Chest pain	Tightness around mouth or chest
Cold, stiff or tingling extremities	Unable to take deep breath
Distended abdomen	Vision blurred
Dizziness	

the commonest is *Pneumocystis carinii* pneumonia; they may develop active pulmonary tuberculosis or a non-tuberculous mycobacterial infection of the lung. The patients are also at increased risk of infection from *Haemophilus influenzae* and other pyogenic organisms, lymphoid interstitial pneumonitis and neoplasms, including Kaposi sarcoma, which are associated with the acquired immune deficiency syndrome (AIDS).

Pneumocystis carinii pneumonia usually presents with fever, dry cough and mild breathlessness on exertion. This is due to impaired lung function and reflects proliferation of the protozoon in alveoli extending out from the hilar regions of the lung. The total lung capacity and all its subdivisions are reduced as are the transfer factor and Kco. There is hypoxaemia which is increased on exercise. The hypoxaemia is due to ventilation–perfusion inequality and is accompanied by some hyperventilation; the latter gives rise to hypocapnia. A reduced transfer factor and exercise hypoxaemia in a person who has symptoms suggestive of pneumonitis and is HIV positive can be an indication for broncho-alveolar lavage.

The susceptibility of HIV positive individuals to all types of infections requires that the respiratory equipment should be sterile. This is necessary to avoid the risk that either the patients may acquire a secondary infection or, if infected that they may give the infection to others. The guiding principles are first that a high level of cleanliness should be maintained at all times and second that high risk patients should be isolated from those parts of the equipment which cannot be sterilised effectively. This can be done using biological filters and Bag-in-box systems with disposable bags (page 54).

Lung disorders of occupational origin

Introduction

Inhaled dust particles deposit on the respiratory tract by the processes of impaction, sedimentation and Brownian diffusion. The impaction occur~ mainly proximally in the nose and at the bifurcations of the larger a rways and leads to the virtual exclusion from the smaller airways of particles having a diameter of more than about $10\,\mu m$, or in the case of fibres, a diameter of about $3-4\,\mu m$. The length and curvature of fibres has an additional exclusive effect due to chance contact with the walls of the airways (interception). The process of sedimentation leads to the deposition in the gas exchanging regions of the lung of a proportion of particles of the size $1-10\,\mu m$. The average retention is of the order of 5%. It varies directly with the time the particles are in the lung and with the lung volume, the tidal volume and functional residual capacity. Small particles less than about $0.5\,\mu m$ may impact on the walls of the alveoli and smaller airways by Brownian diffusion but few are retained.

Narrowing of lung airways leads to the deposition of particles and fibres occurring more proximally than would otherwise be the case;

this is a feature of some patients with chronic bronchitis and some cigarette smokers.

Dust depositing on the walls of the conducting airways is cleared rapidly towards the pharynx by the mucociliary apparatus. Particles depositing on the respiratory epithelium peripherally are removed more slowly by alveolar macrophages either towards the ciliated airways or, by penetrating the epithelium, into the lymphatic system of the lung (page 87).

The acute effect of an inhaled dust is dependent on its size distribution, its nature and its dose. Inert particles impacting on the large airways produce bronchoconstriction, cough, secretion of mucus and a change in the pattern of breathing (page 88). Irritant particles impacting on larger airways can cause bronchoconstriction directly (e.g. SO_2 in smog) or by release of mediators such as histamine (e.g. cotton dust). Constriction of larger airways can result from prior sensitisation to organic particles (e.g. asthma). Inert particles lodging on the gas-exchanging epithelium appear to have no detectable acute effect. Irritant particles can cause alveolitis directly and organic materials can give rise to alveolitis by hyper-sensitivity.

The chronic effect of inhaled dust on the conductive airways may be to produce cough and sputum (bronchitis), airways obstruction or bronchiectasis. The chronic effect on the parenchyma of the lung is usually of minor proportions in the case of inert dusts (e.g. oxides of iron and tin) which may none the less give rise to characteristic appearances on the chest radiograph. The effects on the lung parenchyma of more reactive dusts may be to cause pulmonary fibrosis with characteristic changes in gas transfer and elastic recoil (e.g. asbestos) or granuloma formation (e.g. quartz, berylium or organic dusts) or pulmonary emphysema (e.g. in coalworkers pneumoconiosis or from the inhalation of proteolytic materials). The chronic effects of inhaled dusts can be modified by individual susceptibility (e.g. rheumatoid factor and progressive massive fibrosis) or by superimposed extrinsic factors (e.g. tuberculosis). The effects are often aggravated by smoking.

Pneumoconiosis of coal workers and other occupational groups

Pneumoconiosis is the condition of a subject who has inhaled and retained dust in the lung. In the mineral pneumoconioses the dust usually collects in foci which are adjacent to respiratory bronchioles. The foci gives rise to a characteristic fine mottled appearance on the chest radiograph which is evidence for simple pneumoconiosis. At post-mortem there may be dilatation of respiratory bronchioles which is visible on large lung section. When this change occurs in relation to dust foci without evidence of tissue destruction it is called focal emphysema. However, despite the occurrence of focal emphysema in a proportion of subjects, the presence of dust in the lung does not necessarily give rise to symptoms and there may be no demonstrable impairment of pulmonary function. The majority of men with pneumoconiosis fall

into this category. With prolonged exposure to dust, enough may
accumulate in the lung to induce the changes of progressive massive
fibrosis; this condition is discussed below. Simple pneumoconiosis is
commonly due to inhalation of coal dust but may occasionally occur
with kaolin, Fuller's earth, carbon black, barium, tin oxide, antimony,
iron oxide, diatomaceous earth or other insoluble particulate material.

Any change in lung function due to simple pneumoconiosis needs to
be separated from that due to smoking or bronchitis, which whilst
possibly aggravated by the dust, is not related to the amount present in
the lung. It may be speculated that the absence of an association is due
to the bronchitis increasing the proportion of the dust particles which
deposit in the larger airways but the evidence is meagre. The decline in
forced expiratory volume with age amongst working coal miners has
been investigated by the British National Coal Board amongst others.
For an average miner aged 47 years, the principal additional factors
contributing to the decline were found to be smoking (0.34 l), cumulative
dust exposure (0.1 l) and when present, chronic bronchitis (0.08 l,
rising to 0.24 l if the man has had two or more chest illnesses). There
was no interaction between the effects of smoking and of exposure to
dust; after taking these factors into account there was no additional
effect due to simple pneumoconiosis. The vital capacity and the maximal
expiratory flows can also be reduced, whilst the residual volume is on
average increased. The total lung capacity and the static compliance
are usually within normal limits but can be increased if there is much
focal emphysema. The tension of oxygen in the arterial blood may be
somewhat lower than in subjects without pneumoconiosis but not to
the extent that there is a material reduction in the blood oxygen
saturation. However, the transfer factor for the lung is usually slightly
reduced and the mean pulmonary arterial pressure slightly increased in
those cases where the pneumoconiosis is of the pinhead type (diameter
of opacities up to 1.5 mm). These changes are seldom of sufficient
magnitude to cause breathlessness or to shorten life. In the absence of
emphysema or other complicating factors the remaining indices of lung
function are usually within normal limits.

Progressive massive fibrosis is associated with distinctive changes in
lung function. They are due to the nature of the disease whereby the
dust lesions coalesce and break down by a process of avascular necrosis
to form massive lesions; these are separated from the remaining lung
by fibrous tissue. The regions of coalescence behave as space-occupying
lesions which become denser and slowly enlarge whilst the fibrotic
areas cotract; concurrently the remaining lung tissue becomes stretched
and, in the late stages of the condition, exhibits the changes of compensatory emphysema. The airways become distorted and the necrotic
lesions can erode into the bronchi. These events give rise to bronchitis
and to the changes associated with irreversible airway obstruction.
Pulmonary arteritis on the periphery of the massive lesions reduces the
size of the pulmonary vascular bed and, in conjunction with hypoxaemia,
can progress to congestive cardiac failure.

On assessment of lung function the total lung capacity is often reduced and there is usually evidence for irreversible obstruction to the lung airways. This may be secondary to bronchitis. The transfer factor and its subdivisions are reduced by the loss of functioning lung tissue and by emphysema. In a typical case the airway resistance is increased and the ventilatory capacity is reduced; the $FEV_1\%$ is usually slightly reduced and the residual volume is increased. The indices which reflect the range of the ventilation−perfusion ratios show evidence of impairment. The exercise ventilation when breathing air is normal at first but in later stages of the disease is increased so that the capacity for exercise may be markedly diminished. In this event the exercise ventilation can usually be reduced by breathing oxygen; hence the patient may benefit from portable oxygen therapy (page 639).

Disability in patients with progressive massive fibrosis is determined mainly by the ventilatory capacity; this can be increased by measures directed at relieving the reversible component of the airway obstruction (page 559). Episodes of acute hypoventilation and of congestive cardiac failure may also require treatment. The findings on assessment of lung function in progressive massive fibrosis are illustrated by the case of Mr K. which is summarised in Case Study 16.6.

Case Study 16.6 Lung function in subjects with occupational lung disorders

Complicated pneumoconiosis (PMF)

Mr K. was an ex-coalminer, aged 63 years, who had worked underground for 31 years, first as a collier and then as an overman; he gave a history of shortness of breath on exertion since the age of 45 years. At that time an X-ray revealed the presence of numerous dust foci throughout the lung with superimposed areas of coalescence. A diagnosis was made of progressive massive fibrosis of coal-workers' pneumoconiosis and the patient was transferred to a less dusty occupation. However, his capacity for exercise continued to deteriorate and he developed chronic bronchitis. At the time of assessment the patient was convalescing from an episode of chest illness and was receiving treatment with digoxin and diuretics as well as bronchodilator and antibiotic drugs. On examination of the chest there were few abnormal physical signs, but the breath sounds and the tactile vocal fremitus were reduced. There was no cardiac failure. The X-ray showed progressive massive fibrosis (category 3/B, 2/2 on the International Classification). The ECG showed prominent *P* waves but was otherwise normal. On assessment of lung function the forced expiratory volume was reduced and represented a small proportion of the forced vital capacity; both volumes were labile and increased after the inhalation

Continued on p. 591

Case Study 16.6 *Continued*

of a bronchodilator aerosol. The total lung capacity was on the low side of normal but the residual volume was increased. The patient could expel from his lung by forced expiratory effort a volume of gas which was as large as his vital capacity and there was no evidence of air-trapping on the spirogram. The transfer factor (diffusing capacity) for the lung was reduced on account of a diminution in the membrane component. The lung volume index of uneven ventilation showed evidence of abnormality. The tension of oxygen in the arterial blood was reduced at rest, but the tension of carbon dioxide was normal. However, during exercise when the patient was breathing oxygen the tension of carbon dioxide increased and at this time the ventilation was markedly reduced. The lung was less compliant than normal and the airway resistance was increased.

The findings were evidence for impairment of all aspects of lung function; they were consistent with a space-occupying lesion (i.e. progressive massive fibrosis) plus airway obstruction. However, with a different industrial history, they could have been due to the combination of the latter condition with interstitial pulmonary fibrosis, though a lower value for the transfer factor would then have been expected. The relatively large bronchodilator response suggested that the patient was not receiving adequate therapy at the time of assessment. In addition, in view of the improvement in the capacity for exercise during breathing oxygen the patient was a suitable candidate for portable oxygen therapy.

Hard metal disease

Mr L., aged 64 years, gave a history of working for 20 years in the tungsten carbide industry where he was exposed to cobalt dust. For the first 11 years he was cleaning the insides of the furnaces. Subsequently he developed breathlessness on exertion which was aggravated by recurrent bouts of bronchitis; on this account he was transferred to lighter work in a less dusty atmosphere. At the time of assessment he was breathless on moderate exertion (clinical grade 3) but was otherwise in good health. On examination of the chest a few fine râles were heard at both lung bases and there were some sibilant rhonchi. The chest X-ray showed diffuse nodulation. The ECG was normal. On assessment of lung function the forced expiratory volume and the forced vital capacity were somewhat reduced but the lung volumes were otherwise within normal limits. The $FEV_1\%$ was normal and there was no air-trapping on the spirogram. The transfer factor (diffusing capacity) for the lung was reduced, due mainly to a diminution in the membrane

Continued on p. 592

Case Study 16.6 *Continued*

component. The tensions of oxygen and carbon dioxide in the arterial blood were both low at rest. The Pa,O_2 fell further on exercise when breathing air; at the same time the exercise ventilation was abnormally high. It was somewhat reduced by breathing oxygen. The airway resistance and the compliance were relatively normal.

These findings were evidence for disease affecting the lung parenchyma; in view of the history they were probably occupational in origin.

Table B16.6 Case study measurements

Subject:	Mr K.		Mr L.	Mr N.*
Condition:	PMF	Reference value	Hard metal disease	Byssinosis
Age (yrs)	63	—	64	66
Height (m)	1.63	—	1.76	1.72
Weight (kg)	54	—	79	77
FEV_1 (l)	1.23	2.5	2.03	1.33
Change with bronchodilator (%)	+17	<10	+7	NA
FVC (l)	2.71	3.5	2.90	2.75
FEV_1%	45	68	70	48
TLC (l)	5.01	5.6	5.98	8.23
IVC (l)	2.40	3.5	3.37	4.32
FRC (l)	3.59	3.7	3.73	4.68
RV (l)	2.61	2.0	2.61	3.91
RV%	52	38	44	48
Air-trapping	No	—	No	Yes
Tl† (single breath)	6.7 (20)	7.5 (22)	4.4 (13)	9.3 (28)
Dm† (single-breath)	9.7 (29)	14 (42)	8.0 (24)	NA
Vc (ml)	58	70	43	NA
VA eff/VA	0.64	>0.75	—	0.90
Pa,O_2†	8.3 (62)	12 (89)	9.6 (72)‡	11.2 (84)
Pa,CO_2†	5.6 (42)	<6 (46)	4.3 (32)	5.9 (44)
$\dot{V}E$, ex air (l min^{-1})	32	24	56	43.1
O_2 (l min^{-1})	23	22	35	43.1
Cst, inspn†	1.1 (0.11)	2.2 (0.23)	1.8 (0.18)	1.9 (0.19)
Raw (plethysmograph)†	0.25 (2.5)	0.1 (1.0)	0.14 (1.4)§	0.48 (4.8)

* See Case Study 16.8 (page 600) for details.
† For units see footnote to Table B16.1 (page 533).
‡ On exercise Pa,O_2 fell to 8.3 kPa (62 mmHg).
§ Interrupter method on inspiration.
NA = not available.

Silicosis

Silica dust causes nodular lesions which differ from the dust foci of simple pneumoconiosis by being relatively avascular and in containing more macrophages and fibrous tissue. The lesions occur along lymphatics and in the lung tissue; the latter are numerous in acute silicosis which is a diffuse interstitial pneumonitis caused by inhaling a large quantity of dust. Silicosis also occurs in subacute, progressive and chronic forms and the lesions can coalesce to give rise to massive fibrosis.

The lung function resembles that in pneumoconiosis of coal workers but in simple silicosis the reductions in forced expiratory volume and vital capacity are larger than in simple pneumoconiosis of coal workers and the changes can progress following cessation of exposure. In addition the transfer factor is often reduced, especially in acute silicosis. The pattern of function is then that of disease of the lung parenchyma.

Asbestos-related lung disease

The inhalation of fibres of asbestos and related minerals can cause a cellular reaction throughout the lung including the pleural surfaces and in the walls of the respiratory bronchioles and alveoli. When the intrapulmonary changes progress to diffuse fibrosis the condition is called asbestosis. Fibrous or calcified plaques can form on the parietal pleura. The extent of any diffuse pleural fibrosis can be assessed radiographically by the technique of computer-assisted tomography (CT scans). The pleural fibrosis is of greater functional significance if it involves the costophrenic angles (e.g. Table 16.22) than when confined

Table 16.22 Lung function in three men exposed to asbestos

Details	Diffuse pleural disease		Asbestosis
	Plaques	Fibrosis	
Age (yrs)	60	42	50
Height (m)	1.87	1.80	1.69
Weight (kg)	85	93	59
FEV_1 (l)	3.3 (3.5)*	1.9 (3.8)	1.2 (3.1)
FVC (l)	4.1 (4.8)	2.9 (4.8)	2.1 (4.1)
$FEV_1\%$	81 (69)	64 (76)	57 (73)
TLC (l)	5.9 (7.7)	4.0 (7.1)	4.3 (6.1)
RV (l)	2.0 (2.6)	1.4 (2.1)	1.8 (2.0)
Cst ($1\,kPa^{-1}$)	1.7 (3.1)	1.1 (2.8)	1.0 (2.4)
Pmax (kPa)	5.0 (2.5)	3.5 (2.5)	5.1 (2.5)
Tl ($mmol\,min^{-1}\,kPa^{-1}$)	8.6 (10.5)	7.6 (10.9)	3.4 (9.1)
Kco (Tl/V_A)	1.6 (1.4)	1.9 (1.7)	0.9 (1.5)
$\dot{V}_{E45}$ ($l\,min^{-1}$)	33 (24)	34 (24)	42† (24)
Vt_{30} (l)*	1.0 (1.5)	1.0 (1.5)	0.8 (1.4)
Sao_2 (rest/ex.%)	96/96	NA	91/84

These patients all had a reduced total lung capacity associated with a low compliance and high recoil pressure. The low TLC contributed to reductions in exercise tidal volume (Vt_{30}) and in transfer factor; in asbestos pleural disease the latter effect was associated with an increase in Kco. In all the patients the exercise ventilation was increased, mainly on account of an enlarged physiological deadspace. Exercise hypoxaemia occurred in the patient with asbestosis.
* Reference values are in parentheses: those for Vt_{30} are based on the predicted FVC. The upper limit for Pmax is 3.7 kPa.
† Extrapolated.
(Source: Cotes JE, Steel J. *Work-Related Lung Disorders.* Oxford: Blackwell Scientific Publications, 1987.)

to the costal surface of the pleura. Asbestosis is associated with an increased risk of developing bronchial carcinoma and exposure to one of the straight fibre types of asbestos (e.g. crocidolite) can cause mesothelioma. Thus asbestos can affect the lung in many ways.

Discrete pleural plaques do not usually impair the lung function. However, plaques which are very extensive may do so (Table 16.22) or they may conceal diffuse pulmonary fibrosis. Diffuse pleural fibrosis is associated with a restrictive type of ventilatory defect (page 575). The transfer factor is then reduced only by the change in size of the lung, and the Kco is increased above normal. By contrast in asbestosis the Kco is reduced. In both conditions the lung compliance is low and the recoil pressure increased. With asbestosis the pattern of impaired function is primarily that of interstitial lung disease (page 558); its severity is correlated with the extent of the disease as assessed radiographically from the profusion of small irregular opacities (Fig. 16.18). However, the typical features may be somewhat obscured by the superimposition of irreversible airway obstruction. This is most likely to occur amongst subjects working in a polluted atmosphere. The respiratory impairment is aggravated by smoking (cf. page 482). The change in lung function includes reduction of the vital capacity and transfer factor (diffusing capacity) and an increase in the ventilation during exercise. The residual volume is reduced by the shrinkage of the lung except when the deposited fibres cause air-trapping on account of narrowing of the small lung airways. The lesions mainly affect the lower zones of the lung and in this event the ventilation and perfusion may be redistributed towards the upper zones. If a bronchial cancer or a pleural mesothelioma should develop the additional features of a space-occupying lesion may be found. The lung function of men with extensive plaques, diffuse pleural fibrosis which also involved the costophrenic angles and asbestosis are summarised in Table 16.22. The

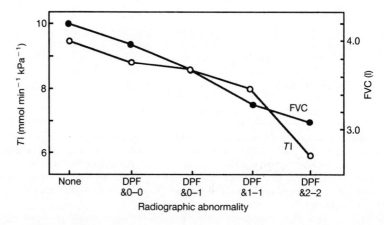

Fig. 16.18 Relationships of forced vital capacity (FVC) and transfer factor (*T*l) to diffuse pleural fibrosis (DPF) and the extent of involvement of the lung parenchyma (graded 0−2) in dockyard workers exposed to asbestos. (Source: Harries P. *Institute of Naval Medicine Report*. CRWP 1/71.)

progressive shrinkage of the lungs which can occur is illustrated in Fig. 16.12 (page 564). Some physiological findings are illustrated in Fig. 16.18.

Beryllium disease

Inhalation of beryllium dust or fumes can given rise to granulomatous lesions in the lung of an acute, sub-acute or chronic type. Heavy exposure causes an acute pneumonitis or pulmonary oedema. The sub-acute form may present with fever, lassitude and loss of weight. Alternatively the lung function can deteriorate and lead to the patient presenting with breathlessness on exertion either during the course of exposure to beryllium or on cessation of exposure or up to several years afterwards; the chest radiograph then shows diffuse small opacities. The impairment of lung function is typical of proliferative disease of the lung parenchyma, including a defect of gas transfer and a ventilatory defect of the restrictive type (page 558). Tachypnoea is sometimes a prominent feature and, except when the condition has progressed to interstitial fibrosis, the symptoms and the changes in lung function are restored towards normal during the administration of corticosteroid drugs (Fig. 16.13, page 566).

Farmer's lung and related conditions

Farmer's lung is an example of extrinsic allergic alveolitis which is a group of disorders caused by an antigen–antibody reaction leading to the formation of multiple granulomata in the lung parenchyma. In this instance the antigen is present on the spores of mouldy hay. In bird handler's lung the antigen is in dust from the feathers or droppings of pigeons, budgerigars or some other birds. Other antigens are listed in Table 16.23.

Repeated exposure to the antigen leads to sensitisation; this is characterised by a rise in the titre of precipitating antibodies in the blood plasma. Subsequent exposure to the antigen can then cause a pulmonary reaction 3–6 hours later. In addition persons who are atopic, and on this account are predisposed to asthma, can develop an immediate attack. An acute episode of extrinsic allergic alveolitis usually presents with breathlessness, fever, malaise, chest pain and the expectoration of a rust-coloured sputum. In the case of farmer's lung the acute episodes usually occur during the winter subsequent to feeding mouldy hay to cattle. The breathlessness appears to be due to both impaired lung function of the type associated with diseases of the lung parenchyma and stimulation of pulmonary juxtacapillary receptors. The latter aggravates a tendency to shallow rapid breathing. The respiratory impairment involves the vital capacity, lung compliance, transfer factor and ventilatory response to exercise. The changes are usually maximal some 10 h after exposure and persist into the next day. On the first occasion the affected person usually recovers completely. At this

Table 16.23 Some causes of extrinsic allergic alveolitis

Source	Condition	Possible cause
(a) *Moulds, other microorganisms and spores*		
Hay	Farmer's lung	*Micropolyspora faeni*
Grain	Thresher's lung	*Sitophilus granaris*
Straw, thatch	Chaffcutter's lung	*Thermoactinomyces vulgaris**
Dry rot		*Merulius lacrymans**
Bagasse	Bagassosis	*Thermactinomyces vulgaris*
Mushroom compost		*Agaricus hortensis**
Cork	Suberosis	*Penicillium frequentans*
Malt dust		*Aspergillus clavatus*
Maple bark		*Cryptostroma corticale*
Redwood dust	Sequoiosis	*Aureobasidium pullulans*
Cheese washings		*Pencillium* sp.
Paprika		*Mucor liemalis*
Air filters	Air conditionitis	*Thermoactinomyces candidus*
Humidifier sludge	Humidifier fever	*Acanthamoeba*

(b) *Animal residues*
Droppings, feathers and serum of pigeons, budgerigars and other birds
bovine and porcine serum and pituitary snuff

(c) *Chemical substances*
Pyrethrum, some resins*
Diisocyanates* etc.

* These agents can also cause occupational asthma.
(Source: Cotes JE, Steel J. *Work-Related Lung Disorders*. Oxford: Blackwell Scientific Publications, 1987.)

stage recurrent episodes can be avoided by removing the source of exposure or, if this is not practicable, by the use of a fine-dust respirator (8800 (3 M)). Repeated mild exposure can lead to the patient becoming progressively more breathless on exertion; the breathlessness is accompanied by the features of diffuse interstitial fibrosis which often affects primarily the upper zones of the lung. The findings on assessment of lung function are those of a defect of gas transfer and a ventilatory defect of the restrictive type. In addition when the subject has a predisposition to asthma, or as a result of bronchitis, the picture can be complicated by the occurrence of airways obstruction. The pattern of lung function during recovery from an acute episode of farmer's lung uncomplicated by bronchitis is illustrated by the case of Mrs M. which is summarised in Case Study 16.7. The role of smoking is discussed on pages 482 and 528.

Byssinosis

A characteristic pattern of respiratory insufficiency is observed in byssinosis which is a condition caused by the inhalation of the dust of cotton, flax and soft hemp (*Cannabis sativa*). It does not occur with jute, manila hemp, sisal or man-made fibres though the exposure to dust of these substances in high concentration may cause cough, expectoration and reduction in ventilatory capacity. The condition differs from other forms of occupational lung disease in that it is not associated with any specific changes in the structure of the lung. The operatives develop symptoms of tightness in the chest which appear first on

---

Case Study 16.7 Illustrative case of farmer's lung

History

The patient and her husband, who was a quarry man, looked after three cows on a smallholding in mid-Wales. One summer, for the first time, they used a bailer for their hay which was subsequently found to be mouldy. The following spring the patient (age 51 years, height 1.57 m) experienced an acute febrile illness with breathlessness and expectoration of some greenish, blood-flecked sputum.

Examination

Coarse inspiratory crepitations were heard at the lung bases. The chest X-ray showed some diffuse mottling of both lung fields, and the ECG showed evidence of left ventricular hypertropy. The blood pressure was 160/105 mmHg.

Lung function

The compliance, total lung capacity and subdivisions were slightly reduced but the ventilatory capacity, FEV_1 and airflow resistance were normal. The transfer factor (Tl) and its membrane component (Dm) were reduced and the exercise ventilation was increased to a greater extent breathing air than oxygen.

Diagnosis

The diagnosis of disease of the lung parenchyma due to farmer's lung was supported by the findings of precipitating antibodies against *M. faeni*.

Subsequent course

The condition cleared up during the summer and the advice to change over to making silage was rejected. However, after an illness the following winter the patient agreed to use a fine dust respirator which was carefully chosen to fit her face. This prevented further episodes.

Continued on p. 598

Case Study 16.7 *Continued*

Table B16.7 Case study measurements

	Subacute	3 months later	Reference value
Forced expiratory voume (FEV$_1$, l)	2.30	2.45	2.25
Forced vital capacity (FVC, l)	2.73	3.05	3.2
FEV$_1$/FVC (%)	84	80	75
Total lung capacity (TLC, l)	4.46	4.94	4.9
Residual volume (RV, l)	1.49	1.65	1.7
Transfer factor (*Tl*)*	4.5 (13)	6.7 (20)	7.7
Diffusing capacity of alv. membrane (*Dm*)*	6.7 (20)	14.4 (43)	15
Vol. of blood in alv. caps. (*Vc*, ml)	43	43	56
Lung compliance (*Cst*, l kPa^{-1})	1.2	1.4	2.0
Airflow resistance (kPa l^{-1} s)	0.11	0.11	1.2
Exercise ventilation ($\dot{V}_{E45}$, l min^{-1})			
Air	39	24	24
O$_2$	30	24	24

* mmol min^{-1} kPa^{-1} (ml min^{-1} mmHg^{-1}).

Mondays after a weekend away from the dust, or on other days after returning from a holiday. The symptoms are associated with a progressive reduction in the ventilatory capacity and a rise in the airway resistance throughout the working day (Fig. 16.19). Indices of uneven distribution of the inspired gas also show evidence of abnormality. Partial or complete recovery occurs during the night. The condition is due to one or more substances associated with cotton but the mechanism has still to be unravelled. The causative agent is present in the bracts of the cotton bols rather than in the cotton linters and seeds; it is active as an extract when inhaled by healthy subjects. The inhalation leads to the release of histamine from the mast cells in the lung. This process, and the subsequent reaccumulation of the histamine, both occur slowly. The acute effects upon the lung airways are illustrated in Fig. 6.9 (page 147).

In addition to the reversible changes, there is evidence from epidemiological studies that exposure to the dust over periods of years causes permanent impairment of lung function of the type associated with chronic obstructive pulmonary disease. This pattern of lung function is illustrated by the case of Mr N. which is summarised in Case Study 16.8.

Other occupational lung diseases

The working environment can contain any of a number of substances present as dusts, vapours or fumes which are capable of damaging the lungs. The majority are sensitising agents which cause occupational asthma (page 548) or extrinsic allergic alveolitis (page 596); some

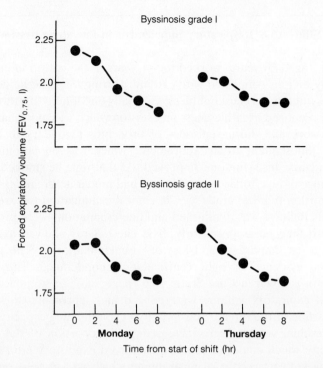

Fig. 16.19 Mean levels of $FEV_{0.75}$ over a working shift for cardroom workers with byssinosis grades I and II. In grade I the decline was most marked on Mondays but in grade II it occurred on other days as well. (Source: McKerrow CB, McDermott M, Gilson JC, Schilling RSF. *Br J Industr Med* 1958; **15**: 75−83.)

agents can cause both types of reaction (Table 16.23). The prevalences of all these conditions appear to be increasing. In westernised countries, by contrast, the prevalences of the traditional occupational diseases due to silica, coal and cotton have decreased dramatically and the prevalence of asbestos-related diseases is beginning to show a similar trend. Other conditions which can affect smaller groups of exposed workers are listed in Table 16.24.

Lung function in cardiac diseases

Introduction

Breathlessness on exertion is a common presenting symptom in many cardiac diseases. The immediate cause is usually a rise in pulmonary venous pressure during exercise; this causes some interstitial oedema which in turn contributes to ventilation−perfusion inequality and leads to stimulation of pulmonary juxta capillary receptors (J receptors). Both factors increase the ventilation during exercise. The congestion also reduces the compliance of the lung and hence lowers the maximal ventilation which the subject can sustain during exercise. The two ventilatory indices are respectively the numerator and the denominator of the dyspnoeic index which is increased (page 392). Breathlessness

Case Study 16.8 Respiratory impairment in late stage byssinosis

Mr N., aged 66 years, worked for 51 years in the cotton industry, mainly on jobs connected with carding. During this time he developed symptoms of chest tightness, especially on Monday afternoons. He also noticed breathlessness on exertion which was most marked after work and during episodes of bronchitis secondary to head colds. Subsequent to his retirement, which was on account of redundancy, his symptoms improved. At that time he smoked half an ounce of pipe tobacco per day and had moderate breathlessness on exertion (clinical grade 3). On clinical examination the area of cardiac dullness was diminished and fine crepitations were present at both lung bases posteriorly. The chest X-ray showed a large lung, a flat diaphragm and loss of vascular markings. The ECG showed evidence of right ventricular preponderance. The lung function is given in Case Study 16.6 (page 590). In summary the forced expiratory volume was reduced and represented a small proportion of the forced vital capacity. The total lung capacity and the residual volume were increased; the proportion of the vital capacity which could be expelled by forced expiratory effort was diminished on account of air-trapping which was present on the spirogram. The transfer factor (diffusing capacity) for the lung, its subdivisions and the tension of oxygen and carbon dioxide in the arterial blood were all within normal limits. The response of ventilation to exercise was increased both when breathing air and when breathing oxygen. The airway resistance was increased but the static lung compliance was within normal limits.

These findings were evidence for chronic obstructive pulmonary disease, though the normal value for the lung volume index of uneven ventilation (V_A eff/V_A) was an inconsistent feature. This was a true finding and not an artefact due to underestimation of the residual volume by the closed circuit method since measurements of lung volume by plethysmography yielded a similar result. The high level of ventilation during exercise, was evidence for enlargement of the physiological deadspace.

increases in consequence. Repeated minor episodes of pulmonary congestion lead to the acute changes persisting; the resulting impairment of lung function interacts with any coexisting lung disease particularly chronic airflow obstruction, and with those types of interstitial or occupational lung disease of which the prevalence increases with age. On this account in epidemiological studies the extent of any respiratory impairment including undue breathlessness on exertion and reductions in forced expiratory volume and vital capacity have been found to presage premature death from ischaemic heart disease as well as from

Table 16.24 Some additional occupational and environmental factors which can damage the lungs

Process or agent	Effect on the lung
Refining aluminium	Pot room asthma
Handling chlorine*	Chronic airflow obstruction
Deep sea diving	See page 411
Enzyme detergents*	Emphysema (if heavy exposure) and asthma
Fire fighting*	Any, depending on exposure
Foundry work*	Asthma, chronic airflow obstruction, silicosis
Producing tungsten carbide	Hard metal disease (Case Study 16.6).
Lipid aerosol	Lipid pneumonia (acute or chronic)
Nitrogen dioxide*	Silo-filler's disease, airflow obstruction
Organophosphates	Parathion poisoning etc. (Table 16.18)
Ozone*	Airflow obstruction, shallow breathing
Paraquat	Respiratory distress syndrome (page 569)
Sulphur dioxide*	Airflow obstruction
Welding steel (especially in shipbuilding)*	Respiratory symptoms, airflow obstruction, ozone poisoning (stainless steel)

* Effects summate or interact with those of smoking.
(Source: Cotes JE, Steel J. *Work-Related Lung Disorders*. Oxford: Blackwell Scientific Publications, 1987.)

lung disease (page 606). This has implications for the study of healthy elderly people (page 487).

Whether or not there is interstitial pulmonary oedema is determined by the pulmonary capillary and osmotic pressure differences across the walls of pulmonary capillaries. The capillary pressure is normally below the level at which there is rupture of the endothelial lining. However, West and colleagues have shown that ruptures occur in rabbits at transmural pressures of or above 40 mmHg; the breaks usually occur at intercellular junctions and affect the endothelium rather than the basement membrane; they often re-unite rapidly when the pressure is reduced. Breaks can also occur in the alveolar epithelium; these ruptures are usually elongated with uneven edges, do not occur at intercellular junctions and appear not to be immediately reversed by a reduction in pressure. Endothelial ruptures often coexist. The transmural pressures at which the ruptures occur are not much above those observed in healthy persons during maximal exercise. Thus the margin of safety is small. It can be breached in some healthy persons during supramaximal effort; a similar effect has been observed in racing greyhound dogs and in galloping racehorses. These animals can develop intrapulmonary haemhorrages during a race. The likelihood of this occurring can be reduced by prophylactic treatment with frusemide. In patients with heart disease a similar mechanism could contribute to acute changes occurring during exercise. However, with persistent pulmonary venous hypertension some protection against interstitial oedema is provided by thickening of the zona densita of the alveolar capillary membrane.

Most chronic lung diseases are associated with pulmonary hypertension, which occurs as a result of both hypoxic pulmonary vaso constriction and loss of pulmonary vascular bed. The hypertension can progress to failure of the right ventricle with congestion of systemic veins, including the hepatic veins (page 541), and dependent oedema (page 623). Hypoxaemia and the enlargement of the right ventricle can interfere with the function of the left ventricle. In addition lung disease can be associated with discomfort on exertion which is sometimes diagnosed as angina of effort. Thus functional interaction between the heart and lungs is a two way process; the association led the Royal College of Physicians to recommend that cardiac and respiratory function laboratories should share common facilities. However, few joint assessments appear to be carried out.

Congenital heart disease

Left-to-right shunt. The passage of blood from the left to the right side of the heart occurs in inter-atrial and inter-ventricular septal defect and in patent ductus arteriosus; in these conditions the flow of blood through the lung is increased. The change can increase the volume of blood in the alveolar capillaries and hence the transfer factor (Tlco). When the shunt is very large there may also be compression of small airways; Englert and colleagues have shown that this leads to diminutions in the forced expiratory flow, total lung capacity and lung compliance and to an increase in the airways resistance.

Right-to-left shunt. The blood passes from the right side to the left side of the heart in Fallot's tetralogy and in the late stages of left-to-right shunt when this is complicated by pulmonary hypertension. The resulting hypoxaemia leads to cyanosis; it also stimulates breathing, except in those subjects in whom the chemoreceptor drive is reduced (page 349). The change might be expected to cause hypocapnia. However, because of the shunt, only part of the cardiac output passes through the lung, and no CO_2 is eliminated from the remainder. Consequently Pa,co_2 is normal or moderately increased.

During exercise, there is an increase in the flow of blood through the alternative pathway which bypasses the lung; the flow through the alveolar capillaries is often relatively constant. Hence, the tension of oxygen in the systemic arterial blood falls during exercise whilst that of carbon dioxide rises. These changes increase the drive to respiration. Additional stimulation to respiration during exercise is provided by a rise in the concentration of hydrogen ions in the arterial blood. This change is partly a result of hypercapnia; it is also due to lactacidaemia secondary to rapid glycolysis which is a consequence of insufficient delivery of oxygen to the active muscles. H. Davies and others have shown that summation of these stimuli to respiration can cause a considerable increase in exercise ventilation in some patients with cyanotic congenital heart disease. The successful correction by surgery of the defect causing the cyanosis leads to a material reduction in the level of ventilation during exercise. This occurs despite an increase

Pulmonary stenosis. In this condition the function of the lung is usually within normal limits, but the stenosis can reduce the outflow of blood from the right ventricle. The volume of blood in the lung capillaries is then reduced and the transfer factor is low in consequence. In addition the delivery of oxygen to the active muscles may not keep pace with its utilisation. The deficit is made good by rapid glycolysis with formation of lactic acid. The consequent rise in the concentration of hydrogen ions in the arterial blood stimulates breathing. This change increases the exercise ventilation and hence the numerator of the dyspnoeic index; the capacity for exercise is reduced in consequence.

Mitral stenosis

Mitral stenosis resembles pulmonary stenosis in causing a reduction in cardiac output, especially during exercise. It also raises the pulmonary venous pressure; this change causes transudation of fluid into the interstitial tissue. There is then passive and active constriction of the pulmonary arterioles and redistribution of blood flow in the pulmonary circulation. These changes impair the function of the lung.

Ventilatory capacity, lung mechanics and ventilation−perfusion relationships. The changes in the pulmonary circulation have the effect of increasing the elastic recoil of the lung tissues and hence of reducing the static compliance. The total lung capacity is reduced in consequence. The residual volume is usually increased except in the presence of marked pulmonary hypertension when it may be moderately reduced. The mechanism is not fully understood. Any reduction in residual volume is usually less than that in total lung capacity so the vital capacity is almost always diminished. The forced expiratory volume is then reduced and the residual volume as a percentage of total lung capacity is on the high side of normal. The energy cost of breathing is also increased with the result that the ventilatory capacity is reduced. The distribution of pulmonary blood flow is affected not only by the raised intravascular pressure but also by the increase in the quantity of lung water. This raises the interstitial pressure. The rise is greatest in dependent parts of the lung, at small lung volumes; it leads to compression of pulmonary arterioles supplying the lower zones of the lung. The perfusion of the upper zones is increased in consequence and this increases the range of the ventilation−perfusion ratios. The alveolar to arterial tension differences for oxygen, carbon dioxide and nitrogen are increased in consequence. For the same reason the arterial oxygen tension is reduced but not usually to a level which materially diminishes the oxygen saturation.

Gas exchange. In the early stages of mitral stenosis the diffusing capacity of the alveolar capillary membrane (Dm) is usually normal. Subsequently the transudation of fluid into the interstitial tissue of the lung increases the path length for diffusion; this reduces Dm. By contrast, the volume of blood in the alveolar capillaries (Vc) is usually increased by the pulmonary venous hypertension distending the alveolar capillaries. Later there is obliteration of part of the pulmonary vascular bed and Vc tends to decline. The combined magnitudes of the diffusing capacity of the alveolar capillary membrane and the volume of blood in the alveolar capillaries determine the size of the transfer factor (diffusing capacity) for the lung. This index is usually increased early in the disease by reason of the increase in the volume of blood in the alveolar capillaries; it is usually decreased in the late stage when both component variables are reduced. In the intermediate stages the changes in Dm and Vc tend to cancel out with the result that the transfer factor can be normal despite abnormalities in both its components (page 297).

Control of respiration and response to exercise. The hypoxaemia increases the resting ventilation and causes mild hypocapnia. At the same time, because of the increased work of breathing, the ventilatory response to breathing carbon dioxide is on average reduced. Episodes of increased ventilation occur in association with tachypnoea and with paroxysmal nocturnal dyspnoea. These conditions are consequences of the pulmonary congestion, which the work of Whitteridge and Paintal have shown to result from activation of the respiratory reticular formation via small unmyelinated nerve fibres in the vagi (page 334).

The physiological response to exercise is affected by all the factors which have been discussed. The pulmonary congestion and the accumulated interstitial fluid reduce the ventilatory capacity. This contributes to breathlessness. The increased work of breathing is mitigated by a change in the pattern of breathing with an increase in respiratory frequency. The resulting tachypnoea is augmented by activation of the juxta capillary receptors of Paintal. The shallow breathing in turn increases the proportion of ventilation which is wasted in ventilating the deadspace and adds to the ventilation–perfusion inequality caused by the retained interstitial fluid. The required level of alveolar ventilation is then dependent on a bigger minute volume than would otherwise be the case. The minute volume is further increased by the hypoxaemia and by the reduced cardiac output both of which augment the chemo-receptor drive to ventilation. Consequently breathing oxygen reduces the ventilation to a greater extent than in healthy subjects, by mechanisms discussed in Chapter 12.

The reduced cardiac output is due to a diminished stroke volume and is partly compensated by an increase in the cardiac frequency. However, the compensation is incomplete and the delivery of oxygen to the muscle tissue is inadequate; the resulting lactacidaemia further increases the ventilation during exercise and reduces the capacity for exercise.

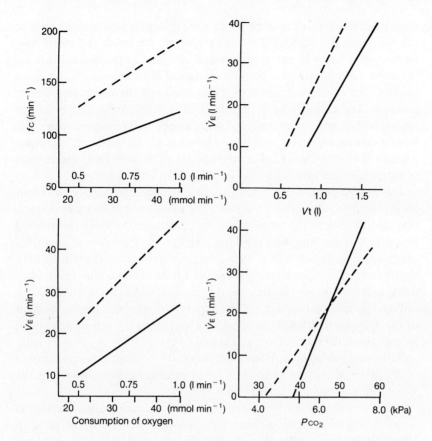

Fig. 16.20 The physiological response to submaximal exercise and to breathing carbon dioxide in female patients with mitral stenosis (– – –) compared with healthy women of the same mean age and size (———). (Source: Reed JW, Ablett M, Cotes JE. *Clin Sci* 1978; **54**: 9–16.)

The findings in patients with mitral stenosis during exercise and whilst breathing carbon dioxide are compared with control subjects in Fig. 16.20. The way in which the response to exercise in these subjects differs from that of patients with lung disease is considered on pages 405 and 432.

Failure of the left ventricle

Acute failure of the left ventricle such as occurs in patients with acute myocardial infarction may be associated with hyperventilation and tachypnoea which is itself an adverse prognostic sign. The tension of oxygen in the arterial blood is usually reduced, whilst the tension in the alveolar gas may be increased. These changes occur to their greatest extent in patients who are in a state of shock. Compared with patients who have uncomplicated myocardial infarction they are more marked in those with evidence of a rise in pulmonary venous pressure causing transudation of fluid into the interstitial tissue of the lung — i.e. with clinical signs of congestion including basal crepitations, and radiographic signs of segmental collapse or pulmonary oedema. The changes reduce the lung compliance and the transfer factor, compress the small lung airways and extra-alveolar vessels and, by raising pulmonary arterial pressure redistribute the pulmonary blood flow (see mitral stenosis above). The closing volume is then increased and there may be alveolar oedema. The changes have the effect of increasing the proportion of alveoli which are underventilated with respect to their perfusion. The venous admixture effect and the proportion of the tidal volume which comprises the physiological deadspace are then increased; the tension of oxygen in the arterial blood is reduced in consequence.

The hypoxaemia, by augmenting the chemoreceptor drive to respiration, increases the minute volume. The associated pulmonary congestion contributes to the tachypnoea via effects on both the mechanical properties of the lung and the lung J receptors. Paroxysmal nocturnal dyspnoea may occur, often with airways obstruction which may then mimic nocturnal asthma. For patients in a state of shock, the respiratory drive can be further augmented by lactacidaemia associated with a reduced peripheral blood flow. The hyperventilation and the component of the hypoxaemia which is due to $\dot{V}_A/\dot{Q}$ inequality can be alleviated by the administration of oxygen (page 615).

Following the acute episode of myocardial infarction the restoration of the arterial oxygen tension is often relatively slow, reflecting the slow re-absorption of the exudates.

Minor degrees of left ventricular failure or transient episodes such as occur during exercise in patients with ischaemic heart disease, have an effect similar but smaller than that observed during the acute episodes. The changes resemble those in mitral stenosis which are described in detail above. They have been shown by S.W. Davies and colleagues to be related to indices of the diastolic function of the heart including the isovolume relaxation time and mitral pressure half time, but not to indices of systolic function such as the ejection fraction, the peak aortic velocity and the aortic acceleration. Chronic left heart failure in which exercise is limited by breathlessness is also associated with respiratory muscle weakness and fatigue. Latent failure can be a cause of unexplained tachypnoea occurring on exertion. The evidence that a reduction in vital capacity is associated with an increased mortality from ischaemic heart disease is referred to above. The association was first observed in the Framingham study where it remained after the effect of all the conventional risk factors had been allowed for.

Pulmonary embolism

Thrombi which sometimes form on the walls of systemic veins can become detached and be carried to the lung where they impact in the pulmonary vascular bed. The consequences are determined by the number and size of the emboli. A large embolus which lodges on the bifurcation of the pulmonary artery obstructs the pulmonary circulation and can be fatal. A small embolus may have no effect.

Recurrent small emboli reduce the quantity of functioning lung tissue and cause pulmonary hypertension by progressively obstructing the pulmonary vascular bed. This process will eventually cause right heart failure. In the intermediate stages the patient usually presents with breathlessness on exertion. This differs from the breathlessness of lung disease in that the lung volumes and ventilatory capacity are relatively normal, and from cardiac dyspnoea because no characteristic cardiac lesion is present. The breathlessness is due to a marked increase in ventilation, especially during exercise; it is accompanied by hypocapnia. The condition superficially resembles overbreathing of psychogenic origin, but can be distinguished by the occurrence of hypoxaemia. This often has a multiple aetiology including ventilation–perfusion inequality, shunting of blood through collapsed regions of lung or through a patent foramen ovale, and a reduced systemic venous oxygen tension secondary to a reduction in cardiac output. The ventilation–perfusion inequality is associated with an enlarged physiological deadspace which can be further increased by breathing oxygen. The obliteration of part of the pulmonary vascular bed reduces the volume of blood in the lung capillaries. The transfer factor is reduced in consequence.

Emboli of intermediate size which are too small to cause immediate death may give rise to infarction of the lung; this condition is characterised by localised chest pain of a pleuritic type, the expectoration of red or rust-coloured sputum, the presence of fever and the physical signs of a local lesion in the chest. There may also be hypoxaemia, and hyperventilation which has the effect of lowering the tension of carbon dioxide in the arterial blood. In addition, Robin and others have pointed out that whereas the impaction of the embolus reduces the circulation in a part of the lung it does not immediately reduce the ventilation. In these circumstances the tension of carbon dioxide in the mixed alveolar gas is reduced relative to that in the arterial blood. The extent of the vascular obstruction can then be deduced from the size of the arterial–alveolar tension difference for carbon dioxide. Robin and colleagues have shown that the proportion of lung which is ventilated but not perfused can be expressed as follows:

$$\% \text{ unperfused lung} = \frac{100\ (P_{a,CO_2} - P_{A,CO_2})}{P_{a,CO_2} - P_{A,CO_2} + P_{E,CO_2}} \qquad (16.3)$$

where P_{a,CO_2}, P_{A,CO_2} and P_{E,CO_2} are the tensions of carbon dioxide respectively in the arterial blood, the end-tidal or alveolar gas and the mixed expired gas. The proportion is normally less than 3%. However, the $a\text{-}AD_{CO_2}$ is also increased in other conditions and, when due to embolism, can be reduced by both the onset of pulmonary infarction and the operation of mechanisms whereby the ventilation and the perfusion of the lung are mutually adjusted (Chapter 7). Thus the index is of limited usefulness and then only soon after an acute episode. It has now been replaced by pulmonary angiography and other scanning techniques (page 230).

Guide to references

The references (Chapter 18) are classified under subject headings of which the following are particularly relevant to the present chapter:

17: Physiological Aspects of Treatment

Tissue hypoxia; causes and means of correction

The proper function of every tissue in the body depends on an adequate supply of oxygen by mechanisms described in earlier chapters. Lack of oxygen has its greatest effect on the central nervous system where the cells are not able to obtain energy by recourse to rapid glycolysis; for these cells complete deprivation of oxygen for as short a time as 2 min can lead to their death, with disastrous consequences for the whole organism. Lesser degrees of hypoxia acting for a longer time can have equally serious effects.

Deficiency of oxygen can be due to a reduction in the partial pressure of oxygen in the inspired gas or to disruption of any stage in the process of transfer of oxygen from the atmosphere to mitochondria in the tissue cells; some of the circumstances in which a deficiency of oxygen can occur are listed in Table 17.1.

Deficiency of oxygen in the inspired gas

A fall in the barometric pressure reduces the partial pressure of oxygen in the inspired gas. This is a feature of ascent to altitude or simulation of an ascent in a decompression chamber. It is, therefore, associated with flight in unpressurised aircraft or balloons, and expeditions to or residence at high altitude. The partial pressure of oxygen in the alveoli is also influenced by the presence of carbon dioxide and water vapour. The water vapour pressure is a function of body temperature and is effectively constant at about 6.3 kPa (47 mmHg). The partial pressure of carbon dioxide is not constant but decreases during hypoxaemia as a result of the increased chemoreceptor drive raising the level of ventilation. The hypocapnia is compensated by renal and other mechanisms which contribute to acclimatisation (page 358). The processes enable a person to sustain a higher ventilation and hence a higher alveolar oxygen tension than would otherwise be the case. Acclimatisation also facilitates the transport of oxygen. Figure 17.1 shows the

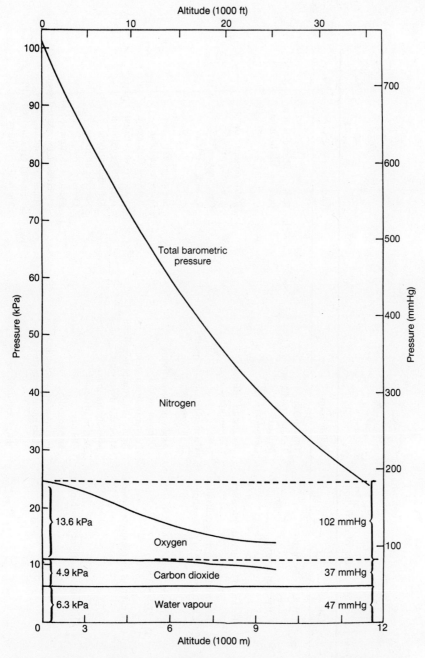

Fig. 17.1 Diagram showing the composition of alveolar gas in unacclimatised subjects under conditions of reduced barometric pressure. The upper line indicates the barometric pressure; this falls exponentially with altitude, the pressure halving every 5.5 km (18 000 ft). The distances between the other lines represent the approximate partial pressures of the alveolar gases. Conditions at sea level are represented by the horizontal lines; the line for oxygen intercepts the curve for barometric pressure at about 10 300 m (34 000 ft). The alveolar oxygen tension of a subject who is breathing oxygen at this altitude is equal to that which obtains while breathing air at sea level.

Table 17.1 Tissue hypoxia: causes and means of correction

Category	Cause	Subdivision	Treatment
Blocked airway	Physical obstruction	Diphtheria	Relieve obstruction or perform tracheotomy
	Laryngeal spasm	Foreign body, etc.	
Deficiency of oxygen in inspired gas	Reduced barometric pressure	Primary	Raise pressure or give oxygen
		Secondary	
		Ascent to altitude	Give oxygen
	Reduced oxygen concentration	Decompression	
	Exhaustion of oxygen supply	—	
		Confined space or results of combustion	Provide fresh air
Hypoventilation	Reduced central drive to respiration	Asphyxia neonatorum	See page 621
		Depressant drugs	Specific antidote
		Lesion in brain stem	Assisted ventilation
	Weakness in respiratory muscles	Acute anterior poliomyelitis	Assisted ventilation
		Muscular dystrophy	Assisted ventilation
		Myasthenia gravis	Specific antidote
		Action of drugs	Specific antidote
	Increased work of breathing	Obesity	Diet
		Kyphoscoliosis	Medical treatment and occasionally assisted ventilation
		Raised airway resistance	
		Pharyngeal obstruction	Nasal continuous positive airway pressure (CPAP)
		Status asthmaticus	Medical treatment

Wide range of $\dot{V}_A/\dot{Q}$ ratios	Abnormality of surface tension	Respiratory distress syndrome (RDS)	Medical treatment supplied by O_2 (be alert for hypoventilation, see page 629. Consider positive end-expiratory pressure (for RDS) and long-term O_2 therapy (for pulmonary hypertension in COPD patients)
	Airflow obstruction	Chronic obstructive pulmonary disease (COPD)	
		Asthma	
		Response to inhaling dust	
		Action of drugs, etc.	
	Reduced lung compliance	Disease of lung parenchyma	
		Pulmonary oedema	
		Action of drugs	
	Reduced lung volume	Anaesthesia	
	Abnormal distribution of pulmonary blood flow	Low cardiac output (q.v.)	
		Mitral stenosis	Mitral valvotomy
	Right-to-left shunt	Intrapulmonary, intracardiac, reversed left-to-right shunt	Treat cause. With reversed shunt O_2 may help
Reduced blood flow	Low cardiac output	Myocardial infarction	Medical treatment supplemented by O_2
		Trauma, burn, haemorrhage, etc.	
	Local disturbance of blood flow	Atherosclerosis, A-V anastomosis injury, etc.	100% or hyperbaric O_2 of limited use
Interference with transport of oxygen	Methaemoglobinaemia	Congenital, reductase defic. haemoglobinopathy m.	Methylene blue
		Acquired from nitrobenzene, etc.	100% O_2
	Carboxyhaemoglobinaemia	Carbon monoxide poisoning	Hyperbaric oxygen, carbogen or assisted ventilation with 100% O_2
Inactivation of cytochromes	Cyanide poisoning		Specific antidote, resuscitation

approximate composition of the alveolar gas in an unacclimatised subject breathing air at different barometric pressures. To ensure normal cerebral function the pressure of oxygen in the alveolar gas should not fall below about 11 kPa (83 mmHg), (page 622); this yields an oxygen saturation of about 95% and occurs at an altitude of approximately 1500 m (5000 ft). At or above this altitude there may be a need for supplementary oxygen (page 616). At approximately 10 300 m (34 000 ft) the barometric pressure less the partial pressures of carbon dioxide and water vapour is only about 14 kPa (105 mmHg); under these circumstances when breathing 100% oxygen the alveolar oxygen tension is no greater than when breathing air at sea level. At higher altitudes in order to prevent hypoxaemia the pressure of the respired gas must be increased.

Apart from hypobaria the inspired oxygen tension can be reduced in the course of study of lung function or during anaesthesia; in such circumstances the means for correction are immediately available. Hypoxia can also occur in a confined space as a result of the utilisation of oxygen by metabolism, combustion or a chemical process such as can occur in a sewer or coal mine, where it gives rise to black damp, or a tank, ship's hold or silo containing grain or similar material. The local environment then contains nitrogen and additional carbon dioxide but little oxygen; entry into it can be fatal. The gas can seep into adjacent closed spaces including overlying buildings. Hypoxia without hypercapnia can occur in empty, but sealed, iron or steel chambers (e.g. floatation tanks of ships) from which the oxygen is removed by rusting of the iron. In order to make the gas safe to breathe, oxygen must be added and, where appropriate, carbon dioxide removed; alternatively the subject can be provided with a source of respirable gas via a compressed air line or closed circuit breathing apparatus.

A wide range of ventilation−perfusion ratios (V$_A$/Q inequality)

An increase in the number of alveoli which are poorly ventilated in relation to their perfusion causes hypoxaemia for the reasons discussed in Chapter 7. The condition constitutes the commonest medical indication for oxygen; some examples are listed in Table 17.1 under the headings 'wide range of V$_A$/Q ratios' and 'low cardiac output'.

Hypoxaemia which is caused by a wide range of ventilation−perfusion ratios can be corrected by the provision of a relatively small amount of additional oxygen. This is due to the shape of the oxygen dissociation curve. Nearly full saturation of the blood with oxygen is achieved at an alveolar oxygen tension of about 12 kPa (90 mmHg) and only sufficient oxygen to achieve this tension need be supplied. Thus for the majority of conditions including almost all cases of chronic lung disease a gas mixture containing oxygen in a fractional concentration of 0.25−0.40 is adequate.* However, where there is latent or overt pulmonary

---

* This concentration, which relates to conditions at sea level, was formerly reported as 25−40% O_2. The equivalent oxygen partial pressures are 25−40 kPa and the equivalent concentration 11−18 mmol l^{-1} (see Table 2.5, page 17).

oedema, for example following acute myocardial infarction, a higher concentration (e.g. $F_{I,O_2} = 0.60$) is usually required. In this and many other circumstances the oxygen is given to correct hypoxaemia which is likely to be of relatively short duration. Oxygen can also be used to treat the complications of chronic hypoxaemia including pulmonary hypertension, congestive heart failure and secondary polycythaemia.

High altitude

Inadequacy or failure of the circulation

A low cardiac output lowers pulmonary arterial pressure and hence gives rise to pulmonary $\dot{V}_A/\dot{Q}$ inequality and consequent hypoxaemia. In the absence of lung disease this can cause hyperventilation (air hunger). Both aspects usually respond to oxygen in the dosage given above. A reduction in blood flow to an organ or tissue causes local hypoxia. This is likely to respond to an increase in the local blood flow if it can be achieved. If not there may be a need to increase the quantity of oxygen dissolved in the blood plasma, which is normally $0.13\,\mathrm{mmol\,l^{-1}}$ (0.3 vol%). It can be raised to $0.9\,\mathrm{mmol\,l^{-1}}$ (2 vol%) by breathing oxygen. The increase ($0.77\,\mathrm{mmol\,l^{-1}}$) can materially improve the tissue oxygen supply. As evidence of this, breathing oxygen materially increases the capacity for exercise of healthy people (page 407). A further increase in the content of oxygen in the plasma can be secured by administering the oxygen under pressure; this hyperbaric oxygen therapy can be used to raise the local tissue oxygen tension in acute myocardial infarction and when there is intractable pain, ulceration, infection with anaerobic organisms or gangrene due to local insufficiency of the circulation (page 638). The tissue oxygen tension is also increased by reducing the rate of metabolism; in appropriate circumstances this can be achieved by hypothermia or by reducing the activity of the thyroid gland.

Other causes of hypoxia

Other causes of hypoxia are listed in Table 17.1. They include hypoventilation particularly that associated with disturbed sleep (page 350), chemical interference with the transport of oxygen (page 625) and a right-to-left shunt across the lungs. The latter is not usually amenable to oxygen therapy since, during breathing air, the blood which transverses the pulmonary capillaries is normally fully saturated with oxygen and a small increase in dissolved oxygen is all that can be supplied. However, when the hypoxaemia is due to the reversal of a left-to-right shunt, oxygen therapy can sometimes contribute to its correction.

High altitude

Passengers in aircraft

Flying personnel and passengers in civil aircraft can be exposed to short periods of hypoxia (page 610). This can be corrected by

615

Table 17.2 Conditions of equivalent alveolar oxygen tension for unacclimatised subjects breathing mixtures of oxygen and nitrogen at altitude and at sea level

Altitude ($\div 1000$)		Barometric pressure		P_{A,O_2} breathing air at altitude		F_{I,O_2} in inspired gas	
						At sea level equivalent to	At altitude equivalent to 1500 m
m	ft	kPa	mmHg	kPa	mmHg	air at altitude	breathing air
0	0	101	760	13.6	102	0.209	—
1.5	5	84	632	10.9	82	0.17	0.209
3.0	10	70	523	8.1	61	0.14	0.26
4.6	15	57	429	5.9	44	0.11	0.32
6.1	20	46	349	4.7	35	0.09	0.41
7.6	25	38	282	4.4	33	0.07	0.52

administration of oxygen; appropriate dosages for different altitudes are listed in Table 17.2 (right hand column).

Passengers who are at increased risk include those in whom the arterial oxygen saturation breathing air at sea level is less than 90%, persons with degenerative arterial disease and those with sickle cell disease. Supplementary oxygen is seldom needed in other circumstances because the pressure in the cabin is usually maintained at above the level of the surrounding atmosphere. An upper limit of 1500 m (5000 ft) is commonly adopted but can be exceeded if there is a technical fault on the aircraft. A normal cabin altitude has an effect upon the subject equivalent to inhaling oxygen at a fractional concentration of 0.17 at sea level. This gas mixture can be used to assess the likely need for supplementary oxygen. If a supplement is needed a convenient dosage is $2 \, l \, STPD \, min^{-1}$ delivered to a properly fitted mask of the type that has an oxygen reservoir bag. For subjects who are seated, this dosage is usually adequate at cabin altitudes of up to 5500 m (18 000 ft); more oxygen is required at higher altitudes. Alternatively or in addition the duration of the flight can be reduced through travelling by supersonic aircraft (for example Concorde).

Visitors to high-altitude. Visitors seldom require supplementary oxygen; however, this possibility can be assessed before the journey by the subject breathing the gas mixtures listed in the 7th column of Table 17.2. The effects of lack of oxygen are most prominent during exercise and at night. During exercise there may be hyperventilation, giddiness and tachycardia. Alternatively during very strenuous exercise, the tachycardia can convert to bradycardia on account of a rise in parasympathetic tone. At night there is insomnia and Cheyne-Stokes respiration in which the subject experiences cyclical fluctuations in the depth of breathing between apnoea and hyperventilation. The condition occurs as part of the sleep apnoea/hypopnoea syndrome and is described on page 359. These effects of hypoxaemia are most often experienced by elderly subjects at altitudes of above 1800 m (6000 ft) but symptoms in relation to strenuous exercise also occur at lower altitudes; they improve with acclimatisation. The nocturnal symptoms can be alleviated by the administration of oxygen at a flow rate of $0.5-1.0\,l\,STPD\,min^{-1}$. For symptoms related to exercise a flow of $2-4\,l\,min^{-1}$ can be administered through a mask fitted with an oxygen reservoir bag. The special case of mountain sickness at very high altitudes is considered under this heading below. Expeditions to above 6000 m (20 000 ft) should be equipped with oxygen for use in emergencies. In addition, at altitudes of over 7600 m (25 000 ft) the use of oxygen during exercise and at night should be considered on medical grounds as well as for its beneficial effect upon performance.

Residents at high altitude. Such persons are fully acclimatised and lead normal lives at altitudes of up to about 5000 m (16 000 ft), although even at lower altitudes their capacity to perform skilled tasks has been shown (by Tichauer) to be considerably reduced. The tolerance to alcohol and carbon monoxide in cigarette smoking is also reduced. Minor degrees of airways obstruction such as can occur during episodes of bronchitis may cause disproportionate hypoxaemia. The hypoxaemia can be aggravated by a loss of the chemoreceptor response to hypoxia (page 360). For these reasons the early stages of chronic obstructive pulmonary disease (COPD) can be more often complicated by pulmonary hypertension and right heart failure than is the case at sea level; subjects with responsive pulmonary vessels are particularly at risk (page 204). Vascular thromboses are also common. In addition, on rapid ascent to an altitude in excess of 3000 m (10 000 ft) from sea level the inhabitants and their visitors are liable to develop mountain sickness.

Mountain sickness. Mountain sickness is due to inappropriately rapid ascent to altitudes in excess of 3000 m and formerly occurred mainly in the Andes. Since the advent of air travel it has become prevalent in other mountainous regions particularly the Himalayas where depending on circumstances, 10−60% of visitors can be affected. Predisposing factors include a relatively young age, a high level of activity and a below average ventilatory response or an above average pulmonary vasoconstrictor response to hypoxia. High altitude residents returning from a visit to low altitudes are at increased risk. The condition typically occurs on the second or third day when it may be precipitated by activity, exposure or a minor respiratory infection.

The cause of mountain sickness is hypoxaemia leading to cerebral vasodilatation with some oedema. These changes cause the initial symptoms of euphoria leading to lethargy, disturbed sleep (often with dreams), dizziness on standing up and headache which does not respond to aspirin. There is conspicuous breathlessness on exertion and often nausea, anorexia, vomiting and general misery. The condition usually responds to rest and leaves no sequelae provided that any further ascent is made at a suitably slow rate. Progression of the condition can take the form of focal neurological lesions affecting particularly the

617

cranial nerves; there may be pulmonary oedema, often with pulmonary vascular thromboses, and oedema of the legs, hands or face. Acute mountain cerebral oedema with hallucinations leading to coma can also occur. However, susceptibility varies widely on account of individual differences in the extent of fluid retention. This in turn reflects the responsiveness of the renin—aldosterone system to hypoxia; the mechanisms have been investigated by Milledge amongst others.

Mountain sickness should be prevented by allowing time for acclimatisation during any ascent to over 3000 m; this can be achieved by not ascending more than 300 m per day and by having a pause after every third day. The process is helped by abstaining from smoking, alcohol and sedative drugs. It can also be helped by prior administration of acetazolamide (Diamox, page 699) or a diuretic such as spironolactone. However, acclimatisation is best achieved in the manner described. The treatment in mild cases is rest in bed; the occurrence of pulmonary oedema or marked cerebral symptoms is an indication for immediate descent towards sea level on a stretcher. Alternatively where appropriate facilities are available, the inspired oxygen tension can be raised by pressurisation using a portable chamber (page 638). Meanwhile the life of the patient can be preserved by the administration of oxygen, diuretics and morphine.

Healthy persons during exercise

A maximal increase in the capacity for exercise is achieved by the inhalation of oxygen in a fractional concentration of about 0.60, whilst an F_{I,O_2} of 0.30 exerts a significant effect. The improvement is greatest for periods of exercise of duration 2−10 min. It is due to both increased delivery of oxygen to the muscles and reduced chemoreceptor drive to breathing. The former is a consequence of additional oxygen carried in solution in the blood plasma. The latter is both a direct effect of hyperoxia (page 342) and secondly to a reduced need for rapid glycosis; this reduces the lactacidaemia which normally accompanies strenuous exercise (page 407). The use of oxygen would appear to be without risk provided the subject does not hold the breath during exercise. However, if this is done the accumulation of carbon dioxide can lead to loss of consciousness. Breathing oxygen before exercise is of no use, except when the gas is stored in the lung by breath holding; its administration afterwards is also of no value, as it does not hasten the repayment of the oxygen debt. Thus for healthy subjects at sea level there is only limited scope for oxygen in relation to exercise. It can have a place in some programmes of athletic training or when a short period of supra-maximal performance is required, for example in order to achieve human flight by muscle power. For this purpose an appropriate oxygen flow rate would be 30−60 l min^{-1} delivered via an Edinburgh mask (page 636). Oxygen for use by patients during exercise is considered subsequently (page 624).

Oxygen in relation to anaesthesia

General anaesthesia greatly affects all aspects of the respiratory system including the control mechanisms, the muscles which serve the upper respiratory tract, the respiratory and accessory muscles and the lungs themselves. Anaesthesia also causes changes in the systemic circulation, reducing the cardiac output and l.ence the oxygen saturation of the mixed venous blood. Other changes that occur are summarised and annotated in Table 17.3. They are influenced by the age and posture of the patient and the type of anaesthetic which is used. The features include a reduction in functional residual capacity (FRC) in a supine but not an upright posture. The reduction is due to summation of the effects of (1) diminished activity of the intercostal muscles; this reduces the cross-sectional area of the thorax, (2) headward displacement of the diaphragm, (3) displacement of some of the blood from the limbs into the thorax. The last two of these tendencies are reversed during application of a positive end-expiratory pressure (PEEP, page 649). In older subjects, in particular, the small FRC predisposes to airway closure, which tends to increase the anatomical blood shunt. Atelectasis

Table 17.3 Effects of general anaesthesia on lung function (for sources, see references)

Soft palate	Moves back; occludes nasopharynx
Intercostal muscles	Activity diminished; thoracic ventilatory excursion reduced except with muscle paralysis
Diaphragm	Usually displaced towards head
Rib-cage volume	Decreased
Thoracic blood volume	Can be increased
Functional residual capacity and expiratory reserve volume	Reduced in supine posture
Regional ventilation	Superior/inferior ratio increased, hence alveolar deadspace increased
Minute volume and tidal volume	Reduced despite increase in frequency
Ventilatory responses to hypercapnia and hypoxia	Reduced
Airway resistance	Little change despite reduced FRC (most anaesthetics are bronchodilators)
Lung compliance	Reduced, recoil pressure increased
Airway closure or atelectasis	Common, hence anatomical shunt increased and compliance reduced
Alveolar blood shunt compartment	Usually normal in young subjects
Cardiac output	Reduced, hence $P\bar{v},o_2$ reduced
Pulmonary vasoconstrictor response to hypoxia	Reduced by inhalation anaesthetics
Arterial blood gases	
Oxygen tension	Reduced in absence of oxygen administration
Carbon dioxide tension	Increased unless ventilation is augmented

can occur in dependent parts of the lung and this augments the shunt; it also reduces the lung compliance. The atelectasis can be visualised by computer-assisted tomography (CT scan) of the lung. It can occur with both inhaled and intravenous anaesthesia, particularly if muscle paralysis is induced, but the mechanism of its formation is not fully understood.

The reduction in activity of the intercostal muscles interacts with the posture of the subject to influence the regional ventilation. Normally the inferior (dependent) regions are the better ventilated. With anaesthesia the proportion of ventilation going to superior, poorly perfused regions and hence the alveolar deadspace is increased. In healthy young and middle aged subjects there does not appear to be a corresponding increase in the proportion of lung units having a low ventilation perfusion ratio. However, the proportion of low $\dot{V}$A$/\dot{Q}$ units is increased by anaesthesia in elderly patients and those with chronic obstructive pulmonary disease (COPD). Thus hypoxaemia occurring during anaesthesia is mainly due to an increased anatomical shunt secondary to airway closure and atelectases, not to a wide scatter of ventilation–perfusion ratios. The hypoxaemia is aggravated by a reduction in the saturation of mixed venous blood (see above); this magnifies the effects of the shunts. In addition in the absence of additional oxygen the reduction in minute volume (which has multiple aetiology) lowers the alveolar oxygen tension. A further factor which could contribute to hypoxaemia during inhalation anaesthesia is inhibition of hypoxic pulmonary vasoconstriction. This might affect persons with existing ventilation perfusion imbalance including the elderly and patients with COPD but the evidence that it does so is incomplete. The hypoxaemia associated with anaesthesia is usually corrected by periodic inflations of the chest to restore the patency of the airways and by maintaining the fractional inspired oxygen concentration in the range 0.25–0.40.

Analgesia for the relief of any post-operative pain can cause sleep apnoea syndrome. This can result in episodes of profound nocturnal hypoxaemia for several nights even in the absence of other predisposing factors (page 352). The mechanism has been investigated by Jones and colleagues amongst others. The principal factor is morphine-induced loss of neural control of the muscles of the upper airways. This prevents the phasic contraction of the pharyngeal muscles which normally precedes diaphragmatic contraction. In its absence the negative pressure generated by the diaphragm leads to collapse of the upper airways at the level of the epiglottis. The morphine also suppresses rapid eye movement sleep (REM sleep). If this is made up during subsequent nights the resulting prolonged REM sleep can itself induce sleep apnoea with maximal effect on the third post-operative night. The resulting hypoxaemia can be relieved by administration of oxygen at the rate of $2 \, l \, min^{-1}$ via nasal prongs, a nasal cannula or simple oxygen mask. The nocturnal hypoxaemia can usually be prevented by substituting regional analgesia with bupivacaine or by using a non-opioid general analgesic.

Oxygen therapy for newborn babies

Asphyxia neonatorum. In this condition normal rhythmic ventilation does not start promptly at birth; instead the baby remains apnoeic or the ventilation is slow and feeble. The condition is most likely to occur following a protracted or difficult delivery. If it persists for more than 2 min from the time of birth, active steps should be taken to secure the ventilation of the lung. The treatment should include first aid and clinical measures; in addition, gentle inflation of the chest should be carried out via a mask and resuscitation bag or, when personnel with the necessary skills are in attendance, an endotracheal catheter.

Respiratory distress in the newborn. This condition is a consequence of prematurity (page 524). Treatment is directed to securing time for the type II alveolar cells to start producing surface-active material. This can now be done by administration of genetically engineered surfactant but some practical problems remain. In addition one should provide the environmental and other conditions which favour spontaneous recovery. To this end, the baby should be nursed in an incubator with high humidity and the temperature should be maintained at 35°C to minimise the consumption of oxygen. The arterial blood gases and pH should be monitored, usually via a catheter in the umbilical artery. However, if there is material right to left shunt, for example through a patent ductus, the systemic arterial blood should be monitored by ear lobe oximetry or sampled directly from a cranial or upper limb artery (page 36). Oxygen should be given in the lowest concentration needed to maintain the systemic arterial oxygen tension at about 13 kPa (100 mmHg) or the umbilical arterial tension in the range 8−12 kPa (60−90 mmHg). To minimise the risk of causing retrolental fibroplasia or oxygen toxicity the oxygen concentration should be reduced to less than 30% as soon as possible (page 630). Acidaemia should be corrected by the intravenous administration of sodium bicarbonate solution. In the event of apnoea, or collapse with gasping respiration and a cardiac frequency of less than 80 per min, the respiration should be stimulated by flicking the soles of the feet or assisted by continuous positive pressure ventilation. Reynolds recommends that the durations of inspiration and expiration are in the ratio 4:1 and the respective pressures approximately 0.75 and 0.25 kPa (7.5 and 2.5 cmH_2O). Alternatively, the incubator can be maintained at a negative pressure of 0.5−1.0 kPa (5−10 cmH_2O) below atmospheric, provided the trachea is connected to atmosphere (see also page 649).

Oxygen therapy for circulatory insufficiency (see page 613)

Oxygen for patients with lung disease

Clinical effects of hypoxaemia. The effects of hypoxaemia vary from minor aberrations of function to gross changes which, whilst they are usually diagnosed correctly, are sometimes attributed to other causes. When compiling a differential diagnosis the possibility that a patient is suffering from the effects of hypoxaemia should always be borne in mind.

The function of the central nervous system is particularly vulnerable to derangement by lack of oxygen. The gross changes include tremor, slurred speech, incoordination and restlessness. There can be variations in mood between euphoria and anxiety. Irritability is a frequent occurrence and the patient may be unusually talkative. The electro-encephalogram shows irregular slow waves and diminished alpha wave activity over the posterior regions. In the presence of a normal tension of carbon dioxide the changes are apparent when the arterial oxygen saturation falls to about 70% $(Pao_2 \approx 5\,kPa)$. Rebuck and his colleagues have shown that a lower saturation can be tolerated in the presence of hypercapnia probably on account of cerebral vasodilatation. In healthy subjects a lesser degree of hypoxaemia for example an alveolar oxygen tension of approximately 9 kPa (67 mmHg) can impair visual discrimination, night vision and performance of complex psycho-motor tasks. Thus even a minor degree of hypoxaemia impairs the function of the brain.

The effects of severe hypoxaemia upon the cardiovascular system include diminished force of ventricular contraction, tachycardia and interference with the conducting system of the heart; this can progress to anoxic cardiac arrest which is a common cause of death in patients with respiratory failure. Moreover with milder hypoxaemia the work which the heart is required to perform is often increased by a rise in pulmonary vascular resistance, an increase in the viscosity of the blood secondary to polycythaemia and a demand for an increase in cardiac output. The superimposition of these changes can precipitate congestive cardiac failure, especially if the pulmonary vascular resistance is already increased on account of chronic lung disease (see also pages 200 and 541).

In the lung the hypoxaemia can give rise to interstitial oedema which interferes with gas exchange and widens of the range of the ventilation—perfusion ratios. The function of the alveolar macrophages is impaired. Intestinal absorption is disturbed and in the liver the parenchymal cells are liable to be damaged by the hypoxaemia and, if the condition persists, by centrilobular fibrosis. The liver function is impaired in consequence. In the kidneys the permeability of the glomeruli can be increased and the tubular function impaired; these changes are aggravated by a coincident reduction in the renal blood flow. Hypoxaemia causes changes in function of the endocrine glands (page 699) and in reproduction. Cellular metabolism is shifted in the direction of rapid glycolysis with consequent lactacidaemia.

Detection of hypoxaemia. Hypoxaemia is difficult to detect clinically since the symptoms and physical signs are not specific. Cyanosis is usually only apparent when the blood contains approximately $5\,g\,dl^{-1}$

of reduced haemoglobin. Thus in anaemia this sign can be absent despite material hypoxaemia, whereas in polycythaemia it can be present when the arterial oxygen tension is within the normal range. Cyanosis should be looked for using daylight or a suitable artificial light (e.g. Philips colour 37 fluorescent lamp); it is present when the tongue and mucous membrane of the inside of the mouth take on a bluish tinge. However, in cases where the result is likely to be important, the saturation or tension of oxygen in the arterial blood should be determined directly (page 39). The measurement should be made early in the course of the acute episode, especially in infants, young children and the elderly, in whom an urgent need for oxygen may not be detectable in other ways.

Indications for oxygen. During the course of an acute chest illness an arterial oxygen tension of less than 6.7 kPa (50 mmHg) which, when the pH is 7.4, is equivalent to a saturation of less than 85%, is usually an indication for immediate therapy. This will normally take the form of the administration of oxygen but if the pH is less than 7.26 (hydrogen ion activity more than $55 \, \text{nmol} \, l^{-1}$) additional respiratory stimulation or support may be required (page 648). If the saturation is between 85% and 92% the administration of oxygen may also be beneficial, particularly in young children and in patients with acute asthma. The indications for its possible use then include a rapid heart rate or frequency of respiration, some evidence of pulmonary hypertension, an electrocardiogram suggesting right heart strain or the presence of congestive cardiac failure. Peripheral oedema which is resistant to treatment with bed rest and diuretic drugs sometimes yields dramatically to the administration of oxygen. Anginal pain arising from the right ventricle or pulmonary conus may also be alleviated. However, the effects of oxygen are not all beneficial and a careful watch should be kept for the complications which may accompany its use; these are discussed on page 629.

During the chronic stages of a chest illness long-term oxygen therapy can be used to relieve congestive cardiac failure secondary to pulmonary hypertension; the treatment also corrects secondary polycythaemia. The method was envisaged by Priestley, introduced by Barach, developed by Bishop and validated by controlled trials in the UK and USA. In patients living at sea level the treatment is given for 15−18 h per day, but for longer in those living at altitude. It has been shown to prolong life in those patients who are not already in the pre-terminal stage of their illness. Thus the treatment should start as soon as possible after the onset of right heart failure. Criteria for long-term oxygen therapy (LTOT) are given in Table 17.4.

In addition to its use at rest, oxygen may be administered to increase the capacity for exercise of some patients. The patients with lung disease who are most likely to benefit have a forced expiratory volume (FEV_1) of less than 1.0 l and are customarily limited on exercise by breathlessness rather than by cough, fatigue or other symptoms.

Table 17.4 Criteria of UK Department of Health for prescribing long-term oxygen in chronic obstructive lung disease (COPD)*

	Criterion	Variability†
Arterial O_2 tension	<7.3 kPa (55 mmHg)	<0.7 kPa (5 mmHg)
Arterial CO_2 tension*	>6 kPa (45 mmHg)	–
Forced expiratory volume	<1.5 (l)	<20%
Forced vital capacity	<2.0 (l)	<20%
Oedema*	One episode sufficient	

* Absence of these features is not a bar to prescription.
† Variability over 3 weeks.

However, not all patients who meet these requirements are able to increase their capacity for exercise by breathing oxygen. Thus before portable oxygen equipment is prescribed, an assessment should be made to confirm that the capacity is increased to a worthwhile extent by breathing oxygen compared with breathing air (e.g. that the walking distance is doubled as in Fig. 17.5, page 640).

Dosage. Short-term oxygen therapy for an acute chest illness will usually be started using an oxygen flow rate of $2 \, l \, min^{-1}$ via nasal prongs or a venturi or Edinburgh mask (page 636). The effects of this regimen should be monitored at 30–60 min after the start. Failure to achieve an arterial oxygen tension of at least 6.7 kPa (50 mmHg) is an indication for increasing the oxygen flow rate. A fall in pH to below 7.26 or an equivalent rise in the arterial carbon dioxide tension is an indication for reducing the oxygen flow rate to $1 \, l \, min^{-1}$ provided that the target oxygen tension can be achieved. If not the respiratory stimulant doxa-pram should be given by intravenous infusion in the dosage $0.5–4 \, mg \, min^{-1}$. This will usually both alleviate the acidaemia and permit adequate oxygenation but if not, the use of assisted ventilation should be considered.

Long-term oxygen therapy is normally directed to maintaining the arterial oxygen tension in excess of 8 kPa (60 mmHg) for 16 hours per day. Administration is via nasal prongs and the flow rate is that which meets the target oxygen tension; it is usually $3 \, l \, min^{-1}$. A humidifier is seldom needed but may help some patients. The oxygen is usually supplied from an oxygen concentrator (page 639) but a source of liquid oxygen can also be used. Cylinder oxygen is not economical. The patient must not smoke whilst taking the oxygen and should preferably have abandoned smoking altogether as part of the treatment.

Oxygen for use during exercise should preferably be delivered via a high efficiency mask with a bag for conserving the oxygen which is delivered during expiration and a non-return valve to prevent re-breathing (page 636). The oxygen flow rate will usually be $2 \, l \, min^{-1}$ but $4 \, l \, min^{-1}$ is often more effective (Fig. 17.5, page 640). The source of the oxygen can be a portable cylinder or liquid oxygen walker. Further details are given on page 639.

Nitrobenzene. Derivatives of aniline and nitrobenzene react with and inactivate oxyhaemoglobin to form methaemoglobin. The presence of this component can give rise to cyanosis. The associated symptoms can include headache, fatigue, breathlessness on exertion and euphoria. Treatment is by withdrawal from exposure when recovery usually occurs over a period of $1-5$ days. During this time the symptoms can be relieved by the use of oxygen. The process of recovery can be hastened by the intravenous infusion of methylene blue in the dosage of up to 1 mg per kilogram of body weight.

Cyanide. Hydrocyanic acid and some of its derivates convert cytochrome into a form which will no longer transport oxygen. The blood is then fully oxygenated but the tissues are acutely short of oxygen. In addition, the cyanide blocks the enzyme chain in the receptor cells of the carotid body; this causes hyperventilation. The patient becomes giddy and confused. There is a sense of constriction in the chest and the breath smells of the oil of bitter almonds. Asphyxial convulsions occur as a pre-terminal event. In addition, if the exposure is to a halogenated cyanide components (CNBr or CNCl) there may be severe irritation of the eyes and respiratory tract. Treatment is with oxygen supplemented by specific antidotes. Cobalt ethylenediaminetetra-acetate (cobalt EDTA, Kelocyanor) can be given intravenously in a dosage of 300 mg, but it is itself quite toxic so should only be administered if the patient is already unconscious. Alternatively sodium nitrite (0.5 g) is infused over 10 min in order to convert some of the patient's own haemoglobin into methaemoglobin, the latter then combines with the cyanide in the blood to form cyanmethaemoglobin. The haemoglobin is subsequently liberated from this compound by the administration of sodium thio-sulphate (25 g); this converts the cyanide radical to thiocyanate. The patient may also require assisted ventilation and measures to sustain the circulation including an infusion of noradrenaline or hydrocortisone.

Carbon monoxide. Carbon monoxide interferes with the transport of oxygen by entering into a reversible combination with haemoglobin (page 291). The resulting carboxyhaemoglobin reduces the capacity of the blood to transport oxygen and displaces the oxygen dissociation curve to the left; the displacement reduces the tension at which oxygen is liberated from the haemoglobin in the tissue capillaries (Fig. 17.2). The carbon monoxide also combines with myoglobin. The changes do not affect the tension of oxygen in the arterial blood so there is no material increase in the chemoreceptor drive to respiration; however, the ventilation can be increased secondary to lactacidaemia. During acute exposure, a rise in the saturation of haemoglobin with carbon monoxide to $20-40\%$ usually causes headache, giddiness and weakness; higher levels of carboxyhaemoglobin cause cerebral oedema. There may then be tachycardia and rapid breathing, a fall in blood pressure

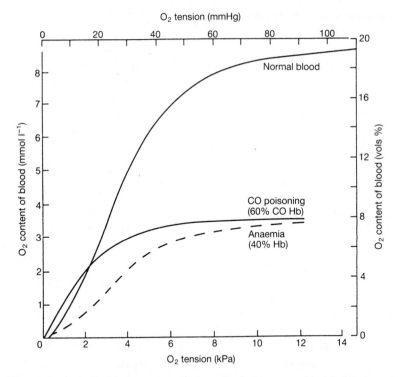

Fig. 17.2 Oxygen dissociation curves showing typical changes associated with anaemia and poisoning by carbon monoxide. In both cases only 40% of the normal quantity of haemoglobin is available for transport of oxygen. In carbon monoxide poisoning the delivery of oxygen to the tissues is impeded by displacement of the curve to the left; this reduces the tension at which the oxygen is liberated into the tissue capillaries. (Source: Roughton FJW, Darling RC. *Am J Physiol* 1944; **141**: 17–31.)

and sudden loss of consciousness. The skin and mucous membranes can have a cherry red appearance due to the presence of carboxy-haemoglobin, but usually the feature is obscured by the circulatory collapse leading to the patient being pale, cold and sweating. In chronic poisoning the subject may present with headache, irritability and dyspepsia. Irritability and depression can also be features of transient minor exposures. There is then an increased risk of dementia and this is increased if the patient is given electro-convulsant therapy. The diagnosis of carbon monoxide poisoning should be confirmed by measurement of the level in blood. This can be done directly by spectrophotometry or indirectly by a gasometric method (page 313).

The treatment of carbon monoxide poisoning is to remove the subject from the contaminated atmosphere and to hasten the dissociation of the carboxyhaemoglobin by administration of oxygen. Depending on circumstances the rate of dissociation can be speeded up by using 5–7% carbon dioxide in oxygen (carbogen) or hyperbaric oxygen therapy (Table 17.5). However, the effectiveness of these procedures has been disputed. Additional treatment may be required for respiratory depression, cardiac arrest or cerebral oedema.

Table 17.5 Mean half-times for elimination of carbon monoxide from dogs to whom oxygen was administered in different ways

Inspired gas	Half-time (min)
21% O_2	210*
100% O_2	29.8
5% CO_2 in O_2	20.6
7% CO_2 in O_2	16.3
O_2 at 2 atmospheres	8.6

* Estimated.
(Source: Douglas TA, Lawson DD, Ledingham I McA *et al. Lancet* 1962; **i**: 68–69.)

Other indications for oxygen

Elimination of nitrogen. The inhalation of oxygen reduces the tension of nitrogen in the alveolar gas relative to that in the blood. Nitrogen then passes from the blood into the gas phase. This process can be used to eliminate gaseous nitrogen from the tissues and from a pneumothorax, pneumoperitoneum or a region of surgical emphysema. Intestinal cysts and flatulence due to paralytic ileus can also be relieved. However, the rate of absorption is slow, and oxygen should be administered continuously as 100% O_2 for a minimal period of 12 h or in a fractional concentration of 0.60 for 6 days in order to have an effect. By contrast gaseous oxygen is rapidly absorbed so should be used instead of air to delineate organs prior to radiography. It should also be used if a small bubble of gas is to be injected into an artery to promote vasodilatation.

In aircrew denitrogenation was formerly used to protect against decompression sickness caused by exposure to reduced barometric pressure following a failure of cabin pressurisation. The condition is a consequence of nitrogen coming out of solution to form bubbles in the blood or some tissues and occurs after rapid ascent from sea level to altitudes in excess of 5500 m (18 000 ft). The conditions favourable for bubble formation include a high partial pressure of nitrogen in the tissues relative to that in the lungs (usually by a factor of at least two), a high nitrogen content (hence obesity) and the presence of trigger factors; these include exercise which increases local turbulence in blood, cosmic rays and anatomical factors. The bubbles affect mainly the limbs where the presenting symptom is pain. Bubbles in the blood can cause cough, breathlessness, chest pain and shock.

The clearance of nitrogen from different tissues varies depending on their blood supply and content of fat, in which nitrogen is five times more soluble than in serum. Older subjects usually have a reduced tissue blood flow but more fat compared with younger ones so their clearance times are prolonged. In young men breathing oxygen, nitrogen is cleared very rapidly from the blood and those organs such as the

627

kidney and the thyroid gland which have a large blood flow in relation to their size (half-time of $1-2$ min). For the abdominal viscera, but not the lumina of the intestines, for the grey matter of the brain and spinal cord and for the organs which are well perfused with blood the half-time is approximately 5 min. The nitrogen in the muscles and the connective tissues of the body is cleared more slowly with a half-time of $25-30$ min, whilst the nitrogen in the depot fat is cleared very slowly with a half-time of $1-4$ h. The use of 90% oxygen in nitrogen for 4 h prior to decompression materially reduces the risk of decompression sickness. One hundred percent oxygen should not be used as it can promote atelectasis (page 631).

In divers and caisson workers decompression sickness is caused by the formation of bubbles from nitrogen which enters the body during the period of pressurisation. The symptoms, colloquially described as the bends and the chokes, come on during, or a few hours after, decompression. In addition the central nervous system and spinal cord can be affected by local bubbles or emboli from the lungs. The condition can present as paraplegia during decompression or be silent and cause damage subsequently. In caisson workers the bubbles can cause aseptic bone necrosis, hence caisson disease. The conditions can be prevented by controlled decompression in which time is allowed for denitrogenation during the decompression; they can also be prevented by breathing an appropriate mixture of helium, oxygen and nitrogen instead of air during the compression and subsequent decompression. Care needs to be taken to avoid oxygen toxicity (page 630) and some nitrogen should be retained to facilitate speech. In addition where the gas is supplied to a diving bell the use of helium can cause hypothermia. This is due to heat loss to the environment on account of the gas having a high thermal conductivity. Additional heat may then need to be provided to the subject. The principal treatment for decompression sickness is recompression. This is usually to 3 atmospheres absolute (3 ATA) with subsequent slow decompression. The prevention and management of decompression sickness is the subject of codes of practise prepared by the Health and Safety Executive and other bodies. Their recommendations should be followed carefully.

Oxygen as a pharmacological agent. Oxygen is a specific remedy for hypoxic pulmonary hypertension (page 200) and for anaerobic and micro-aerophilic infections. For this latter purpose the gas is best administered under pressure (page 638). Hyperbaric oxygen can also be used to restore the radiosensitivity of cells in relatively avascular tumours. The radiosensitivity is reduced by hypoxia ($Po_2 < 4$ kPa equivalent to 30 mmHg). Oxygen can be used to treat infestation of the gastro-intestinal tract by *Ascaris lubricoides* and to induce cerebral vasoconstriction in the dilatation phase of migraine. However, better remedies for migraine are available.

Complications of oxygen therapy

Hypoventilation

Hypoxaemia increases the chemoreceptor drive to respiration. In subjects with healthy lungs, including most infants, children and patients with myocardial infarction, this leads to hyperventilation which is returned towards normal when the hypoxaemia is corrected by the administration of oxygen. By contrast, in patients with chronic lung disease or those with reduced central drive to respiration the increased chemoreceptor drive may be performing the essential role of maintaining an adequate alveolar ventilation. In this circumstance the administration of oxygen, reduces the alveolar ventilation by eliminating the chemoreceptor drive; this leads to retention of carbon dioxide which can then depress the action of the nervous system (Fig. 16.17, page 585). Three patients who were particularly vulnerable to this complication of oxygen therapy are described in Case Study 16.5 (page 581). The following is a hypothetical example:

A patient is admitted to hospital with an acute chest illness. He is anxious and talkative and on examination, in addition to having physical signs related to the chest, is cyanosed and is breathless on slight exertion. The heart rate and the frequency of respiration are increased. The tension of oxygen in the arterial blood is 5.3 kPa (40 mmHg), the tension of carbon dioxide is 8 kPa (60 mmHg) and the blood pH is within the normal limits of 7.45 and 7.35. The patient is prescribed chemotherapy and given oxygen in low dosage. This improves his colour and relieves his anxiety and breathlessness; he relaxes on his pillow apparently greatly improved and is left to sleep undisturbed. It is noted that his colour is a healthy pink, his pulse is full and his hands are warm to touch. Later he is stuporous and difficult to rouse; the tension of carbon dioxide in the arterial blood has risen to 13 kPa (100 mmHg) and the blood pH has fallen to 7.20. The life of the patient is now in jeopardy from carbon dioxide narcosis caused by uncontrolled oxygen therapy.

The risk of carbon dioxide narcosis is reduced by administering the oxygen at the minimal effective concentration. Since the gas exchange is taking place on the steep part of the oxygen dissociation curve (Fig. 9.3, page 280), 24% or 28% oxygen is often sufficient. The oxygen should be given continuously and not intermittently since, during periods when oxygen is withheld, the tension in the blood falls abruptly and may lead to cerebral damage.

The response of the patient should be monitored frequently, usually every 10 min to start with and subsequently at longer intervals; attention should be directed to the state of consciousness, the frequency and depth of respiration, and the oxygenation, tension of carbon dioxide (Fig. 16.2, page 522) and pH of the arterial blood. A way in which the information can be used is given on page 208. The direct measurements can be supplemented using a finger pulse oximeter with a saturation of 92% as the target level. In addition in patients with lung disease all possible steps should be taken to improve the lung function. Some of these are given in Table 16.13 (page 559). The use of hypnotic drugs, derivatives of morphine and some tranquilisers should be avoided except in special circumstances.

The correction of life-threatening hypoxaemia is of paramount importance so if, despite precautions, the patient hypoventilates the ventilation should be increased by active means. Conversation and physical stimulation of the face can help, whilst stimulant drugs such as doxapram or the morphine antagonist naloxone are often effective.

Excessive bronchial secretions should be aspirated using a catheter passed through the larynx via the nose or through an endotracheal catheter. The catheter should be soft and the cuff, depending on its design, may need to be deflated at frequent intervals. If it is likely to be needed for more than a few days a tracheotomy should preferably be performed. The catheter used for aspiration should be of large diameter and have a curved tip to facilitate insertion into the left as well as the right main bronchus (page 225). The air entering the tracheotomy should be humidified. Ways of doing this are reviewed by Hayes and Robinson. If these remedies are unsuccessful the patient should be given assisted ventilation (page 647).

Retrolental fibroplasia

Uncontrolled administration of oxygen to premature infants, including those with respiratory distress syndrome (page 621), can cause spasm of the incompletely developed retinal vessels. The spasm leads to proliferation of connective tissue cells in the retina and subsequently to scarring and blindness. The spasm is reversible in the early stages. The condition can be avoided by restricting the administration of oxygen, in both its concentration and duration, to the minimum which is compatible with resuscitation at birth. For this purpose a fractional concentration of 0.3 appears to be completely safe. If it is necessary to use a higher concentration of oxygen an examination of the retina should be carried out every 12 h or as often as is practicable and the dosage should be reduced or discontinued in the event of spasm, or as soon as the oxygen is no longer essential.

Oxygen toxicity

In experimental animals exposure to oxygen in excess of about 50 kPa (375 mmHg) causes congestion and proliferation of pulmonary capillaries; the changes are secondary to destruction of alveolar endothelium and usually progress to pulmonary oedema and to death within 3–7 days. Similar histological changes have been observed at post-mortem in patients who received prolonged oxygen therapy; the oxygen has usually been given by assisted ventilation. This 'pulmonary respirator syndrome' is a serious complication of respiratory distress in the newborn (page 621) and a cause of the comparable condition in adults (page 569). Oxygen toxicity can also occur in divers exposed to unduly high tensions of oxygen at depth or during decompression following saturation dives.

The early features include cough, retrosternal pain, tracheal inflammation, a reduced velocity of mucus flow and a small diminution in vital capacity. The toxic effects of oxygen are aggravated by a rise in the metabolic rate as a result of exercise, hyperthermia, coexisting viral infection or high blood levels of catecholamines, cortisone and thyroxine; the effects are minimised by adrenergic blockade, anaesthesia and anti-oxidant drugs. Hypercapnia is an additional risk factor whilst the risk is reduced if the exposure to hyperoxia is intermittent.

The present evidence suggests that subjects at sea level can breathe oxygen in a fractional concentration of 0.7 for up to 24 h and at a F_{I,O_2} of 0.5 for a period of months without developing symptoms, though anaemia can occur from suppression of the production of erythropoietin. Since these dosages are more than adequate for most clinical applications the risk to patients is small, provided the treatment is properly supervised.

Oxygen poisoning

Exposure to oxygen at a pressure of 2 bar or above causes oxygen poisoning in which the subject convulses and loses consciousness. This change is preceded by pallor and an ill-defined sense of unease. The incidence of the condition is determined by the pressure applied and the duration of exposure; the predisposing and the ameliorating factors are similar to those for oxygen toxicity. The condition is avoidable.

Oxygen paradox

Some subjects when they are both acutely hypoxic and hypocapnoic react to the administration of oxygen by abruptly becoming unconscious. This paradoxical response is caused by constriction of the cerebral blood vessels which were previously dilated by the deficiency of oxygen. The onset is within half a minute of administering the oxygen and the duration is only a few seconds. The condition can affect aircrew who put on their oxygen masks following sudden loss of cabin pressure. The possible adverse consequences for the aircraft can be avoided by one crew member wearing a mask continuously.

Barotrauma and atelectasis

The constituent gases in an enclosed pocket of air anywhere in the body are in equilibrium with the adjacent tissues; here the sum of the tensions of the oxygen, carbon dioxide, nitrogen and water vapour is less than atmospheric, so the gas in the pocket is gradually absorbed. A closed pocket of oxygen is absorbed more rapidly than one containing air because there is then a larger tension gradient for oxygen between the pocket and its surroundings.

Gas can be absorbed from the para-nasal sinuses and middle ear if the connecting passages are obstructed, but at normal barometric pressures, the absorption is usually slow and incomplete. Complete absorption is more likely while breathing oxygen, especially when this is accompanied by a change in barometric pressure. These circumstances can obtain in relation to hyperbaric oxygen therapy and to aviation. The condition is called delayed barotrauma. Acute barotrauma can occur in a chamber during the application of pressure, in an aeroplane during the descent or a decompression chamber during recompression. The condition is then due to the volume of gas being reduced by compression at a greater rate than it is being replaced by entry of gas from the pharynx. The condition usually arises first in the middle ear when it presents with pain, deafness and a sensation of heaviness on the affected side.

Acute barotrauma is best avoided by adopting a slow rate of pressure change (less than 0.15 bar min^{-1}) and by the subject opening the Eustachian tubes by swallowing, singing or yawning at regular intervals during the time when the pressure is rising. If symptoms develop, the subject should inhale methedrine or a similar decongestant drug, then take a deep breath, shut the mouth, close the nose with one thumb and forefinger and attempt to exhale. The manoeuvre will usually force air into the middle ear or the sinus which is affected. If it is unsuccessful a solution of 0.5% ephedrine in saline should be applied over the ostium of the appropriate sinus by suitably positioning the head. If this treatment fails resort may be made to politzeration or myringotomy.

Alveoli continue to take up oxygen after the airway which serves them has been occluded. On this account a manoeuvre, which when breathing air would cause the temporary closure of a segmental airway can, when breathing oxygen, lead to the absorption of sufficient gas to prolong the occlusion and give rise to atelectasis. This is liable to occur in the lower lobes of military flying personnel when they are exposed to positive acceleration whilst breathing 100% oxygen. Atelectasis can also occur in relation to anaesthesia (page 619) and during the inhalation of 100% oxygen by patients whose breathing is shallow. The condition is prevented by routinely using oxygen in a maximal concentration of 0.7. When closure occurs the patency of the airway can usually be restored by a single deep inspiration.

Overinflation of the lung

Oxygen is usually supplied at a pressure which could rupture the lung or stomach if the outlet from the body were to be occluded. The danger can be avoided by using low pressure equipment or by fitting a relief valve which operates at a maximal pressure of 6 kPa (45 mmHg). Rupture (overdistension) can occur during rapid decompression in a chamber or whilst escaping from a submerged submarine. It can also be caused by a catastrophic loss of cabin pressure in a pressurised aircraft. The condition is rare except when there is coexisting spasm of the glottis or obstruction to a bronchus. In the event of it occurring the subject should be immediately recompressed, or receive other treatment to relieve the tension pneumothorax which develops after rupture.

A moderate increase in the pressure inflating the lung, which is insufficient to cause rupture, can impede the return of venous blood to the thorax and hence reduce the cardiac output. This complication of assisted ventilation is discussed on page 652.

Fire and explosion

Oxygen is not inflammable but it increases the rate at which other objects burn. For this reason the gas should not be used near an open flame, near electrical equipment which is liable to spark or overheat, or in the vicinity of someone who is smoking. Special precautions should be taken during hyperbaric oxygen therapy (page 638). Concentrations of hydrogen, carbon monoxide, acetylene and some other compounds in excess of 2% in oxygen produce an explosive mixture. An explosion can also occur when oxygen under pressure comes in contact with oil or grease; this should not be allowed to happen. The exposure of a plastic fitting on the oxygen line to heat from a table lamp or other equipment can also be dangerous as the fitting is liable to soften and burst if it contains gas under pressure. This danger can be avoided by proper design and location of the equipment. Other precautions, including care in handling oxygen cylinders and the use of non-return valves in the oxygen line, are discussed on page 50.

Oxygen dependency

A patient who is breathless at rest leads a precarious existence. This can be rendered tolerable by the use of oxygen which, in appropriate cases, reduces the breathlessness, improves the appetite and assists sleep. It also provides psychological support to both patient and attendants. In view of these effects of oxygen, it is not surprising that some patients become aware of subjective changes when the supply of the gas is cut off; withdrawal symptoms are commonest if the treatment has been of long duration or if, as a result of a high dosage, the patient has developed oxygen toxicity. However, oxygen dependency is usually psychological in origin. It is best avoided by ensuring that the gas is given only to cases who respond, only at times when it is needed and only in the minimal effective dose. These principles should be explained to the patient and attendants. In addition, in order to overcome the tendency of some patients gradually to increase the dose, it is desirable that the equipment should deliver oxygen at a fixed flow rate.

Methods of administering oxygen

The oxygen is delivered by an oronasal device or via a tent or chamber. The oronasal method is simple to apply, requires inexpensive apparatus, is economical of oxygen, provides some freedom for the patient, constitutes a relatively small fire risk and makes fewer demands on the nursing staff than the other methods. However, an oxygen tent should be used for infants and any adult who is restless or agitated. An oxygen chamber or capsule is used to administer the gas at high pressure.

Oronasal devices for administering oxygen

Oronasal devices for administering oxygen can be classified according to what happens to the flow of oxygen during expiration. In a few devices the flow is cut off completely but usually it continues. The oxygen which flows during expiration is then either lost into the air or stored in a bag which may or may not be protected by a non-return valve to prevent contamination by the gas which the patient exhales.

Devices in which the flow of oxygen is cut off during expiration

In sophisticated equipment, such as that used by flying personnel, the flow of oxygen is cut off during expiration by means of a pressure-compensated demand valve which responds to the pressure difference across the facepiece of the oronasal mask. A demand type of equipment is also used with compressed air in underwater breathing sets. The proper function of the equipment depends on a gas-tight seal between the facepiece and the user. This is difficult to achieve without discomfort and the equipment is relatively expensive and is difficult to sterilise. The method is rarely used in medicine except for patients who require assisted ventilation via an endotracheal tube or tracheotomy.

Alternatively, the flow of oxygen can be synchronised in phase with inspiration using a mechanical device which is controlled by the movement of the thorax or by a thermistor or pressure transducer in the nose. The flow can also be controlled manually as when using a palm breathing device for delivering oxygen inconspicuously during exercise (Fig. 17.5, page 640).

Devices in which oxygen flows to waste during expiration

This category includes oxygen catheters and cannulae, venturi-type masks, the MC and Edinburgh masks and oxygen visors and hoods; the last two are discussed under oxygen tents. These devices are somewhat extravagant of oxygen because approximately half the flow is wasted during expiration. However, they are cheap to buy, comfortable to wear and easy to maintain and operate. The devices are used for low dosage controlled oxygen therapy to relieve hypoxaemia due to ventilation–perfusion inequality. They are not appropriate for high dosages or when there is a need for economy of oxygen as when using portable equipment.

Nasal oxygen. By this method the oxygen is usually delivered via twin plastic tubes (prongs) which are inserted into both nostrils to a depth of 1 cm. Alternatively a single tube, which should be lubricated and changed every 6h, can be inserted into the naso-pharynx. In order not to desiccate the nasal mucosa the gas should preferably be humidified by used of a nebuliser or by bubbling through water in a Woulfe bottle. The equipment should be tested for leaks by pinching the tube with the fingers at regular intervals. Nasal oxygen is simple and reliable and, at low flow rates, the dosage is usually independent of whether or not the patient breathes through the nose. The average relationship of the flow to the concentration in the alveolar gas is shown in Fig. 17.3; the dosage is in the range $0.5-4.01 \text{min}^{-1}$ (usually 2l min^{-1}). Nasal oxygen is the method of choice for use during meals and is acceptable in other circumstances when low dosage oxygen is prescribed.

Venturi-type mask. A venturi device operated by the flow of oxygen provides a constant proportional dilution with air. In this way the concentration of oxygen is independent of the gas flow rate. Provided the flow rate is adequate to meet the peak ventilatory requirements of the patient the dosage of oxygen is also constant. An entrainment ratio of 10:1 provides a fractional concentration of about 0.27 and is recommended for controlled oxygen therapy in patients who are at risk of developing carbon dioxide narcosis. The dosage cannot be exceeded by the patient or his attendant increasing the flow rate of oxygen. The method was pioneered by Campbell. Masks supplying other fractional concentrations are also available, including 0.24 which can be used in an emergency for patients with an acute chest illness whilst they are on their way to hospital.

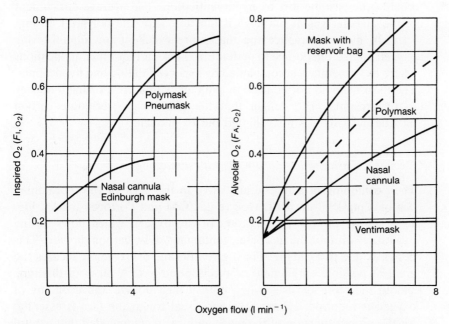

Fig. 17.3 Equivalent inspired and alveolar oxygen concentrations for healthy subjects wearing different types of personal oxygen equipment under resting conditions. The sources are given in the references.

Edinburgh mask. This device is a plastic facepiece with a 5 cm (2 in) diameter orifice through which the patient breathes. The oxygen is delivered into the centre of the orifice; for flow rates of 0.5, 2.0 and $3.0 \, 1 \, min^{-1}$ the fractional concentrations in the inspired gas are respectively about 0.23, 0.30 and 0.35 (Fig. 17.3). Very little carbon dioxide is rebreathed.

MC mask. The Mary Catterall mask is a plastic funnel through which the supply pipe for oxygen protrudes to within a short distance of the lips. The deadspace of the facepiece is about 90 ml. The degree of oxygen enrichment at low flow rates resembles that for nasal cannulae and at high flow rates the polymask (Fig. 17.3).

Oronasal masks which permit rebreathing

In 1938 Boothby, Lovelace and Bulbulian introduced the BLB oronasal mask for use by passengers in civil aircraft. The disposable *polymask* and *pneumask* have similar features. The device consist of a facepiece, an air-mix aperture and a storage bag for oxygen. On inspiration the subject inhales the oxygen from the bag, then makes up the rest of the tidal volume mainly by inhaling air through the aperture. On expiration the gas from the physiological deadspace, which still contains some additional oxygen, passes into the bag together with some carbon dioxide. The remainder is expired through the aperture. By this arrangement there is maximal conservation of oxygen; at the same time when used at altitude, some of the carbon dioxide is retained which would otherwise be lost by hyperventilation. The average enrichment of the alveolar gas at sea level is illustrated for the polymask in Fig. 17.3. In medical practice the masks are excellent for administering oxygen in medium dosage to patients in shock and for other applications where hypoxaemia is accompanied by hyperventilation and hypocapnia. The masks should not be used by patients with a pre-existing tendency to hypercapnia. The danger that the mask may precipitate carbon dioxide narcosis was first pointed out by Barach.

Oronasal masks which do not permit rebreathing

The positioning of a non-return valve in the neck of the rebreathing bag of a mask of the BLB type (e.g. EOM and Portogen masks, Fig. 17.4) allows for the conservation of the oxygen which flows during expiration without the gas being contaminated by carbon dioxide. This design is due to Haldane. For a given dosage of oxygen it secures the greatest possible enrichment of the inspired gas. A mask of this type should therefore be used when both a high dosage and economy of oxygen is required. However, a good seal round the face is essential for the proper function of the mask and it is recommended that careful fitting be carried out using a range of styles of facepiece.

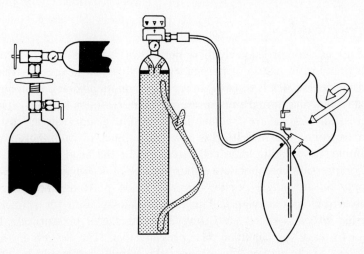

Fig. 17.4 Portable oxygen apparatus (DH170, Kidde) showing the method of charging from a large cylinder. Alternatively a liquid oxygen trolley can be used. The oronasal mask is fitted with an oxygen reservoir bag and valve to prevent rebreathing (Portogen, BOC).

Oxygen tents and visors

The modern oxygen tent differs from the earlier models in providing a controlled environment around the patient in which, when the tent is closed, the concentration of oxygen, the temperature and the humidity are monitored and maintained within specified limits; the concentration of carbon dioxide is effectively zero. Oxygen tents can be used for infants (page 621) and for adults who are restless or semi-conscious, including some cases of head injury and cerebro-vascular accident. The tents provide fractional concentrations of oxygen of up to 0.6, except when they are open. However, they are expensive and cumbersome and a potential fire risk. Some of these disadvantages can be avoided by using a head tent or visor in which a large volume of air enriched with oxygen is directed past the face. The mixture is prepared by a venturi device.

Transtracheal oxygen

A microcatheter which is inserted between the first and second rings of the trachea can be used to deliver oxygen into the airway just above the carina. The method is suitable for patients who are breathing shallowly since much of the deadspace is bypassed. Insertion is under local anaesthesia and can be made from a site on the chest to reduce the risk of local infection over the trachea or of the catheter being displaced. The catheter should be flushed daily to prevent blockage by mucus and the oxygen should be humidified. The method is economical of oxygen and usually very acceptable to the patient.

637

Hyperbaric oxygen

The use of a compression chamber permits the administration of oxygen at a pressure in excess of barometric. This can be of use for treating decompression sickness, gas gangrene, carbon monoxide poisoning and tissue ischaemia from many causes. Thus the treatment has been applied successfully for severe trauma, infected skin ulcers, salivary fistulae and frostbite. Pressurisation is also an adjunct to radiotherapy, for example, for treating large cell carcinoma of the head and neck.

Compression chambers are either capable of accommodating several people or are single person capsules made of transparent Perspex (polymethyl methacrylate). The former can be used for surgical or nursing procedures by staff who are themselves pressurised. They enter or leave the chamber via a pressure lock. The oxygen is usually supplied to the patient via a mask; this should preferably be of the whole-face type. The mask pressure should exceed that of the chamber so that any leaks are outwards. This can be achieved using a pressure compensated demand valve. When using a capsule the pressurising gas can be 100% oxygen; however, there is then a risk of fire. This is minimised by using air to raise the pressure and a mask to dispense the oxygen. The temperature and humidity in the capsule are controlled by air-conditioning and the exhaled carbon dioxide is removed by recirculation of the gas in the capsule through a canister containing soda lime. The physical isolation of the patient is partly overcome by the good visual and oral communication with the operator, and by the continuous monitoring of both the patient's respiration and heart rate and the pressure and composition of the gas in the capsule. At a pressure of 2 bar the duration of each treatment can be up to 2 h with a repeat after 1 h. For radiotherapy a pressure of 3 bar and duration of up to 40 min can be employed. The complications of the therapy are discussed on pages 630–633.

The chambers are expensive to maintain and operate; they usually form part of an underwater diving facility. The capsules are often located in departments of radiotherapy or, for infants, in paediatric departments. Hyperbaric therapy is specific for decompression sickness and can be of spectacular benefit to a few patients with the other disorders listed. Attempts to demonstrate a worthwhile therapeutic role in multiple sclerosis have yielded mainly negative results.

Domiciliary oxygen

A patient may require supplementary oxygen at home as an emergency measure whilst arrangements are made for transfer to hospital, or for the short-term treatment of an acute illness, or for long-term therapy. Oxygen which is required immediately can be contained in portable cylinders of capacity approximately 300 l with flow rates of 2 and 6 l min^{-1} (e.g. BOC). Such cylinders should be widely available. Alternatively a solid state oxygen candle can be used (Scott). For patients with pulmonary oedema or with cardiogenic shock the dosage is usually $61\,min^{-1}$ delivered to a polymask or OEM, Portogen or MC mask.

Oxygen which is required for short-term treatment was formerly supplied in cylinders of medium size (e.g. 48 cuft). However, an oxygen concentrator can be used instead and this device is recommended for long-term oxygen therapy (page 623). The dosage is usually $11\,min^{-1}$ (range $1-41\,min^{-1}$) delivered to nasal cannulae or an Edinburgh or venturi mask. The oxygen concentrator uses the principle of differential absorption to achieve a fractional concentration of oxygen of up to 0.9 by the removal of nitrogen from air. It is quiet, compact and reliable and suitable for long-term therapy. Alternatively, for the latter purpose, oxygen delivery points may be installed and connected to a large cylinder of oxygen (e.g. 250 cuft) or a liquid oxygen tank (Linde). In addition the mobility of the patient about the house can often be increased by using an oxygen line. This is a polyethylene tube of internal diameter 2 or 3 mm and length up to 20 m. The topic is considered further below.

Oxygen for use during exercise

Many patients with advanced lung disease can increase their activity by breathing oxygen during exercise and the quality of their lives can then be improved by portable oxygen equipment. The indications for treatment are outlined on page 623, and the method of assessment in Fig. 17.5. The underlying physiological basis for the treatment is given on page 407. Portable oxygen is also of use for healthy subjects at altitude and occasionally at sea level. The oxygen should be inhaled during exercise and not before or afterwards. The gas is either supplied from a small cylinder which is recharged in the home (Fig. 17.4) or a portable liquid oxygen set (Linde or 3M) is used. The gas should preferably be administerd by a method which does not entail wastage during expiration; in addition, in order that the mask deadspace is as small as possible a rebreathing bag is undesirable. These requirements are met by a mask of the Haldane type with an oxygen reservoir bag and a valve to prevent rebreathing. The optimal flow rate of oxygen is usually $41\,min^{-1}$ (Fig. 17.5). A lower dosage can be used if the patient has been fitted with a transtracheal catheter. For limited activity about the house and garden the oxygen can be supplied from an oxygen concentrator via a long length of tubing. When not in use the tube should be kept on a reel. The treatment should be combined with other measures to improve the exercise capacity, including physical training and weight reduction where appropriate (Table 16.8, page 543). Early expectations that patients might be helped by training the respiratory muscles or by a high fat diet, which on theoretical grounds should reduce the output of carbon dioxide and hence the ventilatory cost of exercise, have not been fulfilled. Ventilatory assistance during exercise could be a help but the equipment is not yet suitable for independent use.

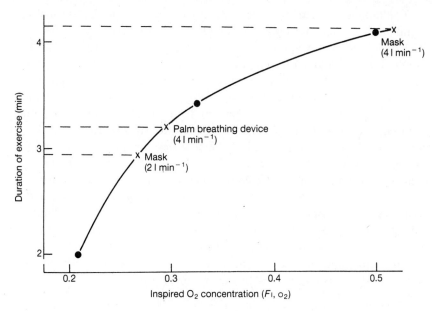

Fig. 17.5 Relationship of the mean duration of exercise to the dosage of oxygen for six patients with COPD. The speed and incline of the treadmill were adjusted so that each patient was obliged to stop on account of incapacitating breathlessness after 2 min when breathing air; most could double their walking time by breathing oxygen (mask, $4 \, l \, min^{-1}$), so were candidates for portable oxygen therapy. The curve is for mixtures of oxygen and nitrogen. The crosses are for a palm breathing device and a mask with reservoir bag and valve to prevent rebreathing; the equivalent concentrations of oxygen are less during exercise than at rest (Fig. 17.3). (Source: Cotes JE, Matthews CR, Tasker PM. *Lancet* 1963; **i**: 1075.)

Bronchodilator therapy

An increase in airway resistance occurs during the acute phase of asthma and is the principal cause of respiratory impairment and disability in patients with chronic bronchitis, asthma and related disorders (page 112). The increase in resistance can often be partly or completely relieved by treatment with bronchodilator drugs. These agents constitute the most frequently used respiratory treatment but they are often administered in an inefficient manner. In addition their effectiveness is often impaired by the patient continuing to smoke or by neglect of some other aspect of treatment. Thus bronchodilator treatment should be part of a therapeutic regimen and not prescribed in isolation. The principles of treatment are given below; the mechanisms in asthma are discussed on page 546 and other aspects of the control of bronchomotor tone on page 198.

Assessment for the need for therapy

The need for bronchodilator therapy should be assessed on clinical grounds and by measurement of the ventilatory capacity or the airway resistance before and after the administration of a potent bronchodilator drug, as described on page 145. The principal indication for therapy is an increase of at least 12% in the forced expiratory volume, forced vital capacity or peak expiratory flow rate, or a corresponding reduction in the airway resistance. The inhalation of the drug should abolish or reduce the intensity of any sibilant rhonchi heard on auscultation of the chest. Subjects in whom bronchodilator therapy does not improve the ventilatory capacity may none the less be able to take more exercise before the onset of breathlessness; thus an increase in exercise capacity can be an additional indication for treatment with this class of drugs.

Bronchodilator drugs

The relaxation of the smooth muscle in the walls of the airways requires energy and is facilitated by an increase in the intra-cellular concentration of cyclic $3',5'$-adenosine monophosphate (AMP). The concentration of this substance is increased by two important classes of bronchodilator drugs, the β adrenergic agonists and the derivatives of methyl xanthine. The former act by raising the activity of adenyl cyclase which increases the formation of cyclic AMP from adenosine triphosphate (ATP). The latter inhibit the action of phosphodiesterase which would otherwise accelerate the breakdown of cyclic AMP to 5-AMP. Since they act on separate parts of the metabolic pathway the actions of the drugs are synergistic and they can usefully be given in combination.

The prototype of the β *adrenergic agonists* is isoprenaline which stimulates the β_2 receptors but has little action on the α receptors so does not cause hypertension; however, as well as stimulating the β_2 receptors in the bronchi, isoprenaline has a pronounced stimulant action on the β_1 receptors in the heart and the blood vessels. Thus its use may lead to tachycardia and to cardiac arrhythmia. It can also dilate pulmonary blood vessels including those supplying regions which are poorly ventilated; this causes hypoxaemia which may require correction by the administration of oxygen. At one time there was an expectation that these complications of treatment might be avoided by the concurrent use of specific β_1 antagonist drugs but on account of side effects and incomplete specificity this has turned out not to be the case. Instead use should be made of β_2 adrenergic drugs which when given locally by inhalation, have a pronounced bronchodilator action but little action on the heart and blood vessels or on the central nervous system. Terbutaline, salbutamol and the long acting analogues salmeterol and fenoterol fall into this category. One of these drugs should be used in preference to adrenaline, ephedrine or other β adrenergic drug. To avoid the occurrence of side effects including tremor, agitation and palpitation, the drugs should preferably not be given orally or parenterally. The dosages for salbutamol and terbutaline are respectively $100-200\,\mu g$ and $0.25-0.5\,mg$ by inhalation every 4 h. The dosage of salmeterol is usually 50 mg taken by mouth before going to bed.

Anticholinergic drugs, such as atropine methonitrate and ipratroprium bromide, can be used to block the access of acetylcholine to smooth muscle receptors; this class of drug inhibits the bronchoconstrictor action of the vagi and can be used to promote bronchodilatation in patients with chronic obstructive pulmonary disease. The drugs are seldom of much help in asthma. The usual dosage of ipratroprium bromide aerosol is 40 μg four times daily often in conjunction with β agonists. Atropine should not be taken by persons who may have glaucoma or prostatic hypertrophy or who are pregnant. The maximal bronchodilator response is achieved after approximately 1 h so the inhalation does not immediately relieve acute bronchospasm, whereas inhaled β agonist drugs act very quickly.

The *xanthine group of drugs*, including choline theophyllinate, provide relief for some patients when taken by mouth; however, aminophylline is usually more effective when administered per rectum as a suppository and is most effective when given as an intravenous infusion in the dosage 250–500 mg. This dosage may be used at night for the immediate relief of acute episodes of wheeze and breathlessness. The effective therapeutic dose approaches that which causes symptoms of toxicity including nausea, vomiting and insomnia. These can be avoided by maintaining the blood concentration at the optimal level of $10-15\,\mathrm{mg\,l^{-1}}$. The hypothesis that theophylline can be used to increase the force of contraction of the diaphragm has not been confirmed.

The *corticosteroid drugs* facilitate the action of the β adrenergic agonists and can be used to initiate a response in many cases of apparently irreversible obstruction. The drugs also reduce the release from mast cells of granules containing substances which mediate delayed onset bronchoconstriction (page 558) and suppress inflammatory reactions; this is effected in part by increasing the migration of macrophages. The drugs are often effective in reducing the bronchial obstruction of patients who are in status asthmaticus; for this purpose hydrocortisone hemisuccinate should be given intravenously in the dosage 200 mg every 2 h or prednisone by mouth in the dosage 15 mg every 6 h for the first day, reducing to 10 mg on the second day. The rate of the subsequent reduction in dosage is determined on clinical grounds. The drug is also effective for the relief of minor degrees of bronchial obstruction in patients who are already receiving a β adrenergic drug. Initially, 40 mg of prednisone may be administered daily as a single dose. Alternatively in patients who tend to retain fluid 32 mg of methyl prednisolone can be used instead. The treatment is monitored using the forced expiratory volume or peak expiratory flow rate and the capacity for exercise. An increase of 25% is evidence of a therapeutic response. At this point the dosage should be gradually reduced to 10 mg daily. Alternatively, if there is no response within 14 days the trial of treatment should be discontinued. If a small dosage has a worthwhile therapeutic action this may be provided locally in the airways by the use of beclomethasone dipropionate as two inhalations each of 50 μg four times in the day or betamethasone valerate in twice this dosage. In order to secure an initial effect the inhalations should be started before the dose of oral prednisone has been tailed off; a watch should be kept for secondary infection with *Candida albicans*.

Sodium cromoglycate and *nedocromil* share with the corticosteroid drugs the property of reducing the degradation of mast cells. In patients with asthma they can be used prophylactically to prevent the development of airways obstruction during exercise or in relation to exposure to a specific allergen. For these purposes the drugs are preferable to steroids because they have almost no important side effects. The dose is 20 mg by inhalation up to six times daily; the drug is usually combined with a β adrenergic drug in order to reduce the bronchoconstrictor effect of the powder, which may be mediated via bronchial irritant receptors. A therapeutic trial of its effectiveness should be undertaken before the drug is prescribed for regular use. In the future other classes of drug including the E series of prostaglandins and derivates of Δ^9tetrahydrocannabinol may also be employed but at present their local irritant effect on the airways and other actions are strong contraindications.

Use of a nebuliser

The majority of bronchodilator drugs are now administered as aerosols in metered doses from pressurised containers; it is essential that instruction should be given in their correct use. To use a nebuliser the patient should exhale to residual volume, insert the nozzle into the open mouth, close the lips around the mouthpiece, activate the mechanism and make a full inspiration through the mouth to total lung capacity; the breath is then to be held for as long as is comfortable. The procedure is repeated once after 1 min. Even using this method of administration some 30% of patients fail to secure maximal benefit due to faulty timing. Such patients are helped by using a spacing device which is a hollow vessel of capacity approximately 750 ml inserted between the dispenser and the mouth. The metered dose is discharged into and then inhaled from the spacer. Alternatively the material is inhaled during regular breathing from a nebuliser which is driven by a supply of compressed gas. This method is suitable for very disabled patients and those requiring a high dosage, but care must be taken to prevent overdose.

Comment

Achieving optimal bronchodilatation reduces wheeze, chest tightness and breathlessness and increases the capacity for exercise of patients with airflow limitation. For these reasons it is usually the principal feature in clinical management and one in which the lung function laboratory can play an important role through assessing reversibility, monitoring the response to treatment and providing instruction on how the nebuliser should be used. The assessment of reversibility is described on page 145 and an example of successful management is given in Fig. 17.6.

643

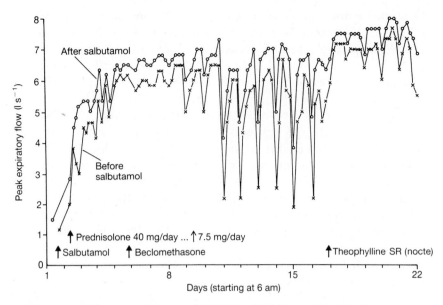

Fig. 17.6 Peak flow chart showing stages in the establishment of a suitable
bronchodilator regimen in a patient with severe airflow limitation. Salbutamol by
inhalation only had a small effect (indicated by distance between the two lines). The
condition responded to oral prednisolone in high dosage. Changing to a maintenance
dose plus inhaled beclomethasone resulted in loss of control, which was re-established
when an evening dose of slow release theophylline was added to the regimen. (Source:
Pearce SJ. In Cotes JE, Steel J, *Work-Related Lung Disorders*. Oxford: Blackwell
Scientific Publications, 1987, p. 408.)

Physiotherapy

Physiotherapy is sometimes effective in clearing secretions, relieving
respiratory symptoms and improving the capacity for exercise, but the
response is variable. It should be continued only in those patients who
appear to benefit.

General exercise

A patient whose activity is reduced or who is confined to bed incurs
penalties on this account. These include muscle wasting, osteoporosis,
reductions in muscle strength and maximal cardiac output and an impairment of the normal circulatory adaptations to exercise and to
alterations in posture. The changes combine to reduce the level of
activity at which there is conspicuous lactacidaemia and hence the
ability of the subject to take exercise. Exercise training can be used to
improve some of the effects of inactivity including the muscle weakness
and incoordination; training can also improve the responses of the
circulation to exercise and to changes in posture. The capacity for
exercise is thus improved. In respiratory patients the improvement is
often accompanied by a change towards a slower deeper pattern of
breathing. The lung function is seldom much affected.

The choice of exercise is likely to be between walking, cycle ergometry and swimming and should take account of the patient's preference. Any medical contraindication should be identified. Prior to the exercise any reversible bronchoconstriction should be relieved by bronchodilator therapy. In very disabled patients the maximal intensity and duration of the training sessions can sometimes be increased by having the patient breathe oxygen instead of air during the exercise (page 623). The exercise should be of sufficient intensity to induce fatigue or breathlessness within a few min and, subject to the patient's tolerance, should be repeated up to a total time of 20 min per session on 3 days in the week. The intensity of the exercise should be increased progressively between sessions and the patient encouraged to give of his best. He should be advised of his performance and it should be explained that becoming breathless does not strain the lungs. Further aspects of physical training are discussed on pages 408 and 472.

Breathing exercises

Breathing exercises can be used to strengthen weak respiratory muscles, reduce undue dynamic compression of airways during expiration and help the patient to acquire an optimal pattern of breathing. There is limited objective evidence for the effectiveness of all these procedures but in individual cases success cannot be assured.

In subjects with healthy lungs, training of the respiratory muscles has been achieved by periods of breathing against an external load; the response has been similar to that in other muscles (cf. page 408). Thus the training could help patients with muscle weakness, but general exercises will usually be better. It has still to be confirmed that a similar training effect can be achieved in patients in whom the work of breathing is already increased on account of lung disease; there is similarly little evidence that in such patients an increase in respiratory muscle strength reduces breathlessness and increases the capacity for exercise.

Breathing exercises have traditionally been used to reduce dynamic compression of airways which is a consequence of forced contraction of the expiratory muscles. The extent of the compression is increased by narrowing of the lumen from any other cause, e.g. a diminution in the elastic recoil pressure. The breathing exercises are directed to reducing the frequency and increasing the depth of breathing, with special emphasis on the excursion of the lower costal margin and on the respiratory movements being performed in a slow relaxed manner. The procedures undoubtedly help some patients but the main use of breathing exercises is probably as an adjunct to postural drainage. Alternatively attention can be directed to increasing the elastic recoil pressure by raising the resting respiratory level; this is done by beginning each inspiration a little earlier than usual in the breathing cycle. Air trapping can be reduced by raising the intrabronchial pressure through pursing the lips during expiration. This is done spontaneously by some patients.

A continuous positive pressure applied throughout the respiratory cycle can exert a similar action.

An abnormal pattern of breathing usually takes the form of shallow rapid breathing which increases the deadspace component of each tidal breath and hence the proportion of the minute volume which is wasted therein. This abnormality increases the exercise ventilation and may aggravate any pre-existing hypoxaemia and hypercapnia. In these circumstances, lowering the frequency of breathing can reduce the ventilatory cost of submaximal exercise, whilst breathing in a relaxed manner can relieve air-trapping and hence increase the maximal ventilation. Both changes contribute to a reduction in breathlessness; they can also improve the matching of ventilation to perfusion and alleviate the hypoxaemia. However, the benefit is likely to be small in patients with severe airflow limitation in whom the patency of airways can depend on breathing at near to total lung capacity.

Clearance of secretions

Secretions in the bronchial tree reduce the ventilatory capacity and interfere with the uniform distribution of the inspired gas; hence their removal improves the function of the lung. Clearance is normally effected by the cilia which propel the material up the airways into the pharynx or to a level at which it can be expectorated. The process can be assisted by a variety of means (Table 17.6). Of these, controlled coughing and posturing are the most useful; where appropriate they should be combined with other measures selected from amongst those listed in Table 17.6. The posture should be that which raises the affected part of the lung above the level of the carina; this is achieved by appropriate positioning of the patient and if necessary by elevating the foot of the bed by up to 0.5 m. The positioning should define the attitude of the patient (prone, supine or lateral), the incline (e.g. with pillows at the back or beneath the abdomen) and the elevation of the foot of the bed. Most upper lobe lesions are treated in an inclining upright posture and most lower lobe lesions by raising the foot of the bed, but there are exceptions. The optimal posture is usually that

Table 17.6 Measures used to increase clearance of secretions

Abandoning smoking	Inhalation of steam, water mist or hypertonic saline
Bronchodilatation, deep breathing	Intermittent positive pressure breathing
Controlled coughing (huffing, page 121)	Mucolytic drugs
Direct suction (page 82)	Percussion or compression of chest
High frequency oscillation	Posturing (gravitational force)*
Hot drinks (e.g. morning tea)	Treating infections

* Patient tolerance can sometimes be increased by administration of oxygen.

which provokes coughing and expectoration in response to the overall treatment. However, overzealous treatment will exhaust the patient and aggravate the hypoxaemia so the measures should be applied with discretion and interspersed with rest pauses. The usefulness of the procedure can be judged by the quantity of sputum which is expectorated, the frequency of coughing and the ventilatory capacity. If postural drainage improves one or more of these indices when the patient is in hospital, treatment should be continued at home.

Assisted ventilation

For a patient with lung disease assistance to respiration is necessary when the alveolar ventilation cannot be maintained at an adequate level by other means. The point at which treatment is required is a matter of clinical judgement; thus a patient who becomes exhausted by the effort of breathing may need help on account of rapid deterioration whilst another with a more severe blood gas abnormality may manage without assistance. In addition the introduction of nasal intermittent positive pressure ventilation (NIPPV) which is not invasive and can be readily applied in the ward or used at home has reduced the need for treatment in an intensive therapy unit. However, NIPPV has blurred the dividing line between normal and controlled breathing and this has increased the risk that failure of medical treatment may occur suddenly and require speedy action. Indications that this point has been reached include a tension of carbon dioxide in arterial blood of more than 10.7 kPa (80 mmHg) and a blood pH of less than 7.25. By contrast an injury to the chest wall or loss of power in the respiratory muscles which has reduced the vital capacity to less than 25% of the initial or expected value is an indication for respiratory assistance, even if the patient is hyperventilating and the tension of carbon dioxide is sub-normal. The respiratory assistance can take the form of *assisted ventilation*, which supplements the patients own respiratory efforts, or *controlled ventilation* in which the respiratory movements are imposed by the equipment.

Methods

Assistance to respiration is usually given during the inspiratory phase of the breathing cycle. Either pressures which are positive with respect to atmospheric are applied directly to the airways, or the excursion of the chest wall and the diaphragm are in some way increased. The simplest of the direct methods is the mouth-to-mouth or mouth-to-nose method of assisted ventilation in which the rescuer uses his own lungs as a bellows. This procedure is simulated by the anaesthetist who applies manual compression to the anaesthetic bag. In clinical practice the source of power is usually either compressed gas or an electrically operated piston. The changes from expiration to inspiration and from inspiration to expiration are referred to as cycling; of these the latter is the more critical. Assisted ventilation which is triggered by the patient's own respiratory excursions is said to be patient-cycled. The signal is usually a change in pressure but a flow or volume signal can be used. When ventilation is externally controlled the tidal volume is regulated by adjusting the magnitude and/or the duration of the pressure which is applied to the airway, or the stroke output of the pump; in the latter event, provision is made for the pressure to be released should it rise above 3.3 kPa (25 mmHg). Otherwise the maximal pressure should not exceed 6.0 kPa (45 mmHg) or 4 kPa (30 mmHg) in those patients with lung disease who are at increased risk of developing a pneumothorax. The equipment may be provided with a negative phase in order to lower the intra-thoracic pressure during expiration. This has the effect of augmenting the return of venous blood to the heart.

The *positive-pressure methods* of ventilation require that there is no material outward leak between the source of pressure and the airway of the subject, also that the tongue does not obstruct the pharynx. These difficulties can be avoided by the insertion of an endotracheal tube or by tracheotomy. The latter is the procedure of choice where the assisted ventilation is likely to be required for more than 48 h. A connection to the patient via a nasal mask is used in the technique of *nasal positive pressure ventilation* (e.g. Prenpac Ltd. or Thomas Respiratory Systems). A comfortable fit without leaks then depends on having a choice of facepieces supplemented by padding, and on careful adjustment of the straps. Alternatively the nosepiece can be made on an individually constructed mould. Intermittent nasal positive pressure ventilation is now widely used for treatment of sleep apnoea/hypnoea syndrome particularly in those cases where upper airway obstruction is a prominent feature. Negative pressure ventilation via a cuirass ventilator is a realistic alternative in other circumstances and for those patients in whom the pressure breathing causes gastric distension.

Negative pressure ventilation simulates normal breathing and is effected by reducing the pressure round the thorax with respect to atmospheric. This is done when the patient is ventilated in a tank or cuirass ventilator or in a breathing jacket. The tank ventilator encloses the subject up to the neck, where there is an airtight seal. This equipment is useful for some patients with neuromuscular and skeletal disorders who are none the less able to swallow normally and in whom secretions are not expected to accumulate in the airways. However, the equipment is bulky. The patient is also rather inaccessible but this disadvantage is minimised by the use of a hinged tank of the alligator type. The cuirass ventilator resembles a shield which makes an airtight seal round the periphery of the abdominal wall; its main function is to increase the excursion of the diaphragm. The seal is effected by constructing the cuirass from a plaster of Paris cast of the patient; the edge is padded and covered with neoprene rubber and the device is held in place with a back strap. Padding may also be needed to protect the back. A cuirass ventilator is of use for patients with kyphoscoliosis and for weaning patients from all types of controlled ventilation. It can

648

be the method of choice for patients requiring assisted nocturnal ventilation particularly those without much upper airway obstruction. The
method is an alternative to nasal positive pressure ventilation if the
latter causes gastric distension. A breathing jacket is a loose fitting
airtight garment on a rigid frame which extends from the head to the
thighs. Unlike the cuirass the jacket does not restrict the movement of
the rib cage and unlike the tank ventilator it carries no risk of pressure
sores. However, the jacket is bulky, difficult to put on and less effective
than a tank ventilator for ill patients. It can be the method of choice
for the domiciliary treatment of patients who were formerly on a tank
ventilator in hospital.

Control of assisted ventilation

The component variables which can contribute to the effectiveness of
assisted ventilation are listed in Table 17.7; not all of them are relevant
at any one time but those that are should be appropriate for the
patient under consideration. Thus the ventilation and the volume−time
profile should resemble those of the patient during normal spontaneous
breathing. The t_I/t_E ratio should be approximately 1:2 in subjects with
healthy lungs and 1:4 in patients with airflow limitation. The provision
of a post-inspiratory pause improves oxygenation whilst a post-expiratory
pause also contributes to the comfort of the patient. Approximately
10% of the time for each breath should normally be used in this way.

During assisted or controlled ventilation for respiratory distress syndrome or pulmonary oedema, positive end-expiratory pressure (PEEP)
is used to raise the functional residual capacity and hence the arterial
oxygen saturation. At the same time the PEEP interferes with the
systemic venous return. The best PEEP can be defined as that which
secures maximal delivery of oxygen to the tissues, where the delivery is
the product of saturation and cardiac output. Alternatively the best
PEEP can be defined in terms of the patient's static volume−pressure
curve. The pressure and the tidal volume should be adjusted so that

Table 17.7 Variables in assisted/controlled ventilation

Ventilation	Tidal volume, respiratory frequency, minute volume
Applied force	Driving pressure, pressure−time profile, volume−time profile
Distending pressure	Continuous positive airway pressure (CPAP), positive end expiratory pressure (PEEP)
Pattern of breathing	Ratio of t_I to t_E, post-inspiratory and post-expiratory pauses
Assistance	Patient triggered, inspiratory pressure support, synchronised intermittent mandatory ventilation (SIMV), mandatory minute ventilation (MMV), high frequency ventilation by jet or oscillator
Monitoring	Carbon dioxide tension in end-tidal gas or arterial or mixed venous blood

inspiration takes place entirely on the linear part of the curve (Fig. 5.7, page 96).

Continuous positive airway pressure (CPAP) is used to improve oxygenation in patients who are breathing spontaneously including those who have respiratory distress syndrome and upper airway obstruction in association with sleep apnoea/hypopnoea. To this end the pressure should be approximately 1 kPa (10 cmHg) and the flow rate generated by the equipment should exceed the maximum achieved by the patient during the respiratory cycle. The comfort of the patient can be improved and the excretion of carbon dioxide increased by the pressure being released intermittently for periods of a minute or two with subsequent reapplication. Alternatively pressure support which is insufficient by itself to inflate the chest, can be given during inspiration but not during expiration. This can be a first step towards controlled ventilation. The next step could be intermittent mandatory ventilation in which a predetermining tidal volume is imposed during spontaneous breathing; the intervention should be synchronised with a spontaneous inspiration (hence SIMV). Mandatory minute ventilation (MMV) imposes a predetermined minute volume. These and other forms of assisted ventilation should normally be directed to maintaining a normal body carbon dioxide tension. In some cases of respiratory distress syndrome this can best be achieved by combining the assistance with an extracorporeal circulation for the removal of carbon dioxide. The various types of assisted ventilation have the advantage over controlled ventilation that weaning the patient from the ventilator when assistance is no longer required is relatively easy and there are few complications.

Weaning from the ventilator

Following discontinuation of controlled ventilation most patients are able to resume normal breathing. However, a few relapse into hypercapnia, exhaustion or panic and require further assistance either continuously or at night. The likelihood of this happening is related to the time on the ventilator and is uncommon if the period is less than 2 days. In some patients the failure to wean is due to previous hyperventilation leading to hypocapnia which cannot be sustained subsequently. This risk is avoided by monitoring the carbon dioxide tension and adjusting the ventilation appropriately. Monitoring can be undertaken by the rebreathing method (page 47). To this end the rebreathing bag is placed in a Donald, Christie box (page 215); the bag is connected to the endotracheal tube and the source of the pressure is connected to the box. The measurement is then made in the manner described. If the respiratory drive is normal the failure to wean may be due to a combination of weak respiratory muscles and an increased work of breathing, caused by either respiratory impairment or the need to breathe through an endotracheal tube or both of these. The weakness is usually a consequence of disuse atrophy due to the ventilator performing all the respiratory work. There is then loss of muscle tissue

Table 17.8 Factors in weaning

Component	Aspects which may need attention
Respiratory drive	Reduced by hypocapnia, drugs etc.
Respiratory muscles	Weakened by controlled ventilation (disuse), under-nutrition, sepsis, hypercapnia (especially plus hypoxaemia), hypophosphataemia etc.
Work of breathing	Increased by stiff lungs, high airway resistance, atelectasis
Ventilation factors	Level of alveolar ventilation Apparatus resistance Valve opening pressures PEEP (lowers Raw but flattens diaphragm)

which can be aggravated by undernutrition. The muscle strength is also reduced by hypercapnia, especially when this is associated with hypoxaemia and by metabolic disturbances including hypophosphataemia. Thus to create the conditions which are favourable for weaning from the ventilator may require attention to several factors (Table 17.8). In the lungs the condition which necessitated ventilation in the first place should so far as possible have been reversed and any residual bronchoconstriction should have been attended to. Any sedative drugs should have been withdrawn. The work of breathing through the apparatus should be low and any superfluous tubing or connectors should have been removed. The respiratory muscles should have been sustained by adequate nutrition.

The strategy for weaning should include retraining of the respiratory muscles: this is usually done by progressively lengthening the periods of spontaneous breathing or by supplementing the spontaneous respiration with mechanical support; the support can be given to individual breaths by synchronous intermittent mandatory ventilation, or to the minute volume by mandatory minute ventilation. The possibility that direct training of the respiratory muscles will be needed can be assessed by measuring inspiratory pressure in the oesophagus* during occlusion of the airway. This manoeuvre can also be used to detect any slowing in the rate of muscle relaxation; the slowing is reflected in the rate at which the oesophageal pressure returns to normal (page 578). These aspects have been reviewed by Goldstone and Moxham.

Avoidance of complications

The likelihood of complications increases with the complexity of the procedure and the time for which it is applied. Complications are uncommon using cuirass ventilation, intermittent nasal positive pressure ventilation or a breathing jacket.

---

* In the pharynx of patients who are not intubated.

651

The use of a tracheotomy tube requires special care in its initial placement and maintenance. Full aseptic precautions should be adopted when the tube is manipulated or used for the aspiration of secretions. To avoid damage to the epithelium, the tube should lie centrally and not obliquely in the trachea and the cuff should not be inflated to a higher pressure than is necessary to secure an air-tight junction; depending on its design the cuff may need to be deflated at frequent intervals during use. The inspired gas should be humidified and warmed to about 37°C before administration. The clearance of secretions should be effected by careful control of the position of the patient, which might need to be adjusted every 2 h, and by aspiration or assisted coughing (page 646); the latter procedures could be needed as often as every 10 min.

The risk that the patient may be overventilated is minimised by monitoring the tension of carbon dioxide; however, a watch should be kept for the clinical manifestations of this condition and for hypoventilation which can cause similar symptoms. These include dizziness, confusion and muscle twitchings. However, with hypoventilation there is usually cyanosis, flushing of the skin, a rise in blood pressure and some additional narrowing of airways but with hyperventilation the skin is pale and there may be paresthesiae. The conditions are treated by making an appropriate adjustment to the level of ventilation. The risk of atelectasis is reduced by positive end expiratory pressure and by periodic increases in tidal volume (sighs). The latter are used in respiratory distress syndrome of the newborn.

In a patient with a low compliance or a high airway resistance good aeration is sometimes achieved only by using a high inflation pressure. This can interfere with the return of venous blood to the thorax, especially in patients who are on the verge of congestive cardiac failure, hypovolaemia or sympathetic paralysis. In such patients assisted ventilation can lower the cardiac output and hence the perfusion of the myocardium. It can also lead to peripheral oedema or thrombosis. These complications of positive pressure ventilation can be avoided by applying a negative pressure to the lung airways during expiration.

Guide to references

The references (Chapter 18) are classified under subject headings of which the following are particularly relevant to the present chapter:

18: Classified Bibliography

Introduction

This chapter provides references to some 2000 articles selected from the many which have contributed to the understanding of lung function. Additional early articles are reproduced or printed in translation in the compilations of Comroe and West which are cited in Section 1 below. The subsequent literature is referenced at length. It is classified under 70 topic headings which are arranged roughly in the order in which the topics are treated in the book. Acquaintance with the order (see below) is a help to using the references effectively. Relevant topic headings are listed at the ends of the chapters and these sections of the references should be consulted in the first instance. Cross references are given to other sections where articles on the same or a closely related topic can be found. Additional references on any topic can be identified via recent citations and general review articles or books (Sections 1 and 5). Articles which are referred to by name in the text can usually be found under the appropriate topic heading or identified via the author index. Sources of diagrams are given in the captions; some of these articles are also referenced under the relevant topic headings.

Format of references

The style of the references is based on that used by *Index Medicus* and most medical journals. This gives the authors up to a total of six followed if appropriate by *et al.*, the title of the article in full, the journal title in abbreviated form, the date, the volume number in bold type, and the first and last page numbers. Only minimal punctuation is used. The present format differs in that if an article has seven authors the seventh has usually been included. However, for indicating the sources of figures the number of authors has been terminated at three or four as appropriate and the title of the article has been omitted.

An historical viewpoint

The present classification covers individual topics in depth and draws attention to related topics. The less obvious links with other apparently unrelated topics can be illuminated by adopting a historical approach. This section indicates some of the paths which might be followed. The journey might start with Hutchinson's description of vital capacity, Jansen, Knipping and Stromberger's accounts of the maximal breathing capacity, then Tiffeneau, Gaensler and Kennedy on what is now the forced vital capacity, and Fry and Hyett on the flow−volume curve. An alternative starting point might be Breuer on the vagal control of tidal volume, followed by Head, Lumsden and Stella on the central control of breathing. These papers could be a lead in to the proceedings of the *Hering−Breuer Centenary Symposium*. The studies of Bohr, Haldane, their contemporaries and colleagues, similarly provide a basis for more recent work on the respective contributions of diffusion and distribution to lung gas exchange. Here Gilson and Hugh Jones' *Lung Function in Coalminers' Pneumoconiosis* (1955) and *The Lung* by Comroe and colleagues link the past with more recent work by Farhi, West, Wagner and others. For respiratory physicians the starting point might be Christie on dyspnoea, Cournand, Richards and colleagues, and Bates and Christie on physiological aspects of respiratory diseases, and Wright and Campbell and Howell on breathlessness. The review of dyspnoea by Adam and Guz would be a logical sequel.

However, browsing need not be chronological. In lung mechanics the starting point could be the studies of Fenn, Otis and Rahn. Their work both led to the rediscovery of many early articles and laid foundations which were built on by Mead and Macklem and their colleagues and successors. The articles make fascinating reading and are likely to instill in the reader an irresistible desire to become involved!

Section headings

Classified references

I GENERAL

American Physiological Society. *Handbook of Physiology*, section 3: *Respiratory System*. Vol 1, Fishman AP, Fisher AB, eds. *Circulation and Nonrespiratory Functions*. Vol 2 (i & ii), Cherniak NS, Widdicombe JG, eds. *Control of Breathing*. Vol 3 (i & ii), Macklem PT, Mead J, eds. *Mechanics of Breathing*. Vol 4, Farhi LE, Tenney SM, eds. *Gas Exchange*. Bethesda: American Physiological Society, 1985–6.

Brewis RAL, Gibson GJ, Geddes DM, eds. *Respiratory Medicine*. London: Baillière Tindall, 1990.

Chang HK, Paiva M, eds. *Respiratory Physiology. Analytical Approach. Lung Biology in Health and Disease 40*. New York: Marcel Dekker, 1989.

Comroe JH Jr, ed. *Pulmonary and Respiratory Physiology. Benchmark Papers in Human Physiology 5–6*. Stroudsberg, Pa: Dowden, Hutchinson & Ross, 1976.

Comroe JH Jr. *Retrospectroscope. Insights into Medical Discovery*. Menlow Park Ca: Von Gehr, 1977.

Crystal RG, West JB, eds. *The Lung: Scientific Foundations*, Vols 1 & 2. New York: Raven Press, 1991.

Murray JF. *The Normal Lung*. 2nd edn. Philadelphia: WB Saunders, 1986.

Nunn JF. *Applied Respiratory Physiology*. 3rd edn. London: Butterworths, 1987. [The gas laws are summarised in an appendix.]

West JB, ed. *Bioengineering Aspects of the Lung. Lung Biology in Health and Disease*, Vol 3. New York: Marcel Dekker, 1977.

West JB, ed. *Translations in Respiratory Physiology*. Stroudsburg, PA: Dowden, Hutchinson & Ross, 1975.

2 GASEOUS ENVIRONMENT

Banks BEC, Vernon CA. The greenhouse effect and human population. *J R Soc Med* 1990; **83**: 284.

Berken LV, Marshall LC. Limitation on oxygen concentration in a primitive planetary atmosphere. *J Atmos Sci* 1966; **23**: 133–143.

Lovelock J. *The Ages of Gaia*. Oxford: Oxford University Press, 1988.

Thomas L. The world's biggest membrane. *New Engl J Med* 1973; 576–577.

Wood HG. Life with CO or CO_2 and H_2 as a source of carbon and energy. *FASEB J* 1991; **5**: 156–163.

3 NUMERICAL ANALYSIS

Altman DG, Gardner MJ. Calculating confidence intervals for regression and correlation. *Br Med J* 1988; **296**: 1238–1242.

Armitage P, Berry G. Statistical methods in medical research. 2nd edn. Oxford: Blackwell Scientific Publications, 1987.

Berry G. Longitudinal observations, their usefulness and limitations with special reference to the forced expiratory volume. *Bull Physiopathol Respir* 1974; **10**: 643–655.

Bland JM, Peacock JL, Anderson HR, Brooke OG, Curtis M de. The adjustment of birthweight for very early gestational ages: two related problems in statistical analysis. *Appl Statist* 1990; **39**: 229–239.

Chatfield C, Collins AJ. *Introduction to Multivariate Analysis*. London: Chapman & Hall, 1980.

Chinn S. The assessment of methods of measurement. *Statistics in Medicine* 1990; **9**: 351–362.

Cole TJ. Linear and proportional regression models in the prediction of ventilatory function. *J Roy Stat Soc, A*, 1975; **138**: 297–328.

Colton T, Freedman LS, Johnson AL, eds. Proceedings of workshop: methods for longitudinal data analysis in epidemiological and clinical studies. *Statistics in Medicine*. 1988; **7**: 1–362.

Defares JG, Sneddon IN, Wise ME. *An Introduction to the Mathematics of Medicine and Biology*. Amsterdam: North-Holland Publ Co, 1973.

Evans SJW. Uses and abuses of multivariate methods in epidemiology. *J Epidemiol Comm Health* 1988; **42**: 311–315.

Feldman HA, Brain JD, Harbison ML. Adjusting for confounded variables: pulmonary function and smoking in a special population. *Environ Res* 1987; **43**: 251–266.

Goldstein H. *The Design and Analysis of Longitudinal Studies. Their Role in the Measurement of Change*. London: Academic Press, 1979.

Matthews JNS, Altman DG, Campbell MJ, Royston P. Analysis of serial measurements in medical research. *Br Med J* 1990; **300**: 230–235.

Oldham PD. A note on the analysis of repeated measurements of the same subjects. *J Chronic Dis* 1962; **15**: 969–977.

Oldham PD. *Measurement in Medicine. The Interpretation of Numerical Data*. London: English University Press, 1968.

Rossiter C. Contribution to discussion. *Scand J Respir Dis* 1976; **57**: 315–316.

Tanner JM. Fallacy of per-weight and per-surface area standards, and their relation to spurious correlation. *J Appl Physiol* 1949; **2**: 1–15.

4 TERMINOLOGY AND UNITS
(*see also* section 5)

Bartels H, Dejours P, Kellogg RH, Mead J. Glossary on respiration and gas exchange. *J Appl Physiol* 1973; **34**: 549–558.

Cotes JE. SI units in respiratory medicine. *Am Rev Respir Dis* 1975; **112**: 753–755.

Denolin H, Arhirii M. Nomenclature and definitions in respiratory physiology and clinical aspects of chronic lung diseases. *Bull Physiopathol Respir* 1975; **11**: 937–959.

Pappenheimer JR, Comroe JH, Cournand A, *et al.* Standardisation of definitions and symbols in respiratory physiology. *Fed Proc* 1950; **9**: 602–605.

Piiper J, Dejours P, Haab P, Rahn H. Concepts and basic quantities in gas exchange physiology. *Respir Physiol* 1971; **13**: 292–304.

5 LUNG FUNCTION TESTING:
GENERAL ASPECTS

American Thoracic Society. Lung function testing; selection of reference values and interpretative strategies. *Am Rev Respir Dis* 1992; **145**: 1202–1218.

Cotes JE, Chinn DJ. Is respiratory function diminished? In: Landrigan PJ, Kazemi H, eds. The third wave of asbestos disease: exposure to asbestos in place. *Ann NY Acad Sci* 1991; **643**: 149–156.

Gardner RM, Clausen JL, Crapo RO, Epler GR, Hankinson JL, Johnson RL Jr, Plumber AL. Quality assurance in pulmonary function laboratories. *Am Rev Respir Dis* 1986; **134**: 625–627.

Kendrick AH. Laboratory Safety. 1. Management. 2. Practice. *Breath* 1988; **33**: 3–8 & **34**: 1–7.

Quanjer PhH, ed. Standardised lung function testing. *Bull Europ Physiopathol Respir* 1983; **19**: suppl 5, 1–95.

Quanjer PhH, Tammeling GJ, Cotes JE, Pedersen OF, Peslin R, Yerneult J-C. Standardised lung function testing: lung volumes and forced ventilatory flows. 1993 update. *Eur Respir J* 1993; **6**: suppl 16: 4–40.

Tablan OC, Williams WW, Martone WJ. Infection control in pulmonary function laboratories. *Infection Control* 1985; **6**: 442–444.

6 MEASUREMENT TECHNIQUES

6.1 Volume, flow and pressure
(*see also* sections on applications)

Askannazi J, Silverberg R, Foster J, Hyman AI, Milic-Emili J, Kinney JM. Effects of respiratory apparatus on breathing pattern. *J Appl Physiol* 1980; **48**: 577–580.

Bentley RA, Griffin OG, Love RG, Muir DCF, Sweetland KF. Acceptable levels for breathing resistance of respiratory apparatus. *Arch Environ Health* 1973; **27**: 273–280.

Blumenfeld W, Turney S, Cowley RA. Mathematical model for flow on the heated Fleisch pneumotachometer. *Med Biol Eng* 1973; **11**: 546–551.

Cole P. Recordings of respiratory air temperature. *J Laryngolotol* 1954; **68**: 295–307.

Finucane KE, Egan BA, Dawson SV. Linearity and frequency response of pneumotachographs. *J Appl Physiol* 1972; **32**: 121–126.

Goldsmith R, Tann GLE, Walker E, Wright BM. Validation of a miniature indicating and sampling electronic respirometer (Miser). *J Physiol (Lond)* 1976; **256**: 102P–103P.

Hankinson JL, Gardner RM. Standard waveforms for spirometer testing. *Am Rev Respir Dis* 1982; **126**: 362–364.

Liese W, Warwick WJ, Cumming G. Water vapour pressure in expired air. *Respiration* 1974; **31**: 252–261.

Madan I, Bright P, Miller MR. Expired air temperature during a maximal forced expiratory manoeuvre. In: Quanjar PhH *et al.* (eds). loc. cit., page 665.

Mead J, Peterson N, Grimby G, Mead J. Pulmonary ventilation measured by body surface movements. *Science* 1967; **156**: 1383–1384.

Milledge JS, Stott FD. Inductive plethysmography – a new respiratory transducer. *J Physiol (Lond)* 1977; **267**: 4P–5P.

Miller MR, Pincock AC. Linearity and temperature control of the Fleisch pneumotachograph. *J Appl Physiol* 1986; **60**: 710–715.

Pedersen OF, Naeraa N, Lyager S, Hilberg C, Larsen L. A device for evaluation of flow recording equipment. *Bull Europ Physiopathol Respir* 1963; **19**: 515–520.

Perks WH, Sopwith T, Brown D, Jones CH, Green M. Effects of temperature on Vitalograph spirometer readings. *Thorax* 1983; **38**: 592–594.

Peslin R. Etude de la response en frequence de pneumotachographies. (English abstract). *Physiopathol Respir* 1972; **8**: 1363–1376.

Petusevsky ML, Lyons LD, Smith AA, Epler GR, Gaensler EA. Calibration of time derivatives of forced vital capacity by explosive decompression. *Am Rev Resp Dis* 1980; **121**: 343–350.

Pincock AC, Miller MR. The effect of temperature on recording spirograms. *Am Rev Respir Dis* 1983; **128**: 894–898.

Sackner JD, Nixon AJ, David B, Atkins N, Sackner MA. Non-invasive measurement of ventilation during exercise using a respiratory inductive plethysmograph. 1. *Am Rev Respir Dis* 1980; **122**: 867–871.

Stembler FW, Craig FN. Effects of respiratory equipment on endurance in hard work. *J Appl Physiol* 1977; **42**: 28–32.

Stott FD. *Instruments in Clinical Medicine.* Oxford: Blackwell Scientific Publications, 1967.

Turney SZ, Blumenfeld W. Heated Fleisch pneumotachometer: a calibration procedure. *J Appl Physiol* 1973; **34**: 117–121.

Verschakelen JA, Deschepper K, Clarysse I, Demedts M. The effect of breath size and posture on calibration of the respiratory inductive plethysmograph by multiple linear regression. *Euro Respir J* 1989; **2**: 71–77.

Von Der Hardt H, Zywietz CH. Reliability in pneumotachographic measurements. *Respiration* 1976; **33**: 416–424.

Wilke CR. Viscosity equation for gas mixtures. *J Chem Phys* 1950; **18**: 517–519.

6.2 Gas analysis

Ammann ECB, Galvin RD. Problems associated with the determination of carbon dioxide by infrared absorption. *J Appl Physiol* 1968; **25**: 333–335.

Bachelard HS. Nomogram for oxygen in gas mixtures at standard atmospheric pressure. *Clin Sci* 1976; **51**: 203–204.

Baker RA, Doerr RC. Methods of sampling and storage of air containing vapors and gases. *Int J Air Pollut* 1959; **2**: 142–158.

Barlett HL, Loomis JL, Deno NS, Kollias J, Hodgson JL, Buskirk ER. A system for automatic end-tidal gas sampling at rest and during exercise. *J Appl Physiol* 1973; **35**: 301–303.

British Occupational Hygiene Society. Carbon monoxide: measurement techniques. *Ann Occup Hyg* 1975; **18**: 37–82.

Chinn DJ, Naruse Y, Cotes JE. Accuracy of gas analysis in lung function laboratories. *Thorax* 1986; **41**: 133–137.

Cormack RS, Heath JR. New techniques for calibrating the Lloyd–Haldane apparatus. *J Physiol (Lond)* 1974; **238**: 627–638.

Croonen F, Binkhorst RA. Oxygen uptake calculated from expiratory volume and oxygen analysis only. *Ergonomics* 1974; **17**: 113–117.

Daines ME. The preparation of standard gas mixtures by a gravimetric technique. *Chem Ind* 1969; **31**: 1047–1053.

Davies CTM, Shirling DS. The rapid sampling, storage and analysis of expired air. *Ergonomics* 1967; **10**: 349–359.

Davies NJH, Denison DM. The uses of long sampling probes in respiratory mass spectrometry. *Respir Physiol* 1979; **37**: 335–346.

Degn H, Balslev I, Brook R, eds. *Measurement of Oxygen*. Amsterdam: Elsevier Scientific Publishing Company, 1976.

Farhi LE, Edwards AWT, Homma T. Determination of dissolved N_2 in blood by gas chromatography and $(a\text{-}A)$ N_2 difference. *J Appl Physiol* 1963; **18**: 97–106.

Frans A, Veriter C, Nullens W, Brasseur L. Préparation de mélanges gazeaux à l'aide pompes Wösthoff. *Bull Physiopathol Respir* 1969; **5**: 409–423.

Gulesian PJ Jr. The design of modern instrumentation for the measurement of gas expired from the lung. *Med Biol Engng* 1971; **9**: 247–254.

Hodgeman CD, West RC, Shankland RS, Selby SM, eds. *Handbook of Chemistry and Physics*. 44th edn. Cleveland, Ohio: Chemical Rubber Co, 1962.

Leighton SB, Kent KM. Precision gas mixing technique for medical applications. *J Appl Physiol* 1973; **34**: 502–503.

Liese W, Warwick WJ, Cumming G. Water vapour pressure in expired air. *Respiration* 1974; **31**: 252–261.

Lohne E, Mohler JG, Armstrong BW. An unusual source of error in measuring V_{O_2}. *Arch Environ Health* 1970; **20**: 264–265.

Meade F, Owen-Thomas JB. A paramagnetic method for measurement of the carbon dioxide content of a

gas mixture. *J Physiol (Lond)* 1973; **234**: 12p.

Musgrove J, Doré C. A nomogram for the calculation of oxygen uptake. *J Appl Physiol* 1974; **36**: 606–607.

Nitta K, Mochizuki M. A continuous method for measuring O_2 and CO_2 in expired gas. *Jap J Physiol* 1969; **19**: 41–54.

Sawin CF, Rummell JA, Michel EL. Automated measurement of respiratory gas exchange by an inert gas dilution method. *J Appl Physiol* 1974; **37**: 608–611.

Scheid P. Respiratory mass spectrometry. In: Laszlo G, ed. *Measurement in Clinical Respiratory Physiology*. London: Academic Press, 1983: 131–166.

6.3 *Blood–gas analysis*

Ali N, Makker H, Cockwell P, Davies P, Rogers S, Gray M *et al*. Radial artery puncture: comparison of three haemostatic techniques. *Thorax* 1989; **44**: 879P.

Bärtschi F, Haab P, Held DR. Reliability of blood P_{CO_2} measurements by the CO_2-electrode, the whole-blood CCO_2/pH method and the Astrup method. *Respir Physiol* 1970; **10**: 121–131.

Bedford RF. Radial arterial function following percutaneous cannulation with 18- and 20-gauge catheters. *Anesthesiology* 1977; **47**: 37–39.

Biswas CK, Ramos JM, Agroyanmis B, Kerr DNS. Blood gas analysis: effect of air bubbles in syringe and delay in estimation. *Br Med J* 1982; **284**: 923–927.

Bouhoutsos J, Morris T. Femoral artery complications after diagnostic procedures. *Br Med J* 1973; **3**: 396–399.

Clark JS, Votteri B, Ariagno RL, Cheung P, Eichhorn JH, Fallat RJ *et al*. Non-invasive assessment of blood gases. *Am Rev Respir Dis* 1992; **145**: 220–232.

Clayton DG, Webb RK, Ralston AC, Duthie D, Runciman WB. A comparison of the performance of 20 pulse oximeters under conditions of poor perfusion. *Anaesthesia* 1991; **46**: 3–10.

Farrell EJ, Siegel JH. Estimation of blood gas contents from expired air under normal and pathologic conditions. *Respir Physiol* 1976; **26**: 303–325.

Fish RG, Lee MR. Technical and experimental errors in the spectroscopic determination of oxygen saturation. *J Clin Pathol* 1963; **16**: 476–478.

Flear CTG, Roberts SW, Hayes S, Stoddart JC, Covington AK. pK_1' and bicarbonate concentration in plasma. *Clin Chem* 1987; **33**: 13–20.

Fletcher G, Barber JL. Effect of sampling technique on the determination of Pa_{O_2} during oxygen breathing. *J Appl Physiol* 1966; **21**: 463–468.

Hannhart B, Haberer J-P, Saunier C, Laxenaire M-C. Accuracy and precision of fourteen pulse oximeters. *Eur Respir J* 1991; **4**: 115–119.

Hulands GH, Nunn JF, Paterson GM. Calibration of polargraphic electrodes with glycerol water mixtures. *Br J Anaesth* 1970; **42**: 9–14.

Hutchison AS, Ralston SH, Dryburgh FJ, Small M, Fogelman I. Too much heparin: possible source of error in blood gas analysis. *Br Med J* 1983; **287**: 1131–1132.

Hutchison DCS, Rocca G, Honeybourne D. Estimation of arterial oxygen tension in adult subjects using a transcutaneous electrode. *Thorax* 1981; **36**: 473–477.

Kelman GR, Nunn JF. *Computer Produced Physiological Tables for Calculations Involving the Relationships Between Blood Oxygen Tension and Content.* London: Butterworths, 1968.

Kelman GR, Nunn JF. Nomograms for correction of blood Po_2, Pco_2, pH and base excess for time and temperature. *J Appl Physiol* 1966; **21**: 1484–1490.

Kelman GR. Digital computer procedure for the conversion of Pco_2 into blood CO_2 content. *Respir Physiol* 1967; **3**: 111–115.

Koch G. The validity of Po_2 measurement in capillary blood as a substitute for arterial Po_2. *Scand J Clin Lab Invest* 1968; **21**: 10–13.

Longmuir IS, Chow J. Rapid method for determining effect of agents on oxyhaemoglobin dissociation curves. *J Appl Physiol* 1970; **28**: 343–345.

Machleder HI, Sweeney JP, Barker WF. Pulseless arm after brachial-artery catheterization. *Lancet* 1972; **i**: 407–409.

McHardy GJR. The relationship between the differences in pressure and content of carbon dioxide in arterial and venous blood. *Clin Sci* 1967; **32**: 299–309.

Peters JP, Van Slyke DD. *Quantitative Clinical Chemistry 2, Methods.* Baltimore: Williams & Wilkins Co, 1932.

Riley RL, Campbell EJM, Shepard RH. A bubble method for estimation of Pco_2 and Po_2 in whole blood. *J Appl Physiol* 1957; **11**: 245–249.

Roberts D, Ostryzniuk P, Loewen E, Shanks A, Wasyluk T, Pronger L *et al.* Control of blood gas measurements in intensive-care units. *Lancet* 1991; **337**: 1580.

Runcie CJ, Ready J. How to perform arterial cannulation. *Br J Hosp Med* 1989; **41**: 378–380.

Scott PV, Horton JN, Mapleson WW. Leakage of oxygen from blood and water samples stored in plastic and glass syringes. *Br Med J* 1971; **3**: 512–516.

Severinghaus JW. Measurements of blood gases: Po_2 and Pco_2. *Ann NY Acad Sci* 1968; **148**: 115–132.

Spiro S, Dowdeswell IRG. Arterialised ear lobe samples for blood gas tensions. *Br J Dis Chest* 1976; **70**: 263–268.

Werner B. A sensitive rapid infra-red method for analysing carbon monoxide in blood. *Scand J Clin Lab Invest* 1976; **36**: 203–205.

Williams T, Shenkin JR. Radial artery puncture and the Allen Test. *Ann Intern Med* 1987; **106**: 164–165.

Zeballos RJ, Weisman IM. Reliability of noninvasive oximetry in black subjects during exercise and hypoxia. *Am Rev Respir Dis* 1991; **144**: 1240–1244.

6.4 Methods using radio-isotopes
(*see also* the sections on applications)

Ball WC Jr, Stewart PB, Newsham LGS, Bates DV. Regional pulmonary function studied with xenon-133. *J Clin Invest* 1962; **41**: 519–531.

Fazio F, Jones T. Assessment of regional ventilation by continuous inhalation of radioactive krypton-8lm. *Br Med J* 1975; **3**: 673–676.

Hughes JMB. Radionuclides and the lung: past, present, and future. *Am J Roentgenol* 1990; **155**: 455–463.

Knipping H, Bolt von H, Venrath H, Valentin H, Ludes H, Endler R. Eine neue Methode zur Prufung der Herz- und Lungenfunktion. *Dtsch Med Wochenschr* 1955; **80**: 1146–1147.

Singleton GJ, Olsen CR, Smith RL. Correction for mechanical deadspace in the calculation of physiological deadspace. *J Clin Invest* 1972; **51**: 2768–2772.

Vaalburg W, Peset R, Beekhuis H, Wolding MG, Tammeling GJ. Recovery of ^{133}Xe from the expired gas in lung function studies. *Int J Appl Radiat* 1971; **22**: 785–786.

6.5 Anthropometric methods
(*see also* sections on exercise and reference values)

Durnin JVGA, Rahaman MM. The assessment of the amount of fat in the human body from measurements of skinfold thickness. *Br J Nutr* 1967; **21**: 681–689.

Durnin JVGA, Womersley J. Body fat assessed from total body density and its estimation from skinfold thickness: measurements on 481 men and women aged from 16 to 72 years. *Br J Nutr* 1974; **32**: 77–97.

Florey C du V. The use and interpretation of ponderal index and other weight-height ratios in epidemiological studies. *J Chron Dis* 1970; **23**: 93–103.

Harrison GA, Weiner JS, Tanner JM, Barnicot NA. *Human Biology: an Introduction to Human Evolution, Variation, Growth and Ecology.* 2nd edn. Oxford: Oxford University Press, 1977.

Jones PRM, Lockett JA, Pearson J, Wyness J. The relationship to age of indices of leg muscle and estimated fat-free mass in adult females. *J Physiol (Lond)* 1974; **238**: 6P–7P.

Norgan NG, Jones PRM. Anthropometry and body composition. In: Collins KJ, ed. *Handbook of Methods for the Measurement of Work Performance, Physical Fitness and Energy Expenditure in Tropical Populations.* Paris: International Union of Biological Sciences, 1990: 95–115.

Slaughter MH, Lohman TG, Boileau RA, Horswill CA, Stillman RJ, van Loan MD, Bemben DA. Skinfold equations for estimation of body fatness in children and youth. *Hum Biol* 1988; **60**: 709–723.

Weiner JS, Lourie JA, eds. *Practical Human Biology.* London: Academic Press, 1981.

Womersley J, Durnin JVGA, Boddy K, Mahaffy M. Influence of muscular development, obesity and age on the fat-free mass of adults. *J Appl Physiol* 1976; **41**: 223–229.

7 LUNG ANATOMY

Angus GE, Thurlbeck WM. Number of alveoli in the human lung. *J Appl Physiol* 1972; **32**: 483–485.

Fillenz M, Widdicombe JG. Receptors of the lungs and airways. In: Neil E, ed. *Handbook of Sensory Physiology*, 3/1 *Enteroceptors*. Berlin: Springer-Verlag, 1972: 81–112.

Fung YC. A model of the lung structure and its validation. *J Appl Physiol* 1988; **64**: 2132–2141.

Hafeli-Bleuer B, Weibel ER. Morphometry of the human pulmonary acinus. *Anal Rec* 1988; **220**: 401–414.

Hansen JE, Ampaya EP, Bryant GH, Navin JJ. Branching pattern of airways and air spaces of a single human terminal bronchiole. *J Appl Physiol* 1975; **38**: 983–989.

Hislop A, Reid L. Pulmonary arterial development during childhood: branching, pattern and structure. *Thorax* 1973; **28**: 129–135.

Horsfield K, Relea FG, Cumming G. Diameter, length and branching ratios in the bronchial tree. *Respir Physiol* 1976; **26**: 351–356.

Horsfield K. Morphology of branching trees related to entropy. *Respir Physiol* 1977; **29**: 179–184.

Lauweryns JM. The juxta-alveolar lymphatics in the human adult lung. *Am Rev Respir Dis* 1970; **102**: 877–885.

Meyrick B, Reid L. The alveolar wall. *Br J Dis Chest* 1970; **64**: 121–140.

Miserocchi G, Mortola J, Sant 'Ambrogio G. Localisation of pulmonary stretch receptors in the airways of the dog. *J Physiol (Lond)* 1973; **235**: 775–782.

Parker H, Horsfield K, Cumming G. Morphology of distal airways in the human lung. *J Appl Physiol* 1971; **31**: 386–391.

Raskin SP, Herman PG. Interacinar pathways in the human lung. *Am Rev Respir Dis* 1975; **111**: 489–495.

Ravin MB, Epstein RM, Malm JR. Contribution of thebesian veins to the physiologic shunt in anaesthetised man. *J Appl Physiol* 1965; **20**: 1148–1152.

Thurlbeck WM, Haines JR. Bronchial dimensions and stature. *Am Rev Respir Dis* 1975; **112**: 142–145.

Weibel ER. *Morphometry of the Human Lung*. Berlin: Springer, 1963.

Whimster WF. The microanatomy of the alveolar duct system. *Thorax* 1970; **25**: 141–149.

Wilson TA, Bachofen H. A model for mechanical structure of the alveolar duct. *J Appl Physiol* 1982; **52**: 1064–1070.

8 RESPIRATORY MUSCLES

(*see also* sections 59, 60, 61, 64 and medical conditions)

Bellemare F, Bigland-Ritchie B. Assessment of human diaphragmatic strength and activation using phrenic nerve stimulation. *Respir Physiol* 1984; **58**: 263–277.

Campbell EJM, Agostoni E, Newsom Davis J, eds. *The Respiratory Muscles: Mechanics and Neural Control*. London: Lloyd-Luke, 1970.

Cook CD, Mead J, Orzalesi MM. Static volume–pressure characteristics of the respiratory system during maximal efforts. *J Appl Physiol* 1964; **19**: 1016–1022.

De Troyer A, Estenne M, Ninane V, Van Gansbeke D, Gorini M. Transversus abdominis muscle function in humans. *J Appl Physiol* 1990; **68**: 1010–1016.

De Troyer A, Estenne M. Functional anatomy of the respiratory muscles. *Clin Chest Med* 1988; **9**: 175–193.

De Troyer A, Loring SH. Action of the respiratory muscles. In: Macklem PT, Mead J, eds. *Handbook of Physiology 3. Mechanics of Breathing, part 2*. Bethesda, MD: American Physiological Society, 1986: 443–461.

De Troyer A, Sampson M, Sigrist S, Macklem PT. The diaphragm: two muscles. *Science* 1981; **213**: 237–238.

De Troyer A. Mechanical role of the abdominal muscles in relation to posture. *Respir Physiol* 1983; **53**: 341–353.

Gandevia SC, McKenzie DK. Human diaphragmatic endurance during different maximal respiratory efforts. *J Physiol (Lond)* 1988; **395**: 625–638.

Gibson GJ, Clark E, Pride NB. Static transdiaphragmatic pressures in normal subjects and in patients with chronic hyperinflation. *Am Rev Respir Dis* 1981; **124**: 685–689.

Green M, Mead J, Sears TA. Muscle activity during chest wall restriction and positive pressure breathing in man. *Respir Physiol* 1978; **35**: 283–300.

Konno K, Mead J. Static volume–pressure characteristics of the rib cage and abdomen. *J Appl Physiol* 1968; **24**: 544–548.

Leith DE, Bradley M. Ventilatory muscle strength and endurance training. *J Appl Physiol* 1976; **41**: 508–516.

Loring SH, Mead J. Action of the diaphragm on the rib cage inferred from a force-balance analysis. *J Appl Physiol* 1982; **53**: 756–760.

Macklem PT, Zocchi L, Agostoni E. Pleural pressure between diaphragm and rib cage during inspiratory muscle activity. *J Appl Physiol* 1988; **65**: 1286–1295.

Mizuno M, Secher Mll. Histochemical characteristics of human expiratory and inspiratory intercostal muscles. *J Appl Physiol* 1989; **67**: 592–598.

Van Lunteren E, Dick TE. Intrinsic properties of pharyngeal and diaphragmatic respiratory motoneurons and muscles. *J Appl Physiol* 1992; **73**: 787–800.

Wade OL. Movements of thoracic cage and diaphragm in respiration. *J Physiol (Lond)* 1954; **124**: 193–212.

Wilson TA, Rehder K, Krayer S, Hoffman EA, Whitney CG, Rodarte JR. Geometry and respiratory displacement of human ribs. *J Appl Physiol* 1987; **62**: 1872–1877.

9.1 General
(*see also* sections 5, 35.3, 44.1)

Bates JHT, Rossi A, Milic-Emili J. Analysis of the behavior of the respiratory system with constant inspiratory flow. *J Appl Physiol* 1985; **58**: 1840–1848.

Demedts M, van de Woestijne KP. Which technique for total lung capacity measurement? *Bull Europ Physiopathol Respir* 1980; **16**: 705–709.

Leith DE, Mead J. Mechanisms determining residual volume of the lungs in normal subjects. *J Appl Physiol* 1967; **23**: 221–227.

Pierce RJ, Brown DJ, Denison DM. Radiographic, scintigraphic and gas-dilution estimates of individual lung and lobar volumes in man. *Thorax* 1980; **35**: 773–780.

9.2 Lung volumes: multibreath methods

Birath G, Swenson EW. A correction factor for helium absorption in lung volume determinations. *Scand J Clin Lab Invest* 1956; **8**: 155–158.

Bründler JP, Lewis CM. Estimation of lung volume from nitrogen washout curves. *Bull Europ Physiopathol Respir* 1982; **18**: 281–289.

Brunner JX, Wolff G, Cumming G, Langenstein H. Accurate measurement of N_2 volumes during N_2 washout requires dynamic adjustment of delay time. *J Appl Physiol* 1985; **59**: 1008–1012.

Darling RC, Cournand A, Richards DW Jr. Studies on the intrapulmonary mixture of gases. III. Open circuit method for measuring residual air. *J Clin Invest* 1940; **19**: 609–618.

Gillespie DJ. Use of an acoustic helium analyzer and microprocessor for rapid measurement of absolute lung volume during mechanical ventilation. *Crit Care Med* 1985; **13**: 118–121.

Hathirat S, Renzetti AD Jr, Mitchell M. Measurement of the total lung capacity by helium dilution in a constant volume system. *Am Rev Respir Dis* 1970; **102**: 760–770.

Jones HA, Davies EE, Hughes JMB. A rapid rebreathing method for measurement of pulmonary gas volume in humans. *J Appl Physiol* 1986; **60**: 311–316.

Larsson A, Linnarsson D, Jonmarker C, Jonson B, Larsson H, Werner O. Measurement of lung volume by sulfur hexafluoride washout during spontaneous and controlled ventilation: further development of a method. *Anesthesiology* 1987; **67**: 543–550.

Rahn H, Fenn WO, Otis AB. Daily variations of vital capacity, residual air and expiratory reserve including a study of the residual air method. *J Appl Physiol* 1949; **1**: 725–736.

Tierney DF, Nadel JA. Concurrent measurements of functional residual capacity by three methods. *J Appl Physiol* 1962; **17**: 871–873.

Wilmore JH. A simplified method for determination of residual lung volumes. *J Appl Physiol* 1969; **27**: 96–100.

9.3 Lung volumes: single breath methods

Loiseau A, Loiseau P, Saumon G. A simple method for correcting single breath total lung capacity for underestimation. *Thorax* 1990; **45**: 873–877.

Nunneley SA, Flynn ET Jr, Camporesi EM. Two-tracer method for rapid determination of residual volume. *J Appl Physiol* 1974; **37**: 286–289.

Rodarte JR, Hyatt RE, Westbrook PR. Determination of lung volume by single- and multiple-breath nitrogen washout. *Am Rev Respir Dis* 1976; **114**: 131–136.

Sterk PJ, Quanjer PhH, van der Maas LLJ, Wise ME, van der Lende R. The validity of the single-breath nitrogen determination of residual volume. *Bull Europ Physiopathol Respir* 1980; **16**: 195–213.

Van Ganse W, Comhaire F, Van der Straeten M. Alveolar volume and transfer factor determined by single breath dilution of a test gas at various apnoea times. *Scand J Resp Dis* 1970; **51**: 82–92.

9.4 Lung volumes: plethysmographic methods
(*see also* sections 9.6, 17.5, 17.7)

DuBois AB, Botelho SY, Bedell GN, Marshall R, Comroe JH Jr. A rapid plethysmographic method for measuring thoracic gas volume; a comparison with a nitrogen washout method for measuring functional residual capacity in normal subjects. *J Clin Invest* 1956; **35**: 322–326.

Bedell GN, Marshall R, DuBois AB, Comroe JH Jr. Plethysmographic determination of the volume of gas trapped in the lungs. *J Clin Invest* 1956; **35**: 664–670.

Begin P, Peslin R. Influence of panting frequency on thoracic gas volume measurements in chronic obstructive pulmonary disease. *Am Rev Respir Dis* 1984; **130**: 121–123.

Bernstein L, Shepard RH Jr. High resolution display for variables in volume-displacement body plethysmography. *J Appl Physiol* 1966; **21**: 721–724.

Bohadana AB, Teculescu D, Peslin R, Jansen da Silva JM, Pino J. Comparison of four methods for calculating the total lung capacity measured by body plethysmography. *Bull Europ Physiopathol Respir* 1980; **16**: 769–776.

Brown R, Hoppin FG Jr, Ingram RH Jr, Saunders NA, McFadden ER Jr. Influence of abdominal gas on the Boyle's law determination of thoracic gas volume. *J Appl Physiol* 1978; **44**: 469–473.

Brown R, Slutsky AS. Frequency dependence of plethysmographic measurement of thoracic gas volume. *J Appl Physiol* 1984; **57**: 1865–1871.

DuBois AB, van de Woestijne KP, eds. *Body Plethysmography. Prog Resp Res*, Vol 4. Basel: Karger, 1969.

Mead J. Volume displacement body plethysmograph

for respiratory measurements in human subjects. *J Appl Physiol* 1960; **15**: 736−740.

Rodenstein DO, Francis C, Stanescu DC. Airway closure in humans does not result in overestimation of plethysmographic lung volume. *J Appl Physiol* 1983; **55**: 1784−1789.

Rodenstein DO, Goncette L, Stanescu DC. Extrathoracic airway changes during plethysmographic measurements of lung volume. *Respir Physiol* 1983; **52**: 217−227.

Skoogh B-E, Rizell S. A high frequency response volume displacement body plethysmograph. *Scand J Clin Lab Invest* 1973; **31**: 419−427.

Wardlaw SC, Kerr HD, Spicer WS Jr. A method for dynamic calibration of the whole-body pressure plethysmographic system. *J Appl Physiol* 1967; **22**: 601−603.

Williams JH Jr, Bencowitz HZ. Differences in plethysmographic lung volumes. Effects of linked vs unlinked spirometry. *Chest* 1989; **95**: 117−123.

9.5 Lung volumes: radiographic and related methods

Barnhard HJ, Pierce JA, Joyce JW, Bates JH. Roentgenographic determination of total lung capacity: a new method evaluated in health, emphysema and congestive heart failure. *Am J Med* 1960; **28**: 51−60.

Bush A, Denison DM. Use of different magnification factors to calculate radiological lung volumes. *Thorax* 1986; **41**: 158−159.

Cooper ML, Friedman PJ, Peters RM, Brimm JE. Accuracy of radiographic lung volume using new equations derived from computed tomography. *Crit Care Med* 1986; **14**: 177−181.

Dull WL, Bonnassis JB, Teculescu D, Sadoul P. Place de la radiographie thoracique dans l'estimation de la capacite pulmonaire totale. *Bull Europ Physiopathol Respir* 1980; **16**: 777−784.

Harris TR, Pratt PC, Kilburn KH. Total lung capacity measured by roentgenograms. *Am J Med* 1971; **50**: 756−763.

Paul JL, Levine MD, Fraser RG, Laszlo CA. The measurement of total lung capacity based on a computer analysis of anterior and lateral radiographic chest images. *IEEE Trans Biomed Eng* 1974; **21**: 444−451.

Pierce RJ, Brown DJ, Holmes M, Cumming G, Denison DM. Estimation of lung volumes from chest radiographs using shape information. *Thorax* 1979; **34**: 726−734.

Reger RB, Young A, Morgan WKC. An accurate and rapid radiographic method for determining total lung capacity. *Thorax* 1972; **27**: 163−168.

Ries AL, Clausen JL, Friedman PJ. Measurement of lung volumes from supine portable chest radiographs. *J Appl Physiol* 1979; **47**: 1332−1335.

Rodenstein DO, Sopwith TA, Denison DM, Stanescu DC. Re-evaluation of the radiographic method for measurement of total lung capacity. *Bull Eur Physiopathol Respir* 1985; **21**: 521−525.

Seeley GW, Mazzeo J, Borgstrom M, Hunter TB, Newell JD, Bjelland JC. Radiologic total lung capacity measurement. Development and evaluation of a computer-based system. *Eur J Radiol* 1986; **6**: 262−265.

9.6 Lung volumes: problems in measurement

Beaupre A, Orehek J. Factors influencing the bronchodilator effect of a deep inspiration in asthmatic patients with provoked bronchoconstriction. *Thorax* 1982; **37**: 124−128.

Brown R, Ingram RH Jr, McFadden ER Jr. Problems in the plethysmographic assessment of changes in total lung capacity in asthma. *Am Rev Respir Dis* 1978; **118**: 685−692.

Burns CB, Taylor WR, Ingram RH Jr. Effects of deep inhalation in asthma: relative airway and parenchymal hysteresis. *J Appl Physiol* 1985; **59**: 1590−1596.

Fairshter RD. Effect of a deep inspiration on expiratory flow in normals and patients with chronic obstructive pulmonary disease. *Bull Eur Physiopathol Respir* 1986; **22**: 119−125.

Gayrard P, Orehek J, Grimaud C, Charpin J. Mechanisms of the bronchoconstrictor effects of deep inspiration in asthmatic patients. *Thorax* 1979; **34**: 234−240.

Gimeno F, Berg WC, Sluiter HJ, Tammeling GJ. Spirometry-induced bronchial obstruction. *Am Rev Respir Dis* 1972; **105**: 68−74.

Hida W, Arai M, Shindoh C, Liu Y-N, Sasaki H, Takishima T. Effect of inspiratory flow rate on bronchomotor tone in normal and asthmatic subjects. *Thorax* 1984; **39**: 86−92.

Malo J-L, L'Archeveque J, Cartier A. Comparative effects of volume history on bronchoconstriction induced by hyperventilation and methacholine in asthmatic subjects. *Eur Respir J* 1990; **3**: 639−643.

Orehek J, Nicoli MM, Delpierre S, Beaupre A. Influence of the previous deep inspiration on the spirometric measurement of provoked bronchoconstriction in asthma. *Am Rev Respir Dis* 1981; **123**: 269−272.

Pare PD, Wiggs BJR, Coppin CA. Errors in the measurement of total lung capacity in chronic obstructive lung disease. *Thorax* 1983; **38**: 468−471.

Pichurko BM, Ingram RH Jr. Effects of airway tone and volume history on maximal expiratory flow in asthma. *J Appl Physiol* 1987; **62**: 1133−1140.

Rodenstein DO, Stanescu DC. Demonstration of failure of body plethysmography in airway obstruction. *J Appl Physiol* 1982; **52**: 949−954.

Shore SA, Huk O, Mannix S, Martin JG. Effect of panting frequency on the plethysmographic determination of thoracic gas volume in chronic obstructive pulmonary disease. *Am Rev Respir Dis* 1983; **128**: 54−59.

Stanescu DC, Rodenstein D, Cauberghs M, van de

Woestijne KP. Failure of body plethysmography in bronchial asthma. *J Appl Physiol* 1982; **52**: 939–948.

Wheatley JR, Pare PD, Engel LA. Reversibility of induced bronchoconstriction by deep inspiration in asthmatic and normal subjects. *Eur Respir J* 1989; **2**: 331–339.

Woolcock AJ, Rebuck AS, Cade JF, Read J. Lung volume changes in asthma measured concurrently by two methods. *Am Rev Respir Dis* 1971; **104**: 703–709.

10 DYNAMIC SPIROMETRY

10.1 FEV$_1$, FVC and related variables
(*see also* sections 5, 17.7 and those on applications and reference values)

ATS Statement. Standardization of spirometry — 1987 update. *Am Rev Respir Dis* 1987; **136**: 1285–1298.

Berry G. Longitudinal observations, their usefulness and limitations with special reference to the forced expiratory volume. *Bull Physiopathol Respir* 1974; **10**: 643–655.

Burki NK, Dent MC. The forced expiratory time as a measure of small airway resistance. *Clin Sci* 1976; **51**: 53–58.

Diem JE, Jones RN, Hendrick DJ, Glindmeyer HW, Dhalmarajan V, Butcher BT *et al.* Five-year longitudinal study of workers employed in new toluene diisocyanate manufacturing plant. *Am Rev Respir Dis* 1982; **126**: 420–428.

Ferris BG Jr, Speizer FE, Bishop Y, Prang G, Weener J. Spirometry for an epidemiologic study: deriving optimum summary statistics for each subject. *Bull Eur Physiopathol Respir* 1978; **14**: 145–166.

Gaensler EA. Analysis of the ventilatory defect by timed vital capacity measurements. *Am Rev Tuberc* 1951; **64**: 256–278.

Gandevia B, Hugh-Jones P. Terminology for measurements of ventilatory capacity. *Thorax* 1957; **12**: 290–293.

Ghio AJ, Castellan RM, Kinsley KB, Hankinson JL. Changes in forced expiratory volume in one second and peak expiratory flow rate across a work shift among unexposed blue collar workers. *Am Rev Respir Dis* 1991; **143**: 1231–1234.

Hutchinson J. On the capacity of the lungs, and on the respiratory movements, with the view of establishing a precise and easy method of detecting disease by the spirometer. *Lancet* 1846; **i**: 630–632.

Kennedy MCS. A practical measure of the maximum ventilatory capacity in health and disease. *Thorax* 1953; **8**: 73–83.

Knudson RJ, Lebowitz MD, Slatin RC. The timing of the forced vital capacity. *Am Rev Respir Dis* 1979; **119**: 315–318.

Kory RC, Hamilton LH. Evaluation of spirometers used in pulmonary function studies. *Am Rev Respir Dis* 1963; **87**: 228–238.

Krowka MJ, Enright PL, Rodarte JR, Hyatt RE. Effect of effort on measurement of forced expiratory volume in one second. *Am Rev Respir Dis* 1987; **136**: 829–833.

Leuallen EC, Fowlor WS. Maximal mid-expiratory flow. *Am Rev Tuberc Pulm Dis* 1953; **72**: 783–800.

McDermott M, McDermott TJ. Digital incremental techniques applied to spirometry. *Proc R Soc Med* 1977; **70**: 169–171.

McKerrow CB, McDermott M, Gilson JC. A spirometer for measuring the forced expiratory volume with a simple calibrating device. *Lancet* 1960; **i**: 149–151.

Minette A, Lavenne F. Reproducibilité des épreuves fonctionnelles pulmonaires applicables en enquêtes épidémiologiques sur la bronchite. *Rev Inst Hyg Mines* 1971; **26**: 63–72.

Ng'ang'a LW, Ernst P, Jaakkola MS, Gerardi G, Hanley JH, Becklake MR. Spirometric lung function. Distribution and determinants of test failure in a young adult population. *Am Rev Respir Dis* 1992; **145**: 48–52.

Olsen CR. The match test. *Am Rev Respir Dis* 1962; **86**: 37–40.

Pennock BE, Rogers RM, McCaffree DR. Changes in measured spirometric indices — what is significant? *Chest* 1981; **80**: 97–99.

Rosner SW, Abraham S, Caceres CA. Observer variation in spirometry. *Dis Chest* 1965; **48**: 265–268.

Segall JJ, Butterworth BA. The maximal midexpiratory flow time. *Br J Dis Chest* 1968; **62**: 139–146.

Sharp JT, Henry JP, Sweany SK, Meadows WR, Pietras RJ. Effects of mass loading the respiratory system in man. *J Appl Physiol* 1964; **19**: 959–966.

Smith AA, Gaensler EA. Timing of forced expiratory volume in one second. *Am Rev Respir Dis* 1975; **112**: 882–885.

Sobol BJ, Weinheimer B. Assessment of ventilatory abnormality in the asymptomatic subject: an exercise in futility. *Thorax* 1966; **21**: 445–449.

Tandon MK, Campbell AH. The relaxed expiratory volume and forced inspiratory volume after bronchodilators. *Br J Dis Chest* 1970; **64**: 73–77.

Tiffeneau R, Pinelli A. Regulation bronchique de la ventilation pulmonaire. *J Fr Med Chir Thorac* 1948; **2**: 221–244.

Townsend MC. Spirometric forced expiratory volumes measured in the standing versus the sitting posture. *Am Rev Respir Dis* 1984; **130**: 123–124.

Tweeddale PM, Merchant S, Leslie M, Alexander F, McHardy GJR. Short term variability in FEV$_1$: relation to pretest activity, level of FEV$_1$, and smoking habits. *Thorax* 1984; **39**: 928–932.

Wever AMJ, Britton MG, Hughes DTD. Evaluation of two spirometers. *Chest* 1976; **70**: 244–250.

10.2 Peak expiratory flow
(*see also* sections 17.7, 35.3, 43.1, 44.1)

Fisher J, Shaw J. Calibration of some Wright peak flow meters. *Br J Anaesth* 1980; **52**: 461–464.

Lunn JN, Hillard EK. The effect of repairs on the performance of the Wright respirometer. *Br J Anaesth* 1970; **42**: 1127−1130.

Milledge JS Re. Calibration of peak expiratory flow (PEF) measuring devices. *Eur Respir J* 1991; **4**: 1152.

Miller MR, Pedersen OF. The characteristics and calibration of devices for recording peak expiratory flow. In: Quanjar PhH *et al.* (eds). loc. cit.

Quanjer PhH, Lebowitz MD, Gregg I. eds. Peak expiratory flow. Draft conclusions and recommendations of a working party of European Respiratory Society. *Eur Respir J* 1993; **6**, suppl: (in press).

Wright BM, McKerrow CB. Maximum forced expiratory flow rate as a measure of ventilatory capacity. *Br Med J* 1959; **2**: 1041−1047.

10.3 Maximal breathing capacity
(*see also* sections 10.1, 64)

Bernstein L, D'Silva JL, Mendel D. Effect of rate of breathing on maximum breathing capacity determined with a new spirometer. *Thorax* 1952; **7**: 255−262.

Cotes JE, Posner V, Reed JW. Estimation of maximal exercise ventilation and oxygen uptake in patients with chronic lung disease. *Bull Eur Physiopathol Respir* 1982; **18**: 221−228.

Cotes JE. Ventilatory capacity at altitude and its relation to mask design. *Proc R Soc Lond (Biol)* 1954; **143**: 32−39.

Freedman S. Sustained maximum voluntary ventilation. *Respir Physiol* 1970; **8**: 230−244.

10.4 Flow−volume curves: MEF$_{50\%}$ FVC and related indices
(*see also* sections 5, 13, 17.7)

Berry RB, Fairshter RD. Partial and maximal expiratory flow−volume curves in normal and asthmatic subjects before and after inhalation of metaproterenol. *Chest* 1985; **88**: 697−702.

Clément J, van de Woestijne KP. Variability of maximum expiratory flow−volume curves and effort independency. *J Appl Physiol* 1971; **31**: 55−62.

Coates AL, Desmond KJ, Demizio D, Allen P, Beaudry PH. Sources of error in flow−volume curves: effect of expired volume measured at the mouth vs that measured in a body plethysmograph. *Chest* 1988; **94**: 976−982.

Dosman J, Bode F, Urbanetti J, Martin R, Macklem PT. The use of a helium−oxygen mixture during maximum expiratory flow to demonstrate obstruction in small airways in smokers. *J Clin Invest* 1979; **55**: 1090−1099.

Fish JE, Peterman VI, Cugell DW. Effect of deep inspiration on airway conductance in subjects with allergic rhinitis and allergic asthma. *J Allergy Clin Immunol* 1977; **60**: 41−46.

Fry DL. Theoretical considerations of the bronchial pressure−flow−volume relationships with particular reference to the maximum expiratory flow−volume curve. *Phys Med Biol* 1958; **3**: 174−194.

Green M, Mead J. Time dependence of flow−volume curves. *J Appl Physiol* 1974; **37**: 793−797.

Guy HJB, Prisk GK, Elliott AR, West JB. Maximum expiratory flow−volume curves during short periods of microgravity. *J Appl Physiol* 1991; **70**: 2587−2596.

Ingram RH, Schilder DP. Effect of thoracic gas compression on the flow−volume curve of the forced vital capacity. *Am Rev Respir Dis* 1966; **94**: 56−63.

Lapp NL, Hyatt RE. Some factors affecting the relationship of maximal expiratory flow to lung volume in health and in disease. *Dis Chest* 1967; **51**: 475−481.

Man SFP, Zamel N. Genetic influence on normal variability of maximum expiratory flow−volume curves. *J Appl Physiol* 1976; **41**: 874−877.

McDonald JB, Cole TJ. The flow−volume loop: reproducibility of air and helium-based tests in normal subjects *Thorax* 1980; **35**: 64−69.

Mialon P, Barthelemy L, Sebert P. Effects of maximal breath holding on maximal expiratory flows. *Eur Respir J* 1989; **2**: 340−343.

Nielsen TM, Pedersen OF. A method to correct for the influence of gas density on maximal expiratory flow rate. *Acta Physiol Scand* 1976; **98**: 123−130.

Peslin R, Bohadana A, Hannhart B, Jardin P. Comparison of various methods for reading maximal expiratory flow−volume curves. *Am Rev Respir Dis* 1979; **119**: 271−277.

Schrader PC, Quanjer PhH, Van Zomeren BC, DeGroodt EG, Wever AMJ, Wise ME. Selection of variables from maximum expiratory flow−volume curves. *Bull Europ Physiopathol Respir* 1983; **19**: 43−49.

Staats BA, Wilson TA, Lai-Fook SJ, Rodarte JR, Hyatt RE. Viscosity and density dependence during maximal flow in man. *J Appl Physiol* 1980; **48**: 313−319.

Teculescu DB, Préfaut C. Why did density dependence of maximal expiratory flows not become a useful epidemiological tool? *Bull Europ Physiopathol Respir* 1987; **23**: 639−648.

Teculescu DB. Density dependence of forced expiratory flows. Methodological aspects. *Bull Europ Physiopathol Respir* 1985; **21**: 193−204.

Webster PM, Zamel N, Bryan AC, Kruger K. Volume dependence of instantaneous time constants derived from the maximal expiratory flow−volume curve. *Am Rev Respir Dis* 1977; **115**: 805−810.

Wellman JJ, Brown R, Ingram RH Jr, Mead J, McFadden ER Jr. Effect of volume history on successive partial expiratory flow−volume maneuvers. *J Appl Physiol* 1976; **41**: 153−158.

Zamel N. Partial flow−volume curves. *Bull Europ Physiopathol Respir* 1985; **20**: 471−475.

10.5 Transit time analysis

Chinn DJ, Cotes JE. Transit time analysis of spirograms: which blow is best? *Bull Europ Physiopathol Respir* 1986; **22**: 461–466.

Meilissinos P, Webster P, Tien Y-K, Mead J. Time dependence of maximum flow as an index of nonuniform emptying. *J Appl Physiol* 1979; **47**: 1043–1050.

Miller MR, Grove DM, Pincock AC. Time domain spirogram indices. Their variability and reference values in nonsmokers. *Am Rev Respir Dis* 1985; **132**: 1041–1048.

Miller MR, Pincock AC. Repeatability of the moments of the truncated forced expiratory spirogram. *Thorax* 1982; **37**: 205–211.

Neuburger N, Levison H, Kruger K. Transit time analysis of the forced expiratory vital capacity in cystic fibrosis. *Am Rev Respir Dis* 1976; **114**: 753–759.

Osmanliev DP, Davies EE, Pride NB. Transit time analysis of the forced expiratory spirogram in male smokers. *Bull Eur Physiopathol Respir* 1984; **20**: 285–293.

Permutt S, Menkes HA. Spirometry. Analysis of forced expiration within the time domain. In: Macklem PT, Permutt S, eds. *The Lung in the Transition Between Health and Disease*. New York, Marcel Dekker 1979; 113–152.

11 WORK OF BREATHING
(*see also* section 8)

Bartlett RG Jr, Bruback HF, Specht H. Oxygen cost of breathing. *J Appl Physiol* 1958; **12**: 413–424.

Bradley ME, Leith DE. Ventilatory muscle training and the oxygen cost of sustained hyperpnea. *J Appl Physiol* 1978; **45**: 885–892.

Campbell EJM, Westlake EK, Cherniack RM. The oxygen consumption and efficiency of the respiratory muscles of young male subjects. *Clin Sci* 1958; **18**: 55–64.

Collett PW, Engel LA. Influence of lung volume on oxygen cost of resistive breathing. *J Appl Physiol* 1986; **61**: 16–24.

Cooper EA. A comparison of the respiratory work done against an external resistance by man and by a sine-wave pump. *Q J Exp Physiol* 1960; **45**: 179–191.

Cournand A, Richards DW, Bader RA, Bader ME, Fishman AP. The oxygen cost of breathing. *Trans Assoc Am Physiol* 1954; **67**: 162–173.

Dodd DS, Yarom J, Loring SH, Engel LA. O_2 cost of inspiratory and expiratory resistive breathing in humans. *J Appl Physiol* 1988; **65**: 2518–2523.

Field S, Sanci S, Grassino A. Respiratory muscle oxygen consumption estimated by the diaphragm pressure–time index. *J Appl Physiol* 1984; **57**: 44–51.

Fritts HN Jr, Filler J, Fishman AP, Cournand A. The efficiency of ventilation during voluntary hyperpnea: studies in normal subjects and in dyspneic patients with either chronic pulmonary emphysema or obesity. *J Clin Invest* 1959; **38**: 1339–1348.

Goldman MD, Grimby G, Mead J. Mechanical work of breathing derived from rib cage and abdominal V-P partitioning. *J Appl Physiol* 1976; **41**: 752–763.

McIlroy MB. Dyspnea and the work of breathing in diseases of the heart and lungs. *Prog Cardiovasc Dis* 1958; **1**: 284–297.

Otis AB. The work of breathing. *Physiol Rev* 1954; **34**: 449–458.

12 AEROSOLS
(*see also* sections 13, 15)

Bennett WD, Smaldone GC. Use of aerosols to estimate mean air-space size in chronic obstructive pulmonary disease. *J Appl Physiol* 1988; **64**: 1554–1560.

Blanchard JD, Heyder J, O'Donnell CR, Brain JD. Aerosol-derived lung morphometry: comparisons with a lung model and lung function indexes. *J Appl Physiol* 1991; **71**: 1216–1224.

Clarke SW, Pavia D, eds. *Aerosols and the Lung: Clinical and Experimental Aspects*. London: Butterworth, 1984.

Emmett PC, Love RG, Hannan WJ, Millar AM, Soutar CA. The relationship between the pulmonary distribution of inhaled fine aerosols and tests of small airway function. *Bull Eur Physiopathol Respir* 1984; **20**: 325–332.

Hankinson JL, Palmes ED, Lapp NL. Pulmonary air space size in coal miners. *Am Rev Respir Dis* 1979; **119**: 391–397.

Love RG, Muir DCF. Aerosol deposition and airway obstruction. *Am Rev Respir Dis* 1976; **114**: 891–897.

Phipps PR, Gonda I, Bailey DL, Borham P, Bautovich G, Anderson SD. Comparisons of planar and tomographic gamma scintigraphy to measure the penetration index of inhaled aerosols. *Am Rev Respir Dis* 1989; **139**: 1516–1523.

13 TESTS OF FUNCTION OF SMALL AIRWAYS
(*see also* sections 10.4, 12, 19.1, 20)

Abboud RT, Morton JW. Comparison of maximal mid-expiratory flow, flow–volume curves, and nitrogen closing volumes in patients with mild airway obstruction. *Am Rev Respir Dis* 1975; **111**: 405–417.

Becklake MR, Permutt S. Evaluation of tests of lung function for screening for early detection of chronic obstructive lung disease. In: Macklem PT, Permutt S, eds. *The Lung in the Transition Between Health and Disease*. New York: Marcel Dekker, 1979: 345–387.

Buist AS, Vollmer WM, Johnson LR, McCamant LE. Does the single-breath N_2 test identify the smoker who will develop chronic airflow limitation? *Am Rev Respir Dis* 1988; **137**: 293–301.

Cochrane GM, Benatar SR, Davis J, Collins JV, Clark TJH. Correlation between tests of small airway function. *Thorax* 1974; **29**: 172–178.

Cotes JE. Lung volume indices of airway obstruction: a suggestion for a new combined index. *Proc R Soc Med* 1971; **64**: 1232–1235.

Dosman J, Bode F, Urbanetti J, Antic R, Martin R, Macklem PT. Role of inertia in the measurement of dynamic compliance. *J Appl Physiol* 1975; **38**: 64–69.

Ligas JR, Primiano FP Jr, Saidel GM, Doershuk CF. Comparison of measures of forced expiration. *J Appl Physiol* 1977; **42**: 607–613.

Macklem PT. Workshop on screening programs for early diagnosis of airway obstruction. Conference report. *Am Rev Respir Dis* 1974; **109**: 567–571.

Martin RR, Lindsay D, Despas P, Bruce D, Leroux M, Anthonisen NR, Macklem PT. The early detection of airway obstruction. *Am Rev Respir Dis* 1975; **111**: 119–125.

McCawley M, Lippmann M. Development of an aerosol dispersion test to detect early changes in lung function. *Am Ind Hyg Assoc J* 1988; **49**: 357–366.

McFadden ER, Kiker R, Holmes B, deGroot WJ. Small airway disease. An assessment of the tests of peripheral airway function. *Am J Med* 1974; **57**: 171–182.

Niewoehner DE, Knoke JD, Kleinerman J. Peripheral airways as a determinant of ventilatory function in the human lung. *J Clin Invest* 1977; **60**: 139–151.

Oxhøj H, Bake B, Wilhelmsen L. Ability of spirometry, flow–volume curves and the nitrogen closing volume test to detect smokers. *Scand J Respir Dis* 1977; **58**: 80–96.

Stanescu DC, Rodenstein DO, Hoeven C, Robert A. 'Sensitive tests' are poor predictors of the decline in forced expiratory volume in one second in middle-aged smokers. *Am Rev Respir Dis* 1987; **135**: 585–590.

Van Muylem A, Vuyst Paul de, Yernault J-C, Paiva M. Inert gas single-breath washout and structural alteration of respiratory bronchioles. *Am Rev Respir Dis* 1992; **146**: 1167–1172.

van de Woestijne KP. Spécificité des tests proposés pour le dépistage de la maladie des petites voies aériennes. *Bull Eur Physiopathol Respir* 1976; **12**: 477–486.

Vollmer WM, McCamant LE, Johnson LR, Buist AS. Long-term reproducibility of tests of small airways function. *Chest* 1990; **98**: 303–307.

Woolcock AJ, Vincent NJ, Macklem PT. Frequency dependence of compliance as a test for obstruction in small airways. *J Clin Invest* 1969; **48**: 1097–1106.

14 UPPER AIRWAYS
(*see also* sections 17.7, 62)

Bartlett D Jr. Respiratory functions of the larynx. *Physiol Rev* 1989; **69**: 33–57.

Boushey HA, Richardson PS, Widdicombe JG, Wise JCM. The response of laryngeal afferent fibres to mechanical and chemical stimuli. *J Physiol (Lond)* 1974; **240**: 153–175.

Butler J. The bronchial circulation. *NIPS* 1991; **6**: 21–25.

Empey DW. Assessment of upper airways obstruction. *Br Med J* 1972; **3**: 503–505.

Gibson GJ, Davis P. Respiratory complications of relapsing polychondritis. *Thorax* 1974; **29**: 726–731.

Harrison BDW. Upper airway obstruction—a report on sixteen patients. *Q J Med* 1976; **45**: 625–645.

Martin TR, Castile RG, Fredberg JJ, Wohl MEB, Mead J. Airway size is related to sex but not lung size in normal adults. *J Appl Physiol* 1987; **63**: 2042–2047.

Mathew OP, Saint 'Ambrogio G, eds. *Respiratory Function of the Upper Airway*. New York: Marcel Dekker, 1988: 87–124.

Proctor DF. Form and function of the upper airways and larynx. In: Macklem PT, Mead J, eds. *Handbook of Physiology*, Section 3, Vol 3, *Mechanics of Breathing*. Bethesda MD: American Physiological Society, 1986: 63–73.

Raphael DT, Epstein MA. Resonance mode analysis for volume estimation of asymmetric branching structures. *Ann Biomed Eng* 1989; **17**: 361–375.

Shim C, Corro P, Park SS, Williams MH. Pulmonary function studies in patients with upper airway obstruction. *Am Rev Respir Dis* 1972; **106**: 233–238.

Stransky A, Szereda-Przestaszewska M, Widdicombe JG. The effects of lung reflexes on laryngeal resistance and motoneurone discharge. *J Physiol (Lond)* 1973; **231**: 417–438.

Tully A, Brancatisano A, Loring SH, Engel LA. Influence of posterior cricoarytenoid muscle activity on pressure–flow relationship of the larynx. *J Appl Physiol* 1991; **70**: 2252–2258.

Wheatley JR, Amis TC, Engel LA. Nasal and oral airway pressure–flow relationships. *J Appl Physiol* 1991; **71**: 2317–2324.

15 LUNG CLEANSING MECHANISMS
(*see also* sections 7, 8, 14)

Barros MJ, Zammattio SJ, Rees PJ. Importance of inspiratory flow rate in the cough response to citric acid inhalation in normal subjects. *Clin Sci* 1990; **78**: 521–525.

Goodman RM, Yergin BM, Landa JF, Golinvaux MH, Sackner MA. Relationship of smoking history and pulmonary function tests to tracheal mucous velocity in nonsmokers, young smokers, ex-smokers and patients with chronic bronchitis. *Am Rev Respir Dis* 1978; **117**: 205–214.

Greenstone M, Rutman A, Dewar A, MacKay I, Cole PJ. Primary ciliary dyskinesia: cytological and clinical features. *Q J Med* 1988; **67**: 405–430.

Heyder J, Blanchard JD, Feldman HA, Brain JD. Convective mixing in human respiratory tract: estimates with aerosol boli. *J Appl Physiol* 1988; **64**:

1273—1278.

Higenbottam T, Jackson M, Woolman P, Lowry R, Wallwork J. The cough response to ultrasonically nebulized distilled water in heart—lung transplantation patients. *Am Rev Respir Dis* 1989; **140**: 58—61.

Jones JG, Clarke SW. Dynamics of cough. *Br J Anaesth* 1970; **42**: 280—285.

Langlands J. The dynamics of cough in health and in chronic bronchitis. *Thorax* 1967; **22**: 88—96.

Lauweryns JM, Baert JH. Alveolar clearance and the role of the pulmonary lymphatics. *Am Rev Respir Dis* 1977; **115**: 625—683.

Lourenço RV, Klimek MF, Borowski CJ. Deposition and clearance of 2μ particles in the tracheobronchial tree of normal subjects — smokers and non-smokers. *J Clin Invest* 1971; **50**: 1411—1420.

Pavia D, Bateman JRM, Lennard-Jones AM, Agnew JE, Clarke SW. Effect of selective and non-selective beta blockade on pulmonary function and tracheobronchial mucociliary clearance in healthy subjects. *Thorax* 1986; **41**: 301—305.

Proctor DF, Reid LM, eds. *Respiratory Defence Mechanisms* Parts 1 & 2. New York: Marcel Dekker, 1977.

Sleigh MA, Blake JR, Liron N. The propulsion of mucus by cilia. *Am Rev Respir Dis* 1988; **137**: 726—741.

Widdicombe JG, Webber SE. Airway mucus secretation. *NIPS* 1990; **5**: p2.

Wong LB, Miller IF, Yeates DB. Stimulation of ciliary beat frequency by autonomic agonists: *in-vivo*. *J Appl Physiol* 1988; **65**: 971—981.

16 PLEURAL SPACE

Agostoni E, D'Angelo E. Pleural liquid pressure. *J Appl Physiol* 1991; **71**: 393—403.

Agostoni E. Mechanics of the pleural space. *Physiol Rev* 1972; **52**: 57—128.

D'Angelo E, Agostoni E. Continuous recording of pleural surface pressure at various sites. *Respir Physiol* 1973; **19**: 356—368.

Lai-Fook SJ, Price DC, Staub NC. Liquid thickness vs. vertical pressure gradient in a model of the pleural space. *J Appl Physiol* 1987; **62**: 1747—1754.

Lai-Fook SJ, Rodarte JR. Pleural pressure distribution and its relationship to lung volume and interstitial pressure. *J Appl Physiol* 1991; **70**: 967—978.

Urmey WF, De Troyer A, Kelly KB, Loring SH. Pleural pressure increases during inspiration in the zone of apposition of diaphragm to rib cage. *J Appl Physiol* 1988; **65**: 2207—2212.

17 LUNG MECHANICS

17.1 General

Brown R, Scharf S, Ingram RH Jr. Nonhomogeneous alveolar pressure swings in the presence of airway closure. *J Appl Physiol* 1980; **49**: 398—402.

Burki NK. The effects of changes in functional residual capacity with posture on mouth occlusion pressure and ventilatory pattern. *Am Rev Respir Dis* 1977; **116**: 895—900.

Clément J, van de Woestijne KP, Pardaens J. A general theory of respiratory mechanics applied to forced expiration. *Respir Physiol* 1973; **19**: 60—79.

De Troyer A, Yernault JC, Rodenstein D. Effects of vagal blockade on lung mechanics in normal man. *J Appl Physiol* 1979; **46**: 217—226.

Fenn WO. Mechanics of respiration. *Am J Med* 1951; **10**: 77—90.

Fry DL, Hyatt RE. Pulmonary mechanics: a unified analysis of the relationship between pressure, volume and gas flow in the lungs of normal and diseased human subjects. *Am J Med* 1960; **29**: 672—689.

Ingram RH Jr, Schilder DP. Effect of gas compression on pulmonary pressure, flow, and volume relationship. *J Appl Physiol* 1966; **21**: 1821—1826.

Macklem PT, Mead J, eds. Mechanics of breathing. *Handbook of Physiology*, Section 3, Vol 3, Parts 1 & 2. Bethesda MD: American Physiological Society, 1986.

Macklem PT. The act of breathing. *NIPS* 1990; **5**: 233—237.

Mead J, Whittenberger JL. Physical properties of human lungs measured during spontaneous respiration. *J Appl Physiol* 1953; **5**: 779—796.

Mead J. Mechanical properties of lungs. *Physiol Rev* 1961; **41**: 281—330.

Milic-Emili J, Orzalesi MM, Cook CD, Turner JM. Respiratory thoraco-abdominal mechanics in man. *J Appl Physiol* 1964; **19**: 217—223.

Otis AB. History of respiratory mechanics. In: Macklem PT, Mead J, eds. *Handbook of Physiology*, Section 3, Vol 3. *Mechanisms of Breathing*. Bethesda MD: American Physiological Society, 1986: 1—12.

Pare PD, Michoud MC, Hogg JC. Lung mechanics following antigen challenge of *Ascaris suum*-sensitive rhesus monkeys. *J Appl Physiol* 1976; **41**: 668—676.

Saunders NA, Betts MF, Pengelly LD, Rebuck AS. Changes in lung mechanics induced by acute isocapnic hypoxia. *J Appl Physiol* 1977; **42**: 413—419.

Wiggs BR, Moreno R, Hogg JC, Hilliam C, Paré PD. A model of the mechanics of airway narrowing. *J Appl Physiol* 1990; **69**: 849—860.

17.2 Lung surface tension
(*see also* sections 17.1, 47, 55)

Bachofen H, Schurch ·S, Urbinelli M, Weibel ER. Relations among alveolar surface tension, surface area, volume, and recoil pressure. *J Appl Physiol* 1987; **62**: 1878—1887.

Clements JA, Hustead RF, Johnson RP, Gribetz I. Pulmonary surface tension and alveolar stability. *J Appl Physiol* 1961; **16**: 444—450.

Clements JA, Tierney DF. Alveolar instability associated with altered surface tension. In: Fenn WO, Rahn H, eds. *Handbook of Physiology*, Section 3,

Respiration, Vol 2. Bethesda MD: American Physiological Society, 1965; 1565−1583.

Davies JM, Veness-Meehan K, Notter RH, Bhutani VK, Kendig JW, Shapiro DL. Changes in pulmonary mechanics after the administration of surfactant to infants with the respiratory distress syndrome. *N Eng J Med* 1988; **319**: 476−479.

Mead J, Whittenberger JL, Radford EP. Surface tension as a factor in pulmonary volume−pressure hysteresis. *J Appl Physiol* 1957; **10**: 191−196.

Pattle RE. Properties, function and origin of the alveolar lining layer. *Nature* 1955; **175**: 1125−1126.

Pattle RE. Surface lining of lung alveoli. *Physiol Rev* 1965; **45**: 48−79.

Radford EP Jr. Recent studies of mechanical properties of mammalian lungs. In: Remington JW, ed. *Tissue Elasticity*. Bethesda MD: American Physiological Society, 1957: 177−190.

Schurch S, Goerke J, Clements JA. Direct determination of volume- and time-dependence of alveolar surface tension in excised lungs. *Proc Nat Acad Sci USA* 1978; **75**: 3417−3421.

Smith JC, Stamenovic D. Surface forces in lungs. 1. Alveolar surface tension−lung volume relationships. *J Appl Physiol* 1986; **60**: 1341−1350.

Van Golde LMG, Batenburg JJ, Robertson B. The pulmonary surfactant system: biochemical aspects and functional significance. *Physiol Rev* 1988; **68**: 374−455.

Wright JR, Clements JA. Metabolism and turnover of lung surfactant. *Am Rev Respir Dis* 1987; **136**: 426−444.

17.3 Lung elastic recoil and compliance

(*see also* sections 5, 17.2, 44.4, 47, 52, 54, 55)

Baydur A, Cha E-J, Sassoon CSH. Validation of esophageal balloon technique at different lung volumes and postures. *J Appl Physiol* 1987; **62**: 315−321.

Bayliss LE, Robertson GW. The visco-elastic properties of the lungs. *Q J Exp Physiol* 1939; **29**: 27−47.

Carson J. On the elasticity of the lungs. *Philos Trans R Soc Lond* 1820; **110**: 29−44.

Colebatch HJH, Greaves IA, Ng CKY. Exponential analysis of elastic recoil and aging in healthy males and females. *J Appl Physiol* 1979; **47**: 683−691.

Colebatch HJH, Ng CKY, Nikov N. Use of an exponential function for elastic recoil. *J Appl Physiol* 1979; **46**: 387−393.

Gibson GJ, Pride NB, Davis J, Schroter RC. Exponential description of the static pressure−volume curve of normal and diseased lungs. *Am Rev Respir Dis* 1979; **120**: 799−811.

Gugger M, Wraith PK, Sudlow MF. A new method of analysing pulmonary quasi-static pressure−volume curves in normal subjects and in patients with chronic airflow obstruction. *Clin Sci* 1990; **78**: 365−369.

Hart A, McKerrow CB, Reynolds JA. A method of using an X−Y recorder in measuring the lung compliance. *J Physiol (Lond)* 1966; **184**: 50P−52P.

Knudson RJ, Mead J, Goldman MD, Schwaber JR, Wohl ME. The failure of indirect indices of lung elastic recoil. *Am Rev Respir Dis* 1973; **107**: 70−82.

Milic-Emili J, Mead J, Turner JM. Topography of esophageal pressure as a function of posture in man. *J Appl Physiol* 1964; **19**: 212−216.

Naimark A, Cherniack RM. Compliance of the respiratory system and its components in health and obesity. *J Appl Physiol* 1960; **15**: 377−382.

Niewoehner DE, Kleinerman J. Morphometric study of elastic fibers in normal and emphysematous human lungs. *Am Rev Respir Dis* 1977; **115**: 15−21.

Permutt S, Martin HB. Static pressure−volume characteristics of lung in normal males. *J Appl Physiol* 1960; **15**: 819−825.

Rahn H, Otis AB, Chadwick LE, Fenn WO. The pressure−volume diagram of the thorax and lung. *Am J Physiol* 1946; **146**: 161−178.

Trop D, Peeters R, van de Woestijne KP. Localisation of recording site in the esophagus by means of cardiac artifacts. *J Appl Physiol* 1970; **29**: 283−287.

Turner JM, Mead J, Wohl ME. Elasticity of human lungs in relation to age. *J Appl Physiol* 1968; **25**: 664−671.

17.4 Distribution of stress in the lung

Budiansky B, Kimmel E. Elastic moduli of lungs. *J Appl Mech* 1990; **54**: 351−358.

Fung YC. Stress, deformation and atelectasis of the lung. *Circ Res* 1975; **37**: 481−496.

Hyatt RE, Bar-Yishay E, Abel MD. Influence of the heart on the vertical gradient of transpulmonary pressure in dogs. *J Appl Physiol* 1985; **58**: 52−57.

Jahed M, Lai-Fook SJ, Bhagat PK, Kraman SS. Propagation of stress waves in inflated sheep lungs. *J Appl Physiol* 1989; **66**: 2675−2680.

Lai-Fook SJ. Pressure−flow behavior of pulmonary interstitium. *J Appl Physiol* 1988; **64**: 2372−2380.

Mead J, Takishima T, Leith D. Stress distribution in lungs: a model of pulmonary elasticity. *J Appl Physiol* 1970; **28**: 596−608.

Menkes H, Linday D, Wood L, Muir A, Macklem PT. Interdependence of lung units in intact dog lungs. *J Appl Physiol* 1972; **32**: 681−686.

Michels DB, Friedman PJ, West JB. Radiographic comparison of human lung shape during normal gravity weightlessness. *J Appl Physiol* 1979; **47**: 851−857.

Parker JC, Allison RC, Taylor AE. Edema affects intra-alveolar fluid pressures and interdependence in dog lungs. *J Appl Physiol* 1981; **51**: 911−921.

Stamenovic D, Wilson TA. A strain energy function for lung parenchyma. *J Biomech Eng* 1985; **107**: 81−86.

Vawter DL, Matthew SFL, West JB. Effect of shape and size of lung and chest wall on stresses in the lung. *J Appl Physiol* 1975; **39**: 9−17.

West JB. Distribution of mechanical stress in the lung, a

possible factor in localisation of pulmonary disease. *Lancet* 1971; **i**: 839−841.

17.5 Lung resistance
(*see also* sections 5, 6.1, 9.4, 9.6, 17.6, 35.3, 44.4)

Clements JA, Sharp JT, Johnson RP, Elam JO. Estimation of pulmonary resistance by repetitive interruption of airflow. *J Clin Invest* 1959; **38**: 1262−1270.

Douma JH. Reynolds similarity law applied to airway resistance. *Bull Physiopathol Respir* 1969; **5**: 385−395.

DuBois AB, Botelho SY, Comroe JH Jr. A new method for measuring airway resistance in man using a body plethysmograph: values in normal subjects and in patients with respiratory disease. *J Clin Invest* 1956; **35**: 327−335.

Frank NR, Mead J, Whittenberger JL. Comparative sensitivity of four methods for measuring changes in respiratory flow resistance in man. *J Appl Physiol* 1971; **31**: 934−938.

Gibson GJ, Pride NB, O'Cain C, Quagliato R. Sex and age differences in pulmonary mechanics in normal nonsmoking subjects. *J Appl Physiol* 1976; **41**: 20−25.

Grimby G, Takishima T, Graham W, Macklem P, Mead J. Frequency dependence of flow resistance in patients with obstructive lung disease. *J Clin Invest* 1968; **47**: 1455−1465.

Hogg JC, Agarawal JB, Gardiner AJS, Palmer WH, Macklem PT. Distribution of airway resistance with developing edema in dogs. *J Appl Physiol* 1972; **32**: 20−24.

Hughes JMB, Hoppin FG Jr, Mead J. Effect of lung inflation on bronchial length and diameter in excised lungs. *J Appl Physiol* 1972; **32**: 25−35.

Hyatt RE, Wilcox RE. The pressure−flow relationship of the intrathoracic airways in man. *J Clin Invest* 1963; **42**: 29−39.

Kaufman J, Wright GW. The effect of nasal and nasopharyngeal irritation on airway resistance in man. *Am Rev Respir Dis* 1969; **100**: 626−630.

Laval P, Feliciano JM, Fondarai J, Kleisbauer JP, Poirier R. Variations de la capacite respiratoire fonctionnelle et des resistances des voies aeriennes chez des sujets normaux en position assise puis couche. *Bull Physiopathol Respir* 1971; **7**: 743−764.

Lisboa C, Wood LDH, Jardim J, Macklem PT. Relationship between flow, curvilinearity, and density dependence of pulmonary pressure−flow curves. *J Appl Physiol* 1980; **48**: 878−885.

Ludwig MS, Dreshaj I, Solowy J, Munoz A, Ingram RH Jr. Partitioning of pulmonary resistance during constriction in the dog: effects of volume history. *J Appl Physiol* 1987; **62**: 807−815.

McDermott M, Collins MM. Acute effects of smoking on lung airways resistance in normal and bronchitic subjects. *Thorax* 1965; **20**: 562−569.

McDermott M. Acute respiratory effects of the inha-lation of coal dust particles. *J Physiol (Lond)* 1962; **162**: 53P.

Nadel JA, Tierney DF. Effect of previous deep inspiration on airway resistance in man. *J Appl Physiol* 1961; **16**: 717−719.

Olive JT Jr, Hyatt RE. Maximal expiratory flow and total respiratory resistance during induced broncho-constriction in asthmatic subjects. *Am Rev Respir Dis* 1972; **106**: 366−376.

Stanescu DC, Pattijn J, Clément J, van de Woestijne KP. Glottis opening and airway resistance. *J Appl Physiol* 1972; **32**: 460−466.

17.6 Respiratory impedance techniques
(*see also* sections 5, 6.1)

Barnas GM, Yoshino K, Stamenovic D, Kikuchi Y, Loring SH, Mead J. Chest wall impedance partitioned into rib cage and diaphragm-abdominal pathways. *J Appl Physiol* 1989; **66**: 350−359.

Cauberghs M, van de Woestijne KP. Effect of upper airway shunt and series properties on respiratory impedance measurements. *J Appl Physiol* 1989; **66**: 2274−2279.

Neild JE, Twort CHC, Chinn S, McCormack S, Jones TD, Burney PGJ *et al*. The repeatability and validity of respiratory resistance measured by the forced oscillation technique. *Respir Med* 1989; **83**: 111−118.

Peslin R, Marchat F, Gallina C, Oswald M, Crance JP. Assessment of thoracic gas volume by low-frequency ambient pressure changes in children. *Eur Respir J* 1988; **1**: 594−599.

Peslin R. Methods for measuring total respiratory impedance by forced oscillations. *Bull Eur Physio-pathol Respir* 1986; **22**: 621−631.

Ying Y, Peslin R, Duvivier C, Gallina C, da Silva JF. Respiratory input and transfer mechanical impedances in patients with chronic obstructive pulmonary disease. *Eur Respir J* 1990; **3**: 1186−1192.

Zwart A, Peslin R, eds. Mechanical respiratory impedance: the forced oscillation method. Contri-butions to the workshop held for the European Commission on 18−19 June, 1990, Antwerp, Belgium. *Eur Respir Rev* 1991; **1**: 131−237.

17.7 Dynamics of forced expiration
(*see also* sections 10.1−10.4, 17.3)

Aldrich TK, Shapiro SM, Sherman MS, Prezant DJ. Alveolar pressure and airway resistance during maximal and submaximal respiratory efforts. *Am Rev Respir Dis* 1989; **140**: 899−906.

Bouhuys A, van de Woestijne KP. Mechanical con-sequences of airway smooth muscle relaxation. *J Appl Physiol* 1971; **30**: 670−676.

Clément J, Stanescu DC, van de Woestijne KP. Glottis opening and effort-dependent part of the isovolume pressure−flow curves. *J Appl Physiol* 1973; **34**: 18−22.

Dawson SV, Elliott EA. Use of the choke point in the prediction of flow limitation in elastic tubes. *Fed Proc* 1980; **39**: 2765–2770.

Dawson SV, Elliott EA. Wave-speed limitation on expiratory flow—a unifying concept. *J Appl Physiol* 1977; **48**: 493–515.

Elad D, Kamm RD, Shapiro AH. Steady compressible flow in collapsible tubes: application to forced expiration. *J Fluid Mech* 1989; **203**: 401–418.

Hoffstein V. Relationship between lung volume, maximal expiratory flow, forced expiratory volume in one second, and tracheal area in normal men and women. *Am Rev Respir Dis* 1986; **134**: 956–961.

Hyatt RE, Schilder DP, Fry DL. Relationship between maximum expiratory flow and degree of lung inflation. *J Appl Physiol* 1958; **13**: 331–336.

Hyatt RE, Wilson TA, Bar-Yishay E. Prediction of maximal expiratory flow in excised human lungs. *J Appl Physiol* 1980; **48**: 991–998.

Hyatt RE. Forced expiration. In: Macklem PT, Mead J, eds. *Handbook of Physiology*, Section 3, Vol 3, *Mechanics of Breathing*. Bethesda, MD: American Physiological Society, 1986: 295–314.

Ingram RH, Pedley TJ. Pressure–flow relationships in the lungs. In: Macklem PT, Mead J, eds. *Handbook of Physiology*, Section 3, Vol 3, *Mechanics of Breathing*. Bethesda MD: American Physiological Society, 1986: 277–293.

Jan DL, Shapiro AH, Kamm RD. Some features of oscillatory flow in a model bifurcation. *J Appl Physiol* 1989; **67**: 147–159.

Lemen RJ, Gerdes CB, Wegmann MJ, Perrin KJ. Frequency spectra of flow and volume events for forced vital capacity. *J Appl Physiol* 1982; **53**: 977–984.

Macklem PT, Wilson NJ. Measurement of intrabronchial pressure in man. *J Appl Physiol* 1965; **20**: 653–663.

Mead J, Turner JM, Macklem PT, Little JB. Significance of the relationship between lung recoil and maximum expiratory flow. *J Appl Physiol* 1967; **22**: 95–108.

Mead J. Dysanapsis in normal lungs assessed by the relationship between maximal flow, static recoil, and vital capacity. *Am Rev Respir Dis* 1980; **121**: 339–342.

Melissinos CG, Mead J. Maximum expiratory flow changes induced by longitudinal tension on trachea in normal subjects. *J Appl Physiol* 1977; **43**: 537–544.

Olafsson S, Hyatt RE. Ventilatory mechanics and expiratory flow limitation during exercise in normal subjects. *J Clin Invest* 1969; **48**: 564–573.

Pedley TJ, Schroter RC, Sudlow MF. Flow and pressure drop in systems of repeatedly branching tubes. *J Fluid Mech* 1971; **46**: 365–383.

Peslin R, Jardin P, Bohadana A, Hannhart B. Contenu harmonique du signal de débit pendant l'expiration forcée chez l'homme normal. (English abstract). *Bull Eur Physiopathol Respir* 1982; **18**: 491–500.

Poiseuille JLM. Recherches experimentales sur le mouvement des liquides dans les tubes de tres petits diametres. *C R Acad Sci* 1840; **11**: 961–967 and 1041–1048.

Pride NB, Permutt S, Riley RL, Bromberger-Barnea B. Determinants of maximal expiratory flow from the lungs. *J Appl Physiol* 1967; **23**: 646–662.

Reynolds O. An experimental investigation of the circumstances which determine whether the motion of water shall be direct or sinuous, and of the law of resistance in parallel channels. *Philos Trans R Soc (Lond)* 1883; **174**: 935–982.

Schroter RC, Sudlow MF. Flow patterns in models of the human bronchial airways. *Respir Physiol* 1969; **7**: 341–355.

Smaldone GC, Bergofsky EH. Delineation of flow-limiting segment and predicted airway resistance by movable catheter. *J Appl Physiol* 1976; **40**: 943–952.

Tsuda A, Kamm R, Fredberg JJ. Periodic flow at airway bifurcations. II. Flow partitioning. *J Appl Physiol* 1990; **69**: 553–561.

van de Woestijne KP, Jacquemin C, Atlan G, eds. Models in ventilatory mechanics. *Bull Physiopathol Respir* 1972; **8**: 179–430.

Wilson TA. The wave speed limit on expiratory flow. In: Chang HK, Paiva M, eds. *Respiratory Physiology: an Analytical Approach*. New York: Marcel Dekker, 1989: 139–166.

18 AIRWAY CALIBRE

18.1 Control mechanisms

Adcock JJ, Schneider C, Smith TW. Effects of codeine, morphine and a novel opioid pentapeptide BW 443C, on cough, nociception and ventilation in the unanaesthetized guinea-pig. *Br J Pharmacol* 1988; **93**: 93–100.

Adcock JJ, Smith TW, Widdicombe JG. Role of the vagus nerves in bronchoconstriction induced by inhaled histamine and capsaicin in normal and hyperreactive airways: irritant versus c-fibre receptors. *Eur Respir J* 1989; **2**(Suppl): 287s.

Bai TR, Lam R, Prasad FYF. Effects of adrenergic agonists and adenosine on cholinergic neurotransmission in human tracheal smooth muscle. *Pulm Pharmacol* 1989; **1**: 193–199.

Barnes PJ. Muscarinic receptors in airways: recent developments. *J Appl Physiol* 1990; **68**: 1777–1785.

Barnes PJ. State of art. Neural control of human airways in health and disease. *Am Rev Respir Dis* 1986; **134**: 1289–1314.

Barnes PJ, Baraniuk JN, Belvisi MG. Neuropeptides in the respiratory tract (pts 1 & 2). *Am Rev Respir Dis* 1991; **144**: 1187–1198, 1391–1399.

Coleridge HM, Coleridge JGG. Reflexes evoked from tracheobronchial tree and lungs. In: Cherniack NS, Widdicombe JG, eds. *Handbook of Physiology*, Section 3, Vol 2, *Control of Breathing*. Part 1.

Bethesda, MD: American Physiological Society, 1986: 395−429.

Fish JE, Ankin MG, Kelly JF, Peterman VI. Regulation of bronchomotor tone by lung inflation in asthmatic and nonasthmatic subjects. *J Appl Physiol* 1981; **50**: 1079−1086.

Fuller RW, Karlsson J-A, Choudry NB, Pride NB. Effect of inhaled and systemic opiates on responses to inhaled capsaicin in humans. *J Appl Physiol* 1988; **65**: 1125−1130.

Fuller RW, Maxwell DL, Dixon CMS, McGregor GP, Barnes VF, Bloom SR *et al*. Effects of substance P on cardiovascular and respiratory function in subjects. *J Appl Physiol* 1987; **62**: 1473−1479.

Jain SK, Subramanian S, Julka DB, Guz A. Search for evidence of lung chemoreflexes in man: study of respiratory and circulatory effects of phenyldiguanide and lobeline. *Clin Sci* 1972; **42**: 163−177.

Josenhans WT, Melville GN, Ulmer WT. Effects of humidity in inspired air, on airway resistance and functional residual capacity in patients with respiratory diseases. *Respiration* 1969; **26**: 435−442.

Kaise A, Freed AN, Mitzner W. Interaction between CO_2 concentration and flow rate on peripheral airway resistance. *J Appl Physiol* 1991; **70**: 2514−2521.

Karlsson J-A, Saint 'Ambrogio G, Widdicombe J. Afferent neural pathways in cough and reflex bronchoconstriction. *J Appl Physiol* 1988; **65**: 1007−1023.

Karlsson J-A. Airway anaesthesia and the cough reflex. *Bull Eur Physiopathol Respir* 1987; **23**(Suppl. 10): 29s−36s.

Lammers J-WJ, Minette P, McCusker M, Barnes PJ. The role of pirenzepine-sensitive (MI) muscarinic receptors in vagally mediated bronchoconstriction in humans. *Am Rev Respir Dis* 1989; **139**: 446−449.

Leff AR. State of the art. Endogenous regulation of bronchomotor tone. *Am Rev Respir Dis* 1988; **137**: 1198−1216.

Libby DM, Briscoe WA, King TKC. Relief of hypoxia-related bronchoconstriction by breathing 30 per cent oxygen. *Am Rev Respir Dis* 1981; **123**: 171−175.

Orehek J, Charpin D, Velardocchio JM, Grimaud C. Bronchomotor effect of bronchoconstriction-induced deep inspirations in asthmatics. *Am Rev Respir Dis* 1980; **121**: 297−305.

Prime FJ, Bianco S, Griffin JP, Kamburoff PL. The effects on airways conductance of alpha-adrenergic stimulation and blocking. *Bull Physiopathol Respir* 1972; **8**: 99−109.

Richardson JB. State of art. Nerve supply to the lungs. *Am Rev Respir Dis* 1979; **119**: 785−802.

Saria A, Martling C-R, Yan Z, Theodorsson-Norheim E, Gamse R, Lundberg JM. Release of multiple tachykinins from capsaicin-sensitive sensory nerves in the lung by bradykinin, histamine, dimethylphenyl piperazinium and vagal nerve stimulation. *Am Rev Respir Dis* 1988; **137**: 1330−1335.

Schultz HD, Pisarri TE, Coleridge HM, Coleridge JCG. Carotid sinus baroreceptors modulate tracheal smooth muscle tension in dogs. *Circ Res* 1987; **60**: 337−345.

Stein JF, Widdicombe JG. The interaction of chemo- and mechanoreceptor signals in the control of airway calibre. *Respir Physiol* 1975; **25**: 363−376.

18.2 Airway hyperreactivity

Belcher NG, Rees PJ, Clark TJH, Lee TH. A comparison of the refractory periods induced by hypertonic airway challenge and exercise in bronchial asthma. *Am Rev Respir Dis* 1987; **135**: 822−825.

Ben-Dov I, Bar-Yishay E, Godfrey S. Exercise-induced asthma without respiratory heat loss. *Thorax* 1982; **37**: 630−631.

Boulet LP, Legris C, Turcotte H, Herbert J. Prevalence and characteristics of late asthmatic response to exercise. *J Allergy Clin Immunol* 1987; **80**: 655−662.

Empey DW, Laitinen LA, Jacobs L, Gold WM, Nadel JA. Mechanisms of bronchial hyperreactivity in normal subjects after upper respiratory tract infection. *Am Rev Respir Dis* 1976; **113**: 131−139.

Fitch KD, Morton AR. Specificity of exercise in exercise-induced asthma. *Br Med J* 1971; **4**: 577−581.

Gilbert IA, Fouke JM, McFadden ER Jr. Intra-airway thermodynamics during exercise and hyperventilation in asthmatics. *J Appl Physiol* 1988; **64**: 2167−2174.

Hopp RJ, Christy J, Bewtra AK, Nair NM, Townley RG. Incorporation and analysis of ultrasonically nebulized distilled water challenges in an epidemiologic study of asthma and bronchial reactivity. *Ann Allergy* 1988; **60**: 129−133.

Jones RS, Buston MH, Wharton MJ. The effect of exercise on ventilatory function in the child with asthma. *Br J Dis Chest* 1962; **56**: 78−86.

Josenhans WT, Melville GN, Ulmer WT. The effect of facial cold stimulation on airway conductance in healthy man. *Can J Physiol Pharmacol* 1969; **47**: 453−457.

Kaliner MA, Barnes PJ, Persson CGA, eds. *Asthma and Bronchial Hyperresponsiveness: Pathogenesis and Treatment*. New York: Marcel Dekker, 1990.

McNeill RS, Nairn JR, Millar JS, Ingram CG. Exercise-induced asthma. *Q J Med* 1966; **35**: 55−67.

O'Connor G, Sparrow D, Taylor D, Segal M, Weiss S. Analysis of dose response curves to methacholine: an approach for population studies. *Am Rev Respir Dis* 1987; **136**: 1412−1417.

Shaw RJ, Anderson SD, Durham SR *et al*. Mediators of hypersensitivity and 'fog'-induced asthma. *Allergy* 1985; **40**: 48−57.

Smith CM, Anderson SD. Inhalation provocation tests using nonisotonic aerosols. *J Allergy Clin Immunol* 1989; **84**: 781−790.

Sterk PJ, Fabbri LM, Quanjer PLH, Cockcroft DW, O'Bryne PM, Anderson SD *et al*. Airway responsiveness: standardized challenge testing with pharmacological, physiological and sensitising stimuli in adults. *Eur Respir J* 1993; 6, suppl 16: 55−86.

Wilson NM, Barnes PJ, Vickers H, Silverman M. Hyperventilation-induced asthma: evidence for two mechanisms. *Thorax* 1982; **37**: 657−662.

Zawadski DK, Lenner KA, McFadden ER Jr. Comparison of intra airway temperatures in normal and asthmatic subjects after hyperpnea with hot, cold and ambient air. *Am Rev Respir Dis* 1988; **138**: 1553−1558

18.3 Bronchodilatation

Afschrift M, Clement J, Peeters R, van de Woestijne KP. Maximal expiratory and inspiratory flows in patients with chronic obstructive pulmonary disease. Influence of bronchodilation. *Am Rev Respir Dis* 1969; **100**: 147−152.

Cotes JE. Reporting the results of tests of lung function. In: Burley DM, Clarke SW, Cuthbert MF, Paterson JW, Shelley JH, eds. *Evaluation of Bronchodilator Drugs, an Asthma Research Council Symposium.* London: Trust for Education and Research in Therapeutics, 1974: 125−135.

Dales RE, Spitzer WO, Tousignant P, Schechter M, Suissa S. Clinical interpretation of airway response to a bronchodilator: epidemiologic considerations. *Am Rev Respir Dis* 1988; **138**: 317−320.

Demedts M. The assessment of reversibility: what physiological tests? *Eur Respir J* 1990; **3**: 1084−1087.

Eliasson O, Degraff AC. The use of criteria for reversibility and obstruction to define patient groups for bronchodilator trials. Influence of clinical diagnosis, spirometric, and anthropometric variables. *Am Rev Respir Dis* 1985; **132**: 858−864.

Lorber DB, Kaltenborn W, Burrows B. Responses to isoproterenol in a general population sample. *Am Rev Respir Dis* 1976; **118**: 855−861.

Meslier N, Racineux JL. Tests of reversibility to airflow obstruction. *Eur Respir Rev* 1991; **1**: 34−40.

Sourk RL, Nugent KM. Bronchodilator testing: confidence intervals derived from placebo inhalations. *Am Rev Respir Dis* 1983; **128**: 153−157.

Tweeddale PM, Alexander F, McHardy GJR. Short term variability in FEV$_1$ and bronchodilator responsiveness in patients with obstructive ventilatory defects. *Thorax* 1987; **42**: 487−490.

Watanabe S, Renzetti AD, Begin R, Bigler AH. Airway responsiveness to a bronchodilator aerosol. *Am Rev Respir Dis* 1974; **109**: 530−537.

Weir DC, Burge PS. Measures of reversibility in response to bronchodilators in chronic airflow obstruction: relation to airway calibre. *Thorax* 1991; **46**: 43−45.

19 DISTRIBUTION OF GAS

19.1 Via airways
(*see also* sections 6.4, 12, 13, 19.2, 20, 44.4)

Amis TC, Jones HA, Hughes JMB. Effect of posture on interregional distribution of pulmonary ventilation in man. *Respir Physiol* 1984; **56**: 145−167.

Briscoe WA, Cournand A. Uneven ventilation of normal and diseased lungs studied by an open-circuit method. *J Appl Physiol* 1959; **14**: 284−290.

Chevrolet JC, Emrich J, Martin RR, Engel LA. Voluntary changes in ventilation distribution in the lateral posture. *Respir Physiol* 1979; **38**: 313−323.

Crawford ABH, Makowska M, Engel LA. Effect of bronchomotor tone on static mechanical properties of lung and ventilation distribution. *J Appl Physiol* 1987; **63**(6): 2278−2285.

Cybulsky IJ, Abel JG, Menon AS, Salerno TA, Lichtenstein SV, Slutsky AS. Contribution of cardiogenic oscillations to gas exchange in constant-flow ventilation. *J Appl Physiol* 1987; **63**: 564−570.

Denison DM, Morgan MDL, Millar AB. Estimation of regional gas and tissue volumes of the lung in supine man using computed tomography. *Thorax* 1986; **41**: 620−628.

Engel LA. Dynamic distribution of gas flow. In: Macklem PT, Mead J, eds. *Handbook of Physiology*, Section 3, Vol 3, *Mechanics of Breathing*. Bethesda, MD: American Physiological Society, 1986: 575−593.

Engel LA. Gas mixing within the acinus of the lung. *J Appl Physiol* 1983; **54**: 609−618.

Gilson JC, Hugh-Jones P, Oldham PD, Meade F. Lung function in coal workers' pneumoconiosis. Gas-distribution and transfer. *Spec Rep Med Res Coun (Lond)* 1955; **290**: 114−124, 150−201.

Greene R, Hughes JMB, Sudlow MF, Milic-Emili J. Regional lung volumes during water immersion to the xiphoid in seated man. *J Appl Physiol* 1974; **36**: 734−736.

Jones RL, Overton TR, Sproule BJ. Frequency dependence of ventilation distribution in normal and obstructed lungs. *J Appl Physiol* 1977; **42**: 548−553.

Krogh A, Lindhard J. The volume of the dead space in breathing and the mixing of gases in the lungs of man. *J Physiol (Lond)* 1917; **51**: 59−90.

Lacquet LM, Van der Linden LP, Paiva M. Transport of H$_2$ and SF$_6$ in the lung. *Respir Physiol* 1975; **25**: 157−173.

Milic-Emili J. Static distribution of lung volumes. In: Macklem PT, Mead J, eds. *Handbook of Physiology*, Section 3, Vol 3, *Mechanics of Breathing*. Bethesda, MD: American Physiological Society, 1986: 561−574.

Otis AB, McKerrow CB, Barlett RA, Mead J, McIlroy MB, Selverstone NJ, Radford EP Jr. Mechanical factors in distribution of pulmonary ventilation. *J*

Appl Physiol 1956; **8**: 427–443.

Paiva M, Engel LA. Gas mixing in the lung periphery. In: Chang HK, Paiva M, eds. *Respiratory Physiology: an Analytical Approach*. New York: Marcel Dekker, 1989; 245–276.

Paiva M, Engel LA. Theoretical studies of gas mixing and ventilation distribution in the lung. *Physiol Rev* 1987; **67**: 750–796.

Pedley TJ, Sudlow MF, Milic-Emili J. A non-linear theory of the distribution of pulmonary ventilation. *Respir Physiol* 1972; **15**: 1–38.

Piiper J, Scheid P. Diffusion and convection in intrapulmonary gas mixing. In: Farhi LE, Tenney SM, eds. *Handbook of Physiology*, Section 3, Vol 4, *Gas Exchange*. Bethesda, MD: American Physiological Society, 1987; 51–70.

Prowse K, Cumming G. Effects of lung volume and disease on the lung nitrogen decay curve. *J Appl Physiol* 1973; **34**: 23–33.

Roussos CS, Siegler DIM, Engel LA. Influence of diaphragmatic contraction and expiratory flow on the pattern of lung emptying. *Respir Physiol* 1976; **27**: 157–167.

Senda M, Murata K, Itoh H, Yonekura Y, Torizuka K. Quantitative evaluation of regional pulmonary ventilation using PET and nitrogen-13 gas. *J Nucl Med* 1986; **27**: 268–273.

Sybrecht G, Landau L, Murphy BG, Engel LA, Martin RR, Macklem PT. Influence of posture on flow dependence of distribution of inhaled 133 Xe boli. *J Appl Physiol* 1976; **41**: 489–496.

Taylor GI. Dispersion of soluble matter in solvent flowing slowly through a tube. *Proc R Soc Lond Ser A* 1953; **219**: 186–193.

West JB, Hugh-Jones P. Patterns of gas flow in the upper bronchial tree. *J Appl Physiol* 1959; **14**: 753–759.

Zwijnenburg A, Klumper A, Roos CM, Jansen HM, van der Schoot JB, van Zandwijk N, et al. Lung volume calculations from 81Krm SPECT for the quantitation of regional ventilation. *Clin Physiol Meas* 1988; **9**: 147–154.

19.2 Collateral ventilation

Frazer DG, Giza A, Stanley CF, Frazer JL, Franz GN, Petson EL. Surface forces and the alveolar pores of Kohn. *FASEB J* 1989; **3**: A547.

Hogg JC, Macklem PT, Thurlbeck WM. The resistance of collateral channels in excised human lungs. *J Clin Invest* 1969; **48**: 421–431.

Kohn HN. Zur histologie der indurirenden fibrinosen pneumonie. *Munch Med Wochenschr* 1893; **8**: 42–45.

Lambert MW. Accessory bronchiole–alveolar communications. *J Pathol Bacteriol* 1955; **70**: 311–314.

Macklem PT. Airway obstruction and collateral ventilation. *Physiol Rev* 1971; **51**: 368–436.

Martin HB. The effect of aging on the alveolar pores of Kohn in the dog. *Am Rev Respir Dis* 1963; **88**: 773–778.

Menkes HA, Macklem PT. Collateral flow. In: *Handbook of Physiology, the Respiratory System* 3. Bethesda MD: American Physiological Society, 1984: 337–353.

Van Allen CM, Lindskog GE, Richter HG. Gaseous interchange between adjacent lung lobules. *Yale J Biol Med* 1930; **2**: 297–300.

20 CLOSING VOLUME
(*see also* sections 6.4, 12, 13, 19.1)

Anthonisen NR, Danson J, Robertson PC, Ross WRD. Airway closure as a function of age. *Respir Physiol* 1970; **8**: 58–65.

Begin R, Renzetti AD Jr, Bigler AH, Watanabe S. Flow and age dependence of airway closure and dynamic compliance. *J Appl Physiol* 1975; **38**: 199–207.

Benson MK, Newberg LA, Jones JG. Nitrogen and bolus closing volumes: differences after histamine-induced bronchoconstriction. *J Appl Physiol* 1975; **38**: 1088–1091.

Bode FR, Dosman J, Martin RR, Ghezzo H, Macklem PT. Age and sex differences in lung elasticity and in closing capacity in nonsmokers. *J Appl Physiol* 1974; **41**: 129–135.

Cooper DM, Doron I, Mansell AL, Bryan AC, Levison H. The relative sensitivity of closing volume in children with asthma and cystic fibrosis. *Am Rev Respir Dis* 1974; **109**: 519–524.

Craig DB, Wahba WM, Don HF, Couture JG, Becklake MR. 'Closing volume' and its relationship to gas exchange in seated and supine positions. *J Appl Physiol* 1971; **31**: 717–721.

DeGroodt EG, Quanjer PhH, Wise ME. Short and long term variability of indices from the single and multibreath nitrogen test. *Bull Eur Physiopathol Respir* 1984; **20**: 271–277.

Demedts M, Clément J, Stanescu DC, van de Woestijne KP. Inflection point on transpulmonary pressure–volume curves and closing volume. *J Appl Physiol* 1975; **38**: 228–235.

Hales CA, Gibbons R, Burnham C, Kazemi H. Determinants of regional distribution of a bolus inhaled from residual volume. *J Appl Physiol* 1976; **41**: 400–408.

Hughes JM. Site of airway closure in dog lungs. *Bull Physiopathol Respir* 1970; **6**: 877–879.

Knudson RJ, Lebowitz MD, Burton AP, Knudson DE. The closing volume test: evaluation of nitrogen and bolus methods in a random population. *Am Rev Respir Dis* 1977; **115**: 423–434.

Leblanc P, Ruff F, Milic-Emili J. Effects of age and body position on 'airway closure' in man. *J Appl Physiol* 1970; **28**: 448–451.

McCarthy DS, Spencer R, Greene R, Milic-Emili J. Measurement of 'closing volume' as a simple and sensitive test for early detection of small airway disease. *Am J Med* 1972; **52**: 747–753.

Make B, Lapp NL. Factors influencing the measurement of closing volume. *Am Rev Respir Dis* 1975; **111**: 749–754.

Marcq M, Minette A. Diurnal variations and reproducibility of the N_2 closing volume test in healthy subjects. *Bull Eur Physiopathol Respir* 1976; **12**: 757–770.

Meyer M, Hook C, Rieke H, Piiper J. Gas mixing in dog lungs studied by single-breath washout of He and SF6. *J Appl Physiol* 1983; **55**: 1795–1802.

National Heart and Lung Institute. *Suggested Standardised Procedures for Closing Volume Determinations (Nitrogen Method)*. Bethesda MD: National Heart and Lung Institute, 1973.

Travis DM, Green M, Don H. Simultaneous comparison of helium and nitrogen expiratory 'closing volumes'. *J Appl Physiol* 1973; **34**: 304–308.

21 PULMONARY BLOOD FLOW

21.1 Measurement

Bate H, Rowlands S, Sirs JA. Influence of diffusion on dispersion of indicators in blood flow. *J Appl Physiol* 1973; **34**: 866–872.

Denison D, Edwards RHT, Jones G, Pope H. Estimates of the CO_2 pressures in systemic arterial blood during rebreathing on exercise. *Respir Physiol* 1971; **11**: 186–196.

Farhi LE, Nesarajah MS, Olszowka AJ, Metildi LA, Ellis AK. Cardiac output determination by simple one-step rebreathing technique. *Respir Physiol* 1976; **28**: 141–159.

Godfrey S, Davies CTM. Estimates of arterial Pco_2 and their effect on the calculated values of cardiac output and deadspace on exercise. *Clin Sci* 1970; **39**: 529–537.

Hysing B, Dahl LE, Varnauskas E. Determination of cardiac output with cardio green in a direct writing colorimeter. *Scand J Clin Lab Invest* 1962; **14**: 430–434.

Jones NL, Campbell EJM, McHardy GJR, Higgs BE, Clode M. The estimation of carbon dioxide pressure of mixed venous blood during exercise. *Clin Sci* 1967; **32**: 311–327.

Jones NL, Robertson DG, Kane JW, Campbell EJM. Effect of Pco_2 level on alveolar–arterial Pco_2 difference during rebreathing. *J Appl Physiol* 1972; **32**: 782–787.

Karatzas NB, Lee G de J. Instantaneous lung capillary blood flow in patients with heart disease. *Cardiovasc Res* 1970; **4**: 265–273.

Kawakami Y, Menkes HA, DuBois AB. A water-filled body plethysmograph for the measurement of pulmonary capillary blood flow during changes of intrathoracic pressure. *J Clin Invest* 1970; **49**: 1237–1251.

Kelman GR. $P\bar{v},o_2$ by nitrogen rebreathing—a critical, theoretical analysis. *Respir Physiol* 1972; **16**: 327–336.

Lane DA, Sirs JA. Indicator dilution measurement of mean transit time and flow in a straight tube. *J Physics E: Sci Instrum* 1974; **7**: 51–55.

Laszlo G, Clark TJH, Pope H, Campbell EJM. Differences between alveolar and arterial Pco_2 during rebreathing experiments in resting human subjects. *Respir Physiol* 1971; **12**: 36–52.

Margaria R, Cerretelli P, Veicsteinas A. Estimation of heart stroke volume from blood hemoglobin and heart rate at submaximal exercise. *J Appl Physiol* 1970; **29**: 204–207.

Murray JF, Davidson FF, Glazier JB. Modified technique for measuring pulmonary shunts using xenon and indocyanine green. *J Appl Physiol* 1972; **32**: 695–700.

Pugh LGCE. A modified acetylene method for the determination of cardiac output during muscular exercise. *Ergonomics* 1972; **15**: 323–335.

Steele P, Davies H. The Swan-Ganz catheter in the cardiac laboratory. *Br Heart J* 1973; **35**: 647–650.

Taplin GV, Johnson DE, Dore EK, Kaplan S. Lung photoscans with macroaggregates of human serum radioalbumin. *Health Phys* 1964; **10**: 1219–1227.

Teichmann J, Adaro F, Veicsteinas A, Cerretelli P, Piiper J. Determination of pulmonary blood flow by rebreathing of soluble inert gases. *Respiration* 1974; **31**: 296–309.

Vliers A. Le principe de la thermodilution. Etude théorique et applications en cardiologie. *Rev Inst Hyg Mines* 1970; **25**: 3–111.

Wessel HU, Paul MH, James GW, Grahn AR. Limitations of thermal dilution curves for cardiac output determinations. *J Appl Physiol* 1971; **30**: 643–652.

West JB, Dollery CT, Hugh-Jones P. The use of radioactive carbon dioxide to measure regional blood flow in the lungs of patients with pulmonary disease. *J Clin Invest* 1961; **40**: 1–12.

Zeidifard E, Godfrey S, Davies EE. Estimation of cardiac output by an N_2O rebreathing method in adults and children. *J Appl Physiol* 1976; **41**: 433–438.

21.2 Pulmonary blood distribution

Banister J, Torrance RW. The effects of the tracheal pressure upon flow: pressure relations in the vascular bed of isolated lungs. *Q J Exp Physiol* 1960; **45**: 352–367.

Burton AC, Stinson RH. The measurement of tension in vascular smooth muscle. *J Physiol (Lond)* 1960; **153**: 290–305.

Dawson CA. Role of pulmonary vasomotion in physiology of the lung. *Physiol Rev* 1984; **64**: 544–616.

Glazier JB, Hughes JMB, Maloney JE, West JB. Measurements of capillary dimensions and blood volume in rapidly frozen lungs. *J Appl Physiol* 1969; **26**: 65–76.

Grant BJB, Davies EE, Jones HA, Hughes JMB. Local regulation of pulmonary blood flow and ventilation−perfusion ratios in the coatimundi. *J Appl Physiol* 1976; **40**: 216−228.

Grant BJB, Schneider AM. Dynamic response of local blood flow to alveolar gas tensions: analysis. *J Appl Physiol* 1983; **54**: 445−452.

Hakim TS, Dean GW, Lisbona R. Effect of body posture on spatial distribution of pulmonary blood flow. *J Appl Physiol* 1988; **64**: 1160−1170.

Hughes JMB, Glazier JB, Maloney JE, West JB. Effect of extra-alveolar vessels on distribution of blood flow in the dog lung. *J Appl Physiol* 1968; **25**: 701−712.

Hughes JMB, Glazier JB, Maloney JE, West JB. Effect of lung volume on the distribution of pulmonary blood flow in man. *Respir Physiol* 1968; **4**: 58−72.

Lai-Fook SJ. A continuum mechanics analysis of pulmonary vascular interdependence in isolated dog lobes. *J Appl Physiol* 1979; **46**: 419−429.

Lopez-Muniz R, Stephens NL, Bromberger-Barnea B, Permutt S, Riley RL. Critical closure of pulmonary vessels analyzed in terms of Starling resistor model. *J Appl Physiol* 1968; **24**: 625−635.

Marshall BE, Marshall C. A model for hypoxic constriction of the pulmonary circulation. *J Appl Physiol* 1988; **64**: 68−77.

Merrill EW. Rheology of blood. *Physiol Rev* 1969; **49**: 863−888.

Pain MCF, West JB. Effect of the volume history of the isolated lung on distribution of blood flow. *J Appl Physiol* 1966; **21**: 1545−1550.

Permutt S, Wise RA. Mechanical interaction of respiration and circulation. In: Macklem PT, Mead J, eds. *Handbook of Physiology*, Section 3, Vol 3, *Mechanisms of Breathing*, Part 2. Bethesda, MD: American Physiological Society, 1986; 647−656.

Read J, Lee JH, Pain MCF. Two groups of subjects with obstructive lung disease, defined by pulmonary vascular reactivity. *Proc Aspen Emphysema Conference*. US Dept Health Education and Welfare 1967; **10**: 229−239.

Rickaby DA, Dawson CA, Linehan JH, Bronikowski TA. Alveolar vessel behavior in the zone 2 lung inferred from indicator-dilution data. *J Appl Physiol* 1987; **63**: 778−784.

Ruiz AV, Bisgard GE, Tyson IB, Grover RF, Will JA. Regional lung function in calves during acute and chronic pulmonary hypertension. *J Appl Physiol* 1974; **37**: 384−391.

Staub NC. Pulmonary edema. *Physiol Rev* 1974; **54**: 678−811.

Tartulier M, Bourret M, Deyrieux F. Pulmonary arterial pressures in normal subjects. Effects of age and exercise. *Bull Physiopathol Respir* 1972; **8**: 1295−1321.

21.3 *Control of pulmonary vasomotor tone*

Archer SL, McMurtry IF, Weir EK. Mechanisms of acute hypoxic and hyperoxic changes in pulmonary vascular reactivity. In: Weir EK, Reeves JT, eds. *Pulmonary Vascular Physiology and Pathophysiology*. New York: Marcel Dekker, 1989.

Archer SL, Peterson D, Nelson DP, DeMaster EG, Kelly B, Eaton JW, Weir EK. Oxygen radicals and antioxidant enzymes alter pulmonary vascular reactivity in the rat lung. *J Appl Physiol* 1989; **66**: 102−111.

Archer SL, Rist K, Nelson DP, DeMaster EG, Cowan N, Weir EK. Comparison of the hemodynamic effects of nitric oxide and endothelium-dependent vasodilators in intact lungs. *J Appl Physiol* 1990; **68**: 735−747.

Barer GR, Cai Y, Russell PC, Emery CJ. Reactivity and site of vasomotion in pulmonary vessels of chronically hypoxic rats: relation to structural changes. *Am Rev Respir Dis* 1989; **140**: 1483−1485.

Barer GR, Howard P, Shaw JW. Stimulus−response curves for the pulmonary vascular bed to hypoxia and hypercapnia. *J Physiol (Lond)* 1970; **211**: 139−155.

Fowler KT, Read J. Cardiac oscillations in expired gas tensions, and regional pulmonary blood flow. *J Appl Physiol* 1961; **16**: 863−868.

Greenberg B, Rhoden K, Barnes PJ. Endothelium-dependent relaxation of human pulmonary arteries. *Am J Physiol* 1987; **253**: H434−H438.

Heymann MA, Soifer SJ. Control of fetal and neonatal pulmonary circulation. In: Weir EK, Reeves FT, eds. *Lung Biology in Health and Disease*, Vol 38. New York: Marcel Dekker, 1988: 33−44.

Kokkola K. Respiratory gas exchange after bronchography. *Scand J Respir Dis* 1972; **53**: 114−119.

Mitzner W, Huang I. Interpretation of pressure-flow curve in the pulmonary vascular bed. In: Will JA, Dawson CA, Weir EK, Buckner CK. *Pulmonary Circulation in Health and Disease*. Orlando, Academic Press, 1987: 215−230.

Rodman DM, Voelkel NF. Regulation of vascular tone. In: Crystal RA, West JB, eds. *The Lung: Scientific Foundations*. New York: Raven Press, 1990: 1105−1119.

Rootwelt K, Vale JR. Pulmonary gas exchange after intravenous injection of ^{99m}Tc-Sulphur-colloid albumin macroaggregates for lung perfusion scintigraphy. *Scand J Clin Lab Invest* 1972; **30**: 17−21.

Said SI, Mutt V. Polypeptide with broad biological activity: isolation from small intestine. *Science* 1970; **169**: 1217−1218.

Schrimshire DA. Theoretical analysis of independent $\dot{V}_A$ and $\dot{Q}$ inequalities upon pulmonary gas exchange. *Respir Physiol* 1977; **29**: 163−178.

West JB. *Ventilation/Blood Flow and Gas Exchange*, 3rd edition. Oxford: Blackwell Scientific Publications, 1977.

Weston AH. Smooth muscle K$^+$ channel openers; their pharmacology and clinical potential. *Pflügers Arch* 1989; **414**: S99−S105.

22.1 General
(*see also* sections 6.4, 12, 13, 19.1, 20, 21.2)

Asmussen E, Nielsen M. Physiological dead space and alveolar gas pressures at rest and during muscular exercise. *Acta Physiol Scand* 1956; **38**: 1–21.

Bradley CA, Harris EA, Seelye ER, Whitlock RML. Gas exchange during exercise in healthy people. (i) The physiological deadspace volume. *Clin Sci* 1976; **51**: 323–333.

Butler C, Kleinerman J. Capillary density: alveolar diameter, a morphometric approach to ventilation and perfusion. *Am Rev Respir Dis* 1970; **102**: 886–894.

Dantzker DR, Wagner PD, West JB. Instability of lung units with low $\dot{V}_A/\dot{Q}$ ratios during O_2 breathing. *J Appl Physiol* 1975; **38**: 886–895.

Ewan PW, Jones HA, Nosil J, Obdrzalek J, Hughes JMB. Uneven perfusion and ventilation within lung regions studied with nitrogen-13. *Respir Physiol* 1978; **34**: 45–59.

Haldane JS. *Respiration*. New Haven, CT: Yale University Press, 1922.

Harf A, Pratt T, Hughes JMB. Regional distribution of $\dot{V}_A/\dot{Q}$ in man at rest and with exercise measured with krypton-81m. *J Appl Physiol* 1978; **44**: 115–123.

Hoffbrand BI. The expiratory capnogram: a measure of ventilation-perfusion equalities. *Thorax* 1966; **21**: 518–523.

Harris EA, Seelye ER, Whitlock RML. Gas exchange during exercise in healthy people. II Venous admixture. *Clin Sci* 1976; **51**: 335–344.

Holland J, Milic-Emili J, Macklem PT, Bates DV. Regional distribution of pulmonary ventilation and perfusion in elderly subjects. *J Clin Invest* 1968; **47**: 81–92.

Hughes JMB. Lung gas tensions and active regulation of ventilation/perfusion ratios in health and disease. *Br J Dis Chest* 1975; **69**: 153–170.

Jones NL, McHardy GJR, Naimark A, Campbell EJM. Physiological deadspace and alveolar–arterial gas pressure differences during exercise. *Clin Sci* 1966; **31**: 19–29.

Kaneko K, Milic-Emili J, Dolovich MB, Dawson A, Bates DV. Regional distribution of ventilation and perfusion as a function of body position. *J Appl Physiol* 1966; **21**: 767–777.

Kety SS. The theory and applications of the exchange of inert gas at the lungs and tissues. *Pharmacol Rev* 1951; **3**: 1–41.

King TKC, Briscoe WA. Blood gas exchange in emphysema: an example illustrating method of calculation. *J Appl Physiol* 1967; **23**: 672–682.

Meade F, Pearl N, Saunders MJ. Distribution of lung function ($\dot{V}_A/\dot{Q}$) in normal subjects deduced from changes in alveolar gas tensions during expiration. *Scand J Respir Dis* 1967; **48**: 354–365.

Michels DB, West JB. Distribution of pulmonary ventilation and perfusion during short periods of weightlessness. *J Appl Physiol* 1978; **45**: 987–998.

Olszowka AJ. Can $\dot{V}_A/\dot{Q}$ distributions in the lung be recovered from inert gas retention data? *Respir Physiol* 1975; **25**: 191–198.

Orphanidou D, Hughes JMB, Meyers MJ, Al-Suhali AR, Henderson B. Tomography of regional ventilation and perfusion using krypton 81m in normal subjects and asthmatic patients. *Thorax* 1986; **41**: 542–551.

Rahn H, Fenn WO. *A Graphical Analysis of the Respiratory Gas Exchange. The O_2–CO_2 Diagram.* Washington, DC: American Physiological Society, 1955.

Riley RL, Cournand A. 'Ideal' alveolar air and the analysis of ventilation–perfusion relationships in the lungs. *J Appl Physiol* 1948–49; **1**: 825–847.

Riley RL, Permutt S. Venous admixture component of the A-aPo_2 gradient. *J Appl Physiol* 1973; **35**: 430–431.

Riley RL, Permutt, S, Said S, Godfrey M, Cheng TO, Howell JBL, Shepard RH. Effect of posture on pulmonary dead space in man. *J Appl Physiol* 1959; **14**: 339–344.

Singleton GJ, Olsen CR, Smith RL. Correction for mechanical deadspace in the calculation of physiological dead space. *J Clin Invest* 1972; **51**: 2768–2772.

22.2 $\dot{V}_A/\dot{Q}$ Multiple inert gas elimination technique (MIGET)
(*see also* sections 32.1, 40 and relevant medical conditions)

Evans JW, Wagner PD. Limits on $\dot{V}_A/\dot{Q}$ distribution from analysis of experimental inert gas elimination. *J Appl Physiol* 1977; **42**: 889–898.

Farhi LE, Olszowka AJ. Analysis of alveolar gas exchange in the presence of soluble inert gases. *Respir Physiol* 1968; **5**: 53–67.

Farhi LE, Yokoyama T. Effects of ventilation–perfusion equality on elimination of inert gases. *Respir Physiol* 1967; **3**: 12–20.

Hlastala MP, Robertson HT. Inert gas elimination characteristics of the normal and abnormal lung. *J Appl Physiol* 1978; **44**: 258–266.

Jaliwala SA, Mates RE, Klocke FJ. An efficient optimization technique for recovering ventilation–perfusion distributions from inert gas data. *J Clin Invest* 1975; **55**: 188–192.

Kapitan KS, Wagner PD. Information content of multiple inert gas elimination measurements. *J Appl Physiol* 1987; **63**: 861–868.

Wagner PD, Laravuso RB, Uhl RR, West JB. Continuous distributions of ventilation–perfusion ratios in normal subjects breathing air and 100% O_2. *J Clin Invest* 1974; **54**: 54–68.

Wagner PD, Saltzman HA, West JB. Measurement of continuous distributions of ventilation–perfusion ratios: theory. *J Appl Physiol* 1974; **36**: 588–599.

Wagner PD. Calculation of the distribution of ventilation–perfusion ratios from inert gas elimination data. *Fed Proc* 1982; **41**: 136–139.

West JB. Ventilation–perfusion inequality and overall gas exchange in computer models of the lung. *Respir Physiol* 1969; **7**: 88–110.

23 ACID–BASE PHYSIOLOGY

(*see also* sections 6.3, 24, 32.1, 40 and medical conditions)

Astrup P, Severinghaus JW. *History of Acid–Base Physiology*. Stockholm: Munksgaard, 1986.

Flenley DC. Another non-logarithmic acid–base diagram? *Lancet* 1971; **i**: 961–965; **ii**: 160–161.

Henderson LJ. *Blood: a Study in General Physiology*. New Haven: Yale University Press, 1928.

Jones NL. *Blood Gases and Acid–Base Physiology*. 2nd ed. New York: Thieme Medical Publishers, 1987.

Peters JP, Van Slyke DD. *Quantitative Clinical Chemistry*, Vol 1, *Interpretations*. Baltimore: Williams & Wilkins, 1931.

Rahn H, Prakash O, eds. *Acid–Base Regulation and Body Temperature*. Boston: Martinus Nijhoff, 1985.

Reeves RB. Temperature-induced changes in blood acid–base status: pH and Pco_2 in a binary buffer. *J Appl Physiol* 1976; **40**: 752–761.

Roughton FJW. Transport of oxygen and carbon dioxide. In: *Handbook of Physiology*, Section 3, *Respiration*, Vol 1. Bethesda MD: American Physiological Society, 1964: 767–825.

Siggaard Andersen O. Blood acid–base alignment nomogram. *Scand J Clin Lab Invest* 1963; **15**: 211–217.

Siggaard Andersen O. The Van Slyke Equation. *Scand J Clin Lab Invest* 1977; **37** Suppl 146: 15–19.

Siggaard Andersen O. The acid–base status of the blood. *Scand J Clin Lab Invest* 1963; **15** Suppl 70: 1–134.

Stewart PA. *How to Understand Acid–Base: a Quantitative Acid–Base Primer for Biology and Medicine*. New York: Elsevier, 1981.

Stewart PA. Modern quantitative acid–base chemistry. *Can J Physiol Pharmacol* 1983; **61**: 1444–1461.

24 EXCHANGE OF GAS WITH BLOOD

(*see also* sections 20, 23, 32.1, 40, 44.4 and medical conditions)

Andersen AM, Ladefoged J. Partition coefficient of [133]Xenon between various tissues and blood *in vivo*. *Scand J Clin Lab Invest* 1967; **19**: 72–78.

Barcroft J. *The Respiratory Function of the Blood. Haemoglobin*, Part 11. London: Cambridge University Press, 1928.

Bencowitz HZ, Wagner PD, West JB. Effect of change in P50 on exercise tolerance at high altitude: a theoretical study. *J Appl Physiol* 1982; **53**: 1487–1495.

Briehl RW, Fishman AP. Principles of the Bohr integration procedure and their application to measurement of diffusing capacity of the lung for oxygen. *J Appl Physiol* 1960; **15**: 337–348.

Chinnard FP, Enn T, Nolan MF. The permeability characteristics of the alveolar capillary barrier. *Trans Assoc Am Physicians* 1962; **75**: 253–261.

di Prampero PE, Lafortuna CL. Breath-by-breath estimate of alveolar gas transfer variability in man at rest and during exercise. *J Physiol* 1989; **415**: 459–475.

Douglas AR, Jones NL, Reed JW. Calculation of whole blood CO_2 content. *J Appl Physiol* 1988; **65**: 473–477.

Effros RM, Mason GR. Measurements of pulmonary epithelial permeability *in vivo*. *Am Rev Respir Dis* 1983; **127**: S59–S65.

Forster RE, Crandall ED. Time course of exchanges between red cells and extracellular fluid during CO_2 uptake. *J Appl Physiol* 1975; **38**: 710–718.

Garby L, DeVerdier C-H. Affinity of human hemoglobin A to 2,3-diphosphoglycerate. Effect of hemoglobin concentration and of pH. *Scand J Clin Lab Invest* 1971; **27**: 345–350.

Gill SJ, Di Cera E, Doyle ML, Bishop GA, Robert CH. Oxygen binding constants for human hemoglobin tetramers. *Biochemistry* 1987; **26**: 3995–4002.

Grant BJB. Influence of Bohr-Haldane effect on steady-state gas exchange. *J Appl Physiol* 1982; **52**: 1330–1337.

Gregory IC. The oxygen and carbon monoxide capacities of foetal and adult blood. *J Physiol (Lond)* 1974; **236**: 625–634.

Hardewig A, Rochester DF, Briscoe WA. Measurement of solubility coefficients of krypton in water, plasma and human blood, using radioactive Kr[85]. *J Appl Physiol* 1960; **15**: 723–725.

Hebbel RP, Eaton JW, Kronenberg RS, Zanjani ED, Moore LG, Berger EM. Human llamas. Adaptation to altitude in subjects with high hemoglobin oxygen affinity. *J Clin Invest* 1978; **62**: 593–600.

Hill EP, Power GG, Longo LD. Mathematical simulation of pulmonary O_2 and CO_2 exchange. *Am J Physiol* 1973; **224**: 904–917.

Hlastala MP. Significance of the Bohr and Haldane effects in the pulmonary capillary. *Respir Physiol* 1973; **17**: 81–92.

Holland RAB, Shibata H, Scheid P, Piiper J. Kinetics of O_2 uptake and release by red cells in stopped-flow apparatus: effects of unstirred layer. *Respir Physiol* 1985; **59**: 71–91.

Holland RAB, van Hezewijk W, Zubzanda J. Velocity of oxygen uptake by partly saturated adult and fetal human red cells. *Respir Physiol* 1977; **29**: 303–314.

Huxley VH, Kutchai H. The effect of the red cell membrane and a diffusion boundary layer on the rate of oxygen uptake by human erythrocytes. *J Physiol* 1981; **316**: 75–83.

Hyde RW, Puy RJM, Raub WF, Forster RE. Rate of disappearance of labelled carbon dioxide from the lungs of humans during breath holding: a method for studying the dynamics of pulmonary CO_2 exchange. *J Clin Invest* 1968; **47**: 1535–1552.

Jameson AG. Gaseous diffusion from alveoli into pulmonary arteries. *J Appl Physiol* 1964; **19**: 448–456.

Kagawa T, Mochizuki M. Numerical solution of partial differential equation describing oxygenation rate of the red blood cell. *Jpn J Physiol* 1982; **32**: 197–218.

Kanber GJ, King FW, Eshchar YR, Sharp JT. The alveolar–arterial oxygen gradient in young and elderly men during air and oxygen breathing. *Am Rev Respir Dis* 1968; **97**: 376–381.

Kelman GR. Digital computer procedure for the conversion of Pco_2 into blood CO_2 content. *Respir Physiol* 1967; **3**: 111–116.

Kelman GR. Digital computer subroutine for the conversion of oxygen tension into saturation. *J Appl Physiol* 1966; **21**: 1375–1376.

Kilmartin JV, Rossi-Bernardi L. Interaction of hemoglobin with hydrogen ions, carbon dioxide, and organic phosphates. *Physiol Rev* 1973; **53**(4): 836–890.

Klocke RA. Carbon dioxide transport. In: Farhi LE, Tenney SM, eds. *Handbook of Physiology*, Section 3, Vol 4, *Gas Exchange*. Bethesda, MD: American Physiological Society, 1987: 173–197.

Kreuzer F, Hoofd L. Facilitated diffusion of oxygen and carbon dioxide. In: Farhi LE, Tenney SM, eds. *Handbook of Physiology*. Section 3, Vol 4, *Gas Exchange*. Bethesda MD: American Physiological Society, 1987: 89–111.

Kvale PA, Davis J, Schroter RC. Effect of gas density and ventilatory pattern on steady-state CO uptake by the lung. *Respir Physiol* 1975; **24**: 385–398.

Lin KM, Cumming G. A model of time-varying gas exchange in the human lung during a respiratory cycle at rest. *Respir Physiol* 1973; **17**: 93–112.

McHardy GJR. The relationship between the differences in pressure and content of carbon dioxide in arterial and venous blood. *Clin Sci* 1967; **32**: 299–309.

Mellemgaard K. The alveolar–arterial oxygen difference: its size and components in normal man. *Acta Physiol Scand* 1966; **67**: 10–20.

Mochizuki M. Oxygenation velocity of the red cell and pulmonary diffusing capacity. In: Hershey D, ed. *Blood Oxygenation*. New York: Plenum Press, 1970: 24–61.

Niizeki K, Mochizuki M, Kagawa T. Secondary CO_2 diffusion following HCO_3^- shift across the red blood cell membrane. *Jpn J Physiol* 1984; **34**: 1003–1013.

Olszowka AJ, Farhi LE. A system of digital computer subroutines for blood gas calculations. *Respir Physiol* 1968; **4**: 270–280.

Perrella M. Intermediate compounds between hemoglobin and CO under equilibrium and kinetic conditions. In: *Symposium on Oxygen Binding Heme Proteins*. Pacific Grove, CA: Alisomar, 1988: PV 1–8.

Perutz MF. Molecular anatomy, physiology, and pathology of hemoglobin. In: Stamatoyannopoulos G, Nienhuis AW, Leder P, Majerus PW, eds. *The Molecular Basis of Blood Disease*. Philadelphia: WB Saunders, 1987: 127–178.

Piiper J. Blood-gas equilibrium of carbon dioxide in lungs: a continuing controversy. *J Appl Physiol* 1986; **60**: 1–8.

Purcell Y, Brozovic B. Red cell 2,3-diphosphoglycerate concentration in man decreases with age. *Nature (Lond)* 1974; **251**: 511–512.

Raine JM, Bishop JM. A-a difference in O_2 tension and physiological dead space in normal man. *J Appl Physiol* 1963; **18**: 284–288.

Robert M. Affinité de l'hémoglobine pour l'oxygène. *Bull Physiopathol Respir* 1975; **11**: 79–170.

Rørth M, Astrup P, eds. *Oxygen Affinity of Hemoglobin and Red Cell Acid Base Status*. Copenhagen: Munksgaard, 1972. See in particular article by FJW Roughton *et al*.

Rotman H, Ikeda I, Chiu CS, Kramer E, Aminoff D. Resistance of red blood cell membrane to oxygen uptake. *J Appl Physiol* 1980: **49**: 306–310.

Schuster KD. Kinetics of pulmonary CO_2 transfer studied by using labelled carbon dioxide $C^{16}O^{18}O$. *Respir Physiol* 1985; **60**: 21–37.

Sirs JA. The egress of oxygen from human HbO_2 in solution and in the erythrocyte. *J Physiol* 1967; **89**: 461–473.

Sirs JA. The Bohr effect on the reaction of carbon monoxide with fully oxygenated haemoglobin. *J Physiol (Lond)* 1976; **263**: 475–488.

Sorbini CA, Grassi V, Solinas E *et al*. Arterial oxygen tension in relation to age in healthy subjects. *Respiration* 1968; **25**: 3–13.

Taylor AE, Gaar KA. Estimation of equivalent pore radii of pulmonary capillary and alveolar membranes. *Am J Physiol* 1970; **218**: 1133–1140.

Weibel ER. Morphological basis of alveolar–capillary gas exchange. *Physiol Rev* 1973; **53**: 419–495.

Whittenberg JB. Myoglobin-facilitated oxygen diffusion: role of myoglobin in oxygen entry into muscle. *Physiol Rev* 1970; **50**: 559–636.

Winslow RM, Samaja M, Winslow NJ, Rossi-Bernardi L, Shrager RI. Simulation of continuous blood O_2 equilibrium curve over the physiological pH, DPG and Pco_2 range. *J Appl Physiol* 1983; **54**: 524–529.

Yamaguchi K, Nguyen-Phu D, Scheid P, Piiper J. Kinetics of O_2 uptake and release by human erythrocytes studied by a stopped-flow technique. *J Appl Physiol* 1985; **58**: 1215–1224.

Zwart A, Kwant G, Oeseburg B, Zijlstra WG. Human whole-blood oxygen affinity: effect of carbon monoxide. *J Appl Physiol* 1984; **57**: 14–20.

25.1 General
(*see also* sections 5, 32.1, 40, 44.3)

Bachofen H, Weber J, Wangensteen D, Weibel ER. Morphometric estimates of diffusing capacity in lungs fixed under zone II and zone III conditions. *Respir Physiol* 1983; **52**: 41–52.

Burrows B, Kasik JE, Niden AH, Barclay WR. Clinical usefulness of the single-breath pulmonary diffusing capacity test. *Am Rev Respir Dis* 1961; **84**: 789–806.

Cassidy SS, Ramanathan M, Rose GL, Johnson RL Jr. Hysteresis in the relation between diffusing capacity of the lung and lung volume. *J Appl Physiol* 1980; **49**: 566–570.

Chinet A, Micheli JL, Haab P. Inhomogeneity effects on O_2 and CO pulmonary diffusing capacity estimates by steady-state methods. Theory. *Respir Physiol* 1971; **13**: 1–22.

Cross CE, Gong H Jr, Kurpershoeck CJ, Gillespie JR, Hyde RW. Alterations in distribution of blood flow to the lung's diffusion surfaces during exercise. *J Clin Invest* 1973; **52**: 414–421.

Federspiel WJ. Pulmonary diffusing capacity: implications of two-phase blood flow in capillaries. *Respir Physiol* 1989; **77**: 119–134.

Finley TN, Swenson EW, Comroe JH Jr. The cause of arterial hypoxaemia at rest in patients with 'alveolar–capillary block syndrome'. *J Clin Invest* 1962; **41**: 618–622.

Forster RE. Exchange of gases between alveolar air and pulmonary capillary blood: pulmonary diffusing capacity. *Physiol Rev* 1957; **37**: 391–452.

Gonzalez Mangado N, Barbera Mir JA, Peces-Barba G, Vallejo Galbete J, Lahoz Navarro F. Pulmonary parenchymal tissue volume and pulmonary capillary blood flow in normal subjects. *Respiration* 1986; **50**: 9–17.

Hyde RW, Marin MG, Rynes RI, Karreman G, Forster RE. Measurement of uneven distribution of pulmonary blood flow to CO diffusing capacity. *J Appl Physiol* 1971; **31**: 605–612.

Kindig NB, Hazlett DR. Temporal effects in the estimation of pulmonary diffusing capacity. *Q J Exp Physiol* 1977; **62**: 121–132.

Kreukniet J, Visser BF. The pulmonary CO diffusing capacity according to Bates and according to Filley in patients with unequal ventilation. *Pflügers Arch* 1964; **281**: 207–211.

Lilienthal J Jr, Riley RL, Proemmel DD, Franke RE. An experimental analysis in man of the oxygen pressure gradient from alveolar air to arterial blood during rest and exercise at sea level and at altitude. *Am J Physiol* 1946; **147**: 199–216.

Michaelson ED, Sackner MA, Johnson RL Jr. Vertical distributions of pulmonary diffusing capacity and capillary blood flow in man. *J Clin Invest* 1973; **52**: 359–369.

Piiper J. Apparent increase of the O_2 diffusing capacity with increased O_2 uptake in inhomogeneous lungs: theory. *Respir Physiol* 1969; **6**: 209–218.

Piiper J. Variations of ventilation and diffusing capacity to perfusion determining the alveolar–arterial O_2 difference: theory. *J Appl Physiol* 1961; **16**: 507–510.

Read J, Read DJC, Pain MCF. Influence of non-uniformity of the lungs on measurement of pulmonary diffusing capacity. *Clin Sci* 1965; **29**: 107–118.

Roughton FJW, Forster RE. Relative importance of diffusion and chemical reaction rates in determining rate of exchange of gases in the human lung, with special reference to true diffusing capacity of pulmonary membrane and volume of blood in the lung capillaries. *J Appl Physiol* 1957; **11**: 290–302.

Scheid P, Piiper J. Blood gas equilibrium in lungs and pulmonary diffusing capacity. In: Chang HK, Paiva M, eds. *Respiratory Physiology an Analytical Approach*. New York: Marcel Dekker, 1989: 453–497.

Staub NC. Alveolar–arterial oxygen tension gradient due to diffusion. *J Appl Physiol* 1963; **18**: 673–680.

Staub N, Bishop JM, Forster RE. Importance of diffusion and chemical reaction rates in O_2 uptake in the lung. *J Appl Physiol* 1962; **17**: 21–27.

Wagner PD. Diffusion and chemical reaction in pulmonary gas exchange. *Physiol Rev* 1977; **57**: 257–312.

25.2 Measurement of transfer factor
(*see also* sections 6.2, 22.2, 24)

Adaro F, Meyer M, Sikand RS. Rebreathing and single breath pulmonary CO diffusing capacity in man at rest and exercise studied by $C^{18}O$ isotope. *Bull Eur Physiopathol Respir* 1976; **12**: 747–756.

American Thoracic Society. Single breath carbon monoxide diffusing capacity (transfer factor). *Am Rev Respir Dis* 1987; **136**: 1299–1307.

Borland C, Cox Y. NO and CO transfer. *Eur Respir J* 1991; **4**: 766–787.

Borland CDR, Cox Y. Effect of varying alveolar oxygen partial pressure on diffusing capacity for nitric oxide and carbon monoxide, membrane diffusing capacity and lung capillary blood volume. *Clin Sci* 1991; **81**: 759–765.

Borland CDR, Higenbottam TW. A simultaneous single breath measurement of pulmonary diffusing capacity with nitric oxide and carbon monoxide. *Eur Respir J* 1989; **2**: 56–63.

Cotes JE, Chinn DJ, Quanjer PhH, Roca J, Yernault J-C. Standardisation of the measurement of transfer factor (diffusing capacity). Report of working party. Standardisation of lung function tests, 1993 update. *Eur Respir J* 1993; **6**, suppl 16: 41–53.

Chinn DJ, Harkawat R, Cotes JE. Standardization of single-breath transfer factor (Tl_{CO}); derivation of breathholding time. *Eur Respir J* 1992; **5**: 492–496.

Cotes JE, Dabbs JM, Elwood PC, Hall AM, McDonald A, Saunders MJ. Iron-deficiency anaemia: its effect on transfer factor for the lung (diffusing capacity) and ventilation and cardiac frequency during submaximal exercise. *Clin Sci* 1972; **42**: 325–335.

Cotes JE, Meade F, Saunders MJ. Effect of volume inspired and manner of sampling the alveolar gas upon components of the transfer factor (diffusing capacity of the lung) by the single breath method. *J Physiol (Lond)* 1965; **181**: 73P–75P.

Crapo RO. Effect of the method of measuring breathholding time on DLCO and DL/VA in normal subjects (abstract). *Am Rev Respir Dis* 1980; **121** (Suppl. 331).

Filley GF, MacIntosh DJ, Wright GW. Carbon monoxide uptake and pulmonary diffusing capacity in normal subjects at rest and during exercise. *J Clin Invest* 1954; **33**: 530–539.

Forster RE, Fowler WS, Bates DV, Van Lingen B. The absorption of carbon monoxide by the lungs during breathholding. *J Clin Invest* 1954; **33**: 1135–1145.

Gaensler EA, Smith AA. Attachment for automated single breath diffusing capacity measurement. *Chest* 1973; **63**: 136–145.

Graham BL, Mink JT, Cotton DJ. Improved accuracy and precision of single-breath CO diffusing capacity measurements. *J Appl Physiol* 1981; **51**: 1306–1313.

Graham BL, Mink JT, Cotton DJ. Overestimation of the single-breath carbon monoxide diffusing capacity in patients with air-flow obstruction. *Am Rev Respir Dis* 1984; **129**: 403–408.

Guenard H, Vuene N, Vaida P. Determination of lung capillary blood volume and membrane diffusing capacity in man by the measurements of NO and CO transfer. *Respir Physiol* 1987; **70**: 113–120.

Hamer NAJ. The effect of age on the components of the pulmonary diffusing capacity. *Clin Sci* 1962; **23**: 85–93.

Hamilton LH, Kersting DJ. A study of gas analysis for measurement of pulmonary diffusing capacity for carbon monoxide by chromatographic techniques. *Am Rev Respir Dis* 1970; **102**: 916–920.

Hammond MD, Hempleman SC. Oxygen diffusing capacity estimates derived from measured $\dot{V}A/\dot{Q}$ distributions in man. *Respir Physiol* 1987; **69**: 129–147.

Hathaway EH, Tashkin DP, Simmons MS. Intra-individual variability in serial measurements of DLCO and alveolar volume over one year in eight healthy subjects using three independent measuring systems. *Am Rev Respir Dis* 1989; **140**: 1818–1822.

Jones RS, Meade F. A theoretical and experimental analysis of anomalies in the estimation of pulmonary diffusing capacity by the single breath method. *Q J Exp Physiol* 1961; **46**: 131–143.

Kreukniet J. Relation between rebreathing CO-diffusing capacity of the lung and unequal ventilation. *Scand J Respir Dis* 1970; **51**: 49–54.

Krogh M. The diffusion of gases through the lungs of man. *J Physiol* 1915; **49**: 271–296.

Leathart GL. Steady-state diffusing capacity determined by a simplified method. *Thorax* 1962; **17**: 302–307.

Leech JA, Martz L, Liben A, Becklake MR. Diffusing capacity for carbon monoxide. The effects of different derivations of breathhold time and alveolar volume and of carbon monoxide back pressure on calculated results. *Am Rev Respir Dis* 1985; **132**: 1127–1129.

Meade F, Saunders MJ, Hyett F, Reynolds JA, Pearl N, Cotes JE. Automatic measurement of lung function. *Lancet* 1965; **ii**: 573–575.

Meyer M, Piiper J. Nitric Oxide (NO), a new test gas for study of alveolar–capillary diffusion. *Eur Respir J* 1989; **2**: 494–496.

Meyer M, Scheid P, Riepl G, Wagner H-J, Piiper J. Pulmonary diffusing capacities for O_2 and CO measured by a rebreathing technique. *J Appl Physiol* 1981; **51**: 1643–1650.

Meyer M, Schuster K-D, Schulz H, Mohr M, Piiper J. Pulmonary diffusing capacities for nitric oxide and carbon monoxide determined by rebreathing in dogs. *J Appl Physiol* 1990; **68**: 2344–2357.

Neville E, Kendrick AH, Gibson GJ. A standardised method of estimating Kco on exercise. *Thorax* 1984; **39**: 823–827.

Ogilvie CM, Forster RE, Blakemore WS, Morton JW. A standardized breathholding technique for the clinical measurement of the diffusing capacity of the lung for carbon monoxide. *J Clin Invest* 1957; **36**: 1–17.

Rosenhamer GJ, Friesen WO, McIlroy MB. A bloodless method for measurement of diffusing capacity of the lungs for oxygen. *J Appl Physiol* 1971; **30**: 603–610.

Sackner MA, Raskin MM, Julien PJ, Aavery WG. Effect of lung volume on steady state pulmonary membrane diffusing capacity and pulmonary capillary blood volume. *Am Rev Respir Dis* 1971; **104**: 408–417.

Van Ganse W, Comhaire F, Van der Straeten M. Residual volume determined by single breath dilution of helium at various apnoea times. *Scan J Respir Dis* 1970; **51**: 73–81.

Zamel N. Use of the RC time constant for CO in the measurement of diffusing capacity. *Am Rev Respir Dis* 1974; **110**: 683–684.

25.3 Some causes of variation in Tl
(see also sections 31, 41, 44.3 and medical conditions, especially 52, 53.4, 54, 57, 63.6)

Bates DV, Varvis CJ, Donevan RE, Christie RV. Variations in the pulmonary capillary blood volume and membrane diffusion component in health and disease. *J Clin Invest* 1960; **39**: 1401–1412.

Bouhuys A, Georg J, Jönsson R, Lundin G, Lindell SE. The influence of histamine inhalation on the pulmonary diffusing capacity in man. *J Physiol (Lond)* 1960; **152**: 176–181.

Cotes JE, Snidal DP, Shepard RH. Effect of negative intra-alveolar pressure on pulmonary diffusing capacity. *J Appl Physiol* 1960; **15**: 372−376.

Danzer LA, Cohn JE, Zechman FW. Relationship of DM and Vc to pulmonary diffusing capacity during exercise. *Respir Physiol* 1968; **5**: 250−258.

Ewan PW, Jones HA, Rhodes CG, Hughes JMB. Detection of intrapulmonary hemorrhage with carbon monoxide uptake. Application in Goodpasture's syndrome. *New Engl J Med* 1976; **295**: 1391−1396.

Freyschuss U, Holmgren A. On the variation of D$_{LCO}$ with increasing oxygen uptake during exercise in healthy ordinarily untrained young men and women. *Acta Physiol Scand* 1965; **65**: 193−206.

Greening AP, Hughes JMB. Serial estimations of carbon monoxide diffusing capacity in intrapulmonary haemorrhage. *Clin Sci* 1981; **60**: 507−512.

Johnson RL, Taylor HF, Lawson WH Jr. Maximal diffusing capacity of the lung for carbon monoxide. *J Clin Invest* 1965; **44**: 349−355.

Kendrick AH, Laszlo G. CO transfer factor on exercise: age and sex differences. *Eur Respir J* 1990; **3**: 323−328.

Kuwahira I, Ide M, Suzuki Y, Ohta Y, Yamabayashi H. Effect of cold pressor test on carbon monoxide diffusing capacity in normal subjects. *Respiration* 1989; **56**: 87−93.

Pande JN, Gupta SP, Guleria JS. Clinical significance of the measurement of membrane diffusing capacity and pulmonary capillary blood volume. *Respiration* 1975; **32**: 317−324.

Reuschlein PS, Reddan WG, Burpee J, Gee JBL, Rankin J. Effect of physical training on the pulmonary diffusing capacity during submaximal work. *J Appl Physiol* 1968; **24**: 152−158.

Riley RL, Shepard RH, Cohn JE, Carroll DG, Armstrong BW. Maximal diffusing capacity of the lungs. *J Appl Physiol* 1954; **6**: 573−587.

Ross JC, Ley GD, Coburn RF, Eller JL, Forster RE. Influence of pressure suit inflation on pulmonary diffusing capacity in man. *J Appl Physiol* 1962; **17**: 259−262.

Stam H, Kreuzer FJA, Versprille A. Effect of lung volume and positional changes on pulmonary diffusing capacity and its components. *J Appl Physiol* 1991; **71**: 1477−1488.

Sundström G. Influence of body position on pulmonary diffusing capacity in young and old men. *J Appl Physiol* 1975; **38**: 418−423.

26 SOME EFFECTS OF CARBON MONOXIDE

Astrup P, Pauli HG. A comparison of prolonged exposure to carbon monoxide and hypoxia in man. *Scand J Clin Lab Invest* 1968; **22**(Suppl. 103): 1−71.

Bartlett D. Pathophysiology of exposure to low concentrations of carbon monoxide. *Arch Environ Health* 1968; **16**: 719−727.

Beard RR, Wertheim GA. Behavioural impairment associated with small doses of carbon monoxide. *Am J Publ Health* 1967; **57**: 2012−2022.

Hogan MC, Bebout DE, Gray AT, Wagner PD, West JB, Haab PE. Muscle maximal O$_2$ uptake at constant O$_2$ delivery with and without CO in the blood. *J Appl Physiol* 1990; **69**: 830−836.

Horvath SM, Raven PB, Dahms TE, Gray DJ. Maximal aerobic capacity at different levels of carboxyhemoglobin. *J Appl Physiol* 1975; **38**: 300−303.

Perrella M, Sabbioneda L, Samaja M, Rossi-Bernardi L. The intermediate compounds between human hemoglobin and carbon monoxide at equilibrium and during approach to equilibrium. *J Biol Chem* 1986; **261**: 8391−8396.

Ramsey JM. Carbon monoxide, tissue hypoxia and sensory psychomotor response in hypoxaemic subjects. *Clin Sci* 1972; **42**: 619−625.

Rawbone RG, Coppin CA, Guz A. Carbon monoxide in alveolar air as an index of exposure to cigarette smoke. *Clin Sci* 1976; **51**: 495−501.

Roughton FJW, Darling RC. The effect of carbon monoxide on the oxyhemoglobin dissociation curve. *Am J Physiol* 1944; **141**: 17−31.

Santiago TV, Edelman NH. Mechanism of the ventilatory response to carbon monoxide. *J Clin Invest* 1976; **57**: 977−986.

Stewart RD. The effect of carbon monoxide on humans. *J Occup Med* 1976; **18**: 304−309.

27 CONTROL OF RESPIRATION

27.1 General
(*see also* sections 14, 31, 34.1)

Bates JHT, Milic-Emili J. Breathing patterns and the concepts of minimum respiratory work and minimum effort. In: von Euler C, Lazercrantz H, eds. *Neurobiology of the Control of Breathing*. New York: Raven Press, 1986: 243−249.

Dejours P. La regulation de la ventilation au cours de l'exercise musculaire chez l'homme. *J Physiol (Paris)* 1959; **51**: 163−261.

Eldridge FL, Millhorn DE, Kiley JP, Waldrop TG. Stimulation by central command of locomotion, respiration and circulation during exercise. *Respir Physiol* 1985; **59**: 313−337.

Fleming PJ, Levine MR, Long AM, Cleave JP. Postneonatal development of respiratory oscillations. *Ann NY Acad Sci* 1988; **533**: 305−313.

Hornbein TF, ed. *Regulation of Breathing. Lung Biology in Health and Disease, 12*. New York: Marcel Dekker, 1981.

Khoo MCK, Yamashiro SM. Models of control of breathing. In: Chang HK, Paiva M, eds. *Respiratory Physiology: an Analytical Approach*. New York: Marcel Dekker, 1989: 799−829.

Longobardo CS, Cherniack NS, Gothe B. Factors affecting respiratory system stability. *Ann Biomed Eng* 1989; **17**: 377−396.

Lourenço RV, ed. Clinical methods for the study of regulation of breathing. *Chest* 1976; **70**: 109−195.

Pallot DJ, ed. *Control of Respiration*. London: Croom Helm, 1983.

Swanson CD, Grodins FS, eds. *Respiratory Control: Modelling Perspective*. New York: Plenum Press, 1990.

Whipp BJ, ed. *The Control of Breathing in Man. Physiological Society Study Guides 3*. Manchester: University Press, 1987.

27.2 Central chemical and thermal mechanisms

Adams M, Chonan T, Cherniack NS, Euler C von. Effects on respiratory pattern of focal cooling in the medulla of the dog. *J Appl Physiol* 1988; **65**: 2004−2010.

Bligh J, Cottle WH, Maskrey M. Influence of ambient temperature on the thermoregulatory responses to 5-hydroxytryptamine, noradrenaline and acetylcholine injected into the lateral cerebral ventricles of sheep, goats and rabbits. *J Physiol* 1971; **212**: 377−392.

Bloom FE. Neurotransmitters: past, present and future directions. *FASEB J* 1988; **21**: 32−41.

Bonora M, Gautier H. Role of dopamine and arterial chemoreceptors in thermal tachypnea in conscious cats. *J Appl Physiol* 1990; **69**: 1429−1434.

Bruce EN, Cherniack NS. Central chemoreceptors. *J Appl Physiol* 1987; **62**: 389−402.

Doblar D, Santiago TV, Edelman NH. Correlation between ventilatory and cerebrovascular responses to inhalation of CO_2. *J Appl Physiol* 1977; **43**: 455−462.

Fencl V, Gabel RA, Wolfe D. Composition of cerebral fluids in goats adapted to high altitude. *J Appl Physiol* 1979; **47**: 508−513.

Frankel H, Kazemi H. Regulation of CSF composition-blocking chloride-bicarbonate exchange. *J Appl Physiol* 1983; **55**: 177−182.

Hutt DA, Parisi RA, Santiago TV, Edelman NH. Brain hypoxia preferentially stimulates genioglossal EMG responses to CO_2. *J Appl Physiol* 1989; **66**: 51−56.

Irsigler GB, Stafford MJ, Severinghaus JW. Relationship of CSF pH, O_2, and CO_2 responses in metabolic acidosis and alkalosis in humans. *J Appl Physiol* 1980; **48**: 355−361.

Javaheri S, Kazemi H. Metabolic alkalosis and hypoventilation in humans. *Am Rev Respir Dis* 1987; **136**: 1011−1016.

Johnson DC, Singer S, Hoop B, Kazemi H. Chloride flux from blood to CSF: inhibition by furosemide and bumetanide. *J Appl Physiol* 1987; **63**: 1591−1600.

Kaminski RP, Forster HV, Bisgard GE, Pan LG, Dorsey SM. Effect of altered ambient temperature on breathing in ponies. *J Appl Physiol* 1985; **58**: 1585−1591.

Kiley JP, Eldridge FL, Milhorn DE. The roles of medullary extracellular and cerebrospinal fluid pH in control of respiration. *Respir Physiol* 1985; **59**: 117−130.

Loeschcke HH. Review lecture: central chemosensitivity and the reaction theory. *J Physiol (Lond)* 1982; **332**: 1−24.

Melton JE, Neubauer JA, Edelman NH. GABA antagonism reverses hypoxic respiratory depression in the cat. *J Appl Physiol* 1990; **69**: 1296−1301.

Millhorn DE, Eldridge FL. Role of ventrolateral medulla in regulation of respiratory and cardiovascular systems. *J Appl Physiol* 1986; **61**: 1249−1263.

Millhorn DE, Hokfelt T. Chemical messengers and their coexistence in individual neurons. *News Physiol Sci* 1988; **3**: 1−5.

Nattie EE, Wood J, Mega A, Goritski W. Rostral ventrolateral medulla muscarinic receptor involvement in central ventilatory chemosensitivity. *J Appl Physiol* 1989; **66**: 1462−1470.

Neubauer JA, Simone A, Edelman NH. Role of brain lactic acidosis in hypoxic depression of respiration. *J Appl Physiol* 1988; **65**: 1324−1331.

Nishimura M, Johnson DC, Hitzig BM, Okunieff P, Kazemi H. Effects of hypercapnia on brain pHi and phosphate metabolite regulation by 31P-NMR. *J Appl Physiol* 1989; **66**: 2181−2188.

Read DJC, Leigh J. Blood−brain tissue P_{CO_2} relationships and ventilation during rebreathing. *J Appl Physiol* 1967; **23**: 53−70.

Santiago TV, Edelman NH. Opioids and breathing. *J Appl Physiol* 1985; **59**: 1675−1685.

Santiago TV, Remolina C, Scoles V, III, Edelman NH. Endorphins and the control of breathing. Ability of naloxone to restore flow-resistive load compensation in chronic obstructive pulmonary disease. *N Engl J Med* 1981; **304**: 1190−1195.

Yamada KA, Norman WP, Hamosh P, Gillis RA. Medullary ventral surface GABA receptors affect respiratory and cardio vascular function. *Brain Res* 1982; **248**: 71−78.

Younes M. The physiologic basis of central apnea and periodic breathing. *Curr Pulmonol* 1989; **10**: 265−326.

27.3 Carotid body mechanisms
(*see also* sections 31.2, 34.2, 40, 54)

Acker H. P_{O_2} chemoreception in arterial chemoreceptors. *Ann Rev Physiol* 1989; **51**: 835−844.

Asmussen E, Nielsen M. Pulmonary ventilation and effect of oxygen breathing in heavy exercise. *Acta Physiol Scand* 1958; **43**: 365−378.

Band DM, Linton RAF, Kent R, Kurer FL. The effect of peripheral chemodenervation on the ventilatory response to potassium. *Respir Physiol* 1985; **60**: 217−225.

Bascom DA, Clement ID, Cunningham DA, Friedland JS, Paterson DJ, Robbins PA. Changes in arterial plasma potassium $[K^+]_a$ and ventilation ($\dot{V}_A$) during exercise in subjects with McArdle's syndrome. *J Physiol (Lond)* 1989; **417**: 141P.

Biscoe TJ, Duchen MR. The cellular basis of transduction in carotid chemoreceptors. *Am J Physiol* 1990; **258**: 271−278.

Biscoe TJ, Purves MJ. Observations on the rhythmic variation in the cat carotid body chemoreceptor activity which has the same period as respiration. *J Physiol (Lond)* 1967; **190**: 389–412.

Bisgard G, Forster HV, Mesina J, Sarazin RG. Role of the carotid body in hyperpnea of moderate exercise in goats. *J Appl Physiol* 1986; **52**: 1216–1222.

Black AMS, Goodman NW, Nail BS, Rao PS, Torrance RW. The significance of the timing of chemoreceptor impulses for their effect upon respiration. *Acta Neurobiol Exp* 1973; **33**: 139–147.

Byrne-Quinn E, Sodal IE, Weil JV. Hypoxic and hypercapnic ventilatory drives in children native to high altitude. *J Appl Physiol* 1972; **32**: 44–46.

Byrne-Quinn E, Weil JV, Sodal IE, Filley GF, Grover RF. Ventilatory control in the athlete. *J Appl Physiol* 1971; **30**: 91–98.

Cosgrove JF, Neuburger N, Bryan MH, Bryan AC, Levison H. A new method of evaluating the chemosensitivity of the respiratory center in children. *Pediatrics* 1975; **56**: 972–980.

Cross BA, Davey A, Guz A, Katona PG, Maclean M, Murphy K *et al*. The pH oscillations in arterial blood during exercise: a potential signal for the ventilatory response in the dog. *J Physiol (Lond)* 1982; **329**: 57–73.

Cummin ARC, Alison J, Jacobi MS, Iyawe VI, Saunders KB. Ventilatory sensitivity to inhaled carbon dioxide around the control point during exercise. *Clin Sci* 1986; **71**: 17–22.

Cunningham DJC, Hey EN, Lloyd BB. The effect of intravenous infusion of noradrenaline on the respiratory response to carbon dioxide. *Q J Exp Physiol* 1958; **43**: 394–399.

Cunningham DJC. The control system regulating breathing in man. *Q Rev Biophys* 1973; **6**: 433–483.

Dahan A, DeGoede J, Berkenbosch AAD, Olievier ICW. The influence of oxygen on the ventilatory response to carbon dioxide in man. *J Physiol (Lond)* 1990; **428**: 485–499.

De Castro F. Sur la structure et l'innervation du sinus carotidien de l'homme et des mammiferes. Nouveaux faits sur l'innervation et la fonction du glomus caroticum. Etudes anatomiques et physiologiques. *Trab Lab Invest Biol Univ Madrid* 1940; **32**: 297–384.

Easton PA, Anthonisen NR. Carbon dioxide effects on the ventilatory response to sustained hypoxia. *J Appl Physiol* 1988; **64**: 1451–1456.

Edstrom H, Choslovsky S, Cherniack RM. The effect of lung volume on the ventilatory response to CO_2 during resistive loading in normal subjects. *Am Rev Respir Dis* 1976; **114**: 761–766.

Eyzaguirre C, Fidone SJ, Fitzgerald RS, Lahiri S, McDonald DM, eds. *Arterial Chemoreception*. New York: Springer-Verlag, 1990.

Forster HV, Pan LG, Bisgard GE, Kaminski RP, Dorsey SM, Busch AM. Hyperpnea of exercise at various P_{I,O_2} in normal and carotid body denervated ponies. *J Appl Physiol* 1983; **54**: 1387–1393.

Gardner WN. The pattern of breathing following step changes of alveolar partial pressure of carbon dioxide and oxygen in man. *J Physiol (Lond)* 1980; **300**: 55–73.

Griffiths TL, Warren SJ, Chant ADB, Holgate ST. Ventilatory effects of hypoxia and adenosine infusion in patients after bilateral carotid endarterectomy. *Clin Sci* 1990; **78**: 25–31.

Lahiri S, Penney DG, Mokashi A, Albertine KH. Chronic CO inhalation and carotid body catecholamines: testing of hypothesis. *J Appl Physiol* 1989; **67**: 239–242.

Leitch AG, Clancy LJ, Costello JF, Flenley DC. Effect of intravenous infusion of salbutamol on ventilatory response to carbon dioxide and hypoxia and on heart rate and plasma potassium in normal man. *Br Med J* 1976; **1**: 365–367.

Linton RAF, Poole-Wilson PA, Davies RJ, Cameron IR. A comparison of the ventilatory response to carbon dioxide by steady-state and rebreathing methods during metabolic acidosis and alkalosis. *Clin Sci* 1973; **45**: 239–249.

Lloyd BB, Jukes MGM, Cunningham DJC. The relation between alveolar oxygen pressure and the respiratory response to carbon dioxide in man. *Q J Exp Physiol* 1958; **43**: 214–227.

Lopez-Barneo J, Lopez-Lopez JR, Urena J, Gonzalez C. Chemotransduction in the carotid body: K^+ current modulated by P_{O_2} in type 1 chemoreceptor cells. *Science* 1988; **241**: 580–582.

McCoy M, Hargreaves M. Potassium and ventilation during incremental exercise in trained and untrained men. *J Appl Physiol* 1992; **73**: 1287–1290.

Matthews AW, Howell JBL. Assessment of the responsiveness to carbon dioxide in patients with chronic airways obstruction by rate of isometric inspiratory pressure development. *Clin Sci* 1976; **50**: 199–205.

Maxwell DL, Clahal P, Nolop KB, Hughes JMB. Somatostatin inhibits the ventilatory response to hypoxia in humans. *J Appl Physiol* 1986; **60**: 997–1002.

Obeso A, Gonzalez C, Dinger B, Fidone S. Metabolic activation of carotid body glomus cells by hypoxia. *J Appl Physiol* 1989; **67**: 484–487.

Paterson DJ. Potassium and ventilation in exercise. *J Appl Physiol* 1992; **72**: 811–820.

Petersen ES, Vejby-Christensen H. Effects of body temperature on ventilatory responses to hypoxia and breathing pattern in man. *J Appl Physiol* 1977; **42**: 492–500.

Powers SK, Beadle RE, Thompson D, Lawler J. Ventilatory and blood gas dynamics at onset and offset of exercise in the pony. *J Appl Physiol* 1987; **62**: 141–148.

Rebuck AS, Campbell EJM. A clinical method for assessing the ventilatory response to hypoxia. *Am Rev Respir Dis* 1974; **109**: 345–350.

Rebuck AS, Rigg JRA, Saunders NA. Respiratory frequency response to progressive isocapnoeic hypoxia. *J Physiol (Lond)* 1976; **258**: 19–31.

Rocher A, Obeso A, Herreros B, Gonzalez C. Activation of the release of dopamine in the carotid body by veratridin. Evidence for the presence of voltage-dependent Na^+ channels in type I cells. *Neurosci Lett* 1988; **94**: 274–278.

Saunders KB. Oscillations of arterial CO_2 tension in a respiratory model: some implications for the control of breathing in exercise. *J Theor Biol* 1980; **84**: 163–179.

Severinghaus JW. Proposed standard determination of ventilatory responses to hypoxia and hypercapnia in man. *Chest* 1976; **70**: 129–131.

Shirahata M, Andronikou S, Lahiri S. Differential effects of oligomycin on carotid chemoreceptor responses to O_2 and CO_2 in the cat. *J Appl Physiol* 1987; **63**: 2084–2092.

Stockley RA, Lee KD. Estimation of the resting reflex hypoxic drive to respiration in patients with diffuse pulmonary infiltration. *Clin Sci* 1976; **50**: 109–114.

Strachova Z, Plum F. Reproducibility of the rebreathing carbon dioxide response test using an improved method. *Am Rev Respir Dis* 1973; **107**: 864–869.

Weil JV, Byrne-Quinn E, Sodal IE, Kline JS, McCullough RE, Filley GF. Augmentation of chemosensitivity during mild exercise in normal man. *J Appl Physiol* 1972; **33**: 813–819.

West JB, Peters RM Jr, Aksnes G, Maret KH, Milledge JS, Schoene RB. Nocturnal periodic breathing at altitudes of 6300 and 8050 m. *J Appl Physiol* 1986; **61**: 280–287.

Whelan RF, Young IM. The effect of adrenaline and noradrenaline infusions on respiration in man. *Br J Pharmacol* 1953; **8**: 98–102.

White DP, Gleeson K, Pickett CK, Rannels AM, Cymerman A, Weil JV. Altitude acclimatisation: influence on periodic breathing and chemoresponsiveness during sleep. *J Appl Physiol* 1987; **63**: 401–412.

27.4 Neurological control mechanisms
(*see also* sections 59, 60, 61, 67)

Adams L, Frankel H, Garlick J, Guz A, Murphy K, Semple SJG. The role of spinal cord transmission in the ventilatory response to exercise in man. *J Physiol (Lond)* 1984; **355**: 85–97.

Aminoff MJ, Sears TA. Spinal integration of segmental, cortical and breathing inputs to thoracic respiratory motoneurones. *J Physiol (Lond)* 1971; **215**: 557–575.

Anthony R, Dowell AR, Buckley CE III, Cohen R, Whalen RE, Sieker HO et al. Cheyne-Stokes respiration: a review of clinical manifestations and critique of physiological mechanisms. *Arch Intern Med* 1971; **127**(2): 712–726.

Aoki M, Fujito Y, Kurosawa Y, Kawasaki H, Kosaka I. Descending inputs to the upper cervical inspiratory neurons from the medullary respiratory neurons and the raphe nuclei in the cat. In: Sieck GC, Gandevia SC, Cameron WE, eds. *Respiratory Muscles and Their Neuromotor Control*. New York: Raven Press, 1987: 73–82.

Brice AG, Forster HV, Pan LG, Funahashi A, Hoffman MD, Murphy CL, Lowry TF. Is the hyperpnea of muscle contractions critically dependent on spinal afferents? *J Appl Physiol* 1988; **64**: 226–233.

Cherniack NS. The central nervous system and respiratory muscle coordination. *Chest* 1990; **97**(Suppl. 3): 525–575.

Clark FJ, Euler C von. On the regulation of depth and rate of breathing. *J Physiol (Lond)* 1972; **222**: 267–295.

Colebatch JG, Gandevia SC, McCloskey DI. Reduction in inspiratory activity in response to sternal vibration. *Respir Physiol* 1977; **29**: 327–338.

Coleridge JCG, Coleridge HM. Afferent C-fibre innervation of the lungs and airways and its functional significance. *Rev Physiol Biochem Pharmacol* 1984; **99**: 1–110.

Cross BA, Guz A, Jain SK, Archer S, Stevens J, Reynolds F. The effect of anaesthesia on the airway in dog and man: a study of respiratory reflexes, sensation and lung mechanics. *Clin Sci* 1976; **50**: 439–454.

Davies A, Saint 'Ambrogio FB, Saint 'Ambrogio G. Control of postural changes of end expiratory volume (FRC) by airways slowly adapting mechanoreceptors. *Respir Physiol* 1980; **41**: 211–216.

Davis JN, Stagg D. Interrelationships of the volume and time components of individual breaths in resting man. *J Physiol (Lond)* 1975; **245**: 481–498.

Euler C von, Lagercrantz H, eds. *Neurobiology of the Control of Breathing*. New York: Raven Press, 1987.

Frazier DT, Revelette WR. Role of phrenic nerve afferents in the control of breathing. *J Appl Physiol* 1991; **70**: 491–496.

Freyschuss U. Respiratory sinus arrhythmia in man: relation to right ventricular output. *Scand J Clin Lab Invest* 1976; **36**: 407–414.

Gautier H, Bonora M, Gaudy JH. Breuer–Hering inflation reflex and breathing pattern in anesthetized humans and cats. *J Appl Physiol* 1981; **51**: 1162–1168.

Getting PA. Emerging principles governing the operation of neural networks. *Annu Rev Neurosci* 1989; **12**: 185–204.

Guz A, Noble MIM, Trenchard D, Cochrane HL, Makey AR. Studies on the vagus nerve in man: their role in respiratory and circulatory control. *Clin Sci* 1964; **27**: 293–304.

Guz A, Trenchard DW. Pulmonary stretch receptor activity in man: a comparison with dog and cat. *J Physiol (Lond)* 1971; **213**: 329–343.

Hamilton RD, Winning AJ, Horner RL, Guz A. The effect of lung inflation on breathing in man during wakefulness and sleep. *Respir Physiol* 1988; **73**: 145–154.

Head H. On the regulation of respiration. *J Physiol (Lond)* 1889; **10**: 1–71.

Hey EN, Lloyd BB, Cunningham DJC, Jukes MGM, Bolton DPG. Effects of various respiratory stimuli on the depth and frequency of breathing in man. *Respir Physiol* 1966; **1**: 193–205.

John WM St, Hwang Q, Nattie EE, Zhou D. Functions of the retrofacial nucleus in chemosensitivity and ventilatory neurogenesis. *Respir Physiol* 1989; **76**: 159–172.

Kalia MP. Anatomical organization of central respiratory neurons. *Annu Rev Physiol* 1981; **43**: 105–120.

Kao FF. The peripheral neurogenic drive: an experimental study. In: Dempsey JA, Reed CE, eds. *Muscular Exercise and the Lung*. Madison, WI: University of Wisconsin Press, 1979: 71–85.

Kay JDS, Petersen ES, Vejby-Christensen H. Mean and breath-by-breath pattern of breathing in man during steady-state exercise. *J Physiol (Lond)* 1975; **251**: 657–669.

Lee L-Y, Kou YR, Frazier DT, Beck ER, Pisarri TE, Coleridge HM. Stimulation of vagal pulmonary C-fibers by a single breath of cigarette smoke in dogs. *J Appl Physiol* 1989; **66**: 2032–2038.

Lei L, Gang S, Wei-Yang L. Studies on the inspiratory generating effect of the dorso-medial area of nucleus facialis. *Respir Physiol* 1989; **75**: 65–74.

Lumsden T. The regulation of respiration. Part I. *J Physiol (Lond)* 1923; **58**: 81–91.

Mitchell RA, Berger AJ. Neural regulation of respiration. *Am Rev Respir Dis* 1975; **111**: 206–224.

Paintal AS. Vagal sensory receptors and their reflex effects. *Physiol Rev* 1973; **53**: 159–227.

Pisarri TE, Yu J, Coleridge HM, Coleridge JCG. Background activity in pulmonary vagal C-fibers and its effect on breathing. *Respir Physiol* 1986; **64**: 29–43.

Plum F, Brown HW. The effect on respiration of central nervous system disease. *Ann NY Acad Sci* 1963; **109**: 915–931.

Porter R, ed. *Breathing: Hering–Breuer Centenary Symposium*. London: Churchill, 1970: 59–71.

Richter DW, Ballantyne D, Remmers JE. How is the respiratory rhythm generated? A model. *News Physiol Sci* 1986; **1**: 109–112.

Saint 'Ambrogio G. Information arising from the tracheobronchial tree of mammals. *Physiol Rev* 1982; **62**: 531–569.

Sears TE. Efferent discharges in alpha and fusimotor fibres of intercostal nerves of the cat. *J Physiol (Lond)* 1964; **174**: 295–315.

Shea SA, Horner RL, Banner NR, McKenzie E, Heaton R, Yacoub MH, Guz A. The effect of human heart–lung transplantation upon breathing at rest and during sleep. *Resp Physiol* 1988; **72**: 131–150.

Stella G. The reflex response of the 'apneustic' centre to stimulation of the chemoreceptors of the carotid sinus. *J Physiol (Lond)* 1939; **95**: 365–372.

Whitteridge D. Multiple embolism of the lung and rapid shallow breathing. *Physiol Rev* 1950; **30**: 475–486.

Widdicombe JG. Upper airway motor systems. In: Cherniack NS, ed. *Respiratory System 2, Control of Breathing*. Bethesda: American Physiological Society, 1986: 223–246.

Wiley RL, Lind AR. Respiratory responses to sustained static muscular contractions in humans. *Clin Sci* 1971; **40**: 221–234.

28 OXYGEN SUPPLY TO SKELETAL MUSCLE

Andersen P, Saltin B. Maximal perfusion of skeletal muscle in man. *J Physiol (Lond)* 1985; **366**: 233–249.

Booth FW. Effect of limb immobilization on skeletal muscle [Brief review]. *J Appl Physiol* 1982; **52**: 1113–1118.

Broberg S, Sahlin K. Adenine nucleotide degradation in human skeletal muscle during prolonged exercise. *Int J Sports Med* 1990; **11**: S62–S67.

Clark PA, Kennedy SP, Clark A Jr. Buffering of muscle tissue Po_2 levels by the superposition of the oxygen field from many capillaries. *Adv Exp Med Biol* 1989; **248**: 165–174.

Cole RP. Myoglobin function in exercising skeletal muscle. *Science* 1982; **216**: 523–525.

Connett RJ, Gayeski TEJ, Honig CR. Lactate efflux is unrelated to intracellular Po_2 in a working red muscle in situ. *J Appl Physiol* 1986; **61**: 402–408.

Connett RJ, Honig CR, Gayeski TEJ, Brooks GA. Defining hypoxia: a systems view of $\dot{V}o_2$, glycolysis, energetics, and intracellular Po_2. *J Appl Physiol* 1990; **68**: 833–842.

Connett RJ, Honig CR. Regulation of $\dot{V}o_2$ in red muscle: do current biochemical hypotheses fit in vivo data? *Am J Physiol* 1989; **256**: R898–R906.

Ellsworth ML, Pittman RN. Arterioles supply oxygen to capillaries by diffusion as well as by convection. *Am J Physiol* 1990; **258**: H1240–H1243.

Federspiel WJ, Popel AS. A theoretical analysis of the effect of the particulate nature of blood on oxygen release in capillaries. *Microvasc Res* 1986; **32**: 164–189.

Folkow B, Halicka HD. A comparison between 'red' and 'white' muscle with respect to blood supply, capillary surface area and oxygen uptake during rest and exercise. *Microvasc Res* 1968; **1**: 1–14.

Gayeski TEJ, Connett RJ, Honig CR. Minimum intracellular Po_2 for maximum cytochrome turnover in red muscle in situ. *Am J Physiol* 1987; **252**: H906–H915.

Gayeski TEJ, Connett RJ, Honig CR. Oxygen transport in rest–work transition illustrates new functions for myoglobin. *Am J Physiol* 1985; **248**: H914–H921.

Gayeski TEJ, Honig CR. Intracellular Po_2 in long axis of individual fibers in working dog gracilis muscle. *Am J Physiol* 1988; **254**: H1179–H1186.

Gayeski TEJ, Honig CR. O_2 gradients from sarcolemma to cell interior in red muscle at maximal $\dot{V}o_2$. *Am J Physiol* 1986; **251**: H789–H799.

Groebe K, Thews G. Effects of red cell spacing and red cell movement upon oxygen release under conditions of maximally working skeletal muscle. *Adv*

Exp Med Biol 1989; **248**: 175−188.

Gutierrez G, Pohil RJ, Strong R. Effect of flow on O_2 consumption during progressive hypoxemia. *J Appl Physiol* 1988; **65**: 601−607.

Hofman E. The significance of phosphofructokinase to the regulation of carbohydrate metabolism. *Rev Physiol Biochem Pharmacol* 1976; **75**: 1−68.

Hogan MC, Roca J, West JB, Wagner PD. Dissociation of maximal O_2 uptake from O_2 delivery in canine gastrocnemius *in situ. J Appl Physiol* 1989; **66**: 1219−1226.

Hoppeler H, Howald H, Conley K, Lindstedt L, Claassen H, Vock P, Weibel ER. Endurance training in humans: aerobic capacity and structure of skeletal muscle. *J Appl Physiol* 1985; **59**: 320−327.

Ivy JL, Withers RT, Van Handel PJ, Elger DH, Costill DL. Muscle respiratory capacity and fiber type as determinants of the lactate threshold. *J Appl Physiol* 1980; **48**: 523−527.

Kety SS. Determinants of tissue oxygen tension. *Fed Proc* 1957; **16**: 666−670.

Kobayashi H, Pelster B, Piiper J, Scheid P. Significance of the Bohr effect for tissue oxygenation in a model with countercurrent blood flow. *Respir Physiol* 1989; **76**: 277−288.

Krogh A. The number and distribution of capillaries in muscles with calculations of the oxygen pressure head necessary for supplying the tissue. *J Physiol (Lond)* 1918; **52**: 391−408.

Laughlin MH. Skeletal muscle blood flow capacity: role of muscle pump in exercise hyperemia. *Am J Physiol* 1987; **253**: H993−H1004.

Mackie BC, Terjung RL. Blood flow to different skeletal muscle fiber types during contraction. *Am J Physiol* 1983; **245**: H265−H275.

Peachey LD, Adrian RH, Geiger SR, eds. *Handbook of Physiology, Section 10: Skeletal Muscle.* Bethesda, MD: American Physiological Society, 1983: 73−112; 555−631.

Popel AS. Theory of oxygen transport to tissue. *Crit Rev Biomed Eng* 1989; **17**: 257−321.

Schumacker PT, Samsel RW. Analysis of oxygen delivery and uptake relationships in the Krogh tissue model. *J Appl Physiol* 1989; **67**: 1234−1244.

Schwerzmann K, Hoppeler H, Kayar SR, Weibel ER. Oxidative capacity of muscle and mitochondria: correlation of physiological, biochemical and morphometric characteristics. *Proc Natl Acad Sci USA* 1989; **86**: 1583−1587.

Tenney SM. A theoretical analysis of the relationship between venous blood and mean tissue oxygen pressures. *Respir Physiol* 1974; **20**: 283−296.

Wasserman K, Hansen JE, Sue DY. Facilitation of oxygen consumption by lactic acidosis during exercise. *NIPS* 1991; **6**: 29−34.

Wilson DF, Rumsey WL. Factors modulating the oxygen dependence of mitochondrial oxidative phosphorylation. *Adv Exp Med Biol* 1988; **222**: 121−131.

Wittenberg BA, Wittenberg JB. Transport of oxygen in muscle. *Annu Rev Physiol* 1989; **51**: 857−878.

Woledge RC, Curtin NA, Homsher E. *Monographs of the Physiological Society. No. 41: Energetic Aspects of Muscle Contraction.* London: Academic Press, 1985.

29 DYSPNOEA
(*see also* sections 10.3, 31, 32, 64)

Adams L, Guz A. Dyspnoa on exertion. In: Whipp BJ, Wassermann K, eds. *Pulmonary Physiology and Pathophysiology of Exercise.* New York: Marcel Dekker, 1991: 449−494.

Bennett ED, Jayson MIV, Rubenstein D, Campbell EJM. The ability of man to detect added non-elastic loads to breathing. *Clin Sci* 1962; **23**: 155−162.

Bleecker ER, Cotton DJ, Fischer SP, Graf PD, Gold WM, Nadel JA. The mechanism of rapid shallow breathing after inhaled histamine aerosol in exercising dogs. *Am Rev Respir Dis* 1976; **114**: 909−916.

Borg G. A category scale with ratio properties for intermodal and interindividual comparisons. In: Geissler HS, Petzold P, eds. *Psychophysical Judgement and the Process of Perceptions. Proceedings of the 22nd International Congress of Psychology.* Amsterdam: North-Holland, 1980: 25−34.

Burns BH, Howell JBL. Disproportionately severe breathlessness in chronic bronchitis. *Q J Med* 1969; **38**: 277−294.

Campbell EJM, Gandevia SC, Killian KJ, Mahutte CK, Rigg JRA. Changes in the perception of inspiratory resistive loads during partial curarization. *J Physiol (Lond)* 1980; **309**: 93−100.

Campbell EJM, Howell JBL. The sensation of breathlessness. *Br Med Bull* 1963; **19**: 36−40.

Christie RV. Dyspnea. *Q J Med* 1938; **7**: 421−454.

Clark TJH, Freedman S, Campbell EJM, Winn RR. The ventilatory capacity of patients with chronic airways obstruction. *Clin Sci* 1969; **36**: 307−316.

Dales RE, Spitzer WO, Schechter MT, Suissa S. The influence of psychological status on respiratory symptom reporting. *Am Rev Respir Dis* 1989; **139**: 1459−1463.

Davies H, Gazetopoulos N. Dyspnoea in cyanotic congenital heart disease. *Br Heart J* 1965; **27**: 28−41.

Edwards RHT, Melcher A, Hesser CM, Wigertz O, Ekelund G. Physiological correlates of perceived exertion in continuous and intermittent exercise with the same average power output. *Eur J Clin Invest* 1972; **2**: 108−114.

Elliott MW, Adams L, Cockcroft A, Macrae KD, Murphy K, Guz A. The language of breathlessness. Use of verbal descriptors by patients with cardiopulmonary disease. *Am Rev Respir Dis* 1991; **144**: 826−832.

Freedman S, Campbell EJM. The ability of normal subjects to tolerate added inspiratory loads. *Respir Physiol* 1970; **10**: 213−235.

Grimby G, Stiksa J. Flow−volume curves and breathing patterns during exercise in patients with obstructive lung disease. *Scand J Clin Lab Invest* 1970; **25**:

303–313.

Guz A, Noble MIM, Widdicombe JG, Trenchard D, Mushin WW, Makey AR. The role of vagal and glossopharyngeal afferent nerves in respiratory sensation, control of breathing and arterial pressure regulation in conscious man. *Clin Sci* 1966; **30**: 161–170.

Hermansen L, Vokac Z, Lereim P. Respiratory and circulatory response to added air flow resistance during exercise. *Ergonomics* 1972; **15**: 15–24.

Howell JBL, Campbell EJM, eds. *Breathlessness*. Oxford: Blackwell Scientific Publications, 1966.

Johnson BD, Reddan WG, Pegelow DF, Seow KC, Dempsey JA. Flow limitation and regulation of functional residual capacity during exercise in a physically activing aging population. *Am Rev Respir Dis* 1991; **143**: 960–967.

King B, Cotes JE. Relationships of lung function and exercise capacity to mood and attitudes to health. *Thorax* 1989; **44**: 402–409.

Lane R, Adams L, Guz A. The effects of hypoxia and hypercapnia on perceived breathlessness during exercise in humans. *J Physiol* 1990; **428**: 579–593.

Leaver DG, Pride NB. Flow–volume curves and expiratory pressures during exercise in patients with chronic airways obstruction. *Scand J Respir Dis* 1971; **52**(Suppl. 77): 23–27.

Manning HL, Basner R, Ringler J, Rand C, Fencl V, Weinberger SE et al. Effect of chest wall vibration on breathlessness in normal subjects. *J Appl Physiol* 1991; **71**: 175–181.

Marshall R, Stone RW, Christie RV. The relationship of dyspnoea to respiratory effort in normal subjects, mitral stenosis and emphysema. *Clin Sci* 1954; **13**: 625–631.

McCloskey DI. The effects of pre-existing loads upon detection of externally applied resistances to breathing in man. *Clin Sci* 1973; **45**: 561–564.

Noble MIM, Eisele JH, Frankel HL, Else W, Guz A. The role of the diaphragm in the sensation of holding the breath. *Clin Sci* 1971; **41**: 275–283.

Patterson JL Jr, Mullinax PF Jr, Bain T, Kreuger JJ, Richardson DW. Carbon dioxide-induced dyspnea in a patient with respiratory muscle paralysis. *Am J Med* 1962; **32**: 811–816.

Raimondi AC, Edwards RHT, Denison DM, Leaver DG, Spencer RG, Siddorn JA. Exercise tolerance breathing a low density gas mixture, 35% oxygen and air in patients with chronic obstructive bronchitis. *Clin Sci* 1970; **39**: 675–685.

Reed JW, Ablett M, Cotes JE. Ventilatory responses to exercise and to carbon dioxide in mitral stenosis before and after valvulotomy; causes of tachypnoea. *Clin Sci* 1978; **54**: 9–16.

Stevens G, ed. *Psychophysics. Introduction to its Perceptual, Neural and Social Aspects*. New York: Wiley-Interscience, 1975.

Wilson RC, Jones PW. Differentiation between the intensity of breathlessness and the distress it evokes in normal subjects during exercise. *Clin Sci* 1991;

80: 65–70.

Wilson RC, Jones PW. Long-term reproducibility of Borg scale estimates of breathlessness during exercise. *Clin Sci* 1991; **80**: 309–312.

Winning AJ, Hamilton RD, Shea SA, Knott C, Guz A. The effect of airway anaesthesia on the control of breathing and the sensation of breathlessness in man. *Clin Sci* 1985; **68**: 215–225.

Wood MM, McCarthy PE, Cotes JE. Perception of airway resistance in relation to breathlessness on exertion in chronic lung disease. *Scand J Respir Dis* 1971; **52**(Suppl. 77): 98–102.

Zechman FW Jr, Wiley RL. Afferent inputs to breathing: respiratory sensation. In: Cherniack NS, Widdicombe JG, eds. *Handbook of Physiology*, Section 3, Vol 2, *Control of Breathing*. Bethesda: American Physiological Society, 1986: 449–474.

30 EXERCISE TESTING: METHODS

Anderson KL, Shephard RJ, Denolin H, Varnauskas E, Masironi R, Bonjer FH et al. *Fundamentals of Exercise Testing*. Geneva: World Health Organization, 1971.

Auchincloss JH Jr, Gilbert R. Estimation of maximum oxygen uptake with a brief progressive stress test. *J Appl Physiol* 1973; **34**: 525–526.

Bassey EJ, Fentem PH, MacDonald IC, Scriven PM. Self-paced walking as a method for exercise testing in elderly and young men. *Clin Sci* 1976; **51**: 609–612.

Beaver WL, Wasserman K, Whipp BJ. A new method for detecting anaerobic threshold by gas exchange. *J Appl Physiol* 1986; **60**: 2020–2027.

Beaver WL, Wasserman K, Whipp BJ. On-line computer analysis and breath-by-breath graphical display of exercise function tests. *J Appl Physiol* 1973; **34**: 128–132.

Bruce RA. Exercise testing for evaluation of ventricular function. *New Engl J Med* 1977; **296**: 671–675.

Clark JH, Greenleaf JE. Electronic bicycle ergometer: a simple calibration procedure. *J Appl Physiol* 1970; **30**: 440–442.

Cotes JE. Response to progressive exercise: a three-index test. *Br J Dis Chest* 1972; **66**: 169–184.

Froelicher VF, Brammell H, Davis G, Noguera I, Stewart A, Lancaster MC. A comparison of the reproducibility and physiological response to three maximal treadmill exercise protocols. *Chest* 1974; **65**: 512–517.

Jones NL. Exercise testing in pulmonary evaluation: rationale, methods, and the normal respiratory response to exercise. *New Engl J Med* 1975; **293**: 541–544.

McGavin CR, Gupta SP, McHardy GJR. Twelve minute walking test for assessing disability in chronic bronchitis. *Br Med J* 1976; **1**: 822–823.

Miller GJ, Martin H de V. Effect of ambient temperatures between 21°C and 35°C on the responses to progressive submaximal exercise in partially acclimated man. *Ergonomics* 1975; **18**: 539–546.

Nagle FJ, Balke B, Naughton JP. Gradational step tests for assessing work capacity. *J Appl Physiol* 1965; **20**: 745−748.

Pollock ML, Bohannon RL, Cooper KH, Ayres JJ, Ward A, White SR, Linnerud AC. A comparative analysis of four protocols for maximal treadmill stress testing. *Am Heart J* 1976; **92**: 39−46.

Sloan AW. The Harvard step test of dynamic fitness. *Triangle (En)* 1962; **5**: 358−363.

Spiro SG, Juniper E, Bowman P, Edwards RHT. An increasing work rate test for assessing the physiological strain of submaximal exercise. *Clin Sci* 1974; **46**: 191−206.

Takano N. Effects of pedal rate on respiratory responses to incremental bicycle work. *J Physiol (Lond)* 1988; **396**: 389−397.

Taylor HL, Wang Y, Rowell L, Blomqvist G. The standardisation and interpretation of submaximal and maximal tests of working capacity. *Pediatrics* 1963; **32**: 703−722.

Wolthuis RA, Froelicher VF, Fischer J, Noguera I, Davis G, Stewart AJ. New practical treadmill protocol for clinical use. *Am J Cardiol* 1977; **39**: 697−700.

31 PHYSIOLOGICAL RESPONSE TO EXERCISE

31.1 General
(*see also* sections 27−30, 32, 33, 39, 64)

Åstrand P-O, Rodahl K. *Textbook of Work Physiology*, 3rd edn. London: McGraw-Hill, 1986.

Cerretelli P, Di Prampero PE. Gas exchange in exercise. In: Farhi LE, Tenney SM, eds. *Handbook of Physiology*, Section 3, Vol 4, *Gas Exchange*. Bethesda, MD: American Physiological Society, 1987: 297−339.

Cotes JE, Berry G, Burkinshaw L, Davies CTM, Hall AM, Jones PRM, Knibbs AV. Cardiac frequency during submaximal exercise in young adults; relation to lean body mass, total body potassium and amount of leg muscle. *Q J Exp Physiol* 1973; **58**: 239−250.

Cotes JE, Davies CTM. Factors underlying the capacity for exercise: a study in physiological anthropometry. *Proc R Soc Med* 1969; **62**: 620−624.

Cotes JE, Reed JW, Elliott C. Breathing and exercise requirements of the work place. In: Whipp BJ, Wassermann K, eds. *Physiology and Pathophysiology of Exercise*. New York: Marcel Dekker, 1991: 495−548.

Jones NL. *Clinical Exercise Testing*, 3rd edn. Philadelphia; Saunders, 1988.

Reeves JT, Dempsey JA, Grover RF. Pulmonary circulation during exercise. In: Weir EK, Reeves JT, eds. *Pulmonary Vascular Physiology and Pathophysiology*, Vol 38. New York: Marcel Dekker, 1989: 107−133.

Reeves JT, Grover RF, Blount SG Jr, Filley GF. Cardiac output response to standing and treadmill walking. *J Appl Physiol* 1961; **16**: 283−288.

Rowell LB. *Human Circulatory Regulation During Physical Stress*. New York: Oxford University Press, 1986.

Taylor CR, Weibel ER. Design of the mammalian respiratory system. *Respir Physiol* 1981; **44**: 1−164.

Wasserman K, Hansen JE, Sue DY, Whipp BJ. *Principles of Exercise Testing and Interpretation*. Philadelphia: Lee Febiger, 1987.

31.2 Exercise transients

Asmussen E. Ventilation at transition from rest to exercise. *Acta Physiol Scand* 1973; **89**: 68−78.

Banner N, Guz A, Heaton R, Innes JA, Murphy K, Yacoub M. Ventilatory and circulatory responses at the onset of exercise in man following heart or heart−lung transplantation. *J Physiol (Lond)* 1988; **399**: 437−449.

Casaburi R, Barstow TJ, Robinson T, Wasserman K. Influence of work rate on ventilatory and gas exchange kinetics. *J Physiol (Lond)* 1989; **67**: 547−555.

di Prampero PE, Mahler PB, Giezendanner D, Cerretelli P. Effects of priming exercise on $\dot{V}_{O_2}$ kinetics and O_2 deficit at the onset of stepping and cycling. *J Appl Physiol* 1989; **66**: 2023−2031.

Krogh A, Lindhard J. The regulation of respiration and circulation during the initial stages of muscular work. *J Physiol (Lond)* 1913; **47**: 112−136.

Lamarra N, Ward SA, Whipp BJ. Model implications of gas exchange dynamics on blood gases in incremental exercise. *J Appl Physiol* 1989; **66**: 1539−1546.

Mellemgaard K. The alveolar-arterial oxygen difference: its size and components in normal man. *Acta Physiol Scand* 1966; **67**: 10−20.

Ren JM, Broberg S, Salhin K. Oxygen deficit is not affected by the rate of transition from rest to submaximal exercise. *Acta Physiol Scand* 1989; **135**: 545−548.

Weissman ML, Jones PW, Oren A, Lamarra N, Whipp BJ, Wasserman K. Cardiac output increase and gas exchange at the start of exercise. *J Appl Physiol* 1982; **52**: 236−244.

Wheatley JR, Amis TC, Engel LA. Oronasal partitioning of ventilation during exercise in humans. *J Appl Physiol* 1991; **71**: 546−551.

31.3 Submaximal exercise: normal responses
(*see also* section 43.2)

Asmussen E, Nielsen M. Alveolo-arterial gas exchange at rest and during work at different O_2 tensions. *Acta Physiol Scand* 1960; **50**: 153−166.

Bannister RG, Cunningham DJC. The effects on the respiration and performance during exercise of adding oxygen to the inspired air. *J Physiol (Lond)* 1954; **125**: 118−137.

Bevegård S, Freyschuss U, Strandell T. Circulatory adaptation to arm and leg exercise in supine and sitting position. *J Appl Physiol* 1966; **21**: 37−46.

Clifford PS, Litzow JT, von Colditz JH, Coon RL. Effect of chronic pulmonary denervation on ventilatory response to exercise. *J Appl Physiol* 1986; **61**: 603−610.

Clode M, Campbell EJM. The relationship between gas exchange and changes in blood lactate concentrations during exercise. *Clin Sci* 1969; **37**: 263−272.

Cole TJ, Miller GJ. Interpretation of the parameters relating oxygen uptake to heart rate and cardiac output during submaximal exercise. *J Physiol (Lond)* 1973; **231**: 12P−13P.

D'Urzo AD, Jhirad R, Jenne H, Avendano MA, Rubenstein I, D'Costa M, Goldstein RS. Effect of caffeine on ventilatory responses to hypercapnia, hypoxia, and exercise in humans. *J Appl Physiol* 1990; **68**: 322−328.

Dempsey JA, Hanson PG, Henderson KS. Exercise-induced arterial hypoxaemia in healthy human subjects at sea level. *J Physiol (Lond)* 1984; **355**: 161−175.

Di Prampero PE, Davies CTM, Cerretelli P, Margaria R. An analysis of O_2 debt contracted in submaximal exercise. *J Appl Physiol* 1970; **29**: 547−551.

Green HJ, Hughson RL, Orr GW, Ranney DA. Anaerobic threshold, blood lactate and muscle metabolites in progressive exercise. *J Appl Physiol* 1983; **54**: 1032−1038.

Hammond MD, Gale GE, Kapitan KS, Ries A, Wagner PD. Pulmonary gas exchange in humans during exercise at sea level. *J Appl Physiol* 1986; **60**: 1590−1598.

Heigenhauser GJF, Sutton JR, Jones NL. Effect of glycogen depletion on the ventilatory response to exercise. *J Appl Physiol* 1983; **54**: 470−474.

Hirsch GL, Sue DY, Wasserman K, Robinson TE, Hansen JE. Immediate effects of cigarette smoking on cardiorespiratory responses to exercise. *J Appl Physiol* 1985; **58**: 1975−1981.

Holmér I. Physiology of swimming man. *Acta Physiol Scand* 1974; **91**, suppl. 407: 1−55.

Hughson RL, Smyth GA. Slower adaptation of $\dot{V}o_2$ steady state of submaximal exercise with β-blockade. *Eur J Appl Physiol* 1983; **52**: 107−110.

Huszczuk A, Whipp BJ, Adams TD, Fisher AG, Crapo RO, Elliott CG *et al*. Ventilatory control during exercise in calves with artificial hearts. *J Appl Physiol* 1990; **68**: 2604−2611.

Katz A, Sahlin K. Regulation of lactic acid production during exercise. *J Appl Physiol* 1988; **65**: 509−518.

Kozlowski J, Brzezinska Z, Nazar K, Kowalski W, Franczyk M. Plasma catecholamines during sustained isometric exercise. *Clin Sci* 1973; **45**: 723−731.

Mador MJ, Acevedo FA. Effect of respiratory muscle fatigue on breathing pattern during incremental exercise. *Am Rev Respir Dis* 1991; **143**: 462−468.

Nielsen B, Savard G, Richter EA, Hargreaves M, Saltin B. Muscle blood flow and muscle metabolism during exercise and heat stress. *J Appl Physiol* 1990; **69**: 1040−1046.

Oldenburg FA, McCormack DW, Morse JLC, Jones NL. A comparison of exercise responses in stair-climbing and cycling. *J Appl Physiol* 1979; **46**: 510−516.

Patil CP, Saunders KB, Sayers B McA. Timing of deep breaths during rest and light exercise in man. *Clin Sci* 1990; **78**: 573−578.

Roth DA, Stanley WC, Brooks GA. Induced lact-acidemia does not affect post-exercise O_2 consumption. *J Appl Physiol* 1988; **65**: 1045−1049.

Rowell LB, Marx HJ, Bruce RA, Conn RD, Kusumi F. Reductions in cardiac output, central blood volume, and stroke volume with thermal stress in normal men during exercise. *J Clin Invest* 1966; **45**: 1801−1816.

Sharraat MT, Henke KG, Aaron EA, Pegelow DF, Dempey JA. Exercise-induced changes in functional residual capacity. *Respir Physiol* 1987; **70**: 313−326.

Wagner PD, Gillespie JR, Landgren GL, Fedde MR, Jones BW, DeBowes RM *et al*. Mechanism of exercise-induced hypoxemia in horses. *J Appl Physiol* 1989; **66**: 1227−1233.

Wasserman K, Whipp BJ, Koyal SN, Beaver WL. Anaerobic threshold and respiratory gas exchange during exercise. *J Appl Physiol* 1973; **35**: 236−243.

Wasserman K, Whipp BJ, Koyal SN, Cleary MG. Effect of carotid body resection on ventilatory and acid−base control during exercise. *J Appl Physiol* 1975; **39**: 354−358.

Wiley RL, Lind AR. Respiratory responses to simultaneous static and rhythmic exercises in humans. *Clin Sci* 1975; **49**: 427−432.

31.4 Submaximal exercise: medical conditions
(*see also* individual conditions)

Cockcroft AE, Beaumont A, Adams L, Guz A. Arterial oxygen desaturation during treadmill exercise and cycle ergometry in patients with chronic obstructive airways disease. *Clin Sci* 1985; **68**: 327−332.

Hagberg JM, King DS, Rogers MA, Montain SJ, Jilka SM, Kohrt WM, Heller SL. Exercise and recovery ventilatory and $\dot{V}o_2$ responses of patients with McArdle's disease. *J Appl Physiol* 1990; **68**: 1393−1398.

Jones NL, Rebuck AS. Tidal volume during exercise in patients with diffuse fibrosing alveolitis. *Bull Eur Physiopathol Respir* 1979; **15**: 321−327.

Paterson DJ, Friedland JS, Bascom DA, Clement ID, Cunningham DA, Painter R *et al*. Changes in arterial K and ventilation during exercise in normal subjects and subjects with McArdle's syndrome. *J Physiol (Lond)* 1990; **429**: 339−348.

Strieder DJ, Mesko ZG, Zaver AG, Gold WM. Exercise tolerance in chronic hypoxia due to right-to-left shunt. *J Appl Physiol* 1973; **34**: 853−858.

Theodore J, Robin ED, Morris AJR, Burke CM, Jamieson SW, Van Kessel A *et al*. Augmented ventilatory response to exercise in pulmonary hypertension. *Chest* 1987: **89**: 39−44.

32.1 Physiological aspects
(see also sections 27–31, 40)

Åstrand P-O, Rodahl K. Textbook of Work Physiology, 3rd edn. London: McGraw-Hill, 1986.

Anderson P, Saltin B. Maximal perfusion of skeletal muscle in man. J Appl Physiol 1985; 366: 233–249.

Babb TG, Viggiano R, Hurley B, Staats B, Rodarte JR. Effect of mild-to-moderate airflow limitation on exercise capacity. J Appl Physiol 1991; 70: 223–230.

Buick FJ, Gledhill N, Froese AB, Spriet L, Meyers EC. Effect of induced erythrocytemia on aerobic work capacity. J Appl Physiol 1980; 48: 636–642.

Fagard R, Bielen E, Amery A. Heritability of aerobic power and anaerobic energy generation during exercise. J Appl Physiol 1991; 70: 357–362.

Hogan MC, Roca J, West JB, Wagner PD. Dissociation of maximal O_2 uptake from O_2 delivery in canine gastrocnemius in situ. J Appl Physiol 1989; 66: 1219–1226.

Holmgren A, Åstrand P-O. DL and the dimensions and functional capacities of the O_2 transport system in humans. J Appl Physiol 1966; 21: 1463–1470.

Hoppeler H, Jones JH, Claassen H, Lindstedt S, Longworth KE, Taylor CR et al. Relating maximal oxygen consumption to skeletal muscle mitochondria in horses. In: Gillespie JR, Robinson NE, eds. Equine Exercise Physiology. Ann Arbor, MI: ICEEP Publications, 1987: 278–289.

Medbø JI, Mohn A-C, Tabata I, Bahr R, Vaage O, Sejersted OM. Anaerobic capacity determined by maximal accumulated O_2 deficit. J Appl Physiol 1988; 64: 50–60.

Powers SK, Lawler J, Dempsey JA, Dodd S, Landry G. Effects of incomplete pulmonary gas exchange on $\dot{V}O_2$ max. J Appl Physiol 1989; 66: 2491–2495.

Reybrouck T, Heigenhauser GF, Faulkner JA. Limitations to maximum oxygen uptake in arm, leg, and combined arm–leg ergometry. J Appl Physiol 1975; 38: 774–779.

Roca J, Hogan MC, Storey D, Bebout DE, Haab P, Gonzalez R et al. Evidence for tissue diffusion limitation of $\dot{V}O_2$ max in normal humans. J Appl Physiol 1989; 67: 291–299.

Rowell LB, Saltin B, Kiens B, Christensen NJ. Is peak quadriceps blood flow in humans even higher during exercise with hypoxemia? Am J Physiol 1986; 251: H1038–H1044.

Rowell LB, Taylor HL, Wang Y, Carlson WS. Saturation of arterial blood with oxygen during maximal exercise. J Appl Physiol 1964; 19: 284–286.

Saltin B. Capacity of blood flow delivery to exercising skeletal muscle in humans. Am J Cardiol 1988; 62: 30E–35E.

Wagner PD. An integrated view of the determinants of maximum oxygen uptake. In: Gonzalez NC, Fedde MR, eds. Oxygen Transfer from Atmosphere to Tissues. Vol 227. New York: Plenum Press, 1988: 245–256.

Weibel ER, Marques LB, Constantinopol M, Doffey F, Gehr P, Taylor CR. Adaptive variation in the mammalian respiratory system in relation to energetic demand. VI. The pulmonary gas exchanger. Respir Physiol 1987; 69: 81–100.

32.2 Effects of age on exercise capacity

Åstrand I. Aerobic work capacity in men and women with special reference to age. Acta Physiol Scand 1960; 169: 169–192.

Åstrand I, Åstrand P-O, Hallbäck I, Kilbom Å. Reduction in maximal oxygen uptake with age. J Appl Physiol 1973; 35: 649–654.

Conway J, Wheeler R, Sannerstedt R. Sympathetic nervous activity during exercise in relation to age. Cardiovasc Res 1971; 5: 577–581.

Fleg JL, Lakatta EG. Role of muscle loss in the age-associated reduction in $\dot{V}O_2$max. J Appl Physiol 1988; 65: 1147–1151.

Higginbotham MB, Morris KG, Williams RS, Coleman E, Cobb FR. Physiologic basis for the age-related decline in aerobic work capacity. Am J Cardiol 1986; 57: 1374–1379.

Hossack KF, Bruce RA. Maximal cardiac function in sedentary normal men and women: comparison of age-related changes. J Appl Physiol 1982; 53: 799–804.

Johnson BD, Reddan WG, Seow KC, Dempsey JA. Mechanical constraints on exercise hyperpnea in a fit aging population. Am Rev Respir Dis 1991; 143: 968–977.

Jones NL, Makrides L, Hitchcock C, Clypchar T, McCartney N. Normal standards for an incremental progressive cycle ergometer test. Am Rev Respir Dis 1985; 131: 700–708.

Jones NL, Summers E, Killian KJ. Influence of age and stature on exercise capacity during incremental cycle ergometry in men and women. Am Rev Respir Dis 1989; 140: 1373–1380.

Julius S, Amery A, Whitlock LS, Conway JL. Influence of age on the hemodynamic response to exercise. Circulation 1967; 36: 222–230.

Kanstrup I-L, Ekblom B. Influence of age and physical activity on central hemodynamics and lung function in active adults. J Appl Physiol 1978; 45: 709–717.

Kohrt WM, Malley MT, Coggan AR, Spina RJ, Ogawa T, Ehsani AA et al. Effects of gender, age, and fitness level on response of $\dot{V}O_{2\ max}$ to training in 60–71 yr olds. J Appl Physiol 1991; 71: 2004–2011.

Norris AH, Shock NW, Yiengst MJ. Age differences in ventilatory and gas exchange responses to graded exercise in males. J Gerontol 1955; 10: 145–155.

Orlander J, Kiessling K-H, Larson L, Karlsson J, Aniasson A. Skeletal muscle metabolism and ultrastructure in relation to age in sedentary man. Acta Physiol Scand 1978; 104: 249–261.

Pugh LGCE. The aerobic capacity of forty British women aged 17–27 years. Ergonomics 1976; 17:

185−192.

Robinson S. Experimental studies of physical fitness in relation to age. *Arbeitsphysiol* 1938; **10**: 251−323.

Rodeheffer RJ, Gerstenblith G, Becker LC, Fleg JL, Weisfeldt ML, Lakatta EG. Exercise cardiac output is maintained with advancing age in healthy human subjects: cardiac dilatation and increased stroke volume compensate for a diminished heart rate. *Circulation* 1984; **69**: 203−213.

Weller JJ, El-Gamal FM, Parker L, Reed JW, Cotes JE. Indirect estimation of maximal oxygen uptake for study of working populations. *Br J Ind Med* 1988; **45**: 532−537.

Wilhelmsen L, Tibblin G, Aurell M, Bjure J, Ekström-Jodal B, Grimby G. Ventilatory function and work performance in a representative sample of 803 men age 54 years. *Chest* 1974; **66**: 506−510.

33 EXERCISE ENERGY EXPENDITURE

Cavagna GA, Kaneko M. Mechanical work and efficiency in level walking and running. *J Physiol (Lond)* 1977; **268**: 467−481.

Cavagna GA, Thys H, Zamboni A. The sources of external work in level walking and running. *J Physiol (Lond)* 1976; **262**: 639−657.

Cotes JE. Relationships of oxygen consumption, ventilation and cardiac frequency to body weight during standardized submaximal exercise in normal subjects. *Ergonomics* 1969; **12**: 415−427.

Cotes JE. The ventilatory cost of activity. *Br J Ind Med* 1975; **32**: 220−223.

Davies CTM, Barnes C. Negative (eccentric) work. II. Physiological responses to walking uphill and downhill on a motor-driven treadmill. *Ergonomics* 1972; **15**: 121−131.

Di Prampero PE, Cortili G, Mognoni P, Saibene F. Energy cost of speed skating and efficiency of work against air resistance. *J Appl Physiol* 1976; **40**: 584−591.

Givoni B, Goldman RF. Predicting metabolic energy cost. *J Appl Physiol* 1971; **30**: 429−433.

Poole DC, Ward SA, Gardner GW, Whipp BJ. Metabolic and respiratory profile on the upper limit for prolonged exercise in man. *Ergonomics* 1988; **31**: 1265−1279.

Pugh LGCE. The influence of wind resistance in running and walking and the mechanical efficiency of work against horizontal or vertical forces. *J Physiol (Lond)* 1971; **213**: 255−276.

Pugh LGCE. The relation of oxygen intake and speed in competition cycling and comparative observations on the cycle ergometer. *J Physiol (Lond)* 1974; **241**: 795−808.

Ramanathan NL, Kamon E. The application of stair-climbing to ergometry. *Ergonomics* 1974; **17**: 13−22.

Schmidt-Nielson K. Locomotion: energy cost of swimming, flying and running. *Science* 1972; **177**: 222−228.

Walt WH van der, Wyndham CH. An equation for prediction of energy expenditure of walking and running. *J Appl Physiol* 1973; **34**: 559−563.

34 RESPIRATORY PHYSIOLOGY OF NEWBORN

34.1 General

Avery ME, ed. *Neonatology. Pathophysiology and Management of the Newborn*, 2nd edn. Philadelphia: JB Lippincott, 1981.

Dawes GS. *Fetal and Neonatal Physiology; a Comparative Study of the Changes at Birth*. Chicago: Year Book Publishers, 1968.

Gluckman PD, Johnston BM, Nathanielsz PW, eds. *Advances in Fetal Physiology*. Ithaca: Perinatology Press, 1989.

34.2 Respiratory control
(*see also* sections 27.1−27.4)

Blanco CE, Hanson MA, McCooke HB, Williams BA. Studies of chemoreceptor resetting after hypoxic ventilation of the fetus *in utero*. In: Ribero JA, Pallot DJ, eds. *Chemoreceptors in Respiratory Control*. Kent, England: Croom Helm, 1987: 369−376.

Boeck C de, Reempts R van, Rigatto H, Chernick V. Naloxone reduces decrease in ventilation induced by hypoxia in newborn infants. *J Appl Physiol* 1984; **56**: 1507−1511.

Chernick V, Warshaw JB, Kiley JP. Development neurobiology of respiratory control. *Am Rev Respir Dis* 1989; **139**: 1295−1301.

Cross KW, Oppe TE. The effect of inhalation of high and low concentrations of oxygen on the respiration of the premature infant. *J Physiol (Lond)* 1952; **117**: 38−55.

Gaultier C, Praud JP, Canet E, Delaperche MF, Allest AM. Paradoxical inward rib cage motion during rapid eye movement sleep in infants and young children. *J Dev Physiol* 1987; **9**: 391−397.

Haddad GG, Mellins RB. Hypoxia and respiratory control in early life. *Annu Rev Physiol* 1984; **46**: 629−643.

Harned HS, Ferreiro J. Initiation of breathing by cold stimulation: effects of change in ambient temperature on respiratory activity of the full-term fetal lamb. *J Pediatr* 1973; **83**: 663−669.

Hasan SU, Lee DS, Gibson DA, Nowaczyk BJ, Cates DB, Sitar DS. Effect of morphine on breathing and behavior in fetal sheep. *J Appl Physiol* 1988; **64**: 2058−2065.

Henderson-Smart DJ, Cohen GL. Chemical control of breathing in early life. *Ann NY Acad Sci* 1988; **533**: 276−288.

Hertzberg T, Lagercrantz H. Postnatal sensitivity of the peripheral chemoreceptors in newborn infants. *Arch Dis Child* 1987; **62**: 1238−1241.

Ioffe S, Jansen AH, Chernick V. Maturation of spontaneous fetal diaphragmatic activity and fetal response to hypercapnia and hypoxemia. *J Appl Physiol* 1987; **63**: 609–622.

Kosch PC, Hutchison AA, Wozniak JA, Carlo WA, Stark AR. Posterior cricoarytenoid and diaphragm activities during tidal breathing in neonates. *J Appl Physiol* 1988; **64**: 1968–1978.

Lagercrantz H, Milerad J, Walker DW. Control of ventilation in the fetus and newborn. In: Crystal RG, West JB, Barnes PJ, Cherniack NS, Weibel ER, eds. *The Lung: Scientific Foundations*. New York: Raven Press, 1990.

Martin-Body RL, Johnston BM. Central origin of the hypoxic depression of breathing in the newborn. *Respir Physiol* 1988; **71**: 25–32.

Mortola JP, Fisher JT, Smith JB, Fox GS, Weeks S, Willis D. Onset of respiration in infants delivered by cesarean section. *J Appl Physiol* 1982; **52**: 716–724.

Natale R, Nasello-Paterson C, Connors G. Patterns of fetal breathing activity in the human fetus at 24 to 28 weeks of gestation. *Am J Obstet Gynecol* 1988; **158**: 317–321.

Rigatto H. Control of ventilation in the newborn. *Annu Rev Physiol* 1984; **46**: 661–674.

Thaler I, Goodman JDS, Dawes GS. Effects of maternal cigarette smoking on fetal breathing and fetal movements. *Am J Obstet Gynecol* 1980; **138**: 282–287.

Trippenbach T. Chest wall reflexes in newborns. *Bull Eur Physiopathol Respir* 1985; **21**: 115–122.

Walker DW. Peripheral and central chemoreceptors in the fetus and newborn. *Annu Rev Physiol* 1984; **46**: 687–703.

34.3 Lung function in neonates and infants

American Thoracic and European Respiratory Societies. Respiratory mechanics in infants: physiologic evaluation in health and disease. *Amer Rev Respir Dis* 1993; **147**: 474–496.

Beardsmore CS, Stocks J, Silverman M. Problems in measurement of thoracic gas volume in infancy. *J Appl Physiol* 1982; **52**: 995–999.

Bissonnette JM, Wickham WK, Drummond WH. Placental diffusing capacities at varied carbon monoxide tensions. *J Clin Invest* 1977; **59**: 1038–1044.

Chapman B, O'Callaghan C, Coxon R, Glover P, Jaroszkiewicz G, Howseman A *et al*. Estimation of lung volume in infants by echo planar imaging and total body plethysmography. *Arch Dis Child* 1990; **65**: 168–170.

Cross KW, Tizard JPM, Trythall DAH. The gaseous metabolism of the newborn infant breathing 15% oxygen. *Acta Paediatr* 1958; **47**: 217–237.

Dezateux CA, Fletcher ME, Rabbette PS, Stranger LJ, Stocks J. *Manual of Infant Lung Function Testing*. London: Institute of Child Health, 1991.

Doershuk GF, Matthews LW. Airway resistance and lung volume in the newborn infant. *Pediat Res* 1969; **3**: 128–134.

Fleming PJ, Levine MR, Goncalves A. Changes in respiratory pattern resulting from the use of facemask to record respiration in newborn infants. *Pediatr Res* 1982; **16**: 1031–1034.

Hanrahan JP, Tager IB, Castile RG, Segal MR, Weiss ST, Speizer FE. Pulmonary function measures in healthy infants. Variability and size correction. *Am Rev Respir Dis* 1990; **141**: 1127–1135.

Hill EP, Power GG, Longo LD. A mathematical model of carbon dioxide transfer in the placenta and its interaction with oxygen. *Am J Physiol* 1973; **224**: 283–299.

Hill JR, Robinson DC. Oxygen consumption in normally grown, small-for-dates and large-for-dates new-born infants. *J Physiol (Lond)* 1968; **199**: 685–703.

Kitterman JA. Physiological factors in fetal lung growth. *Can J Physiol Pharmacol* 1988; **66**: 1122–1128.

Koch G. Alveolar ventilation, diffusing capacity and the A-aPo$_2$ difference in the newborn infant. *Respir Physiol* 1968; **4**: 169–192.

Krauss AN, Auld PAM. Measurement of mixed venous oxygen tension in premature infants by a rebreathing method. *Pediat Res* 1972; **6**: 158–161.

Montgomery GL, Tepper RS. Changes in airway reactivity with age in normal infants and young children. *Am Rev Respir Dis* 1990; **142**: 1372–1376.

Morrow RJ, Ritchie JWK, Bull SB. Maternal cigarette smoking: the effects on umbilical and uterine blood flow velocity. *Am J Obster Gynecol* 1988; **159**: 1069–1071.

Mortola JP, Milic-Emili J, Noworaj A, Smith B, Fox G, Weeks S. Muscle pressure and flow during expiration in infants. *Am Rev Respir Dis* 1984; **129**: 49–53.

Nourse CH, Nelson NM. Uniformity of ventilation in the newborn infant: direct assessment of the arterial–alveolar N$_2$ difference. *Pediatrics* 1969; **43**: 226–232.

Saunders RA, Milner AD. Pulmonary pressure/volume relationships during the last phase of delivery and the first postnatal breaths in human subjects. *J Pediatr* 1978; **93**: 667–673.

Versmold H, Seifert G, Riegel KP. Blood oxygen affinity in infancy: the interaction of fetal and adult hemoglobin, oxygen capacity and red cell hydrogen ion and 2,3-diphosphoglycerate concentration. *Respir Physiol* 1973; **18**: 14–25.

Vyas H, Field D, Milner AD, Hopkins IE. Determinants of the first inspiratory volume and functional residual capacity at birth. *Pediat Pulmonol* 1986; **2**: 189–193.

Wohl MEB, Stigol LC, Mead J. Resistance of the total respiratory system in healthy infants and infants with bronchiolitis. *Pediatrics* 1969; **43**: 495–509.

35 LUNG FUNCTION IN CHILDREN

35.1 General
(*see also* sections 4, 5, 6.1, 6.5)

Godfrey S. *Exercise Testing in Children*. London: Saunders, 1974.

Polgar G, Promadhat V. *Pulmonary Function Testing in Children: Techniques and Standards*. Philadelphia: WB Saunders, 1971.

Polgar G, Weng TR. The functional development of the respiratory system. From the period of gestation to adulthood. *Am Rev Respir Dis* 1979; **120**: 625–695.

Quanjer PhH, Helms P, Bjure J, Gaultier CL, eds. Standardisation of lung function tests in paediatrics. *Eur Respir J* 1989; **2**(Suppl. 4): 121S–122S.

35.2 *Lung physiology*

Anderson SD, Godfrey S. Transfer factor for CO during exercise in children. *Thorax* 1971; **26**: 51–54.

Bar-Yishay E, Shulman DL, Beardsmore CS, Godfrey S. Functional residual capacity in healthy preschool children lying supine. *Am Rev Respir Dis* 1987; **135**: 954–956.

Baran D, Yernault JC, Paiva M, Englert M. Static mechanical lung properties in healthy children. *Scand J Respir Dis* 1976; **57**: 139–147.

Cogswell JJ, Hull D, Milner AD, Norman AP, Taylor B. Lung function in children (iii) measurement of airflow resistance in healthy children. *Br J Dis Chest* 1975; **69**: 177–187.

Gaultier C, Zinman R. Maximal static pressures in healthy children. *Respir Physiol* 1983; **51**: 45–61.

Hardt H von der, Logvinoff MM, Dickreiter J, Geubelle F. Static recoil of the lungs and static compliance in healthy children. *Respiration* 1975; **32**: 325–339.

Hardt H von der, Nowak A. Mechanics of respiration in healthy children 6–15 years of age. *Pneumologie* 1976; **153**: 261–274.

Kagamimori S, Robson JM, Heywood C, Cotes JE. Genetic and environmental determinants of the cardio-respiratory response to submaximal exercise—a six year follow-up study of twins. *Ann Hum Biol* 1984; **11**: 29–38.

Kerr AA. Deadspace ventilation in normal children and children with obstructive airways disease. *Thorax* 1976; **31**: 63–69.

Levison H, Featherby EA, Weng TR. Arterial blood gases, alveolar–arterial oxygen difference and physiologic deadspace in children and young adults. *Am Rev Respir Dis* 1970; **101**: 972–974.

Mansell A, Bryan C, Levison H. Airway closure in children. *J Appl Physiol* 1972; **33**: 711–714.

Mansell A, Levison H, Kruger K, Tripp TL. Measurement of respiratory resistance in children by forced oscillations. *Am Rev Respir Dis* 1972; **106**: 710–714.

Zapletal A, Paul T, Samanek M. Pulmonary elasticity in children and adolescents. *J Appl Physiol* 1976; **40**: 953–961.

Zapletal A, Samanek M, Tuma S, Ruth C, Paul T. Assessment of airway function in children. *Bull Physiopathol Respir* 1972; **8**: 535–544.

35.3 *Reference values in Caucasian children* (*see also* sections 3, 35.1)

Bouhuys A. Maximum expiratory flow–volume curves in children and adolescents. *Bull Physiopathol Respir* 1971; **7**: 113–123.

Brough FK, Schmidt CD, Dickman M, Jackson B. Effect of two instructional procedures on the performance of the spirometry test in children five through seven years of age. *Am Rev Respir Dis* 1972; **106**: 604–606.

Cook CD, Hamann JF. Relation of lung volumes to height in healthy persons between the ages of 5 and 38 years. *J Pediatr* 1961; **59**: 710–714.

Cook CD, Helliesen PJ, Agathon S. Relation between mechanics of respiration. Lung size and body size from birth to young adulthood. *J Appl Physiol* 1958; **13**: 349–352.

Cotes JE, Dabbs JM, Hall AM, Axford AT, Laurence KM. Lung volumes, ventilatory capacity and transfer factor in healthy British boy and girl twins. *Thorax* 1973; **28**: 709–715.

Cotes JE, Dabbs JM, Hall AM, Heywood C, Laurence KM. Sitting height, fat free mass and body fat as reference variables for lung function in healthy British children: comparison with stature. *Ann Hum Biol* 1979; **6**: 307–314.

Dickman ML, Schmidt CD, Gardner RM. Spirometric standards for normal children and adolescents. *Am Rev Respir Dis* 1971; **104**: 680–687.

Dugdale AE, Moeri M. Normal values of forced vital capacity (FVC), forced expiratory volume ($FEV_{1.0}$) and peak flow rate (PFR) in children. *Arch Dis Child* 1968; **43**: 229–234.

Helliesen PJ, Cook CD, Friedlander L, Agathon S. Studies of respiratory physiology in children. I. Mechanics of respiration and lung volumes in 85 normal children 5 to 17 years of age. *Pediatrics* 1958; **22**: 80–93.

Juhl B. Pulmonary function investigations in 1011 school children using Wright's peak flow meter. *Scand J Clin Lab Invest* 1970; **25**: 355–361.

Kjellman B. Ventilatory efficiency, capacity and lung volumes in healthy children. *Scand J Clin Lab Invest* 1969; **23**: 19–29.

Levison H, Kamel M, Weng TR, Kruger K. Expiratory flow rates determined by wedge and water spirometer in children and young adults. *Acta Pediat Scand* 1970; **59**: 648–652.

Pistelli R, Brancato G, Forastiere F, Michelozzi P, Corbo GM, Agabiti N *et al*. Population values of lung volumes and flows in children: effect of sex, body mass and respiratory conditions. *Eur Respir J* 1992; **5**: 463–470.

Robinson M. Peak expiratory flow rate and total thoracic resistance in children aged 2.5 to 5 years. Unpublished, Dept. Child Health, Welsh National School of Medicine, Cardiff, 1973.

Shulman DL, Bar-Yishaw E, Beardsmore CS, Beilin B, Godfrey S. Partial forced expiratory flow–volume

696

curves in young children during ketamine anesthesia. *J Appl Physiol* 1987; **63**: 44−50.

Strang LB. The ventilatory capacity of normal children. *Thorax* 1959; **14**: 305−310.

Van Pelt W, Quanjer PhH, Borsboom G, Paoletti P, Di Pede F, Viegi G *et al*. Comparability of reference populations from Holland and Italy. *Eur Respir J* 1990; **3**: 158S.

Weng TR, Levison H. Standards of pulmonary function in children. *Am Rev Respir Dis* 1969; **99**: 879−894.

Zapletal A, Motoyama EK, van de Woestijne KP, Hunt VR, Bouhuys A. Maximum expiratory flow−volume curves and airway conductance in children and adolescents. *J Appl Physiol* 1969; **26**: 308−316.

36 GROWTH OF THE LUNG
(*see also* sections 35, 39)

Brody JS, Fisher AB, Gocmen A, DuBois AB. Acromegalic pneumonomegaly: lung growth in the adult. *J Clin Invest* 1970; **49**: 1051−1060.

Burri PH, Gehr P, Müller H, Weibel ER. Adaptation of the growing lung to increased $\dot{V}O_2$. I. IDPN as inducer of hyperactivity. *Respir Physiol* 1976; **28**: 129−140.

Cotch MF, Beaty TH, Cohen BH. Path analysis of familial resemblance of pulmonary function and cigarette smoking. *Am Rev Respir Dis* 1990; **142**: 1337−1343.

DeGroodt EG, van Pelt W, Borsboom GJJM, Quanjer PhH, van Zomeren BC. Growth of lung and thorax dimensions during the pubertal growth spurt. *Eur Respir J* 1988; **1**: 102−108.

Dittmer DS, Grebe RM, eds. *Handbook of Respiration*. Philadelphia: WB Saunders Co, 1958.

Hunter C, Barer GR, Shaw JW, Clegg EJ. Growth of the heart and lungs in hypoxic rodents: a model of human hypoxic disease. *Clin Sci* 1974; **46**: 375−391.

Klissouras V. Heritability of adaptive variation. *J Appl Physiol* 1971; **31**: 338−344.

Lebowitz MD, Holberg CJ, Knudson RJ, Burrows B. Longitudinal study of pulmonary function development in childhood, adolescence, and early adulthood. *Am Rev Respir Dis* 1987; **136**: 69−75.

Lebowitz MD, Holberg CJ. Effects of parental smoking and other risk factors on the development of pulmonary function in children and adolescents. Analysis of two longitudinal population studies. *Am J Epidemiol* 1988; **128**: 589−597.

Mearns MB, Simon G. Patterns of lung and heart growth as determined from serial radiographs of 76 children with cystic fibrosis. *Thorax* 1973; **28**: 537−546.

Schrader PC, Quanjer PhH, Olievier ICW. Respiratory muscle force and ventilatory function in adolescents. *Eur Respir J* 1988; **1**: 368−375.

Schwartz J, Katz SA, Fegley RW, Tockman MS. Sex and race differences in the development of lung function. *Am Rev Respir Dis* 1988; **138**: 1415−1421.

Sherrill DL, Camilli A, Lebowitz MD. On the temporal relationships between lung function and somatic growth. *Am Rev Respir Dis* 1989; **140**: 638−644.

Stanley NN, Alper R, Cunningham EL, Cherniack NS, Kefalides NA. Effects of a molecular change in collagen on lung structure and mechanical function. *J Clin Invest* 1975; **55**: 1195−1201.

Thurlbeck WM. Lung growth and alveolar multiplication. *Pathobiol Annu* 1975; **5**: 1−34.

Whimster WF, MacFarlane AJ. Normal lung weights in a white population. *Am Rev Respir Dis* 1974; **110**: 478−483.

37 PREGNANCY

Bayliss DA, Millhorn DE. Central neural mechanisms of progesterone action: application to the respiratory system. *J Appl Physiol* 1992; **73**: 393−401.

Chen H-I, Tang Y-R. Effects of the menstrual cycle on respiratory muscle function. *Am Rev Respir Dis* 1989; **140**: 1359−1362.

Contreras G, Gutiérrez M, Beroiza T, Fantin A, Oddó H, Villarroel L *et al*. Ventilatory drive and respiratory muscle function in pregnancy. *Am Rev Respir Dis* 1991; **144**: 837−841.

Craig DB, Toole MA. Airway closure in pregnancy. *Can Anaesth Soc J* 1975; **22**: 665−672.

Field SK, Bell SG, Cenaiko DF, Whitelaw WA. Relationship between inspiratory effort and breathlessness in pregnancy. *J Appl Physiol* 1991; **71**: 1897−1902.

Gaensler EA, Patton WE, Verstraeten JM, Badger TL. Pulmonary function in pregnancy. *Am Rev Tuberc* 1953; **67**: 779−797.

Gee JBL, Packer BS, Millen JE, Robin ED. Pulmonary mechanics during pregnancy. *J Clin Invest* 1967; **46**: 945−952.

Gilbert R, Auchincloss JH Jr. Dyspnea of pregnancy. Clinical and physiological observations. *Am J Med Sci* 1966; **252**: 270−276.

Hessemer V, Brück K. Influence of menstrual cycle on shivering, skin blood flow, and sweating responses measured at night. *J Appl Physiol* 1985; **59**: 1902−1910.

Knuttgen HG, Emerson K Jr. Physiological response to pregnancy at rest and during exercise. *J Appl Physiol* 1974; **36**: 549−553.

Longo LD. The biological effects of carbon monoxide on the pregnant woman, fetus, and newborn infant. *Am J Obstet Gynecol* 1977; **129**: 69−103.

Lotgering FK, Van Doorn MB, Struijk PC, Pool J, Wallenburg HCS. Maximal aerobic exercise in pregnant women: heart rate, O_2 consumption, CO_2 production, and ventilation. *J Appl Physiol* 1991; **70**: 1016−1023.

Lucius H, Gahlenbeck H, Kleine H-O, Fabel H, Bartels H. Respiratory functions, buffer system and electrolyte concentrations of blood during human pregnancy. *Respir Physiol* 1970; **9**: 311−317.

Pauli BD, Reid RL, Munt PW, Wigle RD, Forkert L. Influence of the menstrual cycle on airway function in asthmatic and normal subjects. *Am Rev Respir Dis* 1989; **140**: 358−362.

Pernoll ML, Metcalfe J, Kovach PA, Wachtel R, Dunham MJ. Ventilation during rest and exercise in pregnancy and postpartum. *Respir Physiol* 1975; **25**: 295−310.

Sady SP, Carpenter MW, Thompson PD, Sady MA, Haydon B, Coustan DR. Cardiovascular response to cycle exercise during and after pregnancy. *J Appl Physiol* 1989; **66**: 336−341.

Schoene RB, Robertson HT, Pierson DJ, Peterson AP. Respiratory drives and exercise in menstrual cycles of athletic and nonathletic women. *J Appl Physiol* 1981; **50**: 1300−1305.

38 CYCLICAL VARIATION IN LUNG FUNCTION

Cinkotai FF, Thomsen ML. Diurnal variation in pulmonary diffusing capacity for carbon monoxide. *J Appl Physiol* 1966; **21**: 539−542.

Guberan E, Williams MK, Walford J, Smith MM. Circadian variation of FEV in shift workers. *Br J Industr Med* 1969; **26**: 121−125.

Kerr HD. Diurnal variation of respiratory function independent of air quality. *Arch Environ Health* 1973; **26**: 144−152.

McDermott M. Diurnal and weekly cyclical changes in lung airways resistance. *J Physiol (Lond)* 1966; **186**: 90P−92P.

McKerrow CB, Rossiter CE. An annual cycle in the ventilatory capacity of men with pneumoconiosis and of normal subjects. *Thorax* 1968; **23**: 340−349.

Reinberg A, Gervais P. Circadian rhythms in respiratory functions, with special reference to human chronophysiology and chronopharmacology. *Bull Physiopathol Respir* 1972; **8**: 663−675.

Spodnik MJ Jr, Cushman GD, Kerr DH, Blide RW, Spicer WS Jr. Effects of environment on respiratory function. *Arch Environ Health* 1966; **13**: 243−254.

Wahlberg I, Åstrand I. Physical work capacity during the day and at night. *Work Environ Health* 1973; **10**: 65−68.

39 ATHLETICS AND PHYSICAL TRAINING
(*see also* sections 32.1, 64)

Akabas SR, Bazzy AR, Di Mauro S, Haddad GG. Metabolic and functional adaptation of the diaphragm to training with resistive loads. *J Appl Physiol* 1989; **66**: 529−535.

Andrew GM, Becklake MR, Guleria JS, Bates DV. Heart and lung functions in swimmers and non-athletes during growth. *J Appl Physiol* 1972; **32**: 245−251.

Bass H, Whitcomb JF, Forman R. Exercise training: therapy for patients with chronic obstructive pulmonary disease. *Chest* 1970; **57**: 116−121.

Bassey EJ, Fentem PH. Extent of deterioration in physical condition during post operative bed rest and its reversal by rehabilitation. *Br Med J* 1974; **4**: 194−196.

Blomqvist CG, Saltin B. Cardiovascular adaptations to physical training. *Ann Rev Physiol* 1983; **45**: 169−189.

Brundin T, Cernigliario C. The effect of physical training on the sympatho-adrenal response to exercise. *Scand J Clin Lab Invest* 1975; **35**: 525−530.

Clausen JP. Effect of physical training on cardiovascular adjustments to exercise in man. *Physiol Rev* 1977; **57**: 779−815.

Ekblom B, Goldbarg AN. The influence of physical training and other factors on the subjective rating of perceived exertion. *Acta Physiol Scand* 1971; **83**: 399−406.

Ekblom B. Effect of physical training on oxygen transport system in man. *Acta Physiol Scand* 1969; **328**(Suppl): 1−45.

Eriksson BO, Lundin A, Saltir B. Cardiopulmonary function in former girl swimmers and the effects of physical training. *Scand J Clin Lab Invest* 1975; **35**: 135−145.

Gollnick PD, Saltin B. Significance of skeletal oxidative enzyme enhancement with endurance training. *Clin Physiol* 1982; **66**: 195−201.

Gonyea WJ. Role of exercise in inducing increases in skeletal muscle fiber number. *J Appl Physiol* 1980; **48**: 421−426.

Hagberg JM, Hickson RC, Ehsani AA, Holloszy JO. Faster adjustment to and recovery from submaximal exercise in the trained state. *J Appl Physiol* 1980; **48**: 218−224.

Jansson E, Sjodin B, Tesch P. Changes in muscle fibre type distribution in man after physical training. *Acta Physiol Scand* 1978; **104**: 235−237.

Pyörälä K, Heinonen AO, Karvonen MJ. Pulmonary function in former endurance athletes. *Acta Med Scand* 1968; **183**: 263−273.

Rasmussen B, Klausen K, Clausen JP, Trop-Jensen J. Pulmonary ventilation, blood gases and blood pH after training of the arms or the legs. *J Appl Physiol* 1975; **38**: 250−256.

Roskamm H, Landry F, Samek L, Schlager M, Weidemann H, Reindell H. Effects of a standardised ergometer training program at three different altitudes. *J Appl Physiol* 1969; **27**: 840−847.

Saltin B, Blomqvist G, Mitchell JH, Johnson RL Jr, Wildenthal K, Chapman CB. Response to exercise after bed rest and after training. *Circulation* 1968; **38**(suppl 7): 1−78.

Shapiro W, Patterson JL Jr. Effects of smoking and athletic conditioning on ventilatory mechanics, including observations on the reliability of the forced expirogram. *Am Rev Respir Dis* 1962; **85**: 191−199.

Taylor HL, Henschel A, Brozek J, Keys A. Effects of bed rest on cardiovascular function and work performance. *J Appl Physiol* 1949; **2**: 223−239.

698

40 HIGH ALTITUDE

(*see also* sections 10, 22.2, 24, 25, 32.1, 41, 43, 66)

Barcroft J, Binger CA, Bock AV, Doggart JH, Forbes HS, Garrop G et al. Observations upon the effect of high altitude on the physiological processes of the human body carried out in the Peruvian Andes chiefly at Cerro de Pasco. *Philos Trans R Soc Lond (Biol)* 1923; 211: 351–480.

Baumgarten RJ von, Baldrighi G, Vogel H, Thumler R. Physiological response to hyper- and hypogravity during rollercoaster flight. *Aviat Space Environ Med* 1980; 51: 145–154.

Beall CM, Baker PT, Baker TS, Haas JD. The effects of high altitude on adolescent growth in Southern Peruvian Amerindians. *Hum Biol* 1977; 49: 109–124.

Bebout DE, Storey D, Roca J, Hogan MC, Poole DC, Gonzalez-Camarena R et al. Effects of altitude acclimatisation on pulmonary gas exchange during exercise. *J Appl Physiol* 1989; 67: 2286–2295.

Bredle DL, Chapler CK, Cain SM. Metabolic and circulatory responses of normoxic skeletal muscle to whole-body hypoxia. *J Appl Physiol* 1988; 65: 2063–2068.

Brody JS, Lahiri S, Simpser M, Motoyama EK, Velasquez T. Lung elasticity and airway dynamics in Peruvian natives to high altitude. *J Appl Physiol* 1977; 42: 245–251.

Cruz JC. Mechanics of breathing in high altitude and sea level subjects. *Respir Physiol* 1973; 17: 146–161.

Fenn WO, Rahn H, Otis AB. A theoretical study of the composition of alveolar air at altitude. *Am J Physiol* 1946; 146: 637–653.

Gale GE, Torre-Bueno JR, Moon RE, Saltzman HA, Wagner PD. Ventilation–perfusion inequality in normal humans at sea level and simulated altitude. *J Appl Physiol* 1985; 58: 978–988.

Guleria JS, Pande JN, Sethi PK, Roy SB. Pulmonary diffusing capacity at high altitude. *J Appl Physiol* 1971; 31: 536–543.

Hartley LH, Vogel JA, Cruz JC. Reduction of maximal exercise heart rate at altitude and its reversal with atropine. *J Appl Physiol* 1974; 36: 362–365.

Hornbein TF, Townes BD, Schoene RB, Sutton JR, Houston CS. The cost to the central nervous system of climbing to extremely high altitude. *N Engl J Med* 1989; 321: 1714–1719.

Lahiri S, Milledge JS, Sørensen SC. Ventilation in man during exercise at high altitude. *J Appl Physiol* 1972; 32: 766–769.

Mazess RB. Exercise performance of Indian and white high altitude residents. *Hum Biol* 1969; 41: 494–518.

Paiva M, Estenne M, Engel LA. Lung volumes, chest wall configuration and pattern of breathing in microgravity. *J Appl Physiol* 1989; 67: 1542–1550.

Pugh LGCE, Gill MB, Lahiri S, Milledge JS, Ward MP, West JB. Muscular exercise at great altitudes. *J Appl Physiol* 1964; 19: 431–440.

Pugh LGCE. Athletes at altitude. *J Physiol (Lond)* 1967; 192: 619–646.

Reeves JT, Groves BM, Sutton JR, Wagner PD, Cymerman A, Malconian MK et al. Operation Everest II: preservation of cardiac function at extreme altitude. *J Appl Physiol* 1987; 63: 531–539.

Regard M, Oelz O, Brugger P, Landis T. Persistent cognitive impairment in climbers after repeated exposure to extreme altitude. *Neurology* 1989; 39: 210–213.

Sutton JR, Reeves JT, Wagner PD, Groves BM, Cymerman A, Malconian MK et al. Operation Everest II: oxygen transport during exercise at extreme simulated altitude. *J Appl Physiol* 1988; 64: 1309–1321.

Tichauer ER. Operation of machine tools at high altitude. *Ergonomics* 1963; 6: 51–73.

Vizek M, Pickett C, Weil JV. Increased carotid body hypoxic sensitivity during acclimatisation to hypobaric hypoxia. *J Appl Physiol* 1987; 63: 2403–2410.

Wagner PD, Gale GE, Moon RE, Torre-Bueno JR, Stolp BW, Saltzman HA. Pulmonary gas exchange in humans exercising at sea level and simulated altitude. *J Appl Physiol* 1986; 61: 260–270.

Wagner PD, Sutton JR, Reeves JT, Cymerman A, Groves BM, Malconian MK. Operation Everest II. Pulmonary gas exchange during a simulated ascent of Mt. Everest. *J Appl Physiol* 1987; 63: 2348–2359.

Ward MP, Milledge JS, West JB, eds. *High Altitude Medicine and Physiology*. Philadelphia: University of Pennsylvania Press, 1989.

Weil JV, Byrne-Quinn E, Sodal IE, Filley GF, Grover RF. Acquired attenuation of chemoreceptor function in chronically hypoxic man at high altitude. *J Clin Invest* 1971; 50: 186–195.

Weil JV, Jamieson G, Brown DW, Grover RF. The red cell mass–arterial oxygen relationship in normal man. *J Clin Invest* 1968; 47: 1627–1639.

Weil JV, Vizek M. Ventilatory response to hypoxia in high altitude acclimatization. In: Lahiri S, Forester RE, Davis RO, Pack AI, eds. *Chemoreceptor and Reflexes in Breathing*. New York: Oxford University Press, 1989: 199–207.

West JB, ed. *High Altitude Physiology. Benchmark Papers in Human Physiology 15*. Stroundsbery, PA: Hutchinson Ross, 1981.

West JB, Hackett PH, Maret KH, Milledge JS, Peters RM Jr, Pizzo CJ, Winslow RM. Pulmonary gas exchange on the summit of Mount Everest. *J Appl Physiol* 1983; 55: 678–687.

Williams DA. Athletic performance at high altitude. *Nature (Lond)* 1966; 211: 753.

Wyndham CH, Strydom NB, Rensberg AJ Van, Rorgers GG. Effects on maximal oxygen uptake of acute changes in altitude in a deep mine. *J Appl Physiol* 1970; 29: 552–555.

41 HYPERBARIC CONDITIONS

Blomqvist G, Johnson RL Jr, Saltin B. Pulmonary diffusing capacity limiting human performance at altitude. *Acta Physiol Scand* 1969; 76: 284–287.

Butler PJ, Jones DR. The comparative physiology of diving in vertebrates. *Adv Comp Physiol Biochem* 1982; **8**: 179−364.

Colebatch HJH, Smith MM, Ng CKY. Increased elastic recoil as a determinant of pulmonary barotrauma in divers. *Respir Physiol* 1976; **26**: 55−64.

Cotes JE, Davey IS, Reed JW, Rooks M. Respiratory effects of a single saturation dive to 300 m. *Br J Ind Med* 1987; **44**: 76−82.

Davey IS, Cotes JE, Reed JW. Relationship of ventilatory capacity to hyperbaric exposure in divers. *J Appl Physiol* 1984; **56**: 1655−1658.

Fagius J, Sundlöf G. The diving response in man: effects on sympathetic activity in muscle and skin nerve fascicles. *J Physiol* 1986; **377**: 429−443.

Fagraeus L. Cardiorespiratory and metabolic functions during exercise in the hyperbaric environment. *Acta Physiol Scand* 1974; **92**(Suppl. 414): 1−40.

Fisher AB, DuBois AB, Hyde RW, Knight CJ, Lambertsen CJ. Effect of 2 months' undersea exposure to N_2-O_2 at 2.2 Ata on lung function. *J Appl Physiol* 1970; **28**: 70−74.

Florio JT, Morrison JB, Butt WS. Breathing pattern and ventilatory response to carbon dioxide in divers. *J Appl Physiol* 1979; **46**: 1076−1080.

Hesser CM, Linnarsson D, Fagraeus L. Pulmonary mechanics and work of breathing at maximal ventilation and raised air pressure. *J Appl Physiol* 1981; **50**: 747−753.

Hickey DD, Lundgren CE, Pasche AJ. Influence of exercise on maximal voluntary ventilation and forced expiratory flow at depth. *Undersea Biomed Res* 1983; **10**: 241−254.

Jarrett AS. Alveolar carbon dioxide tension at increased ambient pressures. *J Appl Physiol* 1966; **21**: 158−162.

Mukhtar MR, Patrick JM. Ventilatory drive during face immersion in man. *J Physiol* 1986; **370**: 13−24.

Thorsen E, Hjelle J, Segadal K, Gulsvik A. Exercise tolerance and pulmonary gas exchange after deep saturation dives. *J Appl Physiol* 1990; **68**: 1809−1814.

Vail EG. Hyperbaric respiratory mechanics. *Aerospace Med* 1971; **42**: 536−546.

Van Liew HD. Mechanical and physical factors in lung function during work in dense environments. *Undersea Biomed Res* 1983; **10**: 255−264.

Vorosmarti J Jr. Influence of increased gas density and external resistance on maximum expiratory flow. *Undersea Biomed Res* 1979; **6**: 339−346.

42 EFFECTS OF AGE ON LUNG FUNCTION
(*see also* sections 32.2, 44.1−44.4)

Begin R, Renzetti JR, Bigler AH, Watanabe S. Flow and age dependence of airway closure and dynamic compliance. *J Appl Physiol* 1975; **38**: 199−207.

Bode FR, Dosman J, Martin RR, Ghezzo H, Macklem PT. Age and sex differences in lung elasticity, and in closing capacity in nonsmokers. *J Appl Physiol* 1976; **41**: 129−135.

Cohn JE, Donoso HD. Mechanical properties of lung in normal men over 60 years old. *J Clin Invest* 1963; **42**: 1406−1410.

Colebatch HJH, Greaves IA, Ng CKY. Exponential analysis of elastic recoil and aging in healthy males and females. *J Appl Physiol* 1979; **47**: 683−691.

Frank NR, Mead J, Ferris BG Jr. The mechanical behavior of the lungs in healthy elderly persons. *J Clin Invest* 1957; **36**: 1680−1687.

Gibson GJ, Pride NB, O'Cain C, Quagliato R. Sex and age differences in pulmonary mechanics in normal nonsmoking subjects. *J Appl Physiol* 1976; **41**: 20−25.

Habib MP, Klink ME, Knudson DE, Bloom JW, Kaltenborn WT, Knudson RJ. Physiologic characteristics of subjects exhibiting accelerated deterioration of ventilatory function. *Am Rev Respir Dis* 1987; **136**: 638−645.

Hamer NAJ. The effect of age on the components of the pulmonary diffusing capacity. *Clin Sci* 1962; **23**: 85−93.

Holland J, Milic-Emili J, Macklem PT, Bates DV. Regional distribution of pulmonary ventilation and perfusion in elderly subjects. *J Clin Invest* 1968; **47**: 81−92.

Knudson RJ, Clark DF, Kennedy TC, Knudson DE. Effect of aging alone on mechanical properties of the normal adult human lung. *J Appl Physiol* 1977; **43**: 1054−1062.

Kronenberg RS, Drage CW. Attenuation of the ventilatory and heart rate responses to hypoxia and hypercapnia with aging in normal men. *J Clin Invest* 1973; **52**: 1812−1819.

Mittman C, Edelman NH, Norris AH, Shock NW. Relationship between chest wall and pulmonary compliance and age. *J Appl Physiol* 1965; **20**: 1211−1216.

Muiesan G, Sorbini CA, Grassi V. Respiratory function in the aged. *Bull Physiopathol Respir* 1971; **7**: 973−1009.

Niewoehner DE, Kleinerman J. Morphologic basis of pulmonary resistance in the human lung and effects of aging. *J Appl Physiol* 1974; **36**: 412−418.

Pierce JA, Ebert RV. Fibrous network of the lung and its change with age. *Thorax* 1965; **20**: 469−476.

Pierce JA, Hocott JB. Studies on the collagen and elastin content of the human lung. *J Clin Invest* 1960; **39**: 8−14.

Pride NB. Pulmonary distensibility in age and disease. *Bull Physiopathol Respir* 1974; **10**: 103−108.

Ranga V, Kleinerman J, Ip MPC, Sorensen J. Age-related changes in elastic fibers and elastin of lung. *Am Rev Respir Dis* 1979; **119**: 369−381.

Sorbini CA, Grassi V, Solinas E, Muiesan G. Arterial oxygen tension in relation to age in healthy subjects. *Respiration* 1968; **25**: 3−13.

Tenney SM, Miller RM. Dead space ventilation in old age. *J Appl Physiol* 1956; **9**: 321−327.

Turner JM, Mead J, Wohl ME. Elasticity of human

lungs in relation to age. *J Appl Physiol* 1968; **25**: 664−671.

Yernault J-C, De Troyer A, Rodenstein D. Sex and age differences in intrathoracic airways mechanics in normal man. *J Appl Physiol* 1979; **46**: 556−564.

43 ETHNIC VARIATION

43.1 Lung function

(*see also* sections 35, 36, 39, 43.2 (Miller *et al.*), 44)

Anderson HR, Anderson JA, Cotes JE. Lung function values in healthy children and adults from highland and coastal areas of Papua New Guinea. *Papua New Guinea Med J* 1974; **17**: 165−167.

Bangham CRM, Veale KEA. Ventilatory capacity in healthy Nepalese. *J Physiol (Lond)* 1977; **265**: 31P−32P.

Bhattacharya AK, Banerjee S. Vital capacity in children and young adults of India. *Indian J Med Res* 1966; **54**: 62−71.

Boyce AJ, Haight JS, Rimmer DB, Harrison GA. Respiratory function in Peruvian Quechua Indians. *Ann Hum Biol* 1974; **1**: 137−148.

Chatterjee S, Saha D, Chatterjee BP. Pulmonary function studies in healthy non-smoking men of Calcutta. *Ann Hum Biol* 1988; **15**: 365−374.

Cotes JE, Dabbs JM, Hall AM, Lakhera SC, Saunders MJ, Malhotra MS. Lung function of healthy young men in India: contributory roles of genetic and environmental factors. *Proc R Soc Lond (Biol)* 1975; **191**: 413−425.

Cotes JE, Saunders MJ, Adam JER, Anderson HR, Hall AM. Lung function in coastal and highland New Guineans: comparison with Europeans. *Thorax* 1973; **28**: 320−330.

Crapo RO, Lockey J, Aldrich V, Jensen RL, Elliott CG. Normal spirometric values in healthy American Indians. *J Occup Med* 1988; **30**: 556−560.

Da Costa JL. Pulmonary function studies in healthy Chinese adults in Singapore. *Am Rev Respir Dis* 1971; **104**: 128−131.

De Hamel FA, Welford B. Lung function in Maoris and Samoans working in New Zealand. *NZ Med J* 1983; **96**: 560−562.

Donnelly PM, Yang T-S, Peat JK, Woolcock AJ. What factors explain racial differences in lung volumes? *Eur Respir J* 1991; **4**: 829−838.

Frisancho AR. Functional adaptation to high altitude hypoxia. *Science* 1975; **187**: 313−319.

Jain SK, Gupta CK. Lung function studies in healthy men and women over forty. *Indian J Med Res* 1967; **55**: 612−619.

Jain SK, Ramiah TJ. Normal standards of pulmonary function tests for healthy Indian men 15−40 years old: comparison of different regression equations (prediction formulae). *Indian J Med Res* 1969; **57**: 1453−1466.

Jones PRM, Baber FM, Heywood C, Cotes JE. Ventilatory capacity in healthy Chinese children: relation to habitual activity. *Ann Hum Biol* 1977; **4**: 155−161.

Kamat SR, Tyahi NK, Rashid SSA. Lung function in Indian adult subjects. *Lung India* 1982; **1**: 11−21.

Lam K-K, Pang S-C, Allan WGL, Hill LE, Snell NJC, Nunn AJ. A survey of ventilatory capacity in Chinese subjects in Hong Kong. *Ann Hum Biol* 1982; **9**: 459−472.

Malik MA, Moss E, Lee WR. Prediction values for the ventilatory capacity in male West Pakistani workers in the United Kingdom. *Thorax* 1972; **27**: 611−619.

Malik SK, Jindal SK, Jindal V, Bausal S. Peak expiratory flow rate in healthy adults. *Indian J Chest Dis* 1975; **17**: 166−171.

Marcus EB, Maclean CJ, Curb JD, Johnson LR, Vollmer WM, Buist AS. Reference values for FEV in Japanese−American men from 45 to 68 years of age. *Am Rev Respir Dis* 1988; **138**: 1393−1397.

Milledge JS. Vital capacity and forced expiratory volume one second in South Indian men. *Indian J Chest Dis* 1965; **2**: 97−103.

Miller GJ, Ashcroft MT, Swan AV, Beadnell HMSG. Ethnic variation in forced expiratory volume and forced vital capacity of African and Indian adults in Guyana. *Am Rev Respir Dis* 1970; **102**: 979−981.

Miller GJ, Ashcroft MT. A community survey of respiratory disease among East Indian and African adults in Guyana. *Thorax* 1971; **26**: 331−338.

Patrick JM, Cotes JE. Anthropometric and other factors affecting respiratory responses to CO_2 in New Guineans. *Philos Trans R Soc Lond (Biol)* 1974; **268**: 363−373.

Patrick JM, Femi-Pearse D. Reference values for $FEV_{1.0}$ and FVC in Nigerian men and women: a graphical summary. *Niger Med J* 1976; **6**: 380−385.

Reed TE. Caucasian genes in American negroes. *Science* 1969; **165**: 762−768.

Rossiter CE, Weill H. Ethnic difference in lung function; evidence for proportional differences. *Int J Epidemiol* 1974; **3**: 55−61.

Singh HD, Abraham DL, Anthony NJ. Expiratory flow rates and timed expiratory capacities in south Indian men. *J Indian Med Assoc* 1970; **54**: 412−415.

Smolej-Narancic N, Pavlovic M, Rudan P. Ventilatory parameters in healthy nonsmoking adults of Adriatic island (Yugoslavia). *Eur Respir J* 1991; **4**: 955−964.

Yang T-S, Peat J, Keena V, Donnelly P, Unger W, Woolcock A. Review of the racial differences in the lung function of normal Caucasian, Chinese and Indian subjects. *Eur Respir J* 1991; **4**: 872−880.

Yokoyama T, Mitsufuji M. Statistical representation of the ventilatory capacity of 2247 healthy Japanese adults. *Chest* 1972; **61**: 655−661.

43.2 Ethnic variation in exercise performance

Cotes JE. Genetic and environmental determinants of the physiological response to exercise. In: Jokl E, Anand RL, Stoboy H, eds. *Advances in Exercise*

Physiology. Proc Int Symp Exercise and Sports Physiology. *Medicine and Sport* **9**: Basel: Karger, 1976: 188–202.

Edwards RHT, Miller GJ, Hearn CED, Cotes JE. Pulmonary function and exercise responses in relation to body composition and ethnic origin in Trinidadian males. *Proc R Soc Lond (Biol)* 1972; **181**: 407–420.

Miller GJ, Cotes JE, Hall AM, Slvosa CB, Ashworth A. Lung function and exercise performance of healthy Caribbean men and women of African ethnic origin. *Q J Exp Physiol* 1972; **57**: 325–341.

Miller GJ, Saunders MJ, Gilson RJC, Ashcroft MT. Lung function of healthy boys and girls in Jamaica in relation to ethnic composition, test exercise performance, and habitual physical activity. *Thorax* 1977; **32**: 486–496.

Patrick JM, Cotes JE. Cardiac output during submaximal exercise in New Guineans: the relation with body size and habitat. *Q J Exp Physiol* 1978; **63**: 277–290.

44 REFERENCE VALUES IN ADULT CAUCASIANS

44.1 Flow rates and volumes measured cross sectionally
(*see also* sections 3, 5)

Amrein R, Keller R, Joos H, Herzog H. Valeurs theoriques nouvelles de l'exploration de la fonction ventilatoire du poumon. *Bull Physiopathol Respir* 1970; **6**: 317–349.

Becklake MR, Fournier-Massey G, McDonald JC, Sliemiatycki J, Rossiter CE. Lung function in relation to chest radiographic changes in Quebec asbestos workers. I. Methods, results and conclusions. *Bull Physiopathol Respir* 1970; **6**: 637–659.

Berglund E, Birath G, Bjure J, Grimby G, Kjellmer I, Sandqvist L, Söderholm B. Spirometric studies of normal subjects. I. Forced expirograms in subjects between 7 and 70 years of age. *Acta Med Scand* 1963; **173**: 185–192.

Birath G, Kjellmer I, Sandqvist L. Spirometric studies in normal subjects, 2. Ventilatory capacity tests in adults. *Acta Med Scand* 1963; **173**: 193–198.

Boren HG, Kory RC, Syner JC. The Veterans Administration-Army Cooperative study of pulmonary function. 2. The lung volume and its subdivisions in normal men. *Am J Med* 1966; **41**: 96–114, 1007–1008.

Burrows B, Lebowitz MD, Camilli AE, Knudson RJ. Longitudinal changes in forced expiratory volume in one second in adults. Methodologic considerations and findings in healthy nonsmokers. *Am Rev Respir Dis* 1986; **133**: 974–980.

Cole TJ. The influence of height on the decline in ventilatory function. *Int J Epidemiol* 1974; **3**: 145–152.

Cotes JE, Rossiter CE, Higgins ITT, Gilson JC. Average normal values for the forced expiratory volume

in white Caucasian males. *Br Med J* 1966; **1**: 1016–1019.

Crapo RO, Morris AH, Gardner RM. Reference spirometric values using techniques and equipment that meet ATS recommendations. *Am Rev Respir Dis* 1981; **123**: 659–664.

de Kroon JPM, Joosting PE, Visser BF. Les valeurs normales de la capacité vitale et du volume expiratoire maximum seconde. *Arch Mal Prof* 1964; **25**: 17–30.

Dickman ML, Schmidt CD, Gardner RM, Marshall HW, Day WL, Warner HR. On-line computerized spirometry in 738 normal adults. *Am Rev Respir Dis* 1969; **100**: 780–790.

Drouet D, Kauffman F, Brille D, Lellouch J. Valeurs spirographiques de référence: Modèles mathématiques et utilisation pratique. *Bull Eur Physiopathol Respir* 1980; **16**: 747–767.

Ericsson P, Irnell L. Spirometric studies of ventilatory capacity in elderly people. *Acta Med Scand* 1969; **185**: 179–184.

Ferris BG Jr, Anderson DO, Zickmantel R. Prediction values for screening tests of pulmonary function. *Am Rev Respir Dis* 1965; **91**: 252–261.

Goldman HI, Becklake MR. Respiratory function tests. Normal values at median altitudes and the prediction of normal results. *Am Rev Tuberc* 1959; **79**: 457–467.

Grimby G, Söderholm B. Spirometric studies in normal subjects. III. Static lung volumes and maximum voluntary ventilation in adults with a note on physical fitness. *Acta Med Scand* 1963; **173**: 199–206.

Hall AM, Heywood C, Cotes JE. Lung function in healthy British women. *Thorax* 1979; **34**: 359–365.

Higgins MW, Keller JB. Seven measures of ventilatory lung function. Population values and a comparison of their ability to discriminate between persons with and without chronic respiratory symptoms and disease, Tecumseh, Michigan. *Am Rev Respir Dis* 1973; **108**: 258–272.

Jouasset D. Normalisation des epreuves fonctionnelles respiratoires dans les pays de la Communaute Europeanne du Charbon et de l'Acier. *Pneumon Coeur* 1960; 1145–1159.

Källqvist I, Taube A, Olafsson O. Peak expiratory flow rate in healthy persons aged 45–65 years. *Scand J Respir Dis* 1970; **51**: 177–187.

Knudson RJ, Lebowitz MD, Holberg CJ, Burrows B. Changes in the normal maximal expiratory flow–volume curve with growth and aging. *Am Rev Respir Dis* 1983; **127**: 725–734.

Kory RC, Callahan R, Boren HG, Syner JC. The Veterans Administration–Army Cooperative study of pulmonary function. I. Clinical spirometry in normal men. *Am J Med* 1961; **30**: 243–258.

Kuperman AS, Riker JB. The predicted normal maximal mid-expiratory flow. *Am Rev Respir Dis* 1973; **107**: 231–238.

Leiner GC, Abramowitz S, Small MJ, Stenby VB, Lewis WA. Expiratory peak flow rate. Standard values for normal subjects. *Am Rev Respir Dis* 1963; **88**: 644–651.

Lindall A, Medina A, Grismer JT. A re-evaluation of normal pulmonary function measurements in the adult female. *Am Rev Respir Dis* 1967; **95**: 1061–1064.

Lundsgaard C, Van Slyke DD. Studies of lung volumes: 1. Relation between thorax size and lung volume in normal adults. *J Exp Med* 1916; **27**: 65–86.

Miller A, Thornton JC, Warshaw R, Berstein J, Selikoff IJ, Teirstein AS. Mean and instantaneous expiratory flows, FVC and FEV_1: prediction equations from a probability sample of Michigan, a large industrial state. *Bull Eur Physiopathol Respir* 1986; **22**: 589–597.

Milne JS, Williamson J. Respiratory function tests in older people. *Clin Sci* 1972; **42**: 371–381.

Morris JF, Koski A, Johnson LC. Spirometric standards for healthy nonsmoking adults. *Am Rev Respir Dis* 1971; **103**: 57–67.

Nunn AJ, Gregg I. New regression equations for predicting peak expiratory flow in adults. *Br Med J* 1989; **298**: 1068–1070.

Paoletti P, Pistelli G, Fazzi P, Viegi G, Di Pede F, Guiliano G *et al*. Reference values for vital capacity and flow–volume curves from a general population study. *Bull Eur Physiopathol Respir* 1986; **22**: 451–459.

Pelzer AM, Thomson ML. Expiratory peak flow. *Br Med J* 1964; **2**: 123.

Quanjer PhH, Dalhuijsen A, Van Zomeren BC. Summary equations of reference values. *Bull Eur Physiopathol Respir* 1983; **19**(Suppl. 5): 45–51.

Quanjer PhH. Interpretation of tests of ventilatory function. In: *The ECSC in Technological and Social Research*. Gijon, 1989; 407–425.

Ringqvist T, Ringqvist I. Respiratory forces and variations of static lung volumes in healthy subjects. *Scand J Clin Lab Invest* 1974; **33**: 269–276.

Roca J, Sanchis J, Agusti-Vidal A, Segarra F, Navajas D, Rodriguez-Roisin R *et al*. Spirometric reference values from a Mediterranean population. *Bull Eur Physiopathol Respir* 1986; **22**: 217–224.

Roberts CM, MacRae KD, Winning AJ, Adams L, Seed WA. Reference values and prediction equations for normal lung function in a non-smoking white urban population. *Thorax* 1991; **46**: 643–650.

Schmidt CD, Dickman ML, Gardner RM, Brough FK. Spirometric standards for healthy elderly men and women. *Am Rev Respir Dis* 1973; **108**: 933–943.

44.2 Longitudinal studies
(*see also* sections 36, 45.1)

Burrows B, Lebowitz MD, Camilli AE, Knudson RJ. Longitudinal changes in forced expiratory volume in one second in adults: methodologic considerations and findings in healthy nonsmokers. *Am Rev Respir Dis* 1986; **133**: 974–980.

Habib MP, Klink ME, Knudson DE, Bloom WJ, Kaltenborn WT, Knudson RJ. Physiologic characteristics of subjects exhibiting accelerated deterioration of ventilatory function. *Am Rev Respir Dis* 1987; **136**: 638–645.

Hurwitz S, Allen J, Liben A, Becklake MR. Lung function in young adults: evidence for differences in the chronological age at which various functions start to decline. *Thorax* 1980; **35**: 615–619.

Lawther PJ, Brooks AGF, Waller RE. Respiratory function measurements in a cohort of medical students: a ten-year follow-up. *Thorax* 1978; **33**: 773–778.

Rosenzweig DY, Arkins JA, Schrock LG. Ventilation studies on a normal population after a seven-year interval. *Am Rev Respir Dis* 1966; **94**: 74–78.

Sherrill DL, Lebowitz MD, Knudson RJ, Burrows B. Continuous longitudinal regression equations for pulmonary function measures. *Eur Respir J* 1992; **5**: 452–462.

Ware JH, Dockery DW, Louis TA, Xu X, Ferris BG Jr, Speizer FE. Longitudinal and cross-sectional estimates of pulmonary function decline in never-smoking adults. *Am J Epidemiol* 1990; **132**: 685–700.

44.3 Reference values for transfer factor (diffusing capacity)

Billiet L, Baiser W, Naedts JP. Effet de la taille, du sexe et de l'age sur la capacité de diffusion pulmonaire de l'adult normal. *J Physiol (Paris)* 1963; **55**: 199–200.

Cohn JE, Carroll DG, Armstrong BW, Shepard RH, Riley RL. Maximal diffusing capacity of the lung in normal male subjects of different ages. *J Appl Physiol* 1954; **6**: 588–597.

Cotes JE, Hall AM. The transfer factor for the lung; normal values in adults. In: Arcangeli P, ed. *Normal Values for Respiratory Function in Man*. Torino: Panminerva Medica, 1970: 327–343.

Crapo RO, Morris AH. Standardized single breath normal values for carbon monoxide diffusing capacity. *Am Rev Respir Dis* 1981; **123**: 185–189.

Donevan RE, Palmer WH, Varvis CJ, Bates DV. Influence of age on pulmonary diffusing capacity. *J Appl Physiol* 1959; **14**: 483–492.

Frans A. Les valeurs normales du volume capillaire pulmonaire (*Vc*) et de la capacite de diffusion de la membrane alveolo-capillaire (*DM*). In: Arcangeli P, ed. *Normal Values for Respiratory Function in Man*. Torino: Panminerva Medica, 1970: 352–363.

Georges R, Saumon G, Loiseau A. The relationship of age to pulmonary membrane conductance and capillary blood volume. *Am Rev Respir Dis* 1978; **117**: 1069–1078.

Gulsvik A, Bakke P, Humerfelt S, Omenaas E, Tosteson T, Weiss ST, Speizer FE. Single breath transfer factor for carbon monoxide in an asymptomatic population of never smokers. *Thorax* 1992;

47: 167–173.

Knudson RJ, Kaltenborn WT, Knudson DE, Burrows B. The single-breath carbon monoxide diffusing capacity. Reference equations derived from a healthy nonsmoking population and effects of hematocrit. *Am Rev Respir Dis* 1987; **135**: 805–811.

Love RG, Seaton A, *also* Quanjer PhH. About the ECCS summary equations. Letters to the Editor. *Eur Respir J* 1990; **3**: 489–490.

Miller A, Thornton JC, Warshaw R, Anderson H, Teirstein AS, Selikoff IJ. Single breath diffusing capacity in a representative sample of the population of Michigan, a large industrial state. *Am Rev Respir Dis* 1983; **127**: 270–277.

Paoletti P, Viegi G, Pistelli G, Di Pede F, Fazzi P, Polato R *et al.* Reference equations for the single-breath diffusing capacity. A cross-sectional analysis and effect of body size and age. *Am Rev Respir Dis* 1985; **132**: 806–813.

Teculescu DB, Stanescu DC. Lung diffusing capacity. Normal values in male smokers and non-smokers using the breath-holding technique. *Scand J Respir Dis* 1970; **51**: 137–149.

Van Ganse WF, Ferris BG, Cotes JE. Cigarette smoking and pulmonary diffusing capacity (transfer factor). *Am Rev Respir Dis* 1972; **105**: 30–40.

44.4 *Other reference values (including mechanics and blood gases)*

Bachofen H, Hobi HJ, Scherrer M. Alveolar–arterial N_2 gradients at rest and during exercise in healthy men of different ages. *J Appl Physiol* 1973; **34**: 137–142.

Black LF, Hyatt RE. Maximal respiratory pressures: normal values and relationship to age and sex. *Am Rev Respir Dis* 1969; **99**: 696–702.

Briscoe WA, DuBois AB. The relationship between airway resistance, airway conductance and lung volume in subjects of different age and body size. *J Clin Invest* 1958; **37**: 1279–1285.

Brody AW, Shenan JJ, Wander HJ, Connolly JJ, Schwertley FW. Tests of ventilatory strength and mechanics; graphs of normal values. *Am Rev Respir Dis* 1964; **89**: 270–276.

Brunes L, Holmgren A. Total airway resistance and its relationship to body size and lung volumes in healthy young women. *Scand J Clin Lab Invest* 1966; **18**: 316–324.

Frank NR, Mead J, Ferris BG Jr. The mechanical behaviour of the lungs in healthy elderly persons. *J Clin Invest* 1957; **36**: 1680–1687.

Frank NR, Mead J, Siebens AA, Storey CF. Measurements of pulmonary compliance in seventy healthy young adults. *J Appl Physiol* 1956; **9**: 38–42.

Hertle FH, George R, Lange HJ. Die arteriellen blutgaspartialdrucke und ih re Beziehungen zu Alter und Anthropometrischen Grössen. *Rev Inst Hyg Mines* 1971; **28**: 1–30.

Vooren PH, van Zomeren BC. Reference values of total respiratory resistance, determined with the 'opening' interruption technique. *Eur Respir J* 1989; **2**: 966–971.

45 SMOKING AND AIR POLLUTION

45.1 *Tobacco smoke*
(*see also* sections 15, 44)

Adams L, Lonsdale D, Robinson M, Rawbone R, Guz A. Respiratory impairment induced by smoking in children in secondary schools. *Br Med J* 1984; **288**: 891–895.

Anderson HR. Respiratory abnormalities and ventilatory capacity in a Papua New Guinea Island Community. *Am Rev Respir Dis* 1976; **114**: 537–548.

Bode FR, Dosman J, Martin RR, Macklem PT. Reversibility of pulmonary function abnormalities in smokers. *Am J Med* 1975; **59**: 43–52.

Brunekreef B, Fischer P, Remijn B, Van der Lende R, Schonten J, Quanjer PhH. Indoor air pollution and its effects on pulmonary function in adult non-smoking women: III. Passive smoking and pulmonary function. *Int J Epidemiol* 1985; **14**: 227–230.

Camilli AE, Burrows B, Knudson RJ, Lyle SK, Lebowitz MD. Longitudinal changes in forced expiratory volume in one second in adults: effect of cigarette smoking and respiratory symptoms. *Am Rev Respir Dis* 1987; **135**: 794–799.

Carey GCR, Dawson TAJ, Merrett JD. Daily changes in ventilatory capacity in smokers and in non-smokers. *Br J Prev Soc Med* 1967; **21**: 86–89.

Da Silva AMT, Hamosh P. Effect of smoking a single cigarette on the 'small airways'. *J Appl Physiol* 1973; **34**: 361–365.

Dockery DW, Speizer FE, Ferris BG Jr, Ware JH, Louis TA, Spiro A, III. Cumulative and reversible effects of lifetime smoking on simple tests of lung function in adults. *Am Rev Respir Dis* 1988; **137**: 286–292.

Frans A, Gerin-Portier N, Veriter C, Brasseur L. Pulmonary gas exchange in asymptomatic smokers and nonsmokers. *Scand J Respir Dis* 1975; **56**: 233–244.

Goldbarg AN, Krone RJ, Resnekov L. Effects of cigarette smoking on hemodynamics at rest and during exercise. I. Normal subjects. *Chest* 1971; **60**: 531–536.

Groth S, Hermansen F, Rossing N. Pulmonary permeability in never-smokers between 21 and 67 yr of age. *J Appl Physiol* 1989; **67**: 422–428.

Helsing KJ, Comstock GW, Speizer FE, Ferris BG, Lebowitz MD, Tockman MS, Burrows B. Comparison of three standardized questionnaires on respiratory symptoms. *Am Rev Respir Dis* 1979; **120**: 1221–1231.

Ingram RH Jr, O'Cain CF. Frequency dependence of compliance in apparently healthy smokers versus non-smokers. *Bull Physiopathol Respir* 1971; **7**: 195–212.

Jaakkola MS, Jaakkola JJK, Ernst P, Becklake MR. Ventilatory lung function in young cigarette smokers: a study of susceptibility. *Eur Respir J* 1991; 4: 643–650.

Jones JG, Minty BD, Lawler P, Hulands G, Crawley JCW, Veall N. Increased alveolar epithelial permeability in cigarette smokers. *Lancet* 1980; i: 66–68.

Knudson RJ, Bloom JW, Knudson DE, Kaltenborn WT. Subclinical effects of smoking. Physiologic comparison of healthy middle-aged smokers and nonsmokers and interrelationships of lung function measurements. *Chest* 1984; 86: 20–29.

Knudson RJ, Kaltenborn WT, Burrows B. The effects of cigarette smoking and smoking cessation on the carbon monoxide diffusing capacity of the lung in asymptomatic subjects. *Am Rev Respir Dis* 1989; 140: 645–651.

Krumholz RA, Chavalier RB, Ross JC. Changes in cardiopulmonary functions related to abstinence from smoking. *Ann Intern Med* 1965; 62: 197–207.

Krzyzanowski M, Sherrill DL, Paoletti P, Lebowitz MD. Relationship of respiratory symptoms and pulmonary function to tar, nicotine, and carbon monoxide yield of cigarettes. *Am Rev Respir Dis* 1991; 143: 306–311.

Marco M, Minette A. Lung function changes in smokers with normal conventional spirometry. *Am Rev Respir Dis* 1976; 114: 723–738.

Martinez FD, Antognoni G, Macri F, Bonci E, Midulla F, de Castro G, Ronchetti R. Parental smoking enhances bronchial responsiveness in nine-year-old children. *Am Rev Respir Dis* 1988; 138: 518–523.

Masi MA, Hanley JA, Ernst P, Becklake MR. Environmental exposure to tobacco smoke and lung function in young adults. *Am Rev Respir Dis* 1988; 138: 296–299.

McCarthy DS, Craig DB, Cherniack RM. The effect of acute, intensive cigarette smoking on maximal expiratory flows and the single breath nitrogen washout trace. *Am Rev Respir Dis* 1976; 113: 301–304.

Michels A, Decoster K, Derde L, Vleurinck C, van de Woestijne KP. Influence of posture on lung volumes and impedance of respiratory system in healthy smokers and nonsmokers. *J Appl Physiol* 1991; 71: 294–299.

Sparrow D, Stefos T, Bossé R, Weiss ST. The relationship of tar content to decline in pulmonary function in cigarette smokers. *Am Rev Respir Dis* 1983; 127: 56–58.

Tager IB, Segal MR, Munoz A, Weiss ST, Speizer FE. The effect of maternal cigarette smoking on the pulmonary function of children and adolescents. *Am Rev Respir Dis* 1987; 136: 1366–1370.

Tager IB, Segal MR, Speizer FE, Weiss ST. The natural history of forced expiratory volumes. Effect of cigarette smoking and respiratory symptoms. *Am Rev Respir Dis* 1988; 138: 837–849.

Taylor RG, Gross E, Joyce H, Holland F, Pride NB. Smoking, allergy and rate of decline in FEV_1. *Thorax* 1984; 39: 695.

Tockman M, Menkes H, Cohen B, Permutt S, Benjamin J, Ball WC Jr et al. A comparison of pulmonary function in male smokers and nonsmokers. *Am Rev Respir Dis* 1976; 114: 711–722.

Van der Lende R, Kok TJ, Peset R, Quanjer PhH, Schouten JP, Orie NGM. Decreases in VC and FEV, with time: indicators for effects of smoking and air pollution. *Bull Eur Physiopathol Respir* 1981; 17: 775–792.

Woolf CR, Suero JT. The respiratory effects of regular cigarette smoking in women. *Am Rev Respir Dis* 1971; 103: 26–37.

Zuskin E, Mitchell CA, Bouhuys A. Interaction between effects of beta blockade and cigarette smoke on airways. *J Appl Physiol* 1974; 36: 449–452.

45.2 *Marijuana and opium*

Da Costa JL, Tock EPC, Boey HK. Lung Disease with chronic obstruction in opium smokers in Singapore. *Thorax* 1971; 26: 555–571.

Tashkin DP, Clark VA, Coulson AH, Bourque LB, Simmons M, Reems C et al. Comparison of lung function in young non-smokers and smokers before and after initiation of the smoking habit. *Am Rev Respir Dis* 1983; 128: 12–16.

Tashkin DP, Coulson AH, Clark VA, Simmons M, Bourque LB, Duann S et al. Respiratory symptoms and lung function in habitual heavy smokers of marijuana alone, smokers of marijuana and tobacco, smokers of tobacco alone, and nonsmokers. *Am Rev Respir Dis* 1987; 135: 209–216.

Tashkin DP, Shapiro BJ, Frank IM. Acute pulmonary physiological effects of smoked marijuana and oral Δ^9 Tetrahydrocannabinol in healthy young men. *New Engl J Med* 1973; 289: 336–341.

45.3 *Air pollution*

Andersen I, Lundqvist GR, Jensen PL, Proctor DF. Human response to controlled levels of sulfur dioxide. *Arch Environ Health* 1974; 28: 31–39.

Becklake MR. Chronic airflow limitation: its relationship to work in dusty occupations. *Chest* 1985; 88: 608–617.

Douglas JWB, Waller RE. Air pollution and respiratory infection in children. *Br J Prev Soc Med* 1966; 20: 1–8.

Frampton MW, Morrow PE, Cox C, Gibb FR, Speers DM, Utell MJ. Effects of nitrogen dioxide exposure on pulmonary function and airway reactivity in normal humans. *Am Rev Respir Dis* 1991; 143: 522–527.

Holtzman MJ, Cunningham JH, Sheller JR, Irsigler GB, Nadel JA, Boushey HA. Effect of ozone on bronchial reactivity in atopic and nonatopic subjects. *Am Rev Respir Dis* 1979; 120: 1059–1067.

Huy T, de Schipper K, Chan-Yeung M, Kennedy SM.

Grain dust and lung function. Dose–response relationships. *Am Rev Respir Dis* 1991; **144**: 1314–1321.

Jones GR, Proudfoot AT, Hall JI. Pulmonary effects of acute exposure to nitrous fumes. *Thorax* 1973; **28**: 61–65.

Kagawa J, Toyama T. Effects of ozone and brief exercise on specific airway conductance in man. *Arch Environ Health* 1975; **30**: 36–39.

Karliner JS, Steinberg AD, Williams MH Jr. Lung function after pulmonary edema associated with heroin overdose. *Arch Intern Med* 1969; **124**: 350–353.

Koenig JQ, Covert DS, Hanley QS, Van Belle G, Pierson WE. Prior exposure to ozone potentiates subsequent response to sulfur dioxide in adolescent asthmatic subjects. *Am Rev Respir Dis* 1990; **141**: 377–380.

Lowe CR, Campbell H, Khosla T. Bronchitis in two integrated steel works. Respiratory symptoms and ventilatory capacity related to atmospheric pollution. *Br J Ind Med* 1970; **27**: 121–129.

McDonnell WF, Horstman DH, Hazucha MJ, Seal E Jr, Haak ED, Salaam SA *et al.* Pulmonary effects of ozone exposure during exercise: dose–response characteristics. *J Appl Physiol* 1983; **54**: 1345–1352.

Mohsenin V. Effect of vitamin C on NO_2-induced airway hyperresponsiveness in normal subjects. *Am Rev Respir Dis* 1987; **136**: 1408–1411.

Olsen HC, Gilson JC. Respiratory symptoms, bronchitis and ventilatory capacity in man. *Br Med J* 1960; **1**: 450–456.

Orehek J, Massari JP, Gayrard P, Grimaud C, Charpin J. Effect of short-term, low-level nitrogen dioxide exposure on bronchial sensitivity of asthmatic patients. *J Clin Invest* 1976; **57**: 301–307.

Silverman F, Folinsbee LJ, Barnard J, Shephard RJ. Pulmonary function changes in ozone-interaction of concentration and ventilation. *J Appl Physiol* 1976; **41**: 859–864.

46 ACID–BASE: CLINICAL PHYSIOLOGY
(*see also* section 23)

Arbus GA, Herbert LA, Levesque PR, Etsten BE, Schwartz WB. Characterisation and clinical application of the 'significance band' for acute respiratory alkalosis. *New Engl J Med* 1969; **280**: 117–123.

Bone JM, Cowie J, Lambie AT, Robson JS. The relationship between arterial Pco_2 and hydrogen ion concentration in chronic metabolic acidosis and alkalosis. *Clin Sci* 1974; **46**: 113–123.

Brackett NC Jr, Cohen JJ, Schwartz WB. Carbon dioxide titration curve of normal man. *New Engl J Med* 1965; **272**: 6–12.

Cohen RD, Iles RA. Lactic acidosis: some physiological and clinical considerations. *Clin Sci* 1977; **53**: 405–410.

Cohen JJ, Schwartz WB. Evaluation of acid–base equilibrium in pulmonary insufficiency. *Am J Med*

1966; **41**: 163–167.

Dulfano MJ, Ishikawa S. Quantitative acid–base relationships in chronic pulmonary patients during the stable state. *Am Rev Respir Dis* 1966; **93**: 251–256.

Goldstein MB, Gennari FJ, Schwartz WB. The influence of graded degrees of chronic hypercapnia on the acute carbon dioxide titration curve. *J Clin Invest* 1971; **50**: 208–216.

Ingram RH, Miller RB, Tate LA. Acid–base response to acute carbon dioxide changes in chronic obstructive pulmonary disease. *Am Rev Respir Dis* 1973; **108**: 225–231.

Pingree BJW. Acid–base and respiratory changes after prolonged exposure to 1% carbon dioxide. *Clin Sci* 1977; **52**: 67–74.

Saunders KB, Band DM, Ebden P, Van der Hoff JP, Maberley DJ, Semple SJG. Acid–base status and gas exchange in the anaesthetized dog breathing pure oxygen. *Respiration* 1972; **29**: 305–316.

Van Ypersele de Strihou C, Brasseur L, de Coninck J. The 'carbon dioxide response curve' for chronic hypercapnia in man. *New Engl J Med* 1966; **275**: 117–122.

47 RESPIRATORY DISTRESS IN THE NEWBORN
(*see also* section 17.2)

Avery ME, Mead J. Surface properties in relation to atelectasis and hyaline membrane disease. *Am J Dis Child* 1959; **97**: 517–523.

Corbet AJS, Ross JA, Beaudry PH, Stern L. Effect of positive-pressure breathing on a-ADN_2 in hyaline membrane disease. *J Appl Physiol* 1975; **38**: 33–38.

Jobe A, Ikegami M. Surfactant for the treatment of respiratory distress syndrome. *Am Rev Respir Dis* 1987; **136**: 1256–1275.

Lamarre A, Linsao L, Reilly BJ, Swyer PR, Levison H. Residual pulmonary abnormalities in survivors of idiopathic respiratory distress syndrome. *Am Rev Respir Dis* 1973; **108**: 56–61.

Petty TL, Hodson LD, eds. Acute pulmonary injury and repair. *Chest* 1974; 65: 1S–67S; **66**: 1S–46S.

Reynolds EO. Hypoxia in the newborn infant. *J Clin Path* 1977; **30**(Suppl 11): 134–141.

48 CYSTIC FIBROSIS
(*see also* section 70)

Corbet A, Ross J, Popkin J, Beaudry P. Relationship of arterial–alveolar nitrogen tension to alveolar–arterial oxygen tension, lung volume, low measurements and diffusing capacity in cystic fibrosis. *Am Rev Respir Dis* 1975; **112**: 513–519.

Corey M, McLaughlin FJ, Williams M, Levison H. A comparison of survival, growth and pulmonary function in patients with cystic fibrosis in Boston and Toronto. *J Clin Epidemiol* 1988; **41**: 383–391.

Godfrey S, Mearns M. Pulmonary function and response to exercise in cystic fibrosis. *Arch Dis Child* 1971; **46**: 144–151.

Mansell A, Dubrawsky C, Levison H, Bryan AC, Crozier DN. Lung elastic recoil in cystic fibrosis. *Am Rev Respir Dis* 1974; **109**: 190–197.

Pryor JA, Webber BA, Hodson ME. Effect of chest physiotherapy on oxygen saturation in patients with cystic fibrosis. *Thorax* 1990; **45**: 77.

Wood RE, Boat TF, Doershuk CF. Cystic fibrosis. *Am Rev Respir Dis* 1976; **113**: 833–878.

49 BRONCHIECTASIS

Bass H, Henderson JAM, Heckscher T, Oriol A, Anthonisen NR. Regional structure and function in bronchiectasis. *Am Rev Respir Dis* 1968; **97**: 598–609.

Bhargava RK, Woolf CR. Changes in diffusing capacity after bronchography. *Am Rev Respir Dis* 1967; **96**: 827–829.

Landau LI, Phelan PD, Williams HE. Ventilatory mechanics in patients with bronchiectasis starting in childhood. *Thorax* 1974; **29**; 304–312.

Lourenço RV, Loddenkemper R, Carton RW. Patterns of distribution and clearance of aerosols in patients with bronchiectasis. *Am Rev Respir Dis* 1972; **106**: 857–866.

Pande JN, Jain BP, Gupta RG, Guleria JS. Pulmonary ventilation and gas exchange in bronchiectasis. *Thorax* 1971; **26**: 727–733.

50 MISCELLANEOUS LUNG DISORDERS

Cate TR, Roberts JS, Russ MA, Pierce JA. Effects of common colds on pulmonary function. *Am Rev Respir Dis* 1973; **108**: 858–865.

Fridy WW, Ingram RH Jr, Hierholzer JC, Coleman MT. Airways function during mild viral respiratory illnesses. *Ann Intern Med* 1974; **80**: 150–155.

Khan AKA, Patra RWT, Banu SA, Rabbee MF. Spirometry in tropical pulmonary eosinophilia. *Br J Dis Chest* 1970; **64**: 107–109.

Lemle A, Viera LOBD, Milward GAF, Miranda JL. Lung function studies in pulmonary South American blastomycosis. *Am J Med* 1970; **48**: 434–442.

McElvaney GN, Wilcox PG, Fairbarn MS, Hilliam C, Wilkins GE, Pare PD *et al*. Respiratory muscle weakness and dyspnea in thyrotoxic patients. *Am Rev Respir Dis* 1990; **141**: 1221–1227.

Olsen GN, Block AJ, Swenson EW, Castle JR, Wynne JW. Pulmonary function evaluation of the lung resection candidate: a prospective study. *Am Rev Respir Dis* 1975; **111**: 379–387.

Phillips MS, Kennear WJM, Shaw D, Shneerson JM. Exercise responses in patients treated for pulmonary tuberculosis by thoracoplasty. *Thorax* 1989; **44**: 268–274.

Pianosi P, D'Souza SJA, Charge TD, Béland MJ, Esseltine DW, Coates AL. Cardiac output and oxygen delivery during exercise in sickle cell anemia. *Am Rev Respir Dis* 1991; **143**: 231–235.

Schuyler MR, Niewoehner DE, Inkley SR, Kohn R. Abnormal lung elasticity in juvenile diabetes mellitus. *Am Rev Respir Dis* 1976; **113**: 37–41.

Vansteenkiste J, Rochette F, Demedts M. Diagnostic tests of hyperventilation syndrome. *Eur Respir J* 1991; **4**: 393–399.

Warrell DA, Pope HM, Parry EHO, Perine PL, Bryceson ADM. Cardiorespiratory disturbances associated with infective fever in man: studies of Ethiopian louse-borne relapsing fever. *Clin Sci* 1970; **39**: 123–145.

51 CHRONIC OBSTRUCTIVE PULMONARY DISEASE

51.1 General

Barker DJP, Godfrey KM, Fall C, Osmond C, Winter PD, Shaheen SO. Relation of birth weight and childhood respiratory infection to adult lung function and death from chronic obstructive airways disease. *Br Med J* 1991; **303**: 671–675.

Burrows B, Knudson RJ, Lebowitz MD. The relationship of childhood respiratory illness to adult obstructive airway disease. *Am Rev Respir Dis* 1977; **115**: 751–760.

Carpenter L, Beral V, Strachan D, Ebi-Kryston KL, Inskip H. Respiratory symptoms as predictors of 27 year mortality in a representative sample of British adults. *Br Med J* 1989; **299**: 357–361.

Fletcher C, Peto R, Tinker C, Speizer FE. *The Natural History of Chronic Bronchitis and Emphysema*. Oxford: Oxford University Press, 1976.

Higgins M, Keller J. Familial occurrence of chronic respiratory disease and familial resemblance in ventilatory capacity. *J Chron Dis* 1975; **28**: 239–251.

Jamal K, Fleetham JA, Thurlbeck WM. Cor pulmonale: correlation with central airway lesions, peripheral airway lesions, emphysema, and control of breathing. *Am Rev Respir Dis* 1990; **141**: 1172–1177.

McSweeney AJ, Grant I. *Chronic Obstructive Pulmonary Disease: a Behavioral Perspective. Lung Biology in Health and Disease*, Vol 36. New York: Marcel Dekker, 1988: 105–121.

Peto R, Speizer FE, Cochrane AL, Moore F, Fletcher CM, Tinker CM *et al*. The relevance in adults of airflow obstruction, but not of mucus hypersecretion, to mortality from chronic lung disease. *Am Rev Respir Dis* 1983; **128**: 491–500.

Sluiter HJ, Koëter GH, de Monchy JGR, Postma DS, de Vries K, Orie NGM. The Dutch hypothesis (chronic non-specific lung disease) revisited. *Eur Respir J* 1991; **4**: 479–489.

Thurlbeck WM, Henderson JA, Fraser RG, Bates DV. Chronic obstructive lung disease. *Medicine* 1970; **49**: 81–145.

Vandenberg E, Clement J, van de Woestijne KP. Course and prognosis of patients with advanced chronic obstructive pulmonary disease. *Am J Med* 1973; **55**: 736–746.

Vermeire PA, Pride NB. A 'splitting' look at chronic

nonspecific lung disease (CNSLD): common features but diverse pathogenesis. *Eur Respir J* 1991; **4**: 490−496.

Wright JL, Cagel P, Churg A, Colby TV, Myers J. Diseases of the small airways. *Am Rev Respir Dis* 1992; **146**: 240−262.

51.2 Airway dynamics
(*see also* sections 17, 18, 51.3)

Astin TW, Penman RWB. Airway obstruction due to hypoxaemia in patients with chronic lung disease. *Am Rev Respir Dis* 1967; **95**: 567−575.

Astin TW. Bronchial sympathetic activity in chronic bronchitis. *Clin Sci* 1972; **43**: 881−889.

Bass H. The flow volume loop: normal standards and abnormalities in chronic obstructive pulmonary disease. *Chest* 1973; **63**: 171−176.

Clark TJH, Freedman S, Campbell EJM, Winn RR. The ventilatory capacity of patients with chronic airways obstruction. *Clin Sci* 1969; **36**: 307−316.

Garshick E, Segal MR, Worobec TG, Salekin CMS, Miller MJ. Alcohol consumption and chronic obstructive pulmonary disease. *Am Rev Respir Dis* 1989; **140**: 373−378.

Hogg JC, Macklem PT, Thurlbeck WM. Site and nature of airway obstruction in chronic obstructive lung disease. *New Engl J Med* 1968; **278**: 1355−1360.

Hughes JMB, Grant BJB, Greene RE, Iliff LD, Milic-Emili J. Inspiratory flow rate and ventilation distribution in normal subjects and in patients with simple chronic bronchitis. *Clin Sci* 1972; **43**: 583−595.

Leaver DG, Tattersfield AE, Pride NB. Contributions of loss of lung recoil and of enhanced airways collapsibility to the airflow obstruction of chronic bronchitis and emphysema. *J Clin Invest* 1973; **52**: 2117−2128.

Macklem PT, Thurlbeck WM, Fraser RG. Chronic obstructive disease of small airways. *Ann Intern Med* 1971; **74**: 167−177.

Potter WA, Olafsson S, Hyatt RE. Ventilatory mechanics and expiratory flow limitation during exercise in patients with obstructive lung disease. *J Clin Invest* 1971; **50**: 910−919.

Sasaki H, Okayama H, Aikawa T, Shimura S, Sekizawa K, Yanai M *et al.* Central and peripheral airways as determinants of ventilatory function in patients with chronic bronchitis, emphysema, and bronchial asthma. *Am Rev Respir Dis* 1986; **134**: 1182−1189.

Simon G, Pride NB, Jones NL, Raimondi AC. Relation between abnormalities in the chest radiograph and changes in pulmonary function in chronic bronchitis and emphysema. *Thorax* 1973; **28**: 15−23.

51.3 Respiratory muscles in COPD
(*see also* sections 8, 60, 64)

Byrd RB, Hyatt RE. Maximal respiratory pressures in chronic obstructive lung disease. *Am Rev Respir Dis* 1968; **98**: 848−856.

Donahoe M, Rogers RM, Wilson DO, Pennock BE. Oxygen consumption of the respiratory muscles in normal and in malnourished patients with chronic obstructive pulmonary disease. *Am Rev Respir Dis* 1989; **140**: 385−391.

King TKC, Yu D. Factors determining the ventilatory response to carbon dioxide in chronic obstructive airways disease. *Clin Sci* 1970; **39**: 653−662.

Martinez FJ, Couser JI, Celli BR. Factors influencing ventilatory muscle recruitment in patients with chronic airflow obstruction. *Am Rev Respir Dis* 1990; **142**: 276−282.

Newell SZ, McKenzie DK, Gandevia SC. Inspiratory and skeletal muscle strength and endurance and diaphragmatic activation in patients with chronic airflow limitation. *Thorax* 1989; **44**: 903−912.

Sanchez J, Derenne JP, Debesse B, Riquet TM, Monod H. Typology of the respiratory muscles in normal men and in patients with moderate chronic respiratory diseases. *Bull Eur Physiopathol Respir* 1982; **18**: 901−914.

51.4 Respiratory control in COPD
(*see also* sections 27, 59−62)

Bradley GW, Crawford R. Regulation of breathing during exercise in normal subjects and in chronic lung disease. *Clin Sci* 1976; **51**: 575−582.

Flenley DC, Franklin DH, Millar JS. The hypoxic drive to breathing in chronic bronchitis and emphysema. *Clin Sci* 1970; **38**: 503−518.

Koo FW, Sax DS, Snider GL. Arterial blood gases and pH during sleep in chronic obstructive pulmonary disease. *Am J Med* 1975; **58**: 663−670.

Lane DJ, Howell JBL. Relationship between sensitivity to carbon dioxide and clinical features in patients with chronic airways obstruction. *Thorax* 1970; **25**: 150−159.

Matthews AW. The relationship between central carbon dioxide sensitivity and clinical features in patients with chronic airways obstruction. *Q J Med* 1977; **46**: 179−195.

51.5 Gas exchange, exercise and other aspects of COPD
(*see also* sections 22, 30−33)

Barbera JA, Ramirez J, Roca J, Wagner PD, Sanchez-Lloret J, Rodriguez-Roisin R. Lung structure and gas exchange in mild chronic obstructive pulmonary disease. *Am Rev Respir Dis* 1990; **141**: 895−901.

Dantzker DR, D'Alonzo GE. The effect of exercise on pulmonary gas exchange in patients with severe chronic obstructive pulmonary disease. *Am Rev Respir Dis* 1986; **134**: 1135−1139.

Gray-Donald K, Gibbons L, Shapiro SH, Martin JG. Effect of nutritional status on exercise performance in patients with chronic obstructive pulmonary disease. *Am Rev Respir Dis* 1989; **140**: 1544−1548.

Kawakami Y, Kishi F, Yamamoto H, Miyamoto K. Relation of oxygen delivery, mixed venous oxygenation, and pulmonary hemodynamics to prognosis in chronic obstructive pulmonary disease. *N Engl J Med* 1983; **308**: 1045–1049.

Lindsay DA, Read J. Pulmonary vascular responsiveness in the prognosis of chronic obstructive lung disease. *Am Rev Respir Dis* 1972; **105**: 242–250.

Marcus JH, McLean RL, Duffell GM, Ingram RH. Exercise performance in relation to the pathophysiologic type of chronic obstructive pulmonary disease. *Am J Med* 1970; **49**: 14–22.

Marthan R, Castaing Y, Manier G, Guenard H. Gas exchange alterations in patients with chronic obstructive lung disease. *Chest* 1985; **87**: 470–475.

Millar AB, Fromson B, Strickland BA, Denison DM. Computed tomography based estimates of regional gas and tissue volume of the lung in supine subjects with chronic airflow limitation or fibrosing alveolitis. *Thorax* 1986; **41**: 932–939.

Refsum HE, Kim BM. The alveolo-arterial oxygen tension difference at varying alveolar ventilation in patients with pulmonary disease breathing air. *Clin Sci* 1967; **33**: 569–576.

Salisbury BG, Metzger LF, Altose MD, Stanley NN, Cherniack NS. Effect of fiberoptic bronchoscopy on respiratory performance in patients with chronic airways obstruction. *Thorax* 1975; **30**: 441–446.

Schaanning J. Ventilatory and heart rate adjustments during submaximal and maximal exercise in patients with chronic obstructive lung disease. *Scand J Respir Dis* 1976; **57**: 63–72.

Segel N, Bishop JM. The circulation in patients with chronic bronchitis and emphysema at rest and during exercise, with special reference to the influence of changes in blood viscosity and blood volume on the pulmonary circulation. *J Clin Invest* 1966; **45**: 1555–1568.

Spiro SG, Hahn HL, Edwards RHT, Pride NB. An analysis of the physiological strain of submaximal exercise in patients with chronic obstructive bronchitis. *Thorax* 1975; **30**: 415–425.

Vandenberg E, Billiet L, van de Woestijne KP, Gyselen A. Relationship between single-breath diffusing capacity and arterial blood gases in chronic obstructive lung disease. *Scand J Respir Dis* 1968; **49**: 92–101.

Wagner PD, Dantzker DR, Dueck R, Clausen JL, West JB. Ventilation–perfusion inequality in chronic obstructive pulmonary disease. *J Clin Invest* 1977; **59**: 203–216.

Watanabe S, Kanner RE, Cutillo AG, Menlove RL, Bachand RT Jr, Szalkowski MB et al. Long-term effect of almitrine bismesylate in patients with hypoxemic chronic obstructive pulmonary disease. *Am Rev Respir Dis* 1989; **140**: 1269–1273.

Wehr KL, Johnson RL Jr, Prengler A. Maximal oxygen consumption in patients with lung disease. *J Clin Invest* 1976; **58**: 880–890.

Young IH, Daviskas E, Keena VA. Effect of low dose nebulised morphine on exercise endurance in patients with chronic lung disease. *Thorax* 1989; **44**: 387–390.

52 EMPHYSEMA
(*see also* sections 17.3, 51, 70)

Baldwin E de F, Cournand A, Richards DW Jr. Pulmonary insufficiency. III. A study of 12 cases of chronic pulmonary emphysema. *Medicine (Baltimore)* 1949; **28**: 201–237.

Fromson BH, Denison DM. Quantitative features in the computed tomography of healthy lungs. *Thorax* 1988; **43**: 120–126.

Fujita J, Nelson NL, Daughton DM, Dobry CA, Spurzem JR, Irino S et al. Evaluation of elastase and antielastase balance in patients with chronic bronchitis and pulmonary emphysema. *Am Rev Respir Dis* 1990; **142**: 57–62.

Gelb AF, Gold WM, Wright RR, Bruch HR, Nadel JA. Physiologic diagnosis of subclinical emphysema. *Am Rev Respir Dis* 1973; **107**: 50–63.

Georg J, Lassen NA, Mellemgaard K, Vinther A. Diffusion in the gas phase of the lungs in normal and emphysematous subjects. *Clin Sci* 1965; **29**: 525–532.

Glazier JB, Hughes JMB, Maloney JE, West JB. Vertical gradient of alveolar size in lungs of dogs frozen intact. *J Appl Physiol* 1967; **23**: 694–705.

Gould GA, Macnee W, McLean A, Warren PM, Redpath A, Best JJK et al. CT measurements of lung density in life can quantitate distal airspace enlargement – an essential defining feature of human emphysema. *Am Rev Respir Dis* 1988; **137**: 380–392.

Gould GA, Redpath AT, Ryan M, Warren PM, Best JJK, Flenley DC et al. Lung CT density correlates with measurements of airflow limitation and the diffusing capacity. *Eur Respir J* 1991; **4**: 141–146.

Greaves IA, Colebatch HJH. Elastic behavior and structure of normal and emphysematous lungs postmortem. *Am Rev Respir Dis* 1980; **121**: 127–136.

Gugger M, Gould G, Sudlow MF, Wraith PK, MacNee W. Extent of pulmonary emphysema in man and its relation to the loss of elastic recoil. *Clin Sci* 1991; **80**: 353–358.

Hofford JM, Milakofsky L, Vogel WH, Sacher RS, Savage GJ, Pell S. The nutritional status in advanced emphysema associated with chronic bronchitis. *Am Rev Respir Dis* 1990; **141**: 902–908.

Hutchison DCS, Barter CE, Cook PJL, Laws JW, Martelli NA, Hugh-Jones P. Severe pulmonary emphysema: a comparison of patients with and without α_1-antitrypsin deficiency. *Q J Med* 1972; **41**: 301–315.

Kim WD, Eidelman DH, Izquierdo JL, Ghezzo H, Saetta MP, Cosio MG. Centrilobular and panlobular emphysema in smokers. Two distinct morphologic and functional entities. *Am Rev Respir Dis* 1991; **144**: 1385–1390.

Kuwano K, Matsuba K, Ikeda T, Murakami J, Araki A, Nishitani H et al. The diagnosis of mild emphysema. *Am Rev Respir Dis* 1990; **141**: 169–178.

Lam S, Abboud RT, Chan-Yeung M, Rushton JM.

Neutrophil elastase and pulmonary function in subjects with intermediate alpha$_1$-antitrypsin deficiency (MZ phenotype). *Am Rev Respir Dis* 1979; **119**: 941–951.

Levine BW, Talamo RC, Shannon DC, Kazemi H. Alteration in distribution of pulmonary blood flow: an early manifestation of alpha, antitrypsin deficiency. *Ann Intern Med* 1970; **73**: 397–401.

McHenry LC. Dr Samuel Johnson's emphysema. *Arch Intern Med* 1967; **119**: 98–105.

Miller RR, Müller NL, Vedal S, Morrison NJ, Staples CA. Limitations of computed tomography in the assessment of emphysema. *Am Rev Respir Dis* 1989; **139**: 980–983.

Mittman C, Lieberman J, Marasso F, Miranda A. Smoking and chronic obstructive lung disease in alpha$_1$-antitrypsin deficiency. *Chest* 1971; **60**: 214–221.

Morrison NJ, Abboud RT, Müller NL, Miller RR, Gibson NN, Nelems B *et al*. Pulmonary capillary blood volume in emphysema. *Am Rev Respir Dis* 1990; **141**: 53–61.

Morrison NJ, Abboud RT, Ramadan F, Miller RR, Gibson NN, Evans KG *et al*. Comparison of single breath carbon monoxide diffusing capacity and pressure–volume curves in detecting emphysema. *Am Rev Respir Dis* 1989; **139**: 1179–1187.

Nicklaus TM, Watanabe S, Mitchell MM, Renzetti AD Jr. Roentgenologic, physiologic and structural estimations of the total lung capacity in normal and emphysematous subjects. *Am J Med* 1967; **42**: 547–553.

Osborne S, Hogg JC, Wright JL, Coppin C, Paré PD. Exponential analysis of the pressure–volume curve. Correlation with mean linear intercept and emphysema in human lungs. *Am Rev Respir Dis* 1988; **137**: 1083–1088.

Petty TL, Silvers GW, Stanford RE. Mild emphysema is associated with reduced elastic recoil and increased lung size but not with air-flow limitation. *Am Rev Respir Dis* 1987; **136**: 867–871.

Pride NB, Barter CE, Hugh-Jones P. The ventilatory of bullae and the effect of their removal on thoracic gas volumes and tests of over-all pulmonary function. *Am Rev Respir Dis* 1973; **107**: 83–98.

Pushpakom R, Hogg JC, Woolcock AJ, Angus AE, Macklem PT, Thurlbeck WM. Experimental papain-induced emphysema in dogs. *Am Rev Respir Dis* 1970; **102**: 778–789.

Ross JC, Copher DE, Teays JD, Lord TJ. Functional residual capacity in patients with pulmonary emphysema. *Ann Int Med* 1962; **57**: 18–28.

Sharp JT, Beard GAT, Sunga M, Kim TW, Modh A, Lind J, Walsh J. The rib cage in normal and emphysematous subjects: a roentgenographic approach. *J Appl Physiol* 1986; **61**: 2050–2059.

Stockley RA. Proteolytic enzymes, their inhibitors and lung diseases. *Clin Sci* 1983; **64**: 119–126.

Supinski GS, Kelsen SG. Effect of elastase induced emphysema on the force-generating ability of the diaphragm. *J Clin Invest* 1982; **70**: 978–988.

Thurlbeck WM. Internal surface area and other measurements in emphysema. *Thorax* 1967; **22**: 483–496.

Thurlbeck WM. Diaphragm and body weight in emphysema. *Thorax* 1978; **33**: 483–487.

Thurlbeck WM, Henderson JA, Fraser RG, Bates DV. Chronic obstructive lung disease. *Medicine* 1970; **49**: 81–145.

Warrell DA, Hughes JMB, Rosenzweig DY. Cardio-pulmonary performance at rest and during exercise in seven patients with increased transradiancy of one lung ('Macleod's syndrome'). *Thorax* 1970; **25**: 587–597.

53 ASTHMA

53.1 General
(*see also* sections 18, 51, 63.3)

Barnes PJ. Inflammatory mediator receptors and asthma. *Am Rev Respir Dis* 1987; **135**: S26–S31.

Braman SS, Kaemmerlen JT, Davis SM. Asthma in the elderly: a comparison between patients with recently acquired and long-standing disease. *Am Rev Respir Dis* 1991; **143**: 336–340.

British Thoracic Society. Guidelines for management of asthma in adults: II – acute severe asthma. *Br Med J* 1990; **301**: 797–800.

Clark TJH, Godfrey S, Lee TH, eds. *Asthma*, 3rd edn. London: Chapman and Hall, 1992.

Djukanovic R, Roche WR, Wilson JW, Beasley CRW, Twentyman OP, Howarth PH, Takishimi T. Mucosal inflammation in asthma. *Am Rev Respir Dis* 1990; **142**: 434–457.

Insel PA, Wasserman SI. Asthma: a disorder of adrenergic receptors? *FASEB J* 1990; **4**: 2732–2736.

Jones RS. Assessment of respiratory function in the asthmatic child. *Br Med J* 1966; **2**: 972–975.

Martin AJ, McLennan LA, Landau LI, Phelan PD. The natural history of childhood asthma to adult life. *Br Med J* 1980; **280**: 1397–1400.

Morgan EJ, Hall DR. Abnormalities of lung function in hay fever. *Thorax* 1976; **31**: 80–86.

Pavia D, Bateman JRM, Sheahan NF, Agnew JE, Clarke SW. Tracheobronchial mucociliary clearance in asthma: impairment during remission. *Thorax* 1985; **40**: 171–175.

Quirk FH, Jones PW. Patients' perception of distress due to symptoms and effects of asthma on daily living and an investigation of possible influential factors. *Clin Sci* 1990; **79**: 17–21.

Svartengren M, Anderson M, Bylin G, Philipson K, Camner P. Regional deposition of 3.6-µm particles and lung function in asthmatic subjects. *J Appl Physiol* 1991; **71**: 2238–2243.

Woolcock AJ, Read J. The static elastic properties of the lungs in asthma. *Am Rev Respir Dis* 1968; **98**: 788–794.

53.2 Airway dynamics in asthma
(*see also* section 70)

Gayrard P, Orehek J, Grimaud C, Charpin J. Bronchoconstrictor effects of a deep inspiration in patients with asthma. *Am Rev Respir Dis* 1975; **111**: 433–439.

Patel P, Mukai D, Wilson AR. Dose–response effects of two sizes of monodisperse isoproterenol in mild asthma. *Am Rev Respir Dis* 1990; **141**: 357–360.

van Schayck CP, Dompeling E, van Herwaarden CLA, Wever AMJ, van Weel C. Interacting effects of atopy and bronchial hyperresponsiveness on the annual decline in lung function and the exacerbation rate in asthma. *Am Rev Respir Dis* 1991; **144**: 1297–1301.

Wagner EM, Liu MC, Weinmann GG, Permutt S, Bleecker ER. Peripheral lung resistance in normal and asthmatic subjects. *Am Rev Respir Dis* 1990; **141**: 584–588.

Weiss ST, Tosteson TD, Segal MR, Tager IB, Redline S, Speizer FE. Effects of asthma on pulmonary function in children. A longitudinal population-based study. *Am Rev Respir Dis* 1992; **145**: 58–64.

Williams SJ, Hartley JPR, Graham JDP. Bronchodilator effect of Δ^1-tetrahydrocannabinol administered by aerosol to asthmatic patients. *Thorax* 1976; **31**: 720–723.

Zamal N, Hughes D, Levison H, Fairshter RD, Gelb AF. Partial and complete maximum expiratory flow-volume curves in asthmatic patients with spontaneous bronchospasm. *Chest* 1983; **83**: 35–39.

Zapletal A, Motoyama EK, Gibson LE, Bouhuys A. Pulmonary mechanics in asthma and cystic fibrosis. *Pediatrics* 1971; **48**: 64–72.

53.3 Bronchial provocation in asthma
(*see also* sections 18.2, 63.3)

Godfrey S. Exercise induced asthma: clinical physiological and therapeutic implications. *J Allergy Clin Immunol* 1975; **56**: 1–17.

McFadden ER Jr, Ingram RH Jr, Haynes RL, Wellman JJ. Predominant site of flow limitation and mechanisms of postexertional asthma. *J Appl Physiol* 1977; **42**: 746–752.

Pepys J, Davies RJ, Breslin ABX, Hendrick DJ, Hutchcroft BJ. The effects of inhaled beclomethasone dipropionate (Becotide) and sodium cromoglycerate on asthmatic reactions to provocation tests. *Clin Allerg* 1974; **4**: 13–24.

Strauss RH, Haynes RL, Ingram RH Jr, McFadden ER Jr. Comparison of arm versus leg work in induction of acute episodes of asthma. *J Appl Physiol* 1977; **42**: 565–570.

53.4 Gas exchange in asthma

Ballester E, Reyes A, Roca J, Guitart R, Wagner PD, Rodriguez-Roisin R. Ventilation–perfusion mis-

matching in acute severe asthma: effects of salbutamol and 100% oxygen. *Thorax* 1989; **44**: 258–267.

Ballester E, Roca J, Ramis L, Wagner PD, Rodriguez-Roisin R. Pulmonary gas exchange in severe chronic asthma. Response to 100% oxygen and salbutamol. *Am Rev Respir Dis* 1990; **141**: 558–562.

McFadden ER, Lyons HA. Arterial blood gas tension in asthma. *N Engl J Med* 1968; **78**: 1027–1032.

Roca J, Ramis LI, Rodriguez-Roisin R, Ballester E, Montserrat JM, Wagner PD. Serial relationships between ventilation–perfusion inequality and spirometry in acute severe asthma requiring hospitalization. *Am Rev Respir Dis* 1988; **137**: 1055–1061.

Rodriguez-Roisin R, Ballester E, Roca J, Torres A, Wagner PD. Mechanisms of hypoxemia in patients with status asthmaticus requiring mechanical ventilation. *Am Rev Respir Dis* 1989; **139**: 732–739.

Valabhji P. Gas exchange in the acute and asymptomatic phases of asthma breathing air and oxygen. *Clin Sci* 1968; **34**: 431–440.

Wagner PD, Dantzker DR, Lacovoni VE, Tomlin WC, West JB. Ventilation–perfusion inequality in asymptomatic asthma. *Am Rev Respir Dis* 1978; **118**: 511–524.

Wagner PD, Hedenstierna G, Bylin G. Ventilation perfusion inequality in chronic asthma. *Am Rev Respir Dis* 1987; **136**: 605–612.

Weitzman RH, Wilson AF. Diffusing capacity and over-all ventilation: perfusion in asthma. *Am J Med* 1974; **57**: 767–774.

Weng TR, Langer HM, Featherby EA, Levison H. Arterial blood gas tensions and acid–base balance in symptomatic and asymptomatic asthma in childhood. *Am Rev Respir Dis* 1970; **101**: 274–282.

53.5 Other aspects of lung function in asthma

Blackie SP, Al-Majed S, Staples CA, Hilliam C, Paré PD. Changes in total lung capacity during acute spontaneous asthma. *Am Rev Respir Dis* 1990; **142**: 79–83.

Colebatch HJH, Finucane KE, Smith MM. Pulmonary conductance and elastic recoil relationships in asthma and emphysema. *J Appl Physiol* 1973; **34**: 143–153.

Peress L, Sybrecht G, Macklem PT. The mechanism of increase in total lung capacity during acute asthma. *Am J Med* 1976; **61**: 165–169.

Wilson AF, Surprenant EL, Beall GN, Siegel SC, Simmons DH, Bennett LR. The significance of regional pulmonary function changes in bronchial asthma. *Am J Med* 1970; **48**: 416–423.

Woolcock AJ, Read J. The static elastic properties of the lungs in asthma. *Am Rev Respir Dis* 1968; **98**: 788–794.

54.1 General

(see also sections 22, 24, 27, 29, 63.2, 63.6, 64)

Agusti AGN, Roca J, Gea J, Wagner PD, Xaubet A, Rodriguez-Roisin R. Mechanisms of gas-exchange impairment in idiopathic pulmonary fibrosis. *Am Rev Respir Dis* 1991; **143**: 219–225.

Arndt H, King TKC, Briscoe WA. Diffusing capacities and ventilation–perfusion ratios in patients with the clinical syndrome of alveolar capillary block. *J Clin Invest* 1970; **49**: 408–422.

Carrington CB, Gaensler EA, Coutu RE, FitzGerald MX, Gupta RG. Natural history and treated course of usual and desquamative interstitial pneumonia. *New Engl J Med* 1978; **298**: 801–809.

Chu SS, Cotes JE. Lung transfer and Kco at cardiac frequency 100 beats/min as a guide to impaired function of lung parenchyma. *Thorax* 1984; **39**: 524–528.

Cohen R, Overfield EM. The diffusion component of arterial hypoxaemia. *Am Rev Respir Dis* 1972; **105**: 532–540.

Corris PA, Best JJK, Gibson GJ. Effects of diffuse pleural thickening on respiratory mechanics. *Eur Respir J* 1988; **1**: 248–252.

Denison D, Al-Hillawi H, Turton C. Lung function in interstitial lung disease. *Seminars in Respiratory Medicine* 1984; **6**: 40–54.

Enson Y, Thomas HM, Bosken CH, Wood JA, LeRoy EC, Blanc WA et al. Pulmonary hypertension in interstitial lung disease; relation of vascular resistance to abnormal structure. *Trans Assoc Am Physicians* 1975; **88**: 248–255.

Fitting J-W, Frascarolo P, Jéquier E, Leuenberger P. Resting energy expenditure in interstitial lung disease. *Am Rev Respir Dis* 1990; **142**: 631–635.

Fulmer JD, Roberts WC, von Gal ER, Crystal RG. Small airways in idiopathic pulmonary fibrosis. Comparison of morphologic and physiologic observations. *J Clin Invest* 1977; **60**: 595–610.

Gibson GJ, Pride NB. Pulmonary mechanics in fibrosing alveolitis. The effects of lung shrinkage. *Am Rev Respir Dis* 1977; **116**: 637–647.

Gross NJ. Pulmonary effects of radiation therapy. *Ann Intern Med* 1977; **86**: 81–92.

Hanley ME, King TE Jr, Schwarz MI, Watters LC, Shen AS, Cherniack RM. The impact of smoking on mechanical properties of the lungs in idiopathic pulmonary fibrosis and sarcoidosis. *Am Rev Respir Dis* 1991; **144**: 1102–1106.

Hempleman SC, Hughes JMB. Estimating exercise $D_{L_{O_2}}$ and diffusion limitation in patients with interstitial fibrosis. *Respir Physiol* 1991; **83**: 167–178.

Hughes JMB, Lockwood DNA, Jones HA, Clark RJ. DLCO/$\dot{Q}$ and diffusion limitation at rest and on exercise in patients with interstitial fibrosis. *Respir Physiol* 1991; **83**: 155–166.

Lord GP, Gazioglu K, Kaltreider N. The maximum expiratory flow–volume in the evaluation of patients with lung disease. *Am J Med* 1969; **46**: 72–79.

Michel RP, Hakim TS, Freeman CR. Distribution of pulmonary vascular resistance in experimental fibrosis. *J Appl Physiol* 1988; **65**: 1180–1190.

Ostrow D, Cherniack RM. Resistance to airflow in patients with diffuse interstitial lung disease. *Am Rev Respir Dis* 1973; **108**: 205–210.

Patton JMS, Freedman S. The ventilatory response to CO_2 of patients with diffuse pulmonary infiltrations or fibrosis. *Clin Sci* 1972; **43**: 55–69.

Schofield N McC, Davies RJ, Cameron IR, Green M. Small airways in fibrosing alveolitis. *Am Rev Respir Dis* 1976; **113**: 729–735.

Turner-Warwick M, Burrows B, Johnson A. Cryptogenic fibrosing alveolitis: clinical features and their influence on survival. *Thorax* 1980; **35**: 171–180.

Yernault JC, De Jonghe M, De Coster A, Englert M. Pulmonary mechanics in diffuse fibrosing alveolitis. *Bull Physiopathol Respir* 1975; **11**: 231–244.

54.2 Sarcoidosis, coeliac disease and systemic sclerosis

Chinet T, Dusser D, Labrune S, Collignon MA, Chrétien J, Huchon GJ. Lung function declines in patients with pulmonary sarcoidosis and increased respiratory epithelial permeability to ^{99m}Tc-DTPA. *Am Rev Respir Dis* 1990; **141**: 445–449.

De Troyer A, Yernault JC, Dierckx P, Englert M, De Coster A. Lung and airway mechanics in early pulmonary sarcoidosis. *Bull Eur Physiopathol Respir* 1978; **14**: 299–310.

Eklund A, Broman L, Broman M, Holmgren A. $\dot{V}/\dot{Q}$ and alveolar gas exchange in pulmonary sarcoidosis. *Eur Respir J* 1989; **2**: 135–144.

Emirgil C, Sobol BJ, Herbert WH, Trout K. The lesser circulation in pulmonary fibrosis secondary to sarcoidosis and its relationship to respiratory function. *Chest* 1971; **60**: 371–378.

Guleria JS, Pande JN, Malik SK, Bhutani LK. Lungs in progressive systemic sclerosis. *Br J Dis Chest* 1970; **64**: 150–160.

Huang CT, Lyons HA. Comparison of pulmonary function in patients with systemic lupus erythematosus, scleroderma, and rheumatoid arthritis. *Am Rev Respir Dis* 1966; **93**: 865–875.

Ingram CG, Reid PC, Johnston RN. Exercise testing in pulmonary sarcoidosis. *Thorax* 1982; **37**: 129–132.

Levinson RS, Metzger LF, Stanley NN, Kelsen SG, Altose MD, Cherniack NS, Brody JS. Airway function in sarcoidosis. *Am J Med* 1977; **62**: 51–59.

Marshall R, Karlish AJ. Lung function in sarcoidosis. *Thorax* 1971; **26**: 402–405.

Miller A, Teirstein AS, Jackler I, Chuang M, Siltzbach LE. Airway function in chronic pulmonary sarcoidosis with fibrosis. *Am Rev Respir Dis* 1974; **109**: 179–189.

Smith MJL, Benson MK, Strickland ID. Coeliac disease and diffuse interstitial lung disease. *Lancet* 1971; **i**: 473–475.

Vale JR. Respiratory function in sarcoidosis and other interstitial lung diseases with similar radiological appearance. *Scand J Respir Dis* 1971; **52**: 1–12.

Winterbauer RH, Hutchinson JF. Clinical significance of pulmonary function tests. Use of pulmonary function tests in the management of sarcoidosis. *Chest* 1980; **78**: 640–647.

Young RC Jr, Carr C, Shelton TG, Mann M, Ferrin A, Laurey JR et al. Sarcoidosis: relationship between changes in lung structure and function. *Am Rev Respir Dis* 1967; **95**: 224–238.

55 ADULT RESPIRATORY DISTRESS SYNDROME
(*see also* sections 17.3, 47, 69)

Ashbaugh DG, Bigelow DB, Petty TL, Levine BE. Acute respiratory distress in adults. *Lancet* 1967; **ii**: 319–323.

Cochrane CG, Spragg R, Revak SD. Pathogenesis of the adult respiratory distress syndrome. *J Clin Invest* 1983; **71**: 754–761.

Dantzker RM. Gas exchange in the adult respiratory distress syndrome. *Clin Chest Med* 1982; **3**: 57–67.

Jefferies AL, Coates G, O'Brodovich H. Pulmonary epithelial permeability in hyaline membrane disease. *N Engl J Med* 1985; **311**: 1075–1080.

Kreuzfelder E, Joka T, Keinecke H-O, Obertacke U, Schmit-Neuerburg K-P, Nakhosteen JA et al. Adult respiratory distress syndrome as a specific manifestation of a general permeability defect in trauma patients. *Am Rev Respir Dis* 1988; **137**: 95–99.

Murray JF, Matthay MA, Luce JM, Flick MR. An expanded definition of the adult respiratory distress syndrome. *Am Rev Respir Dis* 1988; **138**: 720–723.

Pepe PE, Hudson LD, Carrico CJ. Early application of positive end-expiratory pressure in patients at risk for the adult respiratory-distress syndrome. *N Engl J Med* 1984; **311**: 281–286.

Staub NC. Pulmonary edema. *Physiol Rev* 1974; **54**: 678–811.

Tomashefski JF, Davies P, Boggis CJ, Greene R, Zapol WM, Reid LM. The pulmonary vascular lesions of the adult respiratory distress syndrome *Am J Pathol* 1983; **112**: 112–126.

56 LUNG TRANSPLANTATION
(*see also* sections 27, 29 and medical conditions)

Glanville AR, Burke CM, Theodore J, Baldwin JC, Harvey J, Vankessel A, Robin ED. Bronchial hyperresponsiveness after human cardiopulmonary transplantation. *Clin Sci* 1987; **73**: 299–303.

Grossman RF, Frost A, Zamel N, Patterson GA, Cooper JD, Myron PR et al. Results of single-lung transplantation for bilateral pulmonary fibrosis. *New Engl J Med* 1990; **322**: 727–733.

Higenbottam T, Otulana BA, Wallwork J. The physiology of heart–lung transplantation in humans. *NIPS* 1990; **5**: 71–74.

Higenbottam T. Physiology of the transplanted lung and the results. In: Wallwork J, ed. *Heart and Heart–Lung Transplantation*. Philadelphia: WB Saunders, 1989: S33–S44.

Slapak M, Lee HM, Hume DM. Transplant lung—a new syndrome. *Br Med J* 1968; **1**: 80–84.

Stevens PM, Johnson PC, Bell RL, Beall AC, Jenkins DE. Regional ventilation and perfusion after lung transplantation in patients with emphysema. *New Engl J Med* 1970; **282**: 245–249.

Williams TJ, Patterson GA, McClean PA, Zamel N, Maurer JR. Maximal exercise testing in single and double lung transplant recipients. *Am Rev Respir Dis* 1992; **145**: 101–105.

57 HEPATIC AND RENAL DISORDERS

Agusti AGN, Roca J, Rodgriguez-Roisin R, Mastai R, Wagner PD, Bosch J. Pulmonary hemodynamics and gas exchange during exercise in liver cirrhosis. *Am Rev Respir Dis* 1989; **139**: 485–491.

Arndt H, Buchta I, Schomerus H. Analysis of factors determining the resistance to diffusion in patients with liver cirrhosis. *Respiration* 1975; **32**: 21–31.

Cotes JE, Field GB, Brown GJA, Read AE. Impairment of lung function after portacaval anastomosis. *Lancet* 1968; **i**: 952–955.

Crosbie WA, Parsons V. Cardio-pulmonary function of congested lungs. *Q J Med* 1974; **43**: 215–230.

Daoud FS, Reeves JT, Schaefer JW. Failure of hypoxic pulmonary vasoconstriction in patients with liver cirrhosis. *J Clin Invest* 1972; **51**: 1076–1080.

Fawcett S, Hoenich NA, Laker MF, Schorr W Jr, Ward MK, Kerr DNS. Haemodialysis-induced respiratory changes. *Nephrol Dial Transplant* 1987; **2**: 161–168.

Funahashi A, Kutty AVP, Prater SL. Hypoxaemia and cirrhosis of the liver. *Thorax* 1976; **31**: 303–308.

Lee HY, Stretton TB, Barnes AM. The lungs in renal failure. *Thorax* 1975; **30**: 46–53.

Mayer G, Thum J, Graf H. Anaemia and reduced exercise capacity in patients on chronic haemodialysis. *Clin Sci* 1989; **76**: 265–268.

Mélot C, Naeije R, Dechamps P, Hallemans R, Lejeune P. Pulmonary and extrapulmonary contributors to hypoxemia in liver cirrhosis. *Am Rev Respir Dis* 1989; **139**: 632–640.

Pezzagno G, Catenacci G, Salvadeo A, Zelaschi F, Segagni S. Valutazione della capacite di diffusione polmonare per il CO e delle sue componenti in soggetti uremici prima e dopo l'emodialisi e nel periodo interdialitico. *Minerva Nefrol* 1971; **18**: 206–217.

Rodriguez-Roisin R, Roca J, Agusti AGN, Mastai R, Wagner PD, Bosch J. Gas exchange and pulmonary vascular reactivity in patients with liver cirrhosis. *Am Rev Respir Dis* 1987; **135**: 1085–1092.

Ruff F, Hughes JMB, Stanley N, McCarthy D, Greene R, Aronoff A et al. Regional lung function in patients with hepatic cirrhosis. *J Clin Invest* 1971; **50**: 2403–2413.

Stanescu DC, Veriter C, De Plaen JF, Frans A, Van Ypersele De Strihou C, Brasseur L. Lung function in chronic uraemia before and after removal of excess fluid by haemodialysis. *Clin Sci* 1974; **47**: 143–151.

Stanley MN, Woodgate DJ. Mottled chest radiograph and gas transfer defect in chronic liver disease. *Thorax* 1972; **27**: 315–323.

Zidulka A, Despas PJ, Milic-Emili J, Anthonisen NR. Pulmonary function with acute loss of excess lung water by hemodialysis in patients with chronic uremia. *Am J Med* 1973; **55**: 134–141.

58 AIDS

Coleman DL, Dodek PM, Golden JA, Luce JM, Golden E, Gold WM, Murray JF. Correlation between serial pulmonary function tests and fiberoptic bronchoscopy in patients with *Pneumocystis carinii* pneumonia and the acquired immune deficiency syndrome. *Am Rev Respir Dis* 1984; **129**: 491–493.

Rocker GM, Pearson D, Wiseman MS, Shale DJ. Diagnostic criteria for adult respiratory distress syndrome: time for reappraisal. *Lancet* 1989; **i**: 120–123.

Shaw RJ, Roussak C, Forster SM, Harris JRW, Pinching AJ, Mitchell DM. Lung function abnormalities in patients infected with the human immunodeficiency virus with and without overt pneumonitis. *Thorax* 1988; **43**: 436–440.

Stover DE, Greeno RA, Gagliardi AJ. The use of a simple exercise test for the diagnosis of *Pneumocystis carinii* pneumonia in patients with AIDS. *Am Rev Respir Dis* 1989; **139**: 1343–1346.

59 NEUROMUSCULAR AND THORACIC CAGE DISORDERS

Bake B, Bjure J, Kasalichy J, Nachemson A. Regional pulmonary ventilation and perfusion distribution in patients with untreated idiopathic scoliosis. *Thorax* 1972; **27**: 703–712.

Bogaard JM, Hovestadt A, Meerwaldt J, Meché FGA v d, Stigt J. Maximal expiratory and inspiratory flow–volume curves in Parkinson's Disease. *Am Rev Respir Dis* 1989; **139**: 610–614.

Davies JN, Goldman M, Loh L, Casson M. Diaphragm function and alveolar hypoventilation. *Q J Med* 1976; **45**: 87–100.

Evans RJC, Benson MK, Hughes DTD. Abnormal chemoreceptor response to hypoxia in patients with tabes dorsalis. *Br Med J* 1971; **1**: 530–531.

Fluck DC. Chest movements in hemiplegia. *Clin Sci* 1966; **31**: 383–388.

Gacad G, Hamosh P. The lung in ankylosing spondylitis. *Am Rev Respir Dis* 1973; **107**: 286–289.

Gibson GJ, Pride NB, Newsom Davis J, Loh LC. Pulmonary mechanics in patients with respiratory muscle weakness. *Am Rev Respir Dis* 1977; **115**: 389–395.

Goldstein RL, Hyde RW, Lapham LW, Gazioglu K, De Papp ZG. Peripheral neuropathy presenting with respiratory insufficiency as a primary complaint. *Am J Med* 1974; **56**: 443–449.

Harrison BDW, Collins JV, Brown KGE, Clark TJH. Respiratory failure in neuromuscular diseases. *Thorax* 1971; **26**: 579–584.

Kuperman AS, Krieger AJ, Rosomoff HL. Respiratory function after cervical cordotomy. *Chest* 1971; **59**: 128–132.

Littler WA, Brown IK, Roaf R. Regional lung function in scoliosis. *Thorax* 1972; **27**: 420–428.

McCredie M, Lovejoy FW Jr, Kaltreider NL. Pulmonary function in diaphragmatic paralysis. *Thorax* 1962; **17**: 213–217.

Mellins RB, Balfour HH Jr, Turino GM, Winters RW. Failure of automatic control of ventilation (Ondine's curse). *Medicine* 1970; **49**: 487–504.

Obenour WH, Stevens PM, Cohen AA, McCutchen JJ. The causes of abnormal pulmonary function in Parkinson's disease. *Am Rev Respir Dis* 1972; **105**: 382–387.

Ringqvist I, Ringqvist T. Respiratory mechanics in untreated myasthenia gravis with special reference to the respiratory forces. *Acta Med Scand* 1971; **190**: 499–508.

Weg JG, Krumholz RA, Harkleroad LE. Pulmonary dysfunction in pectus excavatum. *Am Rev Respir Dis* 1967; **96**: 936–945.

60 DIAPHRAGM
(*see also* sections 8, 27.4, 61)

Arora NS, Rochester DF. Effect of body weight and muscularity on human diaphragm muscle mass, thickness, and area. *J Appl Physiol* 1982; **52**: 64–70.

Edwards RHT. The diaphragm as a muscle. Mechanisms underlying fatigue. *Am Rev Respir Dis* 1979; **119**(Suppl): 81–84.

Ferguson GT, Irvin CG, Cherniack RM. Relationship of diaphragm glycogen, lactate, and function to respiratory failure. *Am Rev Respir Dis* 1990; **141**: 926–932.

Koulouris N, Mulvey DA, Laroche CM, Sawicka EH, Green M, Moxham J. The measurement of inspiratory muscle strength by sniff esophageal, nasopharyngeal, and mouth pressures. *Am Rev Respir Dis* 1989; **139**: 641–646.

Laroche CM, Cairns T, Moxham J, Green M. Hypothyroidism presenting with respiratory muscle weakness. *Am Rev Respir Dis* 1988; **138**: 472–474.

Leith DE, Bradley M. Ventilatory muscle strength and endurance training. *J Appl Physiol* 1976; **41**: 508–516.

Moxham J. Tests of respiratory muscle function. In: *Problems in Respiratory Care*. Philadelphia: J.B. Lippincott, 1990; **3**: 312–328.

NHLBI Workshop. Respiratory muscle fatigue. *Am Rev Respir Dis* 1990; **142**: 474–480.

Roussos C, Fixley M, Gross D, Macklem PT. Fatigue of inspiratory muscles and their synergic behaviour. *J Appl Physiol* 1979; **46**: 897–904.

Roussos CS, Macklem PT. Diaphragmatic fatigue in man. *J Appl Physiol* 1977; **43**: 189–197.

61 SLEEP
(*see also* sections 27, 51, 59, 60, 62)

Badr MS, Skatrud JB, Dempsey JA, Begle RL. Effect of mechanical loading on expiratory muscle activity during NREM sleep. *J Appl Physiol* 1990; **68**: 1195–1202.

Chapman KR, Bruce EN, Gothe B, Cherniack NS. Possible mechanisms of periodic breathing during sleep. *J Appl Physiol* 1988; **64**: 1000–1008.

Cherniack NS. Respiratory dysrhythmias during sleep. *N Engl J Med* 1981; **305**: 325–330.

Douglas NJ, Flenley DC. Breathing during sleep in patients with obstructive lung disease. *Am Rev Respir Dis* 1990; **141**: 1055–1070.

Edelman NH, Santiago TV, eds. *Breathing Disorders of Sleep*. New York: Churchill Livingstone, 1986: 45–56.

Fletcher EC. Chronic lung disease in patients with sleep apnoea. In: Fletcher EC, ed. *Abnormalities of Respiration During Sleep*. Orlando, Fl: Grune & Stratton, 1986: 181–202.

Gugger W, Molloy J, Gould GA, Whyte KF, Raab GM, Shapiro CM, Douglas NJ. Ventilatory and arousal responses to added inspiratory resistance during sleep. *Am Rev Respir Dis* 1989; **140**: 1301–1307.

Henke KG, Badr MS, Skatrud JB, Dempsey JA. Load compensation and respiratory muscle function during sleep. *J Appl Physiol* 1992; **72**: 1221–1234.

Henke KG, Dempsey JA, Kowitz JM, Skatrud JB. Effects of sleep-induced increases in upper airway resistance on respiratory muscle activity. *J Appl Physiol* 1990; **69**: 617–624.

Ingrassia TS III, Nelson SB, Harris CD, Hubmayr RD. Influence of sleep state on CO_2 responsiveness. *Am Rev Respir Dis* 1991; **144**: 1125–1129.

Kryger MH, Roth T, Dement WC, eds. *Principles and Practice of Sleep Medicine*. Philadelphia: WB Saunders, 1989: 552–559.

Orem J. The nature of the wakefulness stimulus. In: Suratt P, Remmers JE, eds. *Sleep and Respiration*. New York: Alan R Liss, 1990.

Parisi RA, Neubauer JA, Frank MM, Santiago TV, Edelman NH. Linkage between brain blood flow and respiratory drive during rapid-eye-movement sleep. *J Appl Physiol* 1988; **64**: 1457–1465.

Parisi RA, Santiago TV, Edelman NH. Genioglossal and diaphragmatic EMG responses to hypoxia during sleep. *Am Rev Respir Dis* 1988; **138**: 610–616.

Ryan T, Mlynczak S, Erikson T, Paulman SF, Mann GCW. Oxygen consumption during sleep: influence of sleep stage and time of night. *Sleep* 1989; **12**: 201–210.

Sanders MH, Black J, Costantino JP, Kern N, Studnicki K, Coates J. Diagnosis of sleep-disordered breathing by half-night polysomnography. *Am Rev Respir Dis* 1991; **144**: 1256–1261.

Shea SA, Winning AJ, McKenzie E, Guz A. Does the abnormal pattern of breathing in patients with interstitial lung disease persist in deep, non-rapid eye movement sleep? *Am Rev Respir Dis* 1989; **139**: 653–658.

Skatrud JB, Dempsey JA. Interaction of sleep state and chemical stimuli in sustaining rhythmic ventilation. *J Appl Physiol* 1983; **55**: 813–822.

Strohl KP, Cherniack NS, Gothe B. Physiologic basis of therapy for sleep apnea. *Am Rev Respir Dis* 1986; **134**: 791–802.

Suratt PM, McTier RF, Wilhiot SC. Upper airway muscle activation is augmented in patients with obstructive sleep apnea compared with that in normal subjects. *Am Rev Respir Dis* 1988; **137**: 889–894.

White DP. Occlusion pressure and ventilation during sleep in normal humans. *J Appl Physiol* 1986; **61**: 1279–1287.

Whyte KF, Gugger M, Gould GA, Molloy J, Wraith PK, Douglas NJ. Accuracy of respiratory inductive plethysmograph in measuring tidal volume during sleep. *J Appl Physiol* 1991; **71**: 1866–1871.

Zwillich C, Devlin T, White D, Douglas N, Weil J, Martin R. Bradycardia during sleep apnea: characteristics and mechanism. *J Clin Invest* 1982; **69**: 1286–1292.

62 OBESITY: EFFECTS ON LUNG FUNCTION
(*see also* sections 27, 59, 61, 64)

Barrera F, Hillyer P, Ascanio G, Bechtel J. The distribution of ventilation, diffusion and blood flow in obese patients with normal and abnormal blood gases. *Am Rev Respir Dis* 1973; **108**: 819–830.

Barrera F, Reidenberg MM, Winters WL. Pulmonary function in the obese patient. *Am J Med Sci* 1967; **254**: 785–796.

Bedell GN, Wilson WR, Seebohm PM. Pulmonary function in obese persons. *J Clin Invest* 1958; **37**: 1049–1060.

Cotes JE, Gilson JC. Effect of inactivity, weight gain and antitubercular chemotherapy upon lung function in working coal-miners. *Ann Occup Hyg* 1967; **10**: 327–335.

Emirgil C, Sobol BJ. The effects of weight reduction on pulmonary function and the sensitivity of the respiratory center in obesity. *Am Rev Respir Dis* 1973; **108**: 831–842.

Gilbert R, Sipple JH, Auchincloss JH. Respiratory control and work of breathing in obese subjects. *J Appl Physiol* 1961; **16**: 21–26.

Jenkins SC, Moxham J. The effects of mild obesity on lung function. *Respir Med* 1991; **85**: 309–311.

Ray CS, Sue DY, Bray G, Hansen JE, Wasserman K. Effects of obesity on respiratory function. *Am Rev Respir Dis* 1983; **128**: 501–506.

Sharp JT. The chest wall and respiratory muscles in obesity, ascites and pregnancy. In: Roussos C, Macklem PT, eds. *The Thorax, Part B*. New York: Marcel Dekker, 1985: 999–1022.

Walsh RE, Michaelson ED, Harkleroad LE, Zighelboim A, Sackner MA. Upper airway obstruction in obese patients with sleep disturbance and somnolence. *Ann Intern Med* 1972; **76**: 185–192.

Zwillich CW, Sutton FD, Pierson DJ, Creagh EM, Weil JV. Decreased hypoxic ventilatory drive in the obesity-hypoventilation syndrome. *Am J Med* 1975; **59**: 343–348.

63 OCCUPATIONAL DISORDERS OF THE LUNG

63.1 General
(*see also* section 5)

Cotes JE, Steel J. *Work-related Lung Disorders*. Oxford: Blackwell Scientific Publications, 1987.

Morgan WKC, Seaton A. *Occupational Lung Diseases*. Philadelphia: Saunders, 1984.

Parkes WR. *Occupational Lung Disorders*. London: Butterworths, 1982.

63.2 Conditions due to asbestos
(*see also* section 63.1)

Agostoni P, Smith DD, Schoene RB, Robertson HT, Butler J. Evaluation of breathlessness in asbestos workers. Results of exercise testing. *Am Rev Respir Dis* 1987; **135**: 812–816.

Agusti A GN, Roca J, Rodriguez-Roisin R, Xaubet A, Agusti-Vidal A. Different patterns of gas exchange response to exercise in asbestosis and idiopathic pulmonary fibrosis. *Eur Respir J* 1988; **1**: 510–516.

Britton MG, Hughes DTD, Wever AMJ. Serial pulmonary function tests in patients with asbestosis. *Thorax* 1977; **32**: 45–52.

Britton MG. Asbestos pleural disease. *Br J Dis Chest* 1982; **76**: 1–10.

Cotes JE, King B. Relationship of lung function to X-ray reading (ILO) in patients with asbestos-related lung disorders. *Thorax* 1988; **43**: 777–783.

Fournier-Massey G, Becklake MR. Pulmonary function profiles in Quebec asbestos workers. *Bull Physiopathol Respir* 1975; **11**: 429–445.

Fridriksson HV, Hedenström H, Hillerdal G, Malmberg P. Increased lung stiffness in persons with pleural plaques. *Eur J Respir Dis* 1981; **62**: 412–424.

Jodoin G, Gibbs GW, Macklem PT, McDonald JC, Becklake MR. Early effects of asbestos exposure on lung function. *Am Rev Respir Dis* 1971; **104**: 525–535.

Konietzko N, Gerke E, Schlehe H, Matthys H. Verschlussvolumen bei Asbeststaubexponierten (Closing volume in workers exposed to asbestos). *Prax Pneumol* 1974; **28**(Suppl): 828–833.

McDermott M, Bevan MM, Elmes PC, Allardice JT, Bradley AC. Lung function and radiographic change in chrysotile workers in Swaziland. *Br J Ind Med* 1982; **39**: 338–343.

McGavin CR, Sheers G. Diffuse pleural thickening in asbestos workers: disability and lung function abnormalities. *Thorax* 1984; **39**: 604–607.

Seaton D. Regional lung function in asbestos workers. *Thorax* 1977; **32**: 40–44.

63.3 Occupational asthma
(*see also* sections 53, 63.1, 63.6)

Ayres J, Ancic P, Clark TJH. Airways responses to oral ethanol in normal subjects and in patients with asthma. *J R Soc Med* 1982; **75**: 699–704.

Brooks SM. Bronchial asthma of occupational origin. *Scand J Work Environ Health* 1977; **3**: 53–72.

Burge PS, O'Brien IM, Harries MG. Peak flow rate records in the diagnosis of occupational asthma due to colophony. *Thorax* 1979; **34**: 308–316.

Burge PS, O'Brien IM, Harries MG. Peak flow rate records in the diagnosis of occupational asthma due to isocyanates. *Thorax* 1979; **34**: 317–323.

Chan-Yeung M, Vedal S, Kus J, Maclean L, Enarson D, Tse KS. Symptoms, pulmonary function and bronchial hyperreactivity in Western red cedar workers compared with those of office workers. *Am Rev Respir Dis* 1984; **130**: 1038–1041.

Darke CS, Knowelden J, Lacey J, Ward AM. Respiratory disease of workers harvesting grain. *Thorax* 1976; **31**: 294–302.

Do Pico GA, Rankin J, Chosy LW, Reddan WG, Barbee RA, Gee B et al. Respiratory tract disease from thermo setting resins. *Ann Intern Med* 1975; **83**: 177–184.

Dosman JA, Cotton DJ, Graham BL, Li KYR, Froh F, Barnett GD. Chronic bronchitis and decreased forced expiratory flow rates in life-time non-smoking grain workers. *Am Rev Respir Dis* 1980; **121**: 11–16.

Eiser NM, Kerrebijn KF, Quanjer PhH, eds. Guidelines for standardisation of bronchial challenges with (nonspecific) bronchoconstricting agents. *Bull Eur Physiopathol Respir* 1983; **19**: 495–514.

Enarson DA, Vedal S, Chan-Yeung M. Rapid decline in FEV_1 in grain handlers. *Am Rev Respir Dis* 1985; **132**: 814–817.

Hendrick DJ, Fabbri LM, Hughes JM, Banks DE, Barkman HW Jr, Connolly MJ et al. Modification of the methacholine inhalation test and its epidemiologic use in polyurethane workers. *Am Rev Respir Dis* 1986; **133**: 600–604.

Higgs CMB, Laszlo G. Coded peak flow measurement and the perception of asthma. *Thorax* 1982; **37**: 780.

Jones RN, Hughes JM, Lehrer SB, Butcher BT, Glindmeyer HW, Diem JE et al. Lung function consequences of exposure and hypersensitivity in workers who process green coffee beans. *Am Rev Respir Dis* 1982; **125**: 199–202.

McCarthy PE, Cockcroft AE, McDermott M. Lung function after exposure to barley dust. *Br J Ind Med* 1985; **42**: 106−110.

63.4 Beryllium disease
(*see also* section 63.1)

Andrews JL, Kazemi H, Hardy HL. Patterns of lung dysfunction in chronic beryllium disease. *Am Rev Respir Dis* 1969; **100**: 791−800.

Cotes JE, Gilson JC, McKerrow CB, Oldham PD. A long-term follow-up of workers exposed to beryllium. *Br J Ind Med* 1983; **40**: 13−21.

Sprince NL, Kanarek DJ, Weber AL, Chamberlin RI, Kazemi H. Reversible respiratory disease in beryllium workers. *Am Rev Respir Dis* 1978; **117**: 1011−1017.

63.5 Byssinosis
(*see also* section 63.1)

Beck GJ, Schachter EN, Maunder LR. The relationship of respiratory symptoms and lung function loss in cotton textile workers. *Am Rev Respir Dis* 1984; **130**: 6−11.

Berry G, McKerrow CB, Molyneux MKB, Rossiter CE, Tombleson JBL. A study of the acute and chronic changes in ventilatory capacity of workers in Lancashire cotton mills. *Br J Ind Med* 1973; **30**: 25−36.

Bouhuys A, van de Woestijne KP. Respiratory mechanics and dust exposure in byssinosis. *J Clin Invest* 1970; **49**: 106−118.

Bouhuys A, Zuskin E. Chronic respiratory disease in hemp workers. *Ann Intern Med* 1976; **84**: 398−405.

Field GB, Owen P. Respiratory function in an Australian cotton mill. *Bull Eur Physiopathol Respir* 1979; **15**: 455−468.

Rylander R, Haglind P, Lundholm M. Endotoxin in cotton dust and respiratory function decrement among cotton workers in an experimental card room. *Am Rev Respir Dis* 1985; **131**: 209−213.

63.6 Extrinsic allergic alveolitis
(*see also* sections 53, 54, 63.1, 63.3)

Allen DH, Williams GV, Woolcock AJ. Bird breeder's hypersensitivity pneumonitis: progress studies of lung function after cessation of exposure to the provoking antigen. *Am Rev Respir Dis* 1976; **114**: 555−566.

Braun SR, Do Pico GA, Tsiatis A, Horvath E, Dickie HA, Rankin J. Farmer's lung disease: long-term clinical and physiologic outcome. *Am Rev Respir Dis* 1979; **119**: 185−191.

Cockcroft A, Edwards J, Bevan C, Campbell I, Collins G, Houston K *et al*. An investigation of operating theatre staff exposed to humidifier fever antigens. *Br J Ind Med* 1981; **38**: 144−151.

Fink JN, Banaszak EG, Barboriak JJ, Hensley GT, Kurup VP, Scanlon GT *et al*. Interstitial lung disease due to contamination of forced air systems. *Ann Intern Med* 1976; **84**: 406−413.

Friend JAR, Gaddie J, Palmer KNV, Pickering CAC, Pepys J. Extrinsic allergic alveolitis and contaminated cooling water in a factory machine. *Lancet* 1977; **i**: 297−300.

Hapke EJ, Seal RME, Thomas GO, Hayes M, Meek JC. Farmer's lung: a clinical, radiographic, functional and serological correlation of acute and chronic stages. *Thorax* 1968; **23**: 451−468.

Harper LO, Burrell RG, Lapp NL, Morgan WKC. Allergic alveolitis due to pituitary snuff. *Ann Intern Med* 1970; **73**: 581−584.

Jackson E, Welch KMA. Mushroom workers lung. *Thorax* 1970; **25**: 25−30.

Jenkins DE, Malik SK, Figueroa-Casas JC, Eichhorn RD. Sequential observations on pulmonary functional derangements in bagassosis. *Arch Intern Med* 1971; **128**: 535−540.

Kokkarinen JI, Tukiainen HO, Terho EO. Effect of corticosteroid treatment on the recovery of pulmonary function in farmer's lung. *Am Rev Respir Dis* 1992; **145**: 3−5.

Lee TH, Wraith DG, Bennett CO, Bentley AP. Budgerigar fancier's lung: the persistence of budgerigar pecipitins and the recovery of lung function after cessation of avian exposure. *Clin Allergy* 1983; **13**: 197−202.

Lunn JA, Hughes DTD. Pulmonary hypersensitivity to the grain weevil. *Br J Ind Med* 1967; **24**: 158−161.

Morgan DC, Smyth JT, Lister RW, Pethybridge RJ, Gilson JC, Callaghan P *et al*. Chest symptoms in farming communities with special reference to farmer's lung. *Br J Ind Med* 1975; **32**: 228−234.

Weill H, Buechner HA, Gonzalez E, Herbert SJ, Aucoin E, Ziskind MM. Bagassosis: a study of pulmonary function in 20 cases. *Ann Intern Med* 1966; **64**: 737−747.

Williams JV. Pulmonary function studies in patients with farmer's lung. *Thorax* 1963; **18**: 255−263.

Wuthe H, Bergmann K-Ch, Vogel J. Frequency of lung function disturbances and immunological status of industrial poultry farmers. *Eur J Respir Dis* 1981; **62**(Suppl. 113): 38−39.

63.7 Pneumoconiosis due to coal and silica
(*see also* sections 51, 63.1)

Becklake MR, Du Preez L, Lutz W. Lung function in silicosis of the Witwaterstrand gold-miner. *Am Rev Tuberc Pulm Dis* 1958; **77**: 400−412.

Cockcroft AE, Wagner JC, Seal RME, Lyons JP, Campbell MJ. Irregular opacities in coal workers' pneumoconiosis − correlation with pulmonary function and pathology. *Ann Occup Hyg* 1982; **26**: 767−787.

Cotes JE, Field GB. Lung gas exchange in simple pneumoconiosis of coal workers. *Br J Ind Med* 1972; **29**: 268−273.

Frans A, Brasseur L. Les gradients alvéolo-artériels et la capacité de diffusion dans l'anthraco-silicose. *Rev Inst Hyg Mines* 1971; **26**: 73–85.

Gaensler EA, Cadigan JB, Sasahara AA, Fox EO, MacMahon HE. Graphite pneumoconiosis of electrotypers. *Am J Med* 1966; **41**: 864–882.

Gilson JC, Hugh-Jones P, Oldham PD, Meade F. Lung function in coal workers' pneumoconiosis. *Spec Rep Ser Med Res Coun (Lond)* 1955; No. 290.

Glover JR, Bevan C, Cotes JE, Elmwood PC, Hodges NG, Kell RW et al. Effects of exposure to slate dust in North Wales. *Br J Ind Med* 1980; **37**: 152–162.

Graham WGB, O'Grady RV, Dubuc B. Pulmonary function loss in Vermont granite workers. *Am Rev Respir Dis* 1981; **123**: 25–28.

Jones RN, Weill H, Ziskind M. Pulmonary function in sandblasters' silicosis. *Bull Eur Physiopath Respir* 1975; **11**: 589–595.

Lapp NL, Block J, Boehlecke B, Lippmann M, Morgan WKC, Reger RB. Closing volume in coalminers. *Am Rev Respir Dis* 1976; **113**: 155–161.

Lapp NL, Seaton A, Kaplan KC, Hunsaker MR, Morgan WKC. Pulmonary hemodynamics in symptomatic coal miners. *Am Rev Respir Dis* 1971; **104**: 418–426.

Legg SJ, Cotes JE, Bevan C. Lung mechanics in relation to radiographic category of coal workers' simple pneumoconiosis. *Br J Ind Med* 1983; **40**: 28–33.

Morgan WKC, Lapp NL. Respiratory disease in coal miners. *Am Rev Respir Dis* 1976; **113**: 531–559.

Motley HL. Pulmonary function measurements in an industry. A follow-up study of 38 diatomite workers on the job. *Arch Environ Health* 1963; **6**: 166–177.

Musk AW, Cotes JE, Bevan C, Campbell MJ. Relationship between type of simple coal workers' pneumoconiosis and lung function. A nine-year follow-up study of subjects with small rounded opacities. *Br J Ind Med* 1981; **38**: 313–320.

Rogan JM, Attfield MD, Jacobsen M, Rae S, Walker DD, Walton WH. Role of dust in the working environment in development of chronic bronchitis in British coal miners. *Br J Ind Med* 1973; **30**: 217–226.

Seaton A, Lapp NL, Morgan WKC. Relationship of pulmonary impairment in simple coal workers' pneumoconiosis to type of radiographic opacity. *Br J Ind Med* 1972; **29**: 50–55.

Ulmer WT, Reichel G. Epidemiological problems of coal workers bronchitis in comparison with the general population. *Scand J Work Environ Health* 1972; **200**: 211–219.

63.8 Other occupational disorders
(*see also* sections 51, 63.1)

Coates EO, Watson JHL. Diffuse interstitial lung disease in tungsten carbide workers. *Ann Intern Med* 1971; **75**: 709–716.

Davies TAL. *Respiratory Disease in Foundrymen: Report of a Survey*. London: HMSO, 1971.

Flenley DC, Matthew H. Paraquat poisoning. *Q J Med* 1973; **42**: 683–692.

Musk AW, Gandevia B. Loss of pulmonary elastic recoil in workers formerly exposed to proteolytic enzyme (alcalase) in the detergent industry. *Br J Ind Med* 1976; **33**: 158–165.

Scott EG, Hunt WB. Silo filler's disease. *Chest* 1973; **63**: 701–706.

Tolot F, Girard R, Dortit G, Tabourin G, Gaby P, Bourret J. Manifestations pulmonaries des 'métaux durs'. *Arch Mal Prof* 1970; **31**: 453–470.

Weill H, Waggenspack C, DeRouen T, Ziskind M. Respiratory reactions to B Sabtilis enzymes in detergents. *J Occup Med* 1973; **15**: 267–271.

Zuskin E, Bouhuys A. Acute airway responses to hairspray preparations. *New Engl J Med* 1974; **290**: 660–663.

64 REHABILITATION AND ASSESSMENT OF DISABILITY
(*see also* sections 32.1, 39, 63.1)

American Thoracic Society. Evaluation of impairment/disability secondary to respiratory disorders. *Am Rev Respir Dis* 1986; **133**: 1205–1209.

Brundin A. Physical training in severe chronic obstructive lung disease. *Scand J Respir Dis* 1974; **55**: 25–36.

Cockcroft AE, Saunders MJ, Berry G. Randomised controlled trial of rehabilitation in chronic respiratory disability. *Thorax* 1981; **36**: 200–203.

Cotes JE. Rating respiratory disability: a report on behalf of a working group of the European Society for Clinical Respiratory Physiology. *Eur Respir J* 1990; **3**: 1074–1077.

Cotes JE, Zejda J, King B. Lung function impairment as a guide to exercise limitation in work-related lung disorders. *Am Rev Respir Dis* 1988; **137**: 1089–1093.

Casaburi R, Patessio A, Ioli F, Zanaboni S, Donner CF, Wasserman K. Reductions in exercise lactic acidosis and ventilation as a result of exercise training in patients with obstructive lung disease. *Am Rev Respir Dis* 1991; **143**: 9–18.

De Coster A. The assessment of treatments for the respiratory cripple. *J T Soc Med* 1978; **1**: 55–66.

Degre S, Sergysels R, Messin R, Vandermoten P, Salhadin P, Denolin H et al. Hemodynamic responses to physical training in patients with chronic lung disease. *Am Rev Respir Dis* 1974; **110**: 395–402.

Donner CF, Howard P, eds. Pulmonary rehabilitation in chronic obstructive pulmonary disease (COPD) with recommendations for its use. *Eur Respir Rev* 1991; **1**: 463–576.

Lane DJ, Garrard CS. Pulmonary mechanics in relation to breathing exercises. *Bull Physiopathol Respir* 1975; **11**: 182P.

McGavin CR, Artvinli M, Naoe H, McHardy GJR.

Dyspnoea, disability and distance walked: comparison of estimates of exercise performance in respiratory disease. *Br Med J* 1978; **11**: 241–243.

Oren A, Sue DY, Hansen JE, Torrance DJ, Wasserman K. The role of exercise testing in impairment evaluation. *Am Rev Respir Dis* 1987; **135**: 230–235.

Paez PN, Phillipson EA, Masangkay M, Sproule BJ. The physiologic basis of training patients with emphysema. *Am Rev Respir Dis* 1967; **95**: 944–953.

Paul G, Eldridge F, Mitchell J, Fiene T. Some effects of slowing respiration rate in chronic emphysema and bronchitis. *J Appl Physiol* 1966; **21**: 877–882.

Petty TL. *Intensive and Rehabilitative Respiratory Care: a Practical Approach to the Management of Acute and Chronic Respiratory Failure*, 2nd edn. Philadelphia: Lea Febiger, 1974.

Saunders KB, White JE. Controlled trial of breathing exercises. *Br Med J* 1965; **2**: 680–682.

Williams RGA, Johnston M, Willis LA, Bennett AE. Disability: a model and measurement technique. *Br J Prev Soc Med* 1976; **30**: 71–78.

Wright GW. Disability evaluation in industrial pulmonary disease. *JAMA* 1949; **141**: 1218–1222.

65 CARDIOVASCULAR DISORDERS: EFFECTS ON THE LUNG

(*see also* sections 22.1, 27, 29)

Auchincloss JH Jr, Gilbert R, Baule GH. Unsteady state measurement of oxygen transfer in patients with rheumatic heart diseases. *Clin Sci* 1970; **39**: 21–37.

Bishop JM, Harris P, Bateman M, Raine JM. Respiratory gas exchange in mitral stenosis at three levels of inspired oxygen before and after the infusion of acetylcholine. *Clin Sci* 1962; **22**: 53–62.

Bishop JM, Wade OL. Relationships between cardiac output and rhythm, pulmonary vascular pressures and disability in mitral stenosis. *Clin Sci* 1963; **24**: 391–404.

Blackmon JR, Rowell LB, Kennedy JW, Twiss RD, Conn RD. Physiological significance of maximal oxygen intake in 'pure' mitral stenosis. *Circulation* 1967; **36**: 497–510.

Blesa MI, Lahiri S, Rashkind WJ, Fishman AP. Normalisation of the blunted ventilatory response to acute hypoxia in congenital cyanotic heart disease. *New Engl J Med* 1977; **296**: 237–241.

Burgess JH. Pulmonary diffusing capacity in disorders of the pulmonary circulation. *Circulation* 1974; **49**: 541–550.

Collins JV, Clark TJH, Brown DJ. Airway function in healthy subjects and patients with left heart disease. *Clin Sci* 1975; **49**: 217–228.

Dantzker DR, Bower JS. Mechanisms of gas exchange abnormality in patients with chronic obliterative pulmonary vascular disease. *J Clin Invest* 1979; **64**: 1050–1055.

Dawson A, Kaneko K, McGregor M. Regional lung function in patients with mitral stenosis studied with xenon[133] during air and oxygen breathing. *J Clin Invest* 1965; **44**: 999–1008.

De Troyer A, Yernault J-C, Englert M. Mechanics of breathing in patients with atrial septal defect. *Am Rev Respir Dis* 1977; **115**: 413–421.

Demedts M, Sniderman A, Utz G, Palmer WH, Becklake MR. Lung volumes including closing volume and arterial blood gas measurements in acute ischaemic left heart failure. *Bull Physiopathol Respir* 1974; **10**: 11–25.

Ebi-Kryston KL, Hawthorne VM, Rose G, Shipley MJ, Gillis CR, Hole DJ *et al*. Breathlessness, chronic bronchitis and reduced pulmonary function as predictors of cardiovascular disease mortality among men in England, Scotland and the United States. *Int J Epidemiol* 1989; **18**: 84–88.

Edelman NH, Lahiri S, Braudo L, Cherniack NS, Fishman AP. The blunted ventilatory response to hypoxia in cyanotic congenital heart disease. *N Engl J Med* 1970; **202**: 405–411.

Freeman J, Nunn JF. Ventilation–perfusion relationships after haemorrhage. *Clin Sci* 1963; **24**: 135–147.

Friedman GD, Klatsky AL, Siegelaub AB. Lung function and risk of myocardial infarction and sudden cardiac death. *New Engl J Med* 1976; **294**: 1071–1075.

Grant GP, Garofano RP, Mansell AL, Leopold HB, Gersony WM. Ventilatory response to exercise after intracardiac repair of tetralogy of Fallot. *Am Rev Respir Dis* 1991; **144**: 833–836.

Greene R, Zapol WM, Snider MT, Reid L, Snow R, O'Connell RS, Novelline RA. Early bedside detection of pulmonary vascular occlusion during acute respiratory failure. *Am Rev Respir Dis* 1981; **124**: 593–601.

Hales CA, Kazemi H. Small-airways function in myocardial infarction. *New Engl J Med* 1974; **290**: 761–765.

Halmagyi DFJ, Colebatch HJH. Cardiorespiratory effects of experimental lung embolism. *J Clin Invest* 1961; **40**: 1785–1796.

Harris P, Segel N, Bishop JM. The relation between pressure and flow in the pulmonary circulation in normal subjects and in patients with chronic bronchitis and mitral stenosis. *Cardiovasc Res* 1968; **2**: 73–83.

Hughes JMB, Glazier JB, Maloney JE, West JB. Effect of interstitial pressure on pulmonary blood-flow. *Lancet* 1967; **i**: 192–193.

Kapitan KS, Buchbinder M, Wagner PD, Moser KM. Mechanisms of hypoxemia in chronic thromboembolic pulmonary hypertension. *Am Rev Respir Dis* 1989; **139**: 1149–1154.

Malik AB. Pulmonary microembolism. *Physiol Rev* 1983; **63**: 1114–1207.

Marshall R, McIlroy MB, Christie RV. The work of breathing in mitral stenosis. *Clin Sci* 1954; **13**: 137–146.

Nadel JA, Gold WM, Burgess JH. Early diagnosis of chronic pulmonary vascular obstruction. *Am J Med*

1968; **44**: 16−25.

Robin ED, Laman PD, Goris ML, Theodore J. A shunt is (not) a shunt is (not) a shunt. *Am Rev Respir Dis* 1977; **115**: 553−557.

Scharf SM, Cassidy SS, eds. *Heart−Lung Interactions in Health and Disease.* New York: Marcel Dekker, 1989: 339−363.

Schlesinger Z, Goldbourt U, Medalie JH, Neufeld HN, Riss E, Oran D. Ischemic heart disease and pulmonary ventilatory function. *Israel J Med Sci* 1975; **11**: 308−313.

Snashall PD, Chung KF. Airway obstruction and bronchial hyperresponsiveness in left ventricular failure and mitral stenosis. *Am Rev Respir Dis* 1991; **144**: 945−956.

Sorensen SC, Severinghaus JW. Respiratory insensitivity to acute hypoxia persisting after correction of tetralogy of Fallot. *J Appl Physiol* 1968; **25**: 221−223.

Strieder DJ, Mesko ZG, Zaver AG, Gold WM. Exercise tolerance in chronic hypoxemia due to right-to-left shunt. *J Appl Physiol* 1973; **34**: 853−858.

Tattersfield AE, McNicol MW, Sillett RW. Relationship between haemodynamic and respiratory function in patients with myocardial infarction and left ventricular failure. *Clin Sci* 1972; **42**: 751−768.

Vedin A, Wilhelmsen L, Wedel H, Pettersson B, Wilhelmsson C, Elmfeldt D *et al.* Prediction of cardiovascular deaths and non-fatal reinfarctions after myocardial infarction. *Acta Med Scand* 1977; **201**: 309−316.

Wagner PD. Mechanisms of hypoxemia in pulmonary embolism. *Appl Cardiopulm Pathophysiol* 1987; **1**: 63−71.

Wilson JE, Pierce AK, Johnson RL Jr, Winga ER, Harrell WR, Curry GC *et al.* Hypoxemia in pulmonary embolism, a clinical study. *J Clin Invest* 1971; **50**: 481−491.

Wimalaratna H, Farrell J, Lee HY. Measurement of diffusing capacity in pulmonary embolism. *Respir Med* 1989; **83**: 481−485.

Wood TE, McLeod P, Anthonisen NR, Macklem PT. Mechanics of breathing in mitral stenosis. *Am Rev Respir Dis* 1971; **104**: 52−60.

66 AVIATION AND SPACE TRAVEL
(*see also* section 40)

Cottrell JJ. Altitude exposure during aircraft flight. *Chest* 1988; **93**: 81−84.

Guy HJ, Prisk GH, West JB. Pulmonary function in microgravity. *Physiologist* 1992; **35**, Suppl I: 99−102.

Richards PR. The effects of air travel on passengers with cardiovascular and respiratory diseases. *Practitioner* 1973; **210**: 232−241.

Sawin CF, Nicogossian AE, Rummel JA, Michel EL. Pulmonary function evaluation during the Skylab and Apollo-Soyuz missions. *Aviat Space Environ Med* 1976; **47**: 168−172.

67 ANAESTHESIA
(*see also* sections 27.1−27.4)

D'Angelo E, Robatto FM, Calderini E, Tavola M, Bono D, Torri G *et al.* Pulmonary and chest wall mechanics in anesthetised paralysed humans. *J Appl Physiol* 1991; **70**: 2602−2610.

Davies RO, Edwards MW, Lahiri S. Halothane depresses the response of carotid body chemoreceptors to hypoxia and hypercapnia in the cat. *Anesthesiology* 1982; **57**: 153−159.

Dueck R, Prutow RJ, Davies NJH, Clausen JL, Davidson TM. The lung volume at which shunting occurs with inhalation anesthesia. *Anesthesiology* 1988; **69**: 854−861.

Eisenkraft JB. Effects of anaesthetics on the pulmonary circulation. *Br J Anaesth* 1990; **65**: 63−78.

Gerson G. Pre-operative respiratory function tests and post-operative mortality. *Br J Anaesth* 1969; **41**: 967−971.

Hedenstierna G, Tokics L, Strandberg Å, Lundqvist H, Brismar B. Correlation of gas exchange impairment to development of atelectasis during anaesthesia and muscle paralysis. *Acta Anaesthesiol Scand* 1986; **30**: 183−191.

Hedenstierna G, Lundquist H, Lundh B, Tokics L, Strandberg Å, Brismar B, Frostell C. Pulmonary densities during anaesthesia. An experimental study on lung morphology and gas exchange. *Eur Respir J* 1989; **2**: 528−535.

Hedenstierna G, Strandberg Å, Brismar B, Lundquist H, Svensson L, Tokics L. Functional residual capacity, thoraco-abdominal dimensions and central blood volume during general anesthesia with muscle paralysis and mechanical ventilation. *Anesthesiology* 1985; **62**: 247−254.

Hedenstierna G, Tokics L, Strandberg Å, Lundquist H, Brismar B. Correlation of gas exchange impairment to development of atelectasis during anesthesia and muscle paralysis. *Acta Anaesthesiol Scand* 1986; **30**: 183−191.

Hedenstierna G. Gas exchange during anaesthesia. *Br J Anaesth* 1990; **64**: 507−514.

Hirshman CA, Bergman NA. Factors influencing intrapulmonary airway calibre during anaesthesia. *Br J Anaesth* 1990; **65**: 30−42.

Hulands GH, Greene R, Iliff LD, Nunn JF. Influence of anaesthesia on the regional distribution of perfusion and ventilation in the lung. *Clin Sci* 1970; **38**: 451−460.

Jakobson S, Fridriksson H, Hedenström H, Ivarsson I. Effects of intercostal nerve blocks on pulmonary mechanics in healthy man. *Acta Anaesthesiol Scand* 1980; **24**: 482−486.

Jones JG, Faithfull D, Jordan C. Rib cage movement during halothane anesthesia in man. *Br J Anaesth* 1979; **51**: 399−407.

Jones JG, Sapsford DJ, Wheatley RG. Postoperative hypoxaemia: mechanisms and time course. *Anaesthesia* 1990; **45**: 566−573.

Juno P, Marsh M, Knopp TJ, Rehder K. Closing capacity in awake and anesthetized-paralyzed man. *J Appl Physiol* 1978; **44**: 238–244.

Marshall BE. Effects of anesthetics on pulmonary gas exchange. In: Stanley TH, Sperry RJ, eds. *Anesthesia and the Lung.* London: Kluwer Academic Publishers, 1989: 117–125.

Nunn JF. Effects of anaesthesia on respiration. *Br J Anaesth* 1990; **65**: 54–62.

Nunn JF. Factors influencing the arterial oxygen tension during halothane anesthesia with spontaneous respiration. *Br J Anaesth* 1964; **36**: 327–341.

Read DJC, Freedman S, Kafer ER. Pressures developed by loaded inspiratory muscles in conscious and anesthetized man. *J Appl Physiol* 1974; **37**: 207–218.

Rehder K, Knopp TJ, Sessler AD, Didier EP. Ventilation–perfusion relationship in young healthy awake and anesthetized-paralyzed man. *J Appl Physiol* 1979; **47**: 745–753.

Simonneau G, Vivien A, Sartene R, Kunstlinger F, Kamran S, Noviant Y, Duroux P. Diaphragm dysfunction induced by upper abdominal surgery. Role of postoperative pain. *Am Rev Respir Dis* 1983; **128**: 899–903.

Strandberg Å, Tokics L, Brismar B, Lundquist H, Hedenstierna G. Constitutional factors promoting development of atelectasis during anaesthesia. *Acta Anaesthesiol Scand* 1987; **31**: 21–24.

Sullivan TY, Yu PL. Airway anesthesia effects on hypercapnic breathing pattern in humans. *J Appl Physiol* 1983; **55**: 368–376.

Sykes MK, Loh L, Seed RF, Kafer E, Chakrabati MK. The effect of inhalational anaesthetics on hypoxic pulmonary vasoconstriction and pulmonary vascular resistance in the perfused lung of the dog and the cat. *Br J Anaesth* 1972; **44**: 776–788.

Sykes MK, McNicol MW, Campbell EJM. *Respiratory Failure* 2nd edn. Oxford: Blackwell Scientific Publications, 1976.

Tokics L, Hedenstierna G, Brismar B, Strandberg Å, Lundquist H. Thoraco abdominal restriction in supine men. CT and lung function measurements. *J Appl Physiol* 1988; **64**: 599–604.

Tokics L, Hedenstierna G, Strandberg Å, Brismar B, Lundquist H. Lung collapse and gas exchange during general anesthesia: effects of spontaneous breathing, muscle paralysis and positive end-expiratory pressure. *Anesthesiology* 1987; **66**: 157–167.

Tokics L, Strandberg Å, Brismar B, Lundquist H, Hedenstierna G. Computerised tomography of the chest and gas exchange measurements during ketamine anaesthesia. *Acta Anaesthesiol Scand* 1987; **31**: 684–692.

Westbrook PR, Stubbs SE, Sessler AD, Rehder K, Hyatt RE. Effects of anesthesia and muscle paralysis on respiratory mechanics in normal man. *J Appl Physiol* 1973; **34**: 81–86.

68 OXYGEN THERAPY, INCLUDING COMPLICATIONS

68.1 Clinical physiology
(*see also* sections 22, 25, 26, 32.1, 40)

Andersen A, Hillstad L. Hemodynamic responses to oxygen breathing and the effect of pharmacological blockade. *Acta Med Scand* 1970; **188**: 419–424.

Caldwell PRB, Lee WL Jr, Schildkraut HS, Archibald ER. Changes in lung volume, diffusing capacity, and blood gases in men breathing oxygen. *J Appl Physiol* 1966; **21**: 1477–1483.

Chance B, Sies H, Boveris A. Hydrogen peroxide metabolism in mammalian organs. *Physiol Rev* 1979; **59**: 527–605.

Chew HER, Hanson GC, Slack WK. Hyperbaric oxygenation. *Br J Dis Chest* 1969; **63**: 113–139.

Clark JM, Lambertsen CJ. Pulmonary oxygen toxicity: a review. *Pharmacol Rev* 1971; **23**: 37–133.

Crapo JD. Morphologic changes in pulmonary oxygen toxicity. *Annu Rev Physiol* 1986; **48**: 721–731.

Davis WB, Rennard SI, Bitterman PB, Crystal RG. Pulmonary oxygen toxicity. Early reversible changes in human alveolar structures induced by hyperoxia. *N Engl J Med* 1983; **309**: 878–883.

Gonder JC, Proctor RA, Will JA. Genetic differences in oxygen toxicity are correlated with cytochrome P-450 inducibility. *Proc Natl Acad Sci USA* 1985; **82**: 6315–6319.

Halliwell B. Tell me about free radicals, doctor: a review. *J R Soc Med* 1989; **82**: 747–752.

Jamieson D, Chance B, Cadenas E, Boveris A. The relation of free radical production to hyperoxia. *Annu Rev Physiol* 1986; **48**: 703–719.

Sackner MA, Landa J, Hirsch J, Zapata A. Pulmonary effects of oxygen breathing. A 6-hour study in normal men. *Ann Intern Med* 1975; **82**: 40–43.

Sutton JR, Coates G, Remmers JE, eds. *Hypoxia: Tissue Adaptations.* Toronto: BC Dekker, 1990.

Welch HG. Hyperoxia and human performance: a brief review. *Med Sci Sports Exerc* 1982; **14**: 253–262.

Winter PM, Smith G. The toxicity of oxygen. *Anaesthesiology* 1972; **37**: 210–241.

68.2 Clinical applications
(*see also* sections on medical conditions)

Chamberlain DA, Millard FJC. The treatment of polycythaemia secondary to hypoxic lung disease by continuous oxygen administration. *Q J Med* 1963; **32**: 341–350.

Donald KW, Fulton WW, Garry RC, Hutchison JH, McGirr EM, Flenley DC et al. *Uses and Dangers of Oxygen Therapy.* Edinburgh: HMSO, 1969.

Douglas TA, Lawson DD, Ledingham IMcA, Norman JN, Sharp GR, Smith G. Carbon-monoxide poisoning. *Lancet* 1962; **i**: 68–69.

Forgacs P, Wright PH, Wyatt AP. Treatment of intestinal gas cysts by oxygen breathing. *Lancet* 1973; **i**: 579–582.

Kvale PA, Anthonisen NR, Cugell W, Petty TL, Boylen T, Timms RM. Continuous or nocturnal oxygen therapy in hypoxemic chronic obstructive lung disease. *Ann Intern Med* 1980; **93**: 391–398.

Lal S, Savidge RS, Chhabra GP. Oxygen administration after myocardial infarction. *Lancet* 1969; **i**: 381–383.

Levin DC, Neff TA, O'Donohue WJ, Pierson DJ, Petty TL, Snider GL. Conference report: further recommendations for prescribing and supplying long-term oxygen therapy. *Am Rev Respir Dis* 1988; **138**: 745–747.

MacNee W, Wathen CG, Flenley DC, Muir AD. The effects of controlled oxygen therapy on ventricular function in patients with stable and decompensated cor pulmonale. *Am Rev Respir Dis* 1988; **137**: 1289–1295.

Medical Research Council. Long term domiciliary oxygen therapy in chronic hypoxic cor pulmonale complicating chronic bronchitis and emphysema. *Lancet* 1981; **i**: 681–686.

Neff TA, Petty TL. Long-term continuous oxygen therapy in chronic airway obstruction. *Ann Intern Med* 1970; **72**: 621–626.

NHLBI Workshop. Hyperbaric oxygenation therapy. *Am Rev Respir Dis* 1991; **144**: 1414–1421.

Northfield TC. Oxygen therapy for spontaneous pneumothorax. *Br Med J* 1971; **4**: 86–88.

Rudolf M, Banks RA, Semple SJG. Hypercapnia during oxygen therapy in acute exacerbations of chronic respiratory failure. *Lancet* 1977; **ii**: 483–486.

Selinger SR, Kennedy TP, Buescher P, Terry P, Parham W, Godreed D. Effects of removing oxygen from patients with chronic obstructive pulmonary disease. *Am Rev Respir Dis* 1987; **136**: 85–91.

Stark RD, Finnigan P, Bishop JM. Long-term domiciliary oxygen in chronic bronchitis with pulmonary hypertension. *Br Med J* 1973; **3**: 467–470.

Swinburn CR, Mould H, Stone TN, Corris PA, Gibson GJ. Symptomatic benefit of supplemental oxygen in hypoxemic patients with chronic lung disease. *Am Rev Respir Dis* 1991; **143**: 913–915.

Thom SR. Hyperbaric oxygen therapy. *J Intensive Care Med* 1989; **4**: 58–74.

Thurston JGB, Greenwood TW, Bending MR, Connor H, Curwen MP. A controlled investigation into the effects of hyperbaric oxygen on mortality following acute myocardial infarction. *Q J Med* 1973; **42**: 751–770.

Timms RM, Khaja FU, Williams GW. The Nocturnal Oxygen Therapy Trial Group. Hemodynamic response to oxygen therapy in chronic obstructive pulmonary disease. *Ann Intern Med* 1985; **102**: 29–36.

Way JL, Gibbon SL, Sheehy M. Cyanide intoxication: protection with oxygen. *Science* 1966; **152**: 210–211.

Weitzenblum E, Sautegeau A, Ehrhart M, Mammosser M, Pelletier A. Long-term oxygen therapy can reverse the progression of pulmonary hypertension in patients with chronic obstructive pulmonary disease. *Am Rev Respir Dis* 1985; **131**: 493–498.

68.3 Technical aspects

Arlati S, Rolo J, Micaleff E, Sacerdoti C, Brambilla I. A reservoir nasal cannula improves protection given by oxygen during muscular exercise in COPD. *Chest* 1988; **93**: 1165–1169.

Barach AL. Ambulatory oxygen therapy: oxygen inhalation at home and out of doors. *Dis Chest* 1959; **35**: 229–241.

Campbell EJM, Gebbie T. Masks and tent for providing controlled oxygen concentrations. *Lancet* 1966; **i**: 468–469.

Catterall M, Kantantzis G, Hodges M. The performance of nasal catheters and a face mask in oxygen therapy. *Lancet* 1967; **i**: 415–417.

Claiborne RA, Paynter DE, Dutt AK, Rowlands JW. Evaluation of the use of an oxygen conservation device in long-term oxygen therapy. *Am Rev Respir Dis* 1987; **136**: 1095–1098.

Cotes JE, Matthews CR, Tasker PM. Continuous versus intermittent administration of oxygen during exercise in patients with chronic lung disease. *Lancet* 1963; **1**: 1075–1077.

Couser JI Jr, Make BJ. Transtracheal oxygen decreases inspired minute ventilation. *Am Rev Respir Dis* 1989; **139**: 627–631.

Dilworth JP, Higgs CMB, Jones PA, White RJ. Prescription of oxygen concentrators: adherence to published guidelines. *Thorax* 1989; **44**: 576–578.

Gibson RL, Comer PB, Beckham RW, McGraw CP. Actual tracheal oxygen concentrations with commonly used oxygen equipment. *Anesthesiology* 1976; **44**: 71–73.

Green ID. Choice of method for administration of oxygen. *Br Med J* 1967; **3**: 593–596.

Griffin OG, Longson DJ. The hazard due to outward leakage of oxygen from a full face mask. *Ann Occup Hyg* 1969; **12**: 147–149.

Lock SH, Paul EA, Rudd RM, Wedzicha JA. Portable oxygen therapy: assessment and usage. *Respir Med* 1991; **85**: 407–412.

Klein EF, Shah DA, Shah NJ, Modell JH, Desantels D. Performance characteristics of conventional and prototype humidifiers and nebulizers. *Chest* 1973; **64**: 690–696.

Massey LW, Hussey JD, Albert RK. Inaccurate oxygen delivery in some portable liquid oxygen devices. *Am Rev Respir Dis* 1988; **137**: 204–205.

Pflug AE, Cheney FW, Butler J. Evaluation of an intermittent oxygen flow system. *Am Rev Respir Dis* 1972; **105**: 449–452.

Stillwell PC, Quick JD, Munro PR, Mallory JB. Effectiveness of open circuit and oxyhood delivery of helium oxygen. *Chest* 1989; **95**: 1222–1224.

Tiep BL, Lewis MI. Oxygen conservation and oxygen-conserving devices in chronic lung disease. *Chest* 1987; **92**: 263–272.

Veer JBV. The 'pinch test' for oxygen therapy. *New Engl J Med* 1970; **282**: 1269–1270.

Wells RE Jr, Perera RD, Kinney JM. Humidification of oxygen during inhalational therapy. *New Engl J Med* 1963; **268**: 644–647.

69 ASSISTED VENTILATION

69.1 General

Biondi JW, Schulman DS, Matthay RA. Effects of mechanical ventilation on right and left ventricular function. *Clin Chest Med* 1988; **9**: 55–71.

Gazmuri RJ, von Planta M, Weil MH, Rackow EC. Arterial Pco_2 as an indicator of systemic perfusion during cardiopulmonary resuscitation. *Crit Care Med* 1989; **17**: 237–240.

Hunter AR. *Essentials of Artificial Ventilation of the Lungs*, 3rd edn. London: Churchill, 1972.

Johansson H, Löfström JB. Effects on breathing mechanics and gas exchange of different inspiratory gas flow patterns. *Acta Anaesth Scand* 1975; **19**: 8–18, 19–27.

Kolobow T, Moretti MP, Fumagalli R, Mascheroni D, Prato P, Chen V, Joris M. Severe impairment in lung function induced by high peak airway pressure during mechanical ventilation. An experimental study. *Am Rev Respir Dis* 1987; **135**: 312–315.

Larsson A, Jonmarker C, Werner O. Ventilation inhomogeneity during controlled ventilation. Which index should be used? *J Appl Physiol* 1988; **65**: 2030–2039.

Levine M, Gilbert R, Auchincloss JH. A comparison of the effects of sighs, large tidal volumes and positive end expiratory pressure in assisted ventilation. *Scand J Respir Dis* 1972; **53**: 101–108.

MacIntyre NR. Respiratory function during pressure support ventilation. *Chest* 1986; **89**: 677–683.

Marini JJ, Rodriguez RM, Lamb V. The inspiratory workload of patient-initiated mechanical ventilation. *Am Rev Respir Dis* 1986; **134**: 902–909.

Morch ET. History of mechanical ventilation. In: Kirby RR, Smith RA, Desautels DA, eds. *Mechanical Ventilation*. New York: Churchill Livingstone, 1985: 1–58.

Mushin WW, Rendell-Baker L, Thompson PW, Mapleson WW. *Automatic Ventilation of the Lungs*, 3rd edn. Oxford: Blackwell Scientific Publications, 1980.

Toung TJK, Saharia P, Mitzner WA, Permutt S, Cameron JL. The beneficial and harmful effects of positive end expiratory pressure. *Surg Gynecol Obstet* 1978; **147**: 518–524.

Valentine DD, Hammond MD, Downs JB, Sears NJ, Sims WR. Distribution of ventilation and perfusion with different modes of mechanical ventilation. *Am Rev Respir Dis* 1991; **143**: 1262–1266.

Watson JW, Kamm RD, Burwen DR, Brown R, Ingenito E, Slutsky AS. Gas exchange during constant flow ventilation with different gases. *Am Rev Respir Dis* 1987; **136**: 420–425.

Young JD, Sykes MK. Artificial ventilation: history, equipment and techniques. *Thorax* 1990; **45**: 753–758.

69.2 Clinical aspects
(*see also* sections 69.1, 69.3)

Braun SR, Sufit RL, Giavannoni R, O'Connor M, Peters H. Intermittent negative pressure ventilation in the treatment of respiratory failure in progressive neuromuscular disease. *Neurology* 1987; **37**: 1874–1875.

Brochard L, Pluskwa F, Lemaire F. Improved efficacy of spontaneous breathing with inspiratory pressure support. *Am Rev Respir Dis* 1987; **136**: 411–415.

Hamilton-Farrell MR, Hanson GC. General care of the ventilated patient in the intensive care unit. *Thorax* 1990; **45**: 962–969.

Harley HRS. Laryngotracheal obstruction complicating tracheostomy or endotracheal intubation with assisted respiration. *Thorax* 1971; **26**: 493–533.

Malo J, Ali J, Wood LDH. How does positive end-expiratory pressure reduce intrapulmonary shunt in canine pulmonary edema? *J Appl Physiol* 1984; **57**: 1002–1010.

Ponte J. Indications for mechanical ventilation. *Thorax* 1990; **45**: 885–890.

69.3 Technical aspects
(*see also* section 68.3)

Branthwaite MA. Non-invasive and domiciliary ventilation: positive pressure techniques. *Thorax* 1991; **46**: 208–212.

Hayes B, Robinson JS. An assessment of methods of humidification of inspired gas. *Br J Anaesth* 1970; **42**: 94–104.

Shneerson JM. Non-invasive and domiciliary ventilation: negative pressure techniques. *Thorax* 1991; **46**: 131–135.

Slutsky AS. Nonconventional methods of ventilation. *Am Rev Respir Dis* 1988; **138**: 175–183.

Sykes MK. Sterilization of ventilators. *Int Anaesthesiol Clin* 1972; **10**: 131–146.

Weisman IM, Rinaldo JE, Rogers RM, Sanders MH. State of the art: intermittent mandatory ventilation. *Am Rev Respir Dis* 1983; **127**: 641–647.

Whitby JL. Sterilization of pulmonary ventilators. *Proc R Soc Med* 1970; **63**: 909–910.

Younes M. Proportional assisted ventilation, a new approach to ventilatory support theory. *Am Rev Respir Dis* 1992; **145**: 114–120.

69.4 High frequency ventilation

Bryan AC, Slutsky AS. Lung volume during high frequency oscillation. *Am Rev Respir Dis* 1986; **133**: 928−930.

Drazen JM, Kamm RD, Slutsky AS. High-frequency ventilation. *Physiol Rev* 1984; **64**: 505−543.

Permutt S, Mitzner W, Weinmann G. Model of gas transport during high-frequency ventilation. *J Appl Physiol* 1985; **58**: 1956−1970.

Solway J, Rossing TH, Saari AF, Drazen JM. Expiratory flow limitation and dynamic pulmonary hyperinflation during high frequency ventilation. *J Appl Physiol* 1986; **60**: 2071−2078.

The HIFI study group. High-frequency oscillatory ventilation compared with conventional mechanical ventilation in the treatment of respiratory failure in preterm infants. *N Engl J Med* 1989; **320**: 88−93.

69.5 Weaning from ventilator

Brochard L, Harf A, Lorino H, Lemaire F. Inspiratory pressure support prevents diaphragmatic fatigue during weaning from mechanical ventilation. *Am Rev Respir Dis* 1989; **139**: 513−521.

Feeley TW, Hedley-Whyte J. Weaning from controlled ventilation and supplemental oxygen. *New Engl J Med* 1975; **292**: 903−906.

Goldstone J, Moxham J. Weaning from mechanical ventilation. *Thorax* 1991; **46**: 56−62.

Petrof BJ, Legaré M, Goldberg P, Milic-Emili J, Gottfried SB. Continuous positive airway pressure reduces work of breathing and dyspnea during weaning from mechanical ventilation in severe chronic obstructive pulmonary disease. *Am Rev Respir Dis* 1990; **141**: 281−289.

Tomlinson JR, Miller KS, Lorch DG, Smith L, Reines HD, Sahn SA. A prospective comparison of IMV and T-piece weaning from mechanical ventilation. *Chest* 1989; **96**: 348−352.

Torres A, Reyes A, Roca J, Wagner PD, Rodriguez-Roisin R. Ventilation-perfusion mismatching in chronic obstructive pulmonary disease during ventilator weaning. *Am Rev Respir Dis* 1989; **140**: 1246−1250.

70 TREATMENT OF AIRFLOW LIMITATION

70.1 Physical methods
(*see also* sections 15, 64 and medical conditions)

Cochrane GM, Webber BA, Clarke SW. Effects of sputum on pulmonary function. *Br Med J* 1977; **2**: 1181−1183.

Miller WF. Physical therapeutic measures in the treatment of chronic bronchopulmonary disorders. *Am J Med* 1958; **24**: 929−940.

Opie LH, Spalding JMK. Chest physiotherapy during intermittent positive-pressure respiration. *Lancet* 1958; **ii**: 671−674.

Sutton PP, Parker RA, Webber BA, Newman SP, Garland N, Lopez-Vidriere MT *et al.* Assessment of the forced expiration technique, postural drainage and directed coughing in chest physiotherapy. *Eur J Respir Dis* 1983; **64**: 62−68.

Thoman RL, Stoker GL, Ross JC. The efficacy of pursed-lips breathing in patients with chronic obstructive pulmonary disease. *Am Rev Respir Dis* 1966; **93**: 100−106.

70.2 Bronchodilator therapy
(*see also* section 18.3, 19.1)

Ellul-Micallef R, Borthwick RC, McHardy GJR. The time-course of response to prednisolone in chronic bronchial asthma. *Clin Sci* 1974; **47**: 105−117.

Fitzpatrick MF, Mackay T, Driver H, Douglas NJ. Salmeterol in nocturnal asthma: a double blind, placebo controlled trial of a long acting inhaled β_2 agonist. *Br Med J* 1990; **301**: 1365−1368.

Freedman BJ. Trial of a terbutaline aerosol in the treatment of asthma and a comparison of its effects with those of a salbutamol aerosol. *Br J Dis Chest* 1972; **66**: 222−229.

Grant IWB, Turner-Warwick M, Fox W. Sodium cromoglycate in chronic asthma. *Br Med J* 1976; **1**: 361−364.

Paterson JW, Evans RJC, Prime FJ. Selectivity of bronchodilator action of salbutamol in asthmatic patients. *Br J Dis Chest* 1971; **65**: 21−38.

Rebuck AS, Read J. Assessment and management of severe asthma. *Am J Med* 1971; **51**: 788−798.

Saunders KB. Bronchodilator response patterns in patients with chronic airways obstruction: use of peak inspiratory flow rate. *Br Med J* 1967; **2**: 399−402.

Shenfield GM, Paterson JW. Clinical assessment of bronchodilator drugs delivered by aerosol. *Thorax* 1973; **28**: 124−128.

Silverman M, Konig P, Godfrey S. Use of serial exercise tests to assess the efficacy and duration of action of drugs for asthma. *Thorax* 1973; **28**: 574−578.

Wright BM. A new nebuliser. *Lancet* 1958; **ii**: 24−25.

Author Index

Page numbers are given for each page where a name appears one or more times except when the name identifies a procedure or item of equipment; such entries are included in the subject index. *Italics* indicate that the author's material has been included in a table or figure.

Bleecker ER 689, 711
Blesa MI 719
Blide RW 698
Bligh J 685
Block AJ 707
Block J 718
Blomqvist CG 691, 698, 699
Bloom FE 685
Bloom JW 700, 705
Bloom SR 674
Bloom WJ 703
Blount SG Jr 691
Blumenfeld W 660
Boat TF 707
Bock AV 699
Boddy K 662
Bode FR 667, 669, 676, 700, 704
Boeck C de 694
Boehlecke B 718
Boey HK 705
Bogaard JM 714
Boggis CJ 713
Bohadana AB 664, 667, 673
Bohannon RL 424, 691
Bohr C 6, 7, 271, 302, 320
Boileau RA 662
Bolt von H 662
Bolton DPG 688
Bonci E 705
Bone JM 522, 706
Bonjer FH 690
Bonnassis JB 655
Bono D 720
Bonora M 339, 685, 687
Booth FW 688
Boothby WM 636
Borelli GA 5
Boren HG 702
Borg G 390, 689
Borgstrom M 665
Borham P 668
Borland CDR 278, 297, 318, 319, 682
Borowski CJ 670
Borsboom GJJM 697
Borthwick RC 724
Bosch J 713
Bosken CH 712
Bossé R 705
Botelho SY 156, 664, 672
Bouhoutsos J 661
Bouhuys A 223, 672, 683, 696, 697, 705, 711, 717, 718
Boulet LP 674
Bourque LB 705
Bourret J 718
Bourret M 678
Boushey HA 669, 705
Boveris A 721
Bower JS 179
Bowman P 691
Boyce AJ 701
Boyle R 4
Boylen T 722
Brackett NC Jr 522, 706
Bradley AC 716

Bradley CA 679
Bradley GW 708
Bradley ME 663, 668, 714
Bradley RD 240
Brain JD 659, 668, 669
Braman SS 710
Brambilla I 722
Brammell H 690
Brancatisano A 669
Brancato G 696
Branthwaite MA 723
Brasseur L 522, 661, 704, 706, 714, 718
Braudo L 719
Braun SR 717, 723
Bray G 715
Bredle DL 699
Breslin ABX 711
Breuer J 8
Brewis RAL 659
Brice AG 687
Bridges N 467
Briehl RW 680
Bright P 660
Brille D 702
Brimm JE 665
Briscoe WA 190, 511, 674, 675, 679, 680, 704, 712
Brismar B 720, 721
British Occupational Hygiene Society 661
British Thoracic Society 710
Britt AG 354
Britton MG 666, 716
Broberg S 688, 691
Brochard L 723, 724
Brodie TG 5
Brody AW 704
Brody JS 697, 699, 712
Broman L 712
Broman M 712
Bromberger-Barnea B 673, 678
Bronikowski TA 678
Brook R 661
Brooks AGF 703
Brooks GA 688, 692
Brooks OG 659
Brooks SM 716
Brough FK 696
Brown A 409
Brown D 660
Brown DJ 664, 665, 719
Brown DW 699
Brown GJA 713
Brown HW 688
Brown IK 714
Brown KGE 714
Brown R 664, 665, 667, 670, 723
Brozek J 698
Brozovic B 681
Bruback HF 668
Bruce D 669
Bruce EN 685, 715
Bruce RA 690, 692, 693
Bruch HR 709
Brück K 697

Brugger P 699
Brundin A 718
Brundin T 698
Bründler JP 664
Brunekreef B 704
Brunes L 704
Brunner JX 664
Bryan AC 667, 676, 687, 696, 706, 723
Bryan MH 686
Bryant GH 663
Bryceson ADM 707
Brzezinska Z 692
Buchbinder M 719
Buchta I 713
Buckley CE III 687
Budiansky B 671
Buechner HA 717
Buescher P 722
Buick FJ 693
Buist AS 476, 502, 668, 669, 701
Bulbulian AH 636
Bull SB 695
Burdon JGW 390
Burge PS 557, 557, 675, 716
Burgess JH 719
Burke CM 692, 713
Burki NK 666, 670
Burkinshaw L 442, 691
Burney PGJ 672
Burnham C 676
Burns BH 689
Burns CB 665
Burrell RG 717
Burri PH 697
Burrows B 675, 682, 697, 702, 703, 704, 705, 707, 712
Burton AC 677
Burton AP 676
Burwen DR 723
Busch AM 686
Bush A 665
Buskirk ER 661
Buston MH 674
Butcher BT 666, 716
Butler JP 119
Butler C 679
Butler J 669, 716, 722
Butler JP 119
Butler PJ 669
Butt WS 700
Butterworth BA 666
Bylin G 710, 711
Byrd RB 708
Byrne-Quinn E 686, 687, 699

Caceres CA 666
Cade JF 666
Cadenas E 721
Cadigan JB 718
Cagel P 708
Cai Y 678
Cain SM 699
Cairns T 714
Calderini E 720

728

733

Moxham J *578*, 651, 714, 715, 724
Muiesan G 700
Muir A 671
Muir AD 722
Muir DCF *185*, 229, 660, 668
Mukai D 711
Mukhtar MR 700
Müller H 9, 697
Müller NL 710
Mullinax PF Jr 690
Mulvey DA 714
Munoz A 672, 705
Munro PR 722
Munt PW 697
Murakami J 710
Murata K 676
Murphy BG 676
Murphy CL 687
Murphy K 686, 687, 689, 691
Murray J 259
Murray JF 659, 677, 713, 714
Musgrove J 661
Mushin WW 690, 723
Musk AW 718
Mutt V 678
Myers J 708
Myron PR 713

Nachemson A 714
Nadel JA 198, *300*, *550*, 664, 672, 674, 689, 705, 709, 719
Naedts JP 703
Naeije R 713
Naeraa N 660
Nagle FJ 691
Nail BS 686
Naimark A 671, 679
Nair NM 674
Nairn JR 674
Nakhosteen JA 713
Naoe H *388*, 719
Naruse Y *50*, *53*, *311*, 661
Nasello-Paterson C 695
Natale R 695
Nathanielsz PW 694
National Heart and Lung Institute 677
Nattie EE 685, 688
Naughton JP 691
Navajas D 703
Navin JJ 663
Nazar K 692
Neegaard K Von 5
Neff TA 722
Neild JE 672
Nelems B 710
Nelson DP 678
Nelson NL 709
Nelson NM 695
Nelson SB 715
Nesarajah MS 677
Neubauer JA 685, 715
Neuburger N 123, 668, 686
Neufeld HN 720
Neville E 683

Newberg LA 676
Newell JD 665
Newell SZ 708
Newhouse MT 229
Newman SP 724
Newsham LGS 662
Newsom Davis J 337, 378, 663, 714
Ng CKY 671, 700
Ng'ang'a LW 666
Nguyen-Phu D 681
NHLBI Workshop 714, 722
Nicklaus TM 710
Nicogossian AE 720
Nicoli MM 665
Niden AH 682
Nielsen B 692
Nielsen M *192*, *347*, 370, 679, 685, 691
Nielsen TM 9, 667
Niewoehner DE 669, 671, 700, 707
Niizeki K 681
Nikov N 671
Ninane V 663
Nishimura M 685
Nishitani H 710
Nitta K 661
Nixon AJ 660
Noble MIM 687, 690
Noguera I 690, 691
Nolan MF 680
Nolop KB 686
Norgin NG 56, 662
Norman AP 696
Norman JN 721
Norman WP 685
Norris AH *491*, 693, 700
Norris RM 215
Northfield TC 722
Nosil J 679
Notter RH 671
Nourse CH 695
Novelline RA 719
Noviant Y 721
Nowaczyk BJ 694
Nowak A 696
Noworaj A 695
Nugent KM 675
Nullens W 661
Nunn AJ 701, 703
Nunn AT *512*
Nunn JF *43*, *572*, 659, 661, 662, 719, 720, 721
Nunneley SA 664

O'Brien IM 716
O'Brodovich H 713
O'Bryne PM 675
O'Cain CF 672, 700, 704
O'Callaghan C 695
O'Connell RS 719
O'Connor G 176, 674
O'Connor M 723
O'Donnell CR 668
O'Donohue WJ 722
O'Grady RV 718

O'Shea J *156*
Obdrzalek J 679
Obenour WH 714
Obertacke U 713
Obeso A 686, 687
Oddó H 697
Oelz O 699
Oeseburg B 681
Ogawa T 693
Ogilvie CM 307, 683
Ohta Y 243, 684
Okayama H 708
Okunieff P 685
Olafsson O 702
Olafsson S *393*, 673, 708
Oldenburg FA 692
Oldham PD 58, 59, 68, 149, 223, *487*, 659, 675, 717, 718
Olievier ICW 686, 697
Olive JT Jr 672
Olsen CR 662, 666, 679
Olsen GN 707
Olsen HC 706
Olszowka AJ 677, 679, 681
Omenaas E 703
Opie LH 724
Oran D 720
Orehek J 665, 674, 711
Orem J 715
Oren A 691, 719
Orie NGM 705, 707
Oriol A 707
Orlander J 693
Orphanidou D 679
Orr GW 692
Orzalesi MM *91*, 663, 670
Osborne S 710
Oski FA 283
Osmanliev DP 668
Osmond C 707
Ostrow D 712
Ostryzniuk P 662
Oswald M 672
Otis AB 6, 129, 182, *264*, 399, 664, 668, 670, 671, 675, 699
Otulana BA 713
Ou LC 360
Overfield EM 712
Overton TR 675
Owen P 717
Owen-Thomas JB 661
Owles NH 357
Oxhøj H 669

Packer BS 697
Paez PN 719
Pain MCF 678, 682
Paintal AS 604, 688
Painter R 692
Paiva M 184, 219, 229, 528, 659, 675, 676, 696, 699
Pallot DJ 684
Palmer KNV 717
Palmer WH 672, 719
Palmes ED 668
Pan LG 685, 686, 687

739

744

746

Subject Index

This index supplements the list of contents of chapters (page v). Numbers in *italics* refer to figures or tables in the text. The section headings for the classified bibliography are listed on pages 564–8.

alveolar capillaries (*contd*)
    adults *497*, 500
    children *460, 463*
alveolar capillary membrane,
  diffusing capacity of (*D*m) 296–7
    measurement 313–5
    reference values
      adults *497, 501*
      children *460, 463*
    transfer of gas across 270–8, 519, 544
alveolar cells
  type I 85
  type II 85, 97
alveolar deadspace 191, 192, 250
alveolar drive *see* transfer gradient
alveolar ducts 84–5
  expansion 94
alveolar epithelium 84–5, 94, *98*, 270
alveolar gas, composition 265–6
  see also individual gases
alveolar plateau, slope of 211–2
  as epidemiological tool 221–2
    measurement 216–9
alveolar ventilation ($\dot{V}$A) 194, 263, 265–6
alveoli 84, 85–6
  collapse 100
  expansion 94
alveolitis,
  diffuse fibrosing 561–63
  extrinsic allergic 595–6, 597–8
alveolar-arterial tension differences
  for O_2 and CO_2 204–7, *210*, *512*
  for N_2 211
American Thoracic Society, recommendations of 24,
    71, 133, 309, 339, 446, 449, 494
aminophylline 202, 642
ammonia 1
AMP 401–2
amphibians 4
amplifiers 30–1
anaemia, exercise limitation in 407
anaerobic metabolism 384, 400, 402–5, *409*
anaerobic threshold 357, 427, 436
anaesthesia,
  alveolar collapse in 100
  effects on lung function *619*
  oxygen in relation to 619–20
  references 720
anatomical deadspace, *see* deadspace, anatomical
anatomical shunt, *see* shunt, anatomical
anemometers, respiratory 26–7
angina of effort 387, 425, 600
ankylosing spondylitis 575–6
anoxia,
  definition *12*
  see hypoxia
anthropometric measurements 54–6
anticholinergic drugs 641–2
antigens, challenges with 555–8
anxiety 442

Aoki centres 330
aortic baroreceptors 200
aortic bodies 341
apneusis 328
apnoea
  definition *12*
  during sleep 359, 336, 579, 582, 620
apomorphine 339
applications of lung function tests 65, 66, *132*, 446,
    514–20
aqueous vapour pressure *see* water vapour
arm span 55, 492
arterial blood *see* blood and individual constituents
arterial cannulation 36–9, 240, 363
asbestos, lung disease due to 593–5
asphyxia, definition *12*
asphyxia neonatorum 621
assisted ventilation 647
  avoidance of complications 651–2
  control of 649–50
  methods 647–9
  references 723–4
  weaning from 650–1
asthma
  agents causing 548–9
  airway resistance in 113
  bronchial hyperreactivity in 555
  case study 551
  chronic childhood 553
  chronic severe 553
  circadian variation in 555
  control of ventilation in 553
  definition and features 546, 547
  diagnosis 554–8
  exercise-induced 176–7, 549, 555
  extrinsic 548–9
  gas exchange in 553
  lung volumes and ventilatory capacity in 550, 552
  management principles 558, 559
  mechanisms and pathology 546–8, 549
  and menstrual cycle 469
  nocturnal aggravation 548
  references 710–12
  uneven lung function in 552
Astrup technique 45–6
atelectasis 100, 619, 632
athletes 408, 472–4
  at altitude 410, 616
atmosphere,
  evolution 1–3
  pollution *529*
  references 659
atopy 547
ATP 203, 401–3
ATPS 18–20
atropine 198, 199
atropine methonitrate 641–2
autonomic nerve supply, pulmonary 87–8
averaging ratios 62
aviation,

spasmogen 547
specific airway conductance (sGaw) 112
specific compliance of the lung (sC) 102
specific resistance (sRaw) 112, 167
specificity of tests 69, 70
spectrophotometry, for measurement of oxygen
           saturation 40−1
    see also mass spectrometry
spinal cord, role in control of respiration 336−7
spirometers 23−5
    calibration 53
    closed circuit 150
spirometry
    dynamic 134−45
    flow-volume 142−4
    in measurement of lung volume 149
standard deviation (SD) 64, 68, 81, 507, *510*
standard deviation of transit times (SDTT) 132, 141
standard error 51
standardisation, recommendations for
    assessing disability and impairment 439−40
    lung function tests in paediatrics 448, 449
    measurement of volumes and flow rates 24, 27, 71,
       133
    non-specific bronchial hyperreactivity 555
    peak expiratory flow 27
    reference values
       equations 456, 493−4
       inclusion of smokers 446
    single breath nitrogen test 217
    terminology and units 14, 16
    transfer factor (*Tl*co, sb) 309
standing height *see* stature
Starling resistor 188, 189, 201
static compliance *see* compliance
    measurement 162−3
static volume-pressure curve 96, 97, 99, 100−2
stature 491−2
    allowance for in reference values 506
    in childhood 454
    measurement 54, 55
steady state, definition 13, 301, 417
steady state method, for
    carbon monoxide transfer factor 300−1
    exercise testing 385, 422, 438
    uneven lung function 301−2
    ventilatory response to carbon dioxide 380
stepping exercise 367−9, 419, *421*
sterilisation, of equipment 54
sternocleidomastoid muscles 88, 89
Stevens' psychophysical power law 338
STPD 18−20
stretch receptors 199, 331, 335
stroke volume 179, 208, 397
    affecting lung mixing 187
    in childhood 461
    during exercise 397, 398
       and maximal oxygen uptake 436
    measurement of 249
    in mitral stenosis 604

suberosis 594
substance P 87, 198, 203, 204, 342
sudden infant death syndrome 350
suffixes 15−16
sulphur
    atmospheric 2
    oxides of 482
superoxide dismutase 203
surgery, suitability for
    non-thoracic 571−2
    thoracic 572
    transplants 572−3
sustained maximal voluntary ventilation 122
    measurement 134−5
symbols 14−15, 35
symptom questionnaires
    for use at end of exercise 430−2
    interpretation 405
    Medical Research Council 527
syndromes
    defective gas transfer 519−20
    primary alveolar hypoventilation 520
    ventilatory defect,
       obstructive 517−8
       non-obstructive 518−9

tachycardia *442*
tachypnoea 442−3
    hyperthermia causing 339
    in interstitial lung disease 566
    and J receptors (q.v.)
    in mitral stenosis 604
Taylor diffusion/laminar dispersion 269
Taylor plateau at maximal oxygen uptake 435
technetium-99m 233, 238−9
technicans, training 76
temperature *see* ambient, body, cold, heat
terbutaline 641
terminology 12−13
    references 659
tetany 586
Thebesian veins 86
thermal panting 339
thoracic cavity, anatomy 82
thoracic pump 396
three compartment model of ventilation−
           perfusion 250−5
thresher's lung 596
tidal volume 105, 106, 153
    alveolar component 179
    in childhood 461
    during exercise 326−8
       index of (*V*t30) 373
       interpretation of 432
       reference values for *431, 509*
       see also exercise
    in neonates and infants 450
    and pattern of breathing 325−7
    Pendelluft and 183
    see also bradypnoea, tachyponea